Natur
Instru
Patients

For Churchill Livingstone:

Publishing Manager: Inta Ozols
Project Development Manager: Claire Wilson
Project Manager: Gail Wright
Design Direction: Judith Wright

Natural Medicine Instructions for Patients

Lara U. Pizzorno MA(Div) MA(Lit) LMT

Senior Medical Editor, Salugenecists, Inc., Seattle, Washington, USA

Joseph E. Pizzorno, Jr ND

President Emeritus, Bastyr University, Kenmore, Washington, USA;
Co-editor *Textbook of Natural Medicine*

Michael T. Murray ND

Faculty, Bastyr University, Kenmore, Washington, USA;
Co-editor *Textbook of Natural Medicine*

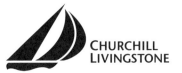

CHURCHILL
LIVINGSTONE

CHURCHILL LIVINGSTONE
An imprint of Elsevier Science Limited

First published 2002

ISBN 0 443 07128 4

British Library Cataloguing in Publication Data
A catalogue record for this book is available from the British Library

Library of Congress Cataloging in Publication Data
A catalog record for this book is available from the Library of Congress

Note
Medical knowledge is constantly changing. As new information becomes available, changes in treatment, procedures, equipment and the use of drugs become necessary. The authors and the publishers have taken care to ensure that the information given in this text is accurate and up to date. However, readers are strongly advised to confirm that the information, especially with regard to drug usage, complies with the latest legislation and standards of practice.

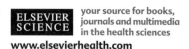

ELSEVIER SCIENCE   your source for books, journals and multimedia in the health sciences
www.elsevierhealth.com

The
publisher's
policy is to use
**paper manufactured
from sustainable forests**

Printed in China by RDC Group Limited

Contents

Preface

Natural Medicine Instructions for Patients has been created as a companion to the *Textbook of Natural Medicine*. It has been written to provide busy clinicians with easily duplicated templates of clearly written, authoritative information and instructions for patients who might suffer from 1 or more of the 76 most common diseases effectively treated with natural medicine. While the *Textbook* provides an in-depth discussion of the pathophysiology, causes, documented natural medicine interventions, and full references for these diseases, *Natural Medicine Instructions for Patients* provides only the patient-centered information that will enable patients to understand the etiology of their particular health concerns and the rationale behind the treatment prescribed.

The astute reader may notice a few inconsistencies between the recommendations found in *Natural Medicine Instructions for Patients* and the *Textbook*. As *Natural Medicine Instructions for Patients* was written three years after the latest edition of the *Textbook*, we have worked to ensure that the latest research has been incorporated.

"The doctor as teacher" is one of the seven cardinal principles upon which naturopathic medicine is based. Naturopathic physicians see themselves as teachers whose primary job is to educate, empower, and motivate patients to become full partners in their own healing. We recognize that the benefits of science-based natural medicine are fully realized only when the patient becomes a true partner with the physician in the healing process. Yet, even during an extended office visit, the most dedicated and perceptive physician may not have time to discuss fully all pertinent considerations, and after leaving the office, even the most proactive and compliant patient may think of additional questions or need a summary of the information presented. *Natural Medicine Instructions for Patients* has been created to meet these needs by providing easy-to-comprehend explanations and instructions, which patients can review at a later time away from your office.

Each handout of *Natural Medicine Instructions for Patients* is composed of the following sections: Description, Frequent Signs and Symptoms, Causes, Risk Increases With, Preventive Measures, Expected Outcomes, and a Treatment section that includes pertinent recommendations for diet, nutritional supplements, botanical medicines, and, where appropriate, drug–herb interaction cautions, topical treatment, and physical medicine. In addition, appendices have been provided that outline the basics of a health-promoting diet and what to look for in a high-quality daily multiple vitamin-and-mineral supplement. Handouts can be easily tailored to the individual patient's needs by simply highlighting relevant diagnostic indicators and associated therapeutic interventions.

We believe *Natural Medicine Instructions for Patients* is a unique work and are aware of no other patient guide that provides patients with an understanding of both the underlying causes of their disease and the mechanisms of action behind the science-based natural therapies with demonstrated efficacy.

We hope *Natural Medicine Instructions for Patients* will be a useful tool that will help you make the most of your time with patients and will help patients receive the maximum benefit from your guidance.

Seattle 2002

Lara U. Pizzorno
Joseph E. Pizzorno, Jr
Michael T. Murray

Acknowledgements

Working with our new co-author, my dear wife Lara, this past year has been an extraordinary pleasure and privilege. Her ability to translate our complex and sophisticated, but at times obtuse, recommendations into easily understood guidance to help patients understand how to get well is remarkable. Despite the long hours, her love and caring for her family have only grown more profound. I am deeply grateful for the honor of her love and companionship.

As ever, this work would not have been possible without the love of Galen and Raven, my beloved children. Thank you for bringing such joy and fullness to my life.

Finally, I would like to thank my dear friend and colleague Michael Murray for his continuing dedication to rigorous science, to advancing the wisdom of natural medicine, and to improving the health and well-being of all.

Joseph E. Pizzorno, Jr

Most of all I would like to acknowledge that inner voice that has guided me in my life, providing me with inspiration, strength, and humility at the most appropriate times. My motivation has been largely the good that I know can come from using natural medicine appropriately. It can literally change people's lives. I know it changed mine.

There are many things that I am thankful for. I am especially thankful for my wife and best friend, Gina. I have also been blessed by having wonderful parents whose support and faith have never waned. I now have the opportunity to carry on their legacy of love with my own children, Alexa and Zachary.

In addition to my family, those people who have truly inspired me include Dr Ralph Weiss, Dr Ed Madison, Dr Bill Mitchell, Dr Gaetano Morello, my classmates and the entire Bastyr University community, and all of the special people I am lucky enough to call friends who have helped me on my life's journey.

And finally, I am deeply honored to have Joe and Lara Pizzorno not only as my co-authors, but also as truly valued friends.

Michael T. Murray

Although I am a writer and words are my trade, I can find none to adequately express my esteem and regard for my daily more beloved husband, Dr Joseph Pizzorno, and a man I am truly blessed to call my friend, Dr Michael Murray. I am forever indebted to you both for your wisdom, integrity, and the vision you share of health and healing, a vision that has inspired and transformed the lives of many thousands besides my own. Thank you for your confidence in my ability to translate the *Textbook of Natural Medicine* into patient-accessible language, and for your unending patience and assistance in this work.

I am so grateful to the Spirit that is the source and substance of all life for gifting me with this opportunity to use my talents to support the health of others. Writing *Natural Medicine Instructions for Patients* has taught me so much, not only about our incredible potential for healing, but about the joy that working for Good brings.

While this format is standard, the depth of the love I feel for my family cannot be circumscribed in any form. Joe, my dearest soul mate, Galen, my wonderful son, Raven, the daughter of my heart, and my faithful felines, Catnip and Smudge, your existence is a constant source of joy in my life. Whenever I have needed an infusion of spiritual good sense, I have always been able to rely on my amazing mother. Thank you for being my dearest friends as well as my loving family.

If I were to thank all those who have blessed me with their support and faith and have inspired me to strive towards the highest vision I can conceive of Who We Really Are, this would become a book in itself. While I cannot list every name here, please know I am truly grateful and that you are always in my prayers.

Lara U. Pizzorno

Finally, we all wish to acknowledge the exceptional professional staff at Elsevier Science, whose expertise, thoughtfulness, and meticulous attention to detail have not only ensured the highest standards were met in the publishing process, but have made the publishing of this book a delight for all its authors. Many thanks are owed, especially to Inta Ozols, Claire Wilson, and Isobel Black.

Abbreviations

Dosage frequencies

q.d.   (quaque die)   = daily
b.i.d. (bis in die)   = twice a day
t.i.d. (ter in die)   = three times a day
q.i.d. (quarter in die) = four times a day

Method of drug administration

IM   = intramuscularly
IV   = intravenously

Natural medicine concentrations

IU   = International Units   a quantity that produces a particular biological effect agreed upon as an international standard

GDU = Gelatin-digesting Units   these units are used to measure enzyme activity. Unit weights cannot be used
MCU = Milk Clotting Units   as different preparations differ in activity. (1 GDU approx. = 1.5 MCU)

Acne

DESCRIPTION

A chronic inflammatory skin condition characterized by skin eruptions on the face, chest, back and shoulders, acne is the most common of all skin problems. *Acne vulgaris*, the least severe form, is a superficial disease that affects the skin's oil-secreting glands and hair follicles and manifests as blackheads, whiteheads and redness. *Acne conglobata*, a more severe form, is characterized by the formation of pustules and cysts with the potential for subsequent scarring. Both forms are more common among males than females with onset typically at or shortly after puberty.

FREQUENT SIGNS AND SYMPTOMS

- **Blackheads:** dilated skin follicles with central dark, horny plugs, pinhead size
- **Whiteheads:** red, swollen follicles with or without white pustules
- **Pustules:** tender nodules of pus deep in the skin that discharge to the surface
- **Cysts:** deep firm nodules that fail to discharge contents to the surface
- **Inflammation:** redness and tenderness around eruptions

CAUSES

- **Hormonal shifts during puberty:**
  - acne originates in the skin's pores, each of which contains a hair follicle and sebaceous glands. The sebaceous glands are connected to the skin by the follicular canal through which the hair shaft passes. During puberty, increases in levels of testosterone cause the sebaceous glands to enlarge and produce more sebum.
  - in addition, testosterone stimulates the cells lining the follicular canal to produce keratin, a fibrous protein that is the main component of the skin's outermost layer.
  - overproduction of either keratin or sebum can result in blocked pores.
  - if the blockage is incomplete, allowing the sebum to reach the surface, a blackhead will form. If the blockage is complete, bacteria normally present in the canal overgrow, releasing enzymes that break down sebum and promote inflammation.
  - if the bacterial overgrowth and resulting inflammation are severe, the wall of the hair canal ruptures, damaging surrounding tissue. If this happens at the skin's surface, the result is superficial redness and pimples. If the rupture occurs deep within the skin, a cyst may form, leading to more significant damage and possible scar formation.
  - although excessive secretion of male hormones is typically thought to be the cause of acne, studies show a poor correlation between blood levels of testosterone and the severity of acne. What is probably more important is the level of the enzyme 5-alpha-reductase, which converts the normal form of testosterone to a more potent form called dihydrotestosterone, and is found in higher levels in the skin of acne patients.
- **Poor intestinal health:** increased blood levels of toxins absorbed from the intestines are frequently found in patients with severe acne.
- **Agents producing acne-like lesions:**
  - drugs: corticosteroids, halogens, isonicotinic acid, diphenylhydantoin, lithium carbonate, oral contraceptives, progesterone, drugs containing bromides or iodides
  - industrial pollutants: machine oils, coal tar derivatives, chlorinated hydrocarbons
  - some cosmetics, pomades
  - overwashing, repetitive rubbing.

RISK INCREASES WITH

- Puberty
- Treatment with long-term, broad-spectrum antibiotics can result in intestinal overgrowth of the yeast *Candida albicans*, which can damage the intestinal wall leading to increased absorption of toxins into the bloodstream.

PREVENTIVE MEASURES

- Avoid exposure to agents noted above which can produce acne-like lesions.
- Avoid long-term use of broad-spectrum antibiotics.
- Wash the pillowcase regularly in "chemical-free" detergents (no added colors or fragrances).
- Wash areas with acne lesions twice daily to remove excess sebum and oil.
- Follow the dietary recommendations provided below.

Expected outcomes

Significant improvement should be seen within 4–6 weeks.

TREATMENT

Diet

- **Consume a diet high in protein:** a high-protein diet (44% protein, 35% carbohydrate, 21% fat) decreases 5-alpha reductase activity. A high carbohydrate diet (10% protein, 70% carbohydrate, 20% fat) has the opposite effect.
- **Eliminate all refined and/or concentrated simple sugars from the diet:** the skin cells of acne patients have been found to be insulin insensitive and to utilize sugar so poorly that one researcher has referred to acne as "skin diabetes".
- **Limit intake of high-fat foods:** also eliminate foods containing *trans* fatty acids (margarine, shortening, and other synthetically hydrogenated oils) or oxidized fatty acids (fried oils). Milk consumption should also be limited because of its high hormone content.
- **Eliminate high-iodine foods:** those who are iodine sensitive should eliminate foods high in iodine, including foods with a high salt content as most salt is iodized.

Nutritional supplements

- **Chromium:** improves glucose tolerance and enhances insulin sensitivity; dosage: 200–400 µg q.d.
- **Vitamin A:** reduces sebum production and the buildup of keratin in the follicle:
  - dosage: no more than 5,000 IU q.d. for sexually active women of childbearing age; for all others, no more than 25,000 IU q.d.
  - **caution:** higher doses may be toxic. Early warning signs of impending toxicity: chapped lips and dry skin. Signs of vitamin A toxicity: headache followed by fatigue, emotional instability, and muscle and joint pain.
  - women of childbearing age should use effective birth control during vitamin A treatment and for at least 1 month after discontinuation.
- **Zinc:** involved in vitamin A function, wound healing, immune system activity, inflammation control, and tissue regeneration:
  - zinc levels are lower in 13- and 14-year-old males than in any other age group.
  - low zinc levels increase 5-alpha reductase conversion of testosterone to dihydrotestosterone.
  - certain forms of zinc have been found more effective. Specifically, zinc gluconate and effervescent zinc sulfate have produced excellent results after 12 weeks of supplementation.
  - dosage: 45–60 mg q.d.
- **Vitamin E:** necessary for proper functioning of vitamin A and selenium; dosage: 400 IU q.d.
- **Selenium:** a trace mineral integral to the enzyme glutathione peroxidase, which is important in preventing the inflammation of acne; dosage: 200 µg q.d.
- **Pyridoxine (B$_6$):** a deficiency of this B vitamin causes both increased uptake of and sensitivity to testosterone; dosage: 25 mg t.i.d.
- **Pantothenic acid (B$_5$):** important in fat metabolism; when given in a study of 100 Chinese patients with acne, it significantly decreased sebum secretion and acne lesions within 2 weeks; dosage: 2.5 g q.i.d. for up to 2 weeks.

Topical medicines

- **Tea tree oil and azelaic acid:** both are natural skin antiseptics and have been shown to lower the bacteria level and inflammation of acne as effectively as benzoyl peroxide or Retin-A, without these drugs' negative side effects of dry skin, redness and peeling:
  - choose a gel, ointment or cream featuring either tea tree oil (5–15% preparations) or azelaic acid (20% preparations).

Affective disorders: depression, dysthymia

DESCRIPTION

A mood disorder in which feelings of sadness, despondency or hopelessness dominate an individual's outlook most of every day for at least 2 weeks with accompanying symptoms. Depression ranges from mild feelings of sadness, known as *dysthymia*, to major or unipolar depression, which may include serious consideration of suicide. Major depression occurs in about 1 in 10 Americans and more than 28 million take antidepressant or antianxiety drugs. By the year 2020, depression is estimated to become the second leading cause of disability in the world.

FREQUENT SIGNS AND SYMPTOMS

Depression

- Poor appetite accompanied by weight loss, or increased appetite accompanied by weight gain
- Insomnia or hypersomnia (excessive sleep)
- Physical hyperactivity or inactivity
- Loss of interest or pleasure in usual activities, or decrease in sex drive
- Loss of energy, feelings of fatigue
- Feelings of worthlessness, self-reproach, or inappropriate guilt
- Diminished ability to think or concentrate
- Recurrent thoughts of suicide

Dysthymia

- Low self-esteem or lack of self-confidence
- Pessimism, hopelessness, or despair
- Lack of interest in ordinary pleasures and activities
- Withdrawal from social activities
- Fatigue or lethargy
- Guilt or ruminating about the past
- Irritability or excessive anger
- Lessened productivity
- Difficulty in concentrating or making decisions

CAUSES

Modern psychiatry focuses on using drugs to manipulate levels of brain neurotransmitters – chemical messengers that transmit information from one nerve cell to another – such as serotonin, dopamine and gamma-amino-butyric acid (GABA). Imbalances among neurotransmitters are frequently the proximate trigger for depression, but the imbalances themselves are often due to an underlying organic (chemical) or physiological cause. These simple organic factors must be ruled out since failure to address such underlying causes of depression will make any antidepressant therapy less successful.

Organic and physiological causes of depression

- **Food allergies:** food allergens damage the intestines, resulting in inadequate absorption of needed nutrients and increased leakage of brain toxins into the circulation.
- **Environmental toxins:** heavy metals (lead, mercury, cadmium, arsenic, nickel, aluminum), solvents (cleaning materials, formaldehyde, toluene, benzene, etc.), pesticides, and herbicides have an affinity for, and disrupt normal function of, nervous tissue.
- **Hypoglycemia:** low blood sugar significantly disrupts normal brain function; the brain utilizes more blood sugar than any other organ and requires a constant supply to function properly.
- **Hypothyroidism:** depression is often an early manifestation of thyroid disease.
- **Microbial factors:** by-products of unfriendly microbe metabolism may be neurotoxic.
- **Nutritional deficiency:** a deficiency of even a single nutrient can alter brain function; nutrient deficiencies are common in depressed individuals, particularly deficiencies of folic acid, vitamins B_{12} and B_6, and omega-3 essential fatty acids:
  - *folic acid and vitamin B_{12}* function together as methyl donors, carrying and donating methyl molecules to important brain compounds, including

neurotransmitters. Without the donation of a methyl group, both the manufacture and the activity of neurotransmitters such as serotonin and dopamine are disrupted.

- *vitamin B_6* has numerous vital functions in the brain (e.g., it is essential to the manufacture of serotonin). B_6 is frequently low in women on birth control pills or Premarin.
- nerve cell membranes, which regulate the passage of molecules into and out of each cell, are largely composed of fatty acids. *Omega-3 fatty acids*, found primarily in cold water fish and flaxseed, make fluid, permeable cell membranes – unlike saturated, animal and *trans* fats, all of which form cell membranes that are much less fluid. Nerve cell function is critically dependent on proper membrane fluidity, which directly influences neurotransmitter synthesis, signal transmission, the uptake of serotonin and other neurotransmitters, and the activity of monoamine oxidase – the enzyme that breaks down serotonin, epinephrine, dopamine and norepinephrine. Disruption of any of these activities may contribute to depression.

- **Nutrient excess:** excessive consumption, particularly of foods detrimental to health such as sugar, saturated fats, cholesterol, salt, and food additives, can negatively impact on brain chemistry and function.
- **Pre-existing physical conditions:** cancer; chronic inflammation; chronic pain; diabetes; diseases of the heart, liver and lung; multiple sclerosis; rheumatoid arthritis.
- **Premenstrual syndrome:** hormonal fluctuations are known to influence mood.
- **Prescription drugs:** antihistamines, antihypertensives, anti-inflammatory agents, birth control pills, corticosteroids, tranquilizers and sedatives can affect brain chemistry and function.
- **Illicit drugs:** disrupt normal brain chemistry.
- **Legal drugs:** alcohol, caffeine, nicotine (smoking):
  - *alcohol*, a brain depressant, increases adrenal hormone output, interferes with many brain cell processes, disrupts normal sleep cycles, and leads to hypoglycemia.
  - *caffeine* intake, particularly when combined with refined sugar, has been correlated with depression in numerous studies, which show that people prone to depression tend to be highly sensitive to adverse effects from caffeine.
  - *nicotine* (smoking) stimulates secretion of the stress hormone cortisol, which lowers both the amount of serotonin produced and its uptake by brain receptors. In addition, the process of detoxifying cigarette smoke dramatically lowers vitamin C

levels; low levels of vitamin C in the brain can result in depression and hysteria.

- **Sleep disturbances:** normal sleep cycles are essential for healthy brain function.
- **Stress/low adrenal function:** defects in adrenal regulation of the stress hormone cortisol can cause depression, mania, nervousness, insomnia and, at high levels, schizophrenia:
  - cortisol affects mood because it shunts the amino acid tryptophan away from the pathway through which it is used to make serotonin and melatonin, a hormone that regulates normal sleep patterns.
- **Sedentary lifestyle/inactivity:** regular exercise increases beta-endorphin levels and has been shown in more than 100 clinical studies to improve self-esteem, lower levels of cortisol and perceived stress, and relieve depression as effectively as antidepressant drugs and psychotherapy.

RISK INCREASES WITH

- A disease-promoting diet, i.e., a diet high in sugar, saturated fats, cholesterol, salt, food additives, and processed foods
- Smoking
- Alcohol
- Caffeine
- Prescription drug use
- Illegal drug use
- Lack of regular exercise

PREVENTIVE MEASURES

- Stop smoking.
- Limit consumption of alcohol to no more than one drink per day for women, two for men. (One drink equals 350 ml (12 US fl oz) of beer, 140 ml (4–5 US fl oz) of wine, or 45 ml (1.5 US fl oz) of distilled spirits.)
- Avoid caffeine.
- Identify and control food allergies.
- Identify and minimize environmental toxins.
- Exercise regularly – a minimum of 30 min, at least three times a week. The best exercises are strength training (weight lifting) and/or aerobic activities such as walking briskly, jogging, bicycling, cross-country skiing, swimming, aerobic dance, and racquet sports.
- A health-promoting diet rich in whole, preferably organic, unprocessed foods, and especially high in plant foods – fruits, vegetables, whole grains, beans, seeds and nuts – and cold-water fish (for more detailed information, see Appendix 1).

- A high-potency, multiple vitamin and mineral supplement including 400 µg of folic acid, 400 µg of vitamin B_{12}, and 50–100 mg of vitamin B_6. (Folic acid supplementation should always be accompanied by vitamin B_{12} supplementation to prevent folic acid from masking a vitamin B_{12} deficiency.)
- Increase consumption of omega-3 essential fatty acids by consuming flaxseed oil (1 tbsp q.d.) and/or eating cold-water fish – salmon, mackerel, tuna, herring (110 g [4 oz] at least three times a week).

Expected outcomes

Significant improvement should be seen within 1–2 weeks.

TREATMENT

Diet
- See Preventive Measures above.
- To avoid hypoglycemia, try eating several small meals interspersed with snacks throughout the day instead of two or three big meals. Divide carbohydrate fairly evenly over the day, consuming carbohydrates with protein-rich foods and health-promoting fats such as flaxseed oil and olive oil.

Nutritional supplements
- **High-potency multiple vitamin and mineral supplement:** (see Appendix 2).
- **Folic acid and vitamin B_{12}:** necessary for neurotransmitter manufacture and activity; dosage: 800 µg of each q.d.
- **Vitamin C:** low levels of vitamin C in the brain have been linked to depression; dosage: 500–1,000 mg t.i.d.
- **Vitamin E:** necessary for brain cell membrane function; dosage: 200–400 IU mixed tocopherols q.d.
- **Flaxseed oil:** supplies omega-3 essential fatty acids necessary for brain cell membrane fluidity; dosage: 1 tbsp q.d.

Natural neurotransmitter precursors
As explained above, a number of lifestyle and dietary factors can lead to an alteration in brain chemistry (primarily a reduction in serotonin levels) that produces depression. All of these factors share a common pathway: they lower serotonin levels by impairing the conversion of tryptophan to serotonin.

Of all the body's chemicals, none has a more widespread effect on the brain and physiology than serotonin. It plays a key role in regulating temperature, blood pressure, blood clotting, immunity, pain, digestion, sleep, and circadian (daily) rhythms. In the brain,
serotonin inhibits the firing of brain cells (neurons), producing a relaxing effect on mood, and is often referred to as the body's own mood-altering drug.

The preceding list of preventive measures will gradually normalize serotonin levels, thus relieving depression but, in the interim, the following natural agents offer effective alternatives to antidepressant drugs and can provide the necessary serotonin boost to support integration of the preventive measures into both diet and lifestyle.

- **5-Hydroxytryptophan (5-HTP):** made by the body from the essential amino acid tryptophan, and then converted into serotonin, 5-HTP has been found in numerous studies to be as effective as drugs such as Prozac, paroxetine and sertraline. It is also less expensive than these drugs, with fewer and much milder side effects. To facilitate uptake into the brain, 5-HTP should be taken with a carbohydrate snack such as a wholegrain cracker, apple or banana; dosage: 100–200 mg t.i.d.
- **Vitamin B_6:** ensures the timely conversion of 5-HTP into serotonin; dosage: 50–100 mg b.i.d.
- **Phenylalanine and tyrosine:** found in high concentrations in chocolate (which may explain chocolate's mood-lifting effects), phenylalanine, a precursor to tyrosine, has been shown in some clinical trials to offer an effective alternative to tricyclic and monoamine oxidase inhibitor drugs:
  - unlike tryptophan and 5-HTP, which are part of the serotonin pathway, phenylalanine and tyrosine are precursors for and part of another chemical pathway – catecholamine pathway – which gives rise to the neurotransmitters dopamine, norepinephrine, and epinephrine. In addition to their powerful antidepressant effects, these neurotransmitters support arousal, alertness, optimism, zest for life, and sex drive.
  - in patients who initially respond well to 5-HTP, but tend to relapse after 1 month despite achieving higher levels of serotonin, supplemental tyrosine has been found to raise levels of dopamine and norepinephrine, thus relieving depression.
  - dosage: 75–400 mg q.d.
- **S-Adenosyl-methionine (SAM):** involved in the methylation of neurotransmitters and phospholipids (fats necessary for brain cell membrane fluidity), SAM is normally manufactured in adequate amounts in the brain. In depressed patients, however, SAM synthesis is impaired. Supplementing with SAM increases levels of serotonin and dopamine, improves their binding to receptor sites and therefore their activity, and improves brain cell membrane fluidity. A very effective natural antidepressant, SAM is better tolerated and

faster acting than tricyclic drugs:

- dosage: gradually increase the dosage to avoid a possible initial response of nausea and vomiting. Start at 200 mg b.i.d. for days 1 and 2, increase to 400 mg b.i.d. on days 3–9, 400 mg t.i.d. on days 10–20, then 400 mg q.i.d. after 20 days.
- **caution:** bipolar (manic) patients should not take SAM as it may induce mania or hypomania in these individuals.

Botanical medicines

- ***Hypericum perforatum* (St John's wort):** in numerous double-blind placebo-controlled studies, extracts of St John's wort standardized for hypericin content (although this might not be the most active constituent) have been extensively researched and found to produce improvements in psychological symptoms comparable to antidepressant drugs, with a significant advantage in terms of lack of side effects (the major side effect is mild stomach irritation in some patients), excellent patient tolerance and much lower cost:
  - dosage: extract standardized to 0.3% hypericin, 300 mg t.i.d.
  - in severe cases, St John's wort can be used with 5-HTP.
  - if over the age of 50, use of *Ginkgo biloba* is preferable.
- ***Ginkgo biloba*:** a standardized extract of *Ginkgo biloba* leaf exerts excellent antidepressant effects in patients over age 50:
  - with age, blood supply to the brain diminishes, and synthesis of serotonin receptors declines. *Ginkgo biloba* improves blood supply to the brain, increases protein synthesis, and is a potent antioxidant. The result is a better-nourished brain with a higher number of serotonin receptors, plus less free radical damage to brain cell membranes.
  - in severe cases, *Ginkgo biloba* can be used in combination with St John's wort and/or 5-HTP.
  - dosage: extract standardized to 24% ginkgo flavonglycosides, 80 mg t.i.d.

- ***Piper methysticum* (Kava):** approved in Germany, UK, Switzerland and Austria for the treatment of nervous anxiety, insomnia, depression, and restlessness, kava extract (standardized for kavalactone content) compares favorably to benzodiazepine drugs in effectiveness, without these drugs' major drawbacks (impaired mental acuity, addictiveness).
  - kava is especially useful for depression with severe anxiety.
  - dosage: 45–70 mg kavalactones t.i.d.

Drug–herb interaction cautions

- ***Hypericum perforatum* (St John's wort):**
  - plus *monoamine oxidase inhibitors (MAO inhibitors)*: possible additive effects of St John's wort with these drugs, so physician monitoring is advised.
  - plus *selective serotonin reuptake inhibitors (SSRIs)*: possible additive effects of St John's wort with these drugs, so physician monitoring is advised. When replacement of an SSRI is desirable, either of two physician-supervised approaches may be used: (1) a trial for several weeks combining a reduced dose of St John's wort or the SSRI prior to withdrawal of the pharmaceutical medication, or (2) a 3-week wash-out period for the SSRI before switching to St John's Wort.
- ***Ginkgo biloba*:**
  - plus *aspirin*: may induce spontaneous bleeding when combined with chronic use of aspirin. Increased bleeding potential reported after *Ginkgo biloba* usage in a chronic user (2 years) of aspirin.
- ***Piper methysticum* (Kava):**
  - plus *CNS depressants*: due to the general sedative and muscle-relaxant activity of kava resin, the action of CNS depressants such as the benzodiazepine, alprazolam and the barbiturate, phenobarbital may be enhanced.

Affective disorders: bipolar (manic) depression

DESCRIPTION

An affective disorder characterized by extreme mood swings unrelated to what is actually happening in the person's life. Periods of inexplicable elation and over-activity (*mania*) alternate on an irregular, but cyclical, basis with deep depression. Periods of normal behavior (lasting for a short time or for years) occur in between the mania and depression. If the elevated mood swings are relatively mild and the episodes last 4 days or less, the disorder is called *hypomania*. Mania lasts longer and is more intense. Patients experiencing a full-blown manic attack usually require hospitalization to prevent impulsive and aggressive behavior from ruining their careers or causing injury to themselves or others.

FREQUENT SIGNS AND SYMPTOMS

Mania
- Accelerated energy levels; euphoric mood
- Reduced need to sleep (some may not sleep at all for 3–4 days)
- Increase in social or work-oriented activities, often with a 60–80-hour workweek
- Inability to concentrate; easily distracted and restless
- May have a very high opinion of own abilities and exaggerated thinking (grandiosity)
- Extreme talkativeness; speech becomes very rapid, wild, illogical
- Poor judgment, as evidenced by sprees of uncontrolled spending, sexual promiscuity, and misguided financial decisions
- May forget to eat, may lose weight and become exhausted
- Often irritable, with attacks of intense anger or rage

Depression
- May become increasingly withdrawn
- Disturbed sleep, late rising becomes a habit
- May stay in own room, afraid to face the world; lacks self-esteem
- Self-neglect

- Decreased sex drive
- Slowing of speech and movement
- Excessive worrying; imagined problems multiply

CAUSES

- Biological, psychological, and hereditary factors may all play a part.
- Extreme stress or a death may trigger a sudden episode of mania or depression.
- Many of the causative principles outlined in the chapter on Affective disorders: depression, apply to bipolar depression.

RISK INCREASES WITH

- A disease-promoting diet, i.e., a diet high in sugar, saturated fats, cholesterol, salt, food additives, and processed foods
- Hypoglycemia
- Food allergies
- Exposure to environmental toxins
- Nutritional deficiency
- Premenstrual syndrome
- Sleep disturbances
- Smoking
- Alcohol
- Caffeine
- Prescription drug use
- Illegal drug use
- Lack of regular exercise
- Extreme stress or a death may trigger a sudden episode of mania or depression

PREVENTIVE MEASURES

- Stop smoking.
- Limit consumption of alcohol to no more than one drink per day for women, two for men. (One drink

equals 350 ml (12 US fl oz) of beer, 140 ml (4–5 US fl oz) of wine, or 45 ml (1.5 US fl oz) of distilled spirits.)
- Avoid caffeine.
- Identify and control food allergies.
- Identify and minimize environmental toxins.
- Exercise regularly – a minimum of 30 min, at least three times a week. The best exercises are strength training (weight lifting) and/or aerobic activities such as walking briskly, jogging, bicycling, cross-country skiing, swimming, aerobic dance, and racquet sports.
- A health-promoting diet rich in whole, unprocessed, preferably organic foods, especially high in plant foods – fruits, vegetables, whole grains, beans, seeds and nuts – and cold-water fish.
- A high-potency multiple vitamin and mineral supplement including 400 µg of folic acid, 400 µg of vitamin B_{12} and 50–100 mg of vitamin B_6. (Folic acid supplementation should always be accompanied by vitamin B_{12} supplementation to prevent folic acid from masking a vitamin B_{12} deficiency.)
- Increase consumption of omega-3 essential fatty acids by consuming flaxseed oil (1 tbsp q.d.) and/or eating cold-water fish – salmon, mackerel, tuna, herring (110 g [4 oz] at least three times a week).

Expected outcomes

Significant improvement should be seen within 1–2 weeks.

TREATMENT

Due to the seriousness of bipolar depression, manic patients are typically hospitalized for 2 weeks under sedation with antipsychotic drugs until blood levels of the mineral lithium, the drug of choice for this condition, have reached acceptable levels.

The natural treatment adjunctive therapy plan below can be used in combination with lithium instead of serotonin uptake inhibitor drugs such as Prozac, sertraline and paroxetine, thus avoiding the negative side effects of these drugs.

Diet

- See Preventive Measures above.
- To avoid hypoglycemia, try eating several small meals interspersed with snacks throughout the day instead of two or three big meals. Divide carbohydrate fairly evenly over the day, consuming carbohydrates with protein-rich foods and health-promoting fats such as flaxseed oil and olive oil.

Nutritional supplements

- **High-potency multiple vitamin and mineral supplement:** (see Appendix 2).
- **Folic acid and vitamin B_{12}:** necessary for neurotransmitter manufacture and activity; dosage: 800 µg of each q.d.
- **Vitamin C:** low levels of vitamin C in the brain have been linked to depression; dosage: 500–1,000 mg t.i.d.
- **Vitamin E:** necessary for brain cell membrane function; dosage: 200–400 IU mixed tocopherols q.d.
- **Flaxseed oil:** supplies omega-3 essential fatty acids necessary for brain cell membrane fluidity; dosage: 1 tbsp q.d.
- **5-Hydroxytryptophan (5-HTP):** the immediate precursor to serotonin, 5-HTP has been found in numerous studies to be as effective as drugs such as Prozac, paroxetine and sertraline. It is also less expensive than these drugs, with fewer and much milder side effects:
  - dosage: 100 mg t.i.d., in addition to lithium
  - **caution:** do not self-medicate with 5-HTP. Due to the seriousness of this condition, and the fact that antidepressant drugs can occasionally induce mania and hypomania, even natural supportive antidepressant therapies should only be used under the supervision of a qualified psychiatrist or physician.
- **Phosphatidylcholine (PC):** the major fat in cell membranes, as well as in soy lecithin, PC has shown good results in the treatment of mania because it raises the levels and brain activity of an important neurotransmitter, acetylcholine; dosage: 15–30 g q.d. in both pure form and as lecithin.
- **Vanadium:** elevated levels of this trace mineral are found in hair samples from manic patients; these levels normalize upon recovery. In depressed patients, hair concentrations of vanadium are normal, while whole blood and serum levels are elevated; once again, levels normalize upon recovery. Vanadium is a strong inhibitor of energy production; lithium reduces this inhibition. Natural therapies to reduce vanadium levels include:
  - vitamin C (3 g q.d.), either alone or in combination with EDTA (a chelating or binding agent that binds to the vanadium and other heavy metals and promotes their excretion).
  - a low-vanadium diet. Foods with the lowest levels of vanadium (1–5 ng/g) include fats, oils, fresh fruits and vegetables. Foods in the range of 5–30 ng/g include whole grains, seafood, meat, and dairy products. Foods with the highest amounts of vanadium (11–93 ng/g) include prepared foods such as peanut butter, white bread and breakfast cereals.

Botanical medicines

■ *Hypericum perforatum* (St John's wort): in numerous double-blind placebo-controlled studies, extracts of St John's wort standardized for hypericin content have been extensively researched and found to produce improvements in psychological symptoms comparable to antidepressant drugs, with a significant advantage in terms of lack of side effects (the major side effect is mild stomach irritation in some patients), excellent patient tolerance, and much lower cost:

 ■ dosage: extract standardized to 0.3% hypericin, 300 mg t.i.d., in addition to lithium. In severe cases, 5-HTP can also be used.

 ■ **caution:** do not self-medicate with St John's wort or any other herbal medicines. Due to the seriousness of this condition, and the fact that antidepressant drugs can occasionally induce mania and hypomania, even natural supportive antidepressant therapies should only be used under the supervision of a qualified psychiatrist or physician.

Drug–herb interaction cautions

■ *Hypericum perforatum* (St John's wort):

 ■ plus *monoamine oxidase inhibitors (MAO inhibitors)*: possible additive effects of St John's wort with these drugs, so physician monitoring is advised.

 ■ plus *selective serotonin reuptake inhibitors (SSRIs)*: possible additive effects of St John's wort with these drugs, so physician monitoring is advised. When replacement of an SSRI is desirable, either of two physician-supervised approaches may be used: (1) a trial for several weeks combining a reduced dose of St John's wort or the SSRI prior to withdrawal of the pharmaceutical medication, or (2) a 3-week wash-out period for the SSRI before switching to St John's wort.

Physical medicine

■ **Phototherapy (light therapy):** manic-depressive patients have a disturbed daily or circadian rhythm of hormonal release that tends to be worse in winter, and find bright light is hard on their eyes. These findings suggest that light therapy, which is simply controlled exposure to bright light, can help to restore proper circadian rhythm:

 ■ specially designed light boxes equipped with a set of full-spectrum fluorescent tubes, a metal reflector, and a protective plastic screen are designed to emit light that closely resembles full-spectrum sunlight, while downplaying the more harmful UV and blue rays.

 ■ a typical light box provides 10,000 lux of bright indoor lighting (one-third the intensity of sunshine).

 ■ patients should position themselves 3 feet away from the light box from 5AM to 8AM and again from 5.30PM to 8.30PM. Activities can be undertaken while glancing at the light at least once per minute.

 ■ some patients find that 30 min of exposure in the morning improves mood, while other individuals require longer exposure – from 2 to the full 6 hours.

 ■ should the above protocol be too difficult to work into a lifestyle, replacing standard light bulbs with full-spectrum bulbs may help.

© 2002, Elsevier Science Ltd Pizzorno L U, Pizzorno, Jr J E, Murray M T   Natural Medicine Instructions for Patients

Affective disorders: seasonal affective disorder

DESCRIPTION

A seasonal disruption of mood that typically occurs during the winter months, SAD symptoms usually begin in September when days begin to shorten and last until March when the days begin to lengthen again. Individuals with SAD feel depressed, slow down, overeat, and crave carbohydrates in the winter. In the summer, these same individuals feel elated, active and energetic. Both adults and children can be affected. In individuals intolerant to heat, SAD symptoms may occur in summer.

FREQUENT SIGNS AND SYMPTOMS

The following can be experienced at the start of winter:
- depression
- tiredness
- sluggishness
- increased appetite (especially for carbohydrates)
- weight gain
- irritability
- increased need for sleep
- feeling less cheerful
- socializing less
- difficulty in coping with life as a result of these changes.

CAUSES

- **Lessened exposure to full-spectrum natural light:**
  - the shortening of daylight hours in winter causes a shift in normal circadian rhythms; specifically, it leads to increased production of melatonin by the pineal gland and increased secretion of cortisol by the adrenal glands.
  - since the body uses serotonin, a mood-elevating neurotransmitter, to produce melatonin, an increase in melatonin production could lead to a decrease in serotonin, reducing to below adequate levels in sensitive individuals.

- this shift from normal circadian rhythms, particularly when combined with an elevation in levels of the stress hormone, cortisol, may produce symptoms associated with SAD.
- the critical factor appears to be the amount of light coming in through the eyes. Light receptor cells in the retina transmit information to a cluster of cells in the hypothalamus – the control center of the brain that regulates mood, appetite and menstrual cycles. In winter, when people are light deprived, the hypothalamus does not regulate and balance mood as smoothly as during the light-rich summer months.

RISK INCREASES WITH

- **Geographical location:** in northern latitudes, daylight hours are significantly shortened in winter, and the geographic distribution of SAD parallels this lack of sun. In the United States, SAD affects 1.4% of Floridians but almost 10% of the population of New Hampshire.
- **Other depressive illness**

PREVENTIVE MEASURES

- Keep drapes and blinds open in the home.
- Sit near windows and gaze outside frequently.
- Turn on bright lights on cloudy days; even though artificial light is not full-spectrum light, it can help.
- Get outside as much as possible, especially in the early morning light. Try to spend 1 hour in the sun each day:
  - winter sunlight is far less intense than summer sunlight; however, it is still best to avoid exposure between 10AM and 2PM when the sun's rays are strongest, and to use proper sunscreen protection, especially if at risk for skin cancer or living in a southern state of the US.
- Exercise regularly – a minimum of 30 min, at least three times a week:
  - regular exercise increases beta-endorphin levels and has been shown in more than 100 clinical studies to

improve self-esteem, lower levels of cortisol and perceived stress, and relieve depression as effectively as antidepressant drugs and psychotherapy.

- the best exercises are strength training (weight lifting) and/or aerobic activities such as walking briskly, jogging, bicycling, cross-country skiing, swimming, aerobic dance, and racquet sports.
- Try to take a vacation to a sunny place in the winter months.
- Avoid alcohol consumption: alcohol, a brain depressant, increases adrenal hormone output, interferes with many brain cell processes, disrupts normal sleep cycles, and leads to hypoglycemia.
- Limit caffeine intake: caffeine, particularly when combined with refined sugar, has been correlated with depression in numerous studies, which show that people prone to depression tend to be highly sensitive to adverse effects from caffeine.
- Stop smoking:
  - nicotine stimulates secretion of the stress hormone, cortisol, which lowers both the amount of serotonin produced and its uptake by brain receptors.
  - the process of detoxifying cigarette smoke dramatically lowers vitamin C levels in the brain, which can result in depression.

Expected outcomes
Significant improvement should be seen within 1 week.

TREATMENT

Nutritional supplements
- **Melatonin:** night-time supplementation may prevent conversion of serotonin to melatonin, thus helping to restore higher serotonin levels and improving mood; dosage: 3 mg 45 min before bedtime.
- **5-Hydroxytryptophan (5-HTP):** the immediate precursor to serotonin, 5-HTP has been found in numerous double-blind studies to raise serotonin levels as effectively as the antidepressant drugs Prozac, paroxetine and sertraline, at significantly less cost and with much fewer and milder side effects:
  - to facilitate uptake into the brain, take 5-HTP with a carbohydrate snack such as a wholegrain cracker, apple or banana.
  - dosage: 50–100 mg b.i.d.
- **Vitamin B$_6$:** ensures the timely conversion of 5-HTP into serotonin; dosage: 50–100 mg b.i.d.

Botanical medicines
- ***Hypericum perforatum* (St John's wort):** in numerous double-blind placebo-controlled studies, extracts of St John's wort standardized for hypericin content have been found to produce improvements in psychological symptoms comparable to antidepressant drugs, with a significant advantage in terms of lack of side effects (the major side effect is mild stomach irritation in some patients), excellent patient tolerance, and much lower cost:
  - in SAD patients, St John's wort extract is more effective when used together with light therapy.
  - dosage: extract standardized to 0.3% hypericin, 300 mg t.i.d.

Drug–herb interaction cautions
- ***Hypericum perforatum* (St John's wort):**
  - plus *monoamine oxidase inhibitors (MAO inhibitors):* possible additive effects of St John's wort with these drugs, so physician monitoring is advised.
  - plus *selective serotonin reuptake inhibitors (SSRIs):* possible additive effects of St John's wort with these drugs, so physician monitoring is advised. When replacement of an SSRI is desirable, either of two physician-supervised approaches may be used: (1) a trial for several weeks combining a reduced dose of St John's wort or the SSRI prior to withdrawal of the pharmaceutical medication, or (2) a 3-week wash-out period for the SSRI before switching to St John's wort.

Physical medicine
- **Phototherapy (light therapy):** controlled exposure to bright light has been shown to help restore proper circadian rhythm.
  - specially designed light boxes equipped with a set of full-spectrum fluorescent tubes, a metal reflector, and a protective plastic screen are designed to emit light that closely resembles full-spectrum sunlight, while downplaying the more harmful UV and blue rays.
  - a typical light box provides 10,000 lux of bright indoor lighting (one-third the intensity of sunshine).
  - patients should position themselves 3 feet away from the light box from 5AM to 8AM and again from 5.30PM to 8.30PM. Activities can be undertaken while glancing at the light at least once per minute.
  - some patients find that 30 min of exposure in the morning is all that is needed to improve mood and reduce SAD symptoms, while other individuals require longer exposure – from 2 to the full 6 hours.
  - should the above protocol be too difficult to work into a lifestyle, replacing standard light bulbs with full-spectrum bulbs may help.

Alcoholism

DESCRIPTION

Psychological and physiological dependence on alcohol, resulting in chronic disease and disruption of interpersonal family and work relationships. The negative consequences of alcoholism are numerous and significant, both to the individual and to society. For the individual, these negative consequences include significantly increased mortality: double the usual death rate in men, triple in women; a 10–12 year decrease in life expectancy; six times the suicide rate. Alcohol is a major factor in the four leading causes of death in men aged 25–44 (accidents, homicides, suicides, cirrhosis). In addition to, at the very least, doubling the risk of early death, alcoholism, which inflicts metabolic damage on every cell, causes numerous health problems including: acne rosacea; brain atrophy and psychiatric disorders; esophagitis, gastritis, ulcer; increased incidence of cancer of the mouth, pharynx, larynx, esophagus; fatty degeneration and cirrhosis of the liver; heart disease, angina, increased serum and liver triglyceride levels, high blood pressure; hypoglycemia; decreased protein synthesis, muscle wasting; decreased testosterone levels; nutritional deficiency diseases; osteoporosis; pancreatitis; psoriasis; spider veins. Should an alcoholic woman become pregnant, the fetus, affected with fetal alcohol syndrome, may suffer birth defects, growth retardation, and mental retardation.

FREQUENT SIGNS AND SYMPTOMS

Initial stages
- Daily consumption of more than two drinks containing alcohol (one drink equals a beer, glass of wine, or mixed drink)
- Increased tolerance to the effects of alcohol
- Need for alcohol at the beginning of the day, to get going or at times of stress
- Inability to stop drinking once started
- Frequent Monday-morning hangovers and/or frequent absences from work
- Preoccupation with obtaining alcohol and hiding drinking from family and friends
- Feeling guilt or remorse after drinking
- Alcohol stigmas: alcohol odor on the breath, flushed face, tremor

- Failure to fulfill normal family or work obligations because of drinking
- Frequent accidents, falls or injuries of vague origin; in smokers, cigarette burns on the hands or chest
- Inability to remember what happened the night before as a result of drinking
- A relative, friend, doctor or other health worker expresses concern about immoderate alcohol consumption

Late stages
- Frequent blackouts, memory loss
- Delirium tremens (tremors, hallucinations, confusion, sweating, rapid heartbeat – these occur most often with alcohol withdrawal)
- Liver disease (yellow skin or eyes)
- Neurological impairment (numbness and tingling in hands and feet, declining sexual interest and potency, confusion, coma)
- Congestive heart failure (shortness of breath, swelling of feet and ankles)

CAUSES

Although alcoholism is a complex, multifactorial condition, recent research indicates genetic basis as a primary contributing factor:
- Genealogical studies show that alcoholism is a family condition.
- Alcoholism is four to five times more common in the biological children of alcoholic parents than in those of non-alcoholic parents.
- Biological children of alcoholic parents who are raised by adoptive parents demonstrate a continued higher risk of alcoholism.
- Twin studies show differences between identical and non-identical twins.
- Genetic markers are associated with alcoholism.
- Biochemical studies show that the levels of enzymes required to detoxify alcohol are lower in people prone to alcoholism.

Other possible contributing factors include:
- personality dynamics – dependency, anger, mania, depression or introversion

- social and cultural pressure to drink
- dysfunctional family life.

RISK INCREASES WITH

- Cultural factors – some ethnic groups have high alcoholism rates for social or biological reasons
- Use of recreational drugs
- Crisis situations including unemployment, frequently moving house, loss of friends or family
- Environmental factors including ready availability, affordability, and social acceptance of alcohol in the group
- Lack of purpose, too much free time, as with retirement

PREVENTIVE MEASURES

- If at risk, admit it to yourself.
- Avoid alcohol, substituting sparkling waters, de-alcoholized wines, or "virgin" mixed drinks when socializing.
- Never drink alone. Set limits; never consume more than one alcoholic drink; dilute your drink and sip slowly. After one alcoholic drink, switch to something non-alcoholic.
- Get educated about the physical and psychosocial effects of alcoholism.
- Get involved in a treatment program such as Alcoholics Anonymous (AA), or work with counselors, and through religious affiliations.
- Replace alcohol addiction with a health-promoting addiction that is non-chemical, time-consuming, and supported by family, friends, and/or peers; for example, AA, involvement in religious, charity or community service work, or in some physical sport or hobby you find absorbing.

Expected outcomes

Taking responsibility and choosing a better life is a daily challenge that grows easier as the social, physical and spiritual rewards of continued freedom from alcohol accumulate.

TREATMENT

Diet

A hypoglycemic diet that stabilizes blood sugar levels is critical to successful treatment. Alcohol consumption often results in reactive hypoglycemia – a rapid rise in blood sugar levels followed by a rapid drop in blood sugar,

which produces a craving for foods that quickly elevate blood sugar, such as sugar and alcohol. Hypoglycemia aggravates the mental and emotional problems of the withdrawing alcoholic, causing symptoms such as sweating, tremor, anxiety, hunger, dizziness, headache, visual disturbance, brain fog, confusion, and depression.

The most important dietary guidelines for hypoglycemia are:

- elimination of all simple sugars (foods that contain added sucrose, fructose, or glucose), fruit juice, dried fruit, and low-fiber fruits (such as grapes and citrus fruits)
- limitation of processed carbohydrates (products made from refined flour, instant potatoes, white rice, etc.)
- increased consumption of complex carbohydrates (whole grains, vegetables, beans)
- keeping blood sugar levels stable by eating several small meals interspersed with snacks throughout the day instead of two or three big meals. Carbohydrates should be consumed evenly over the day, mixing complex carbohydrates with protein-rich foods and health-promoting fats such as those found in cold-water fish (e.g., salmon, tuna), nuts and seeds, flaxseed oil and olive oil.

Nutritional supplements

- **5-Hydroxytryptophan (5-HTP):** depression is common among alcoholics and is known to lead to their high suicide rate. Many alcoholics drink because they are depressed, others develop a depressive condition in the context of their alcoholism. In either case, alcoholics tend to have severely depleted levels of the essential amino acid tryptophan, which may explain both the depression and sleep disturbances common to alcoholics. Tryptophan is converted by the body to 5-HTP and then to serotonin:
  - in numerous studies, 5-HTP has been shown to be an antidepressant as effective as drugs such as Prozac, paroxetine and sertraline; in addition, it is less expensive and has fewer and much milder side effects than these drugs.
  - to facilitate uptake into the brain, 5-HTP should be taken with a complex carbohydrate snack such as a wholegrain cracker, apple or banana.
  - dosage: 100–200 mg t.i.d.
- ***Lactobacillus acidophilus***: the intestinal microflora are severely deranged in alcoholics, leaving the intestines vulnerable to colonization by unfriendly bacteria including the ulcer-causing *Helicobacter pylori*:
  - this disturbance in gut flora leads to malabsorption of fats, carbohydrates, protein, folic acid, and vitamin B_{12}.
  - alcohol ingestion also increases intestinal permeability to toxins and macromolecules, thus

promoting the development of food allergies that may also contribute to cravings for alcohol.

- *Lactobacillus acidophilus* is a friendly bacterium, which supplants unfriendly microbes and whose metabolic by-products provide nutrients necessary for the health of intestinal cells.
- dosage: one to two billion live bacteria q.d.

- **High-potency multiple vitamin and mineral formula:** this should include 400 µg of folic acid, 400 µg of vitamin B_{12}, and 50–100 mg of vitamin B_6. (Folic acid supplementation should always be accompanied by vitamin B_{12} supplementation to prevent folic acid from masking a vitamin B_{12} deficiency.) A daily multiple provides a basic foundation of known vitamins and minerals upon which to build an individualized health promotion program.

- **Zinc:** a key nutrient in the breakdown of alcohol, zinc is typically deficient in alcoholics:
  - low zinc levels are associated with numerous complications of alcohol abuse including impaired alcohol metabolism, a predisposition to cirrhosis (severe damage to the liver), and impaired testicular function.
  - dosage: 30 mg q.d.

- **Vitamin A:** vitamin A deficiency works with zinc deficiency to produce the major complications of alcoholism including night blindness, hormonal disturbances, poor immune function, cirrhosis, decreased testicular function, and skin disorders:
  - **caution:** although vitamin A supplementation has been shown to be of significant benefit to alcoholics, great care must be employed in its use. A liver damaged by excessive alcohol consumption loses much of its ability to store vitamin A, so an alcoholic who continues to drink or shows evidence of impaired liver function is at high risk of vitamin A toxicity if the vitamin is given at dosages above the recommended dietary allowance of 5,000 IU q.d.
  - dosage: 25,000 IU q.d. – only if the person is not drinking and has normal liver function.

- **Vitamin C:** alcohol consumption increases the production of free radicals, and alcoholics are typically deficient in key antioxidants including vitamin C:
  - the higher the levels of free radicals and the lower the levels of antioxidants, the greater the degree of liver damage in alcoholism.
  - higher levels of vitamin C in white blood cells have been directly linked to a faster rate of alcohol detoxification from the blood.
  - dosage: 1,000 mg t.i.d.

- **Vitamin E:** while vitamin C is the primary water-soluble antioxidant, vitamin E plays this role in the fat-soluble areas; dosage: 400–800 IU q.d.

- **Carnitine:** A *lipotropic* agent (nutritional compound that promotes the flow of fat to and from the liver), carnitine significantly inhibits alcohol-induced fatty liver disease. Carnitine, which is normally made in the body when levels of several nutrients (including vitamin B_6 and vitamin C) are adequate, facilitates fatty acid transport and breakdown, lowers triglyceride levels and improves liver function:
  - alcoholics are typically deficient in the nutrients necessary for carnitine production, resulting in low carnitine levels, a problem exacerbated by alcohol consumption increasing the production of fatty acids.
  - dosage: 300 mg t.i.d.

- **Branched chain amino acids:** blood levels of amino acids (the building blocks of protein molecules) are reduced in alcoholics; not surprising as the liver is the primary site for amino acid metabolism. Supplementation with the branched chain amino acids (valine, isoleucine and leucine) greatly aids the alcoholic with cirrhosis; dosage: 3–5 g q.d.

- **B vitamins:** alcoholics are almost always deficient in at least one of the B vitamins, with a thiamin (B_1) deficiency being the most common and most serious:
  - recent evidence indicates that a thiamin deficiency is a predisposing factor for alcoholism.
  - a functional B_6 deficiency is also common because alcohol inhibits the conversion of B_6 to its active form while increasing its degradation and urinary excretion.
  - daily dosages: vitamin B_1 (thiamin) 10–100 mg; vitamin B_2 (riboflavin) 10–50 mg; vitamin B_3 (niacin) 10–100 mg; vitamin B_5 (pantothenic acid) 25–100 mg; vitamin B_6 (pyridoxine) 25–100 mg; vitamin B_{12} (cobalamin) 400 µg; niacinamide 10–30 mg; biotin 100–600 µg; folic acid 400–800 µg; choline 10–100 mg; inositol 10–100 mg.

- **Magnesium:** low magnesium levels, present in as many as 60% of alcoholics and strongly linked to delirium tremens, are thought to be a major contributing factor to the increased incidence of cardiovascular disease in alcoholics; dosage: 200–300 mg of magnesium bound to a Krebs cycle intermediate such as citrate, t.i.d.

- **Essential fatty acids:** alcohol interferes with essential fatty acid (EFA) metabolism and may therefore produce symptoms of EFA deficiency:
  - inadequate EFAs are a significant factor in atherosclerosis, multiple sclerosis, psoriasis, eczema, menstrual cramps, rheumatoid arthritis, and many other allergic or inflammatory conditions.
  - dosage: flaxseed oil 1 tbsp q.d.; gamma-linolenic acid from evening primrose, blackcurrant or borage oil, 180–360 mg q.d.

- **Glutamine:** a non-essential amino acid, glutamine is the preferred fuel for intestinal cells:
  - glutamine supplementation has been shown to significantly improve intestinal function and, by preventing the influx of toxins that occurs when the intestinal wall is damaged, to improve immune function.
  - in preliminary human studies, glutamine supplementation has reduced voluntary alcohol consumption.
  - dosage: 1 g q.d.

Botanical medicines

- ***Silybum marianum* (milk thistle) extract:** the flavonoid complex of milk thistle (*Silybum marianum*) has been shown to be effective in treating the full spectrum of alcohol-related liver disease; dosage: 70–210 mg t.i.d. of a 70–80% silymarin extract; use higher dosages if there is significant liver involvement.

Drug–herb interaction cautions

None.

Physical medicine

- **Exercise:** regular exercise – a minimum of 30 min, at least three times a week – has been shown to be effective in alleviating anxiety and depression, and enables individuals to respond better to stress:
  - improved fitness also promotes improved self-respect, and therefore reduces the likelihood of alcohol abuse, a serious disrespect for oneself.
  - the best exercises are strength training (weight lifting) and/or aerobic activities such as walking briskly, jogging, bicycling, cross-country skiing, swimming, aerobic dance, and racquet sports.

Alzheimer's disease

DESCRIPTION

Functionally, Alzheimer's disease signifies a progressive loss of memory and cognitive performance, eventually leading to a state of mental incapacity commonly referred to as *dementia*, when the individual is no longer able to carry out the activities of daily life. Physically, Alzheimer's disease is characterized by distinctive degenerative changes in the brain, primarily the formation of neurofibrillary tangles and plaques (the equivalent of brain scar tissue), composed of cellular debris. The end result is massive loss of brain cells, especially in key areas that control mental function. A rapidly progressive form of Alzheimer's disease begins in adults around 36–45 years of age. A more gradual form, in which symptoms develop slowly, begins around 65–70 years. In the United States, among the over-65 population, 10% suffer from mild to moderate dementia, and 5% exhibit severe dementia. Risk for dementia increases with age; 25% of people over the age of 80 suffer from dementia.

FREQUENT SIGNS AND SYMPTOMS

Early stages
- Forgetfulness of recent events
- Increasing difficulty performing normal mental tasks, such as adding up a restaurant bill or balancing a checkbook
- Personality changes, including poor impulse control and poor judgment

Later stages
- Difficulty with simple tasks, such as choosing clothing
- Failure to recognize familiar persons
- Disinterest in personal hygiene or appearance
- Difficulty in feeding self
- Belligerence and denial that anything is wrong
- Loss of usual sexual inhibitions
- Wandering away
- Anxiety and insomnia

Advanced stages
- Complete loss of memory, speech and muscle function (including bladder and bowel control), necessitating total care and supervision
- Extreme belligerence and hostility

CAUSES

- **Reversible causes for diagnosed dementia:** these should be ruled out and/or treated. They include: drug toxicity, metabolic and nutritional disorders (hypoglycemia; thyroid disturbances; deficiencies of vitamin B_{12}, folate or thiamin), neurosyphilis, Huntington's disease, cerebral vascular disease, normal pressure hydrocephalus, and intracranial masses.

- **Reduced activity of the enzyme acetyltransferase:** this enzyme synthesizes acetylcholine, a key neurotransmitter especially important for memory.

- **Genetic factors:** several genes have been linked to Alzheimer's disease, including the amyloid precursor gene on chromosome #21, presenilin genes on #14, the apolioprotein E (ApoE) gene on #19, and mutations on #21, 14, and 1. The most significant genetic link for increased risk of developing Alzheimer's disease is with the ApoE of e4 type. In contrast, the ApoE of e2 type has been found to be protective.

- **Environmental factors:** traumatic head injury, chronic exposure to aluminum and/or silicon, exposure to neurotoxins from environmental sources, and free radical/oxidative damage have all been implicated as causative factors.

- **Aluminum:** attention has focussed on aluminum since it is concentrated in the neurofibrillary tangles of persons with Alzheimer's disease, although whether it initiates or is deposited in response to the tangles' formation is not yet clear. Regardless, aluminum does contribute significantly to the progression of Alzheimer's disease:
  - greater aluminum concentrations could explain why symptoms worsen with increasing age. Even in healthy people, aluminum concentration increases with age, but aluminum levels in Alzheimer's sufferers are significantly higher than those of either healthy people or patients with other types of dementia, e.g., from stroke, alcohol or atherosclerosis.
  - in patients whose disease is not yet well established, aluminum removal, via the use of a chelating agent that binds to aluminum and promotes its excretion in the urine, has been shown to significantly slow the rate of decline.

■ primary sources of aluminum appear to be the water supply, food, antacids, deodorants and aluminum cookware. *Drinking water* is the most significant source as the aluminum in water is in a more bioavailable and thus potentially toxic form. When researchers put a tiny amount of soluble aluminum in tap water in animals' stomachs, the trace amounts of aluminum from this single exposure immediately entered the animals' brain tissue.

RISK INCREASES WITH

■ Exposure to neurotoxins, especially aluminum.

■ A diet low in fresh fruits and vegetables, whole grains, nuts and seeds, and therefore low in the protective antioxidants and magnesium these foods supply.

■ Abnormal fingerprint patterns: fingerprints showing an increased number of ulnar loops, along with a decrease in whorls, radial loops and arches, are associated with both Alzheimer's disease and Down's syndrome. Appearance of this abnormal fingerprint pattern warrants an immediate aggressive preventive approach.

PREVENTIVE MEASURES

■ **Avoid all known sources of aluminum:** antacids, antiperspirants that contain aluminum, aluminum pots and pans, aluminum foil as food wrapping, and non-dairy creamers. Aluminum is also added to baking powder and table salt to prevent them from becoming lumpy.

■ **Check aluminum levels in the domestic water supply:** a home water filtration system will reduce aluminum levels in drinking and shower water.

■ **Avoid citric acid and calcium citrate supplements:** both increase the efficiency of aluminum absorption from water and food.

■ **Eat magnesium-rich foods:** magnesium competes with aluminum for absorption, not only in the intestines but also at the blood/brain barrier:
  ■ good food sources of magnesium include vegetables, whole grains, nuts and seeds.
  ■ a magnesium supplement or a multiple vitamin and mineral formula that contains 250–500 mg of magnesium should also be taken daily.

■ **Ensure adequate nutrition (see Appendix 1):**
  ■ particularly in the elderly, a group in which nutrient deficiencies are prevalent, cognitive function is directly related to nutritional status.

■ a growing body of evidence confirms that a high percentage of the geriatric population is deficient in one or more of the B vitamins as well as in zinc, nutrient deficiencies that have been suggested as major factors in the development of Alzheimer's disease.

Expected outcomes
Progression can be significantly slowed and cognitive function improved within 4–6 weeks.

TREATMENT

Diet
Follow the health-promoting diet guidelines provided in Appendix 1. This diet is rich in magnesium, the B vitamins and zinc.

Nutritional supplements
■ **High-potency multiple vitamin and mineral supplement:** this should include 400 µg of folic acid, 400 µg of vitamin B_{12}, and 50–100 mg of vitamin B_6. (Folic acid supplementation should always be accompanied by vitamin B_{12} supplementation to prevent folic acid from masking a vitamin B_{12} deficiency.) A daily multiple providing all of the known vitamins and minerals serves as a foundation upon which to build an individualized health promotion program.

■ **Thiamin:** one of the B vitamins, thiamin is essential for cardiovascular and brain function:
  ■ in the brain, thiamin mimics and potentiates acetylcholine, an important neurotransmitter in memory, which is low in individuals with Alzheimer's disease.
  ■ high-dose thiamin supplementation is without side effects and has been shown to improve mental function in patients with Alzheimer's and age-related impaired mental function.
  ■ dosage: 3–8 g q.d.

■ **Vitamin B_{12}:** a deficiency of B_{12} results in impaired nerve function, which can cause numbness, pins-and-needles sensations, or a burning feeling in the feet, as well as impaired mental function that, in the elderly, can mimic Alzheimer's disease:
  ■ the level of B_{12} declines with age; 42% of persons aged 65 and older are deficient in B_{12}.
  ■ if caught early, B_{12} deficiency is easily treated but, left untreated, can lead to impaired neurological and cognitive function. Best clinical responders to B_{12} supplementation are those who have been showing signs of impaired mental function for less than 6 months.
  ■ in Alzheimer's patients, B_{12} levels are typically quite low, and supplementation of B_{12} and/or folic

acid has resulted in complete reversal in some patients who have had Alzheimer's symptoms for less than 6 months.

- to ensure its utilization, vitamin B_{12} should be taken in its active form, methylcobalamin.
- dosage: methylcobalamin 1,000 µg b.i.d.

- **Vitamin C:** oxidative damage plays a major role in the development and progression of Alzheimer's disease, and vitamin C is one of the most important water-soluble antioxidants; dosage: 500–1,000 mg t.i.d.

- **Vitamin E:** a fat-soluble antioxidant, vitamin E is another critical defender against oxidative damage; dosage: 400–800 IU mixed tocopherols q.d.

- **Flaxseed oil:** an excellent source of omega-3 essential fatty acids, which play a major role in the integrity and fluidity of brain cell membranes:
  - cell membranes can be thought of as the gatekeepers of the cell, allowing in what is needed while sending out what is not. When cell membranes are dysfunctional, toxic debris remains in the cell while needed nutrients cannot gain access.
  - dosage: 1 tbsp q.d.
  - **caution:** flaxseed oil is extremely perishable. It should be sold in an opaque bottle, always kept refrigerated, and never heated.

- **Phosphatidylserine:** another critical component essential for brain cell membrane integrity and fluidity, phosphatidylserine is normally manufactured in the brain when levels of folic acid, vitamin B_{12}, and essential fatty acids are adequate. Should any of these nutrients be deficient, the brain may not be able to make sufficient phosphatidylserine:
  - good results have been obtained in 11 double-blind studies in which phosphatidylserine was used in the treatment of age-related cognitive decline, Alzheimer's disease, and depression.
  - dosage: 100 mg t.i.d.

- **L-Acetylcarnitine:** a special form of carnitine (a vitamin-like compound that transports long-chain fatty acids into the mitochondria, the cellular factories where energy is produced), L-acetylcarnitine (LAC) mimics acetylcholine and benefits not only patients with early-stage Alzheimer's disease, but also elderly patients who are depressed or have impaired memory.
  - LAC stabilizes cell membranes, acts as a powerful antioxidant within brain cells, improves energy production in brain cells, and mimics the function of acetylcholine.
  - well-controlled, extremely thorough studies using LAC to delay the progression of Alzheimer's disease have had uniformly outstanding results.

- dosage: 500 mg t.i.d.
- **Dehydroepiandrosterone (DHEA):** the most abundant hormone in the bloodstream, DHEA is found in extremely high concentrations in the brain:
  - levels of DHEA decline dramatically with age, a drop that has been linked not only to impaired mental function, but also to age-related conditions including diabetes, obesity, elevated cholesterol levels, heart disease, and arthritis.
  - DHEA, from which the body makes all its other steroid hormones, appears to supply the means to maintain optimal levels and balance among all the steroid hormones that regulate the body's activities.
  - dosage: men over age 50: 25–50 mg q.d.; women over age 50: 15–25 mg q.d. Over age 70, higher levels – 50–100 mg q.d. – may be needed.
  - **caution:** too much DHEA can cause acne. Should this occur, decrease the dosage.

Botanical Medicines

- ***Ginkgo biloba* extract (GBE):** In addition to GBE's ability to increase the functional capacity of the brain, it has also been shown to normalize acetylcholine receptors in the hippocampus (the area of the brain most affected by Alzheimer's disease) of aged animals, to increase cholinergic transmission, and to address other major elements of Alzheimer's disease.
  - in studies involving human patients, GBE has been found to help reverse or significantly delay mental deterioration during the early stages of Alzheimer's disease and to cause no side effects.
  - in addition, if the mental deficit is due to vascular insufficiency or depression rather than Alzheimer's disease, GBE will usually be effective in reversing the deficit.
  - GBE should be taken consistently for at least 12 weeks to determine effectiveness. Although some people with Alzheimer's disease note benefits within 2–3 weeks, most need to take GBE for a longer period (e.g., up to 6 months) before seeing results, and GBE must be continued indefinitely to maintain the improvement.
  - dosage: *Ginkgo biloba* extract, 24% ginkgo flavonglycosides, 80 mg t.i.d.

Drug–herb interaction cautions

- ***Ginkgo biloba*:**
  - plus *aspirin*: may induce spontaneous bleeding when combined with chronic use of aspirin. Increased bleeding potential reported after *Ginkgo biloba* usage in a chronic user (2 years) of aspirin.

Angina

DESCRIPTION

A squeezing or pressure-like pain in the chest caused by an insufficient supply of oxygen to the heart, angina usually occurs immediately after exertion, but may be triggered by emotional stress, cold weather, or large meals – all of which increase the heart muscle's need for oxygen. Angina is almost always the body's way of sounding an alarm for the presence of atherosclerosis – a build-up of cholesterol-containing plaque that progressively narrows and ultimately blocks the coronary arteries (the blood vessels supplying the heart). Blood vessels contain no nerves, so atherosclerosis is painless, until it causes either angina or a heart attack. Hypoglycemia can also cause angina. Pain, which typically lasts for 1–20 min, may radiate to the left shoulder blade, left arm or jaw.

Angina is a serious condition that requires careful treatment and monitoring since it frequently precedes a heart attack. Initially, prescription medication may be necessary, but it should eventually be possible to control angina with natural measures.

Another type of angina unrelated to atherosclerosis is *Prinzmetal's variant angina*. Caused by a spasm of the coronary artery, Prinzmetal's angina is more apt to occur at rest, may occur at odd times during the day or night, and is more common in women under the age of 50. Prinzmetal's angina usually responds well to magnesium supplementation. In men, coronary artery spasm induced by magnesium insufficiency is an important cause of heart attack and a significant factor in angina.

FREQUENT SIGNS AND SYMPTOMS

- Tightness, squeezing, pressure or ache in the chest
- Chest pain similar to indigestion
- A choking feeling in the throat
- Chest pain that radiates to the jaw, teeth or earlobes
- Heaviness, numbness, tingling or ache in the chest, arm, shoulder, elbow or hand, usually on the left side
- Pain between the shoulder blades
- Sudden difficulty breathing (sometimes)

CAUSES

- **Atherosclerosis:** the build-up of cholesterol-containing plaque that progressively narrows and ultimately blocks the coronary arteries (the blood vessels supplying the heart).
- **Coronary artery spasm:** the coronary arteries deliver blood to the heart; a spasm in these arteries abruptly interrupts the flow of blood to the heart.
- **Hypoglycemia:** when blood glucose levels drop below normal range, all body systems, including the heart muscle, suffer from lack of necessary fuel.
- **Hyperthyroidism:** hormones produced by the thyroid gland regulate the metabolic rate in every cell in the body. An overactive thyroid increases the metabolic rate and thus the need for oxygen in all organs, including the heart.

RISK INCREASES WITH

- **Stress, overwork, anxiety:** all are associated with increased risk of heart attack. When researchers assessed the impact of worrying, an important component of anxiety, they found that men who worried about social conditions (political, economic, environmental) over which a person has little, if any, control, had a 241% increased risk of developing heart disease.
- **Type A personality:** a predominantly aggressive (hostile), angry coping style doubles an individual's risk of coronary artery disease.
- **Smoking:** this decreases the oxygen carried by red blood cells throughout the body and significantly increases the risk of heart and cardiovascular disease including high blood pressure, coronary artery disease, and heart attack.
- **Obesity:** this contributes significantly to the development of diabetes mellitus, high cholesterol levels, and coronary artery disease.
- **Diabetes mellitus:** in diabetics, both hyper- and hypoglycemia are frequent complications:
  - *hypoglycemia* is a state of low blood sugar in which all systems, including the cardiovascular system, are deprived of adequate fuel, while in

hyperglycemia, excessive blood sugar levels cause damage to arterial walls.

- a diabetic has a two to three times higher risk of dying prematurely of atherosclerosis than a non-diabetic individual.

- **Presence of any of the following risk factors for arteriosclerosis:** excessive intake of fat or salt, high blood pressure, high cholesterol levels, high fibrinogen levels, increased platelet aggregation, elevated levels of homocysteine, elevated levels of C-reactive protein (for explanations of these risk factors, see the chapter on Atherosclerosis).

- **Low levels of magnesium and potassium:** both minerals are essential to the proper functioning of the entire cardiovascular system.

- **Inadequate intake of omega-3 essential fatty acids:** both population and autopsy studies show that individuals who consume the least omega-3 oils have the most heart disease:

  - omega-3 fatty acids protect the heart by lowering levels of low density lipoprotein (bad) cholesterol and triglycerides, inhibiting excessive platelet aggregation, lowering fibrinogen levels and lowering blood pressure in individuals with high blood pressure.

- **Family history of coronary artery disease:** elevations of blood cholesterol and/or triglycerides can be due to genetic factors; such familial tendencies affect about 1:500 people. Atherosclerosis is also directly related to diet and lifestyle, both of which are greatly influenced by learned family behaviors.

PREVENTIVE MEASURES

- Stop smoking.
- Limit consumption of alcohol to no more than one drink per day for women, two for men. (One drink equals 350 ml (12 US fl oz) of beer, 140 ml (4–5 US fl oz) of wine, or 45 ml (1.5 US fl oz) of distilled spirits.)
- Avoid caffeine, a vasoconstrictor.
- Avoid saturated fats, margarine and other foods containing *trans* fatty acids. Extensive research links these fats to heart disease, strokes and cancer.
- Exercise regularly – a minimum of 30 min, at least three times a week. A carefully graded, progressive aerobic exercise program is essential. Walking is a good exercise with which to start.
- Learn how to cope effectively with stress. Use stress-management techniques such as abdominal breathing, progressive relaxation, meditation or guided imagery.

- Consume a heart-healthy diet rich in whole, unprocessed, preferably organic foods, especially plant foods (fruits, vegetables, whole grains, beans, seeds and nuts), and cold-water fish (for more detailed information, see Appendix 1).
- A high-potency multiple vitamin and mineral supplement including 400 µg of folic acid, 400 µg of vitamin B_{12}, and 50–100 mg of vitamin B_6. (Folic acid supplementation should always be accompanied by vitamin B_{12} supplementation to prevent folic acid from masking a vitamin B_{12} deficiency.) A daily multiple providing all of the known vitamins and minerals serves as a foundation upon which to build an individualized health-promotion program.
- Increase consumption of omega-3 essential fatty acids by consuming flaxseed oil (1 tbsp q.d.) and/or eating cold-water fish – salmon, mackerel, tuna, herring (110 g [4 oz] at least three times a week).

Expected outcomes

Significant improvement should occur within 2–3 weeks, but resolution of angina requires reversal of the underlying disease, atherosclerosis.

TREATMENT

Diet

- Increase dietary fiber, especially the soluble fiber found in high amounts in flaxseed, oat bran, pectin and legumes, since it is very effective in lowering cholesterol levels. A daily intake of 35 g of fiber from fiber-rich foods is the aim.
- Increase intake of onions and garlic, both of which have numerous beneficial effects on cholesterol, triglycerides and fibrinogen.
- Increase intake of colorful vegetables and fruits. The colors of fruits and vegetables are due to the presence of heart-protective carotenoids and flavonoids.
- Increase intake of cold-water fish such as salmon, mackerel, herring and halibut. These fish are particularly good sources of omega-3 fatty acids, which lower cholesterol and triglyceride levels.
- For cooking, as salad dressing, or on bread, use olive oil. This monounsaturated oil, composed mainly of oleic acid, is less susceptible to free radical damage. Population studies routinely show decreased risk of heart disease when intake of oleic acid is high.
- Reduce consumption of saturated fats, animal protein, and cholesterol.
- Avoid refined sugar, which may appear on food labels as sucrose, glucose, maltose, lactose, fructose, corn syrup, or white grape juice concentrate.

- Avoid alcohol and coffee.
- Avoid fried foods and food allergens.
- Those with episodic hypoglycemia should eat small frequent meals and avoid all simple carbohydrates (sugar, honey, dried fruit, fruit juice, etc.).

Nutritional supplements

- **Carnitine:** a vitamin-like compound, carnitine transports fatty acids into the mitochondria – the energy-production factories in every cell – where they are converted into energy:
  - carnitine levels quickly drop when the supply of oxygen to the heart is decreased, as in angina.
  - without adequate carnitine, unused fatty acids accumulate within the heart muscle, making it extremely susceptible to cellular damage, which ultimately leads to a heart attack.
  - supplementation normalizes heart carnitine levels and allows the heart muscle to use its limited supply of oxygen more effectively.
  - dosage: L-carnitine: 500 mg t.i.d.
- **Coenzyme Q_{10}:** essential for energy production, CoQ_{10} is important in the heart, one of the most metabolically active tissues in the body:
  - the need for CoQ_{10} increases in cardiovascular diseases such as angina, with the result that this nutrient has been found to be deficient in 50–75% of patients with various heart diseases.
  - dosage: 150–300 mg q.d.
- **Pantethine:** formed in the body from the B vitamin pantothenic acid, pantethine is used to synthesize coenzyme A (CoA), which is involved in the transport of fatty acids to the mitochondria and to and from cells. By accelerating the breakdown of fatty acids in the mitochondria, pantethine lowers serum cholesterol and triglyceride levels:
  - like carnitine, heart pantethine levels decrease during times of reduced oxygen supply, so supplementation is advised.
  - pantethine's lipid-lowering ability is impressive when its toxicity (virtually none) is compared with that of conventional lipid-lowering drugs.
  - dosage: 900 mg q.d.
- **Magnesium:** deficiency has been shown to produce spasms of the coronary arteries and may be a cause of non-occlusive heart attacks. Men who die suddenly of heart attacks have significantly lower levels of heart magnesium than matched controls:
  - magnesium relaxes the arteries, which improves the ability of the coronary arteries to deliver oxygen to the heart, reduces the effort with which the heart must pump, and normalizes heart rate, lessening arrhythmias.
  - magnesium also inhibits platelets from aggregating and forming blood clots.
  - magnesium bound to aspartate, citrate, or other intermediate of the Krebs cycle (a part of the energy production process in the mitochondria) is more effectively assimilated and utilized.
  - dosage: 200–400 mg t.i.d.

Botanical medicines

- ***Crataegus* (hawthorn):** flavonoids found in both the berry and flowering tops of the hawthorn tree are widely used in Europe for their beneficial effects on cardiovascular health:
  - hawthorn flavonoids dilate the coronary blood vessels, increasing the supply of blood and oxygen to the heart; they also interact with key enzymes, enhancing the heart's ability to contract.
  - studies have demonstrated that hawthorn's actions are effective in reducing angina attacks and in lowering blood pressure and serum cholesterol levels.
  - dosage: choose one of the following forms and take the recommended dosage t.i.d.:
    - berries or dried flowers: 3–5 g or as a tea
    - tincture (1 : 5): 4–6 ml (1–1.5 tsp)
    - fluid extract (1 : 1): 1–2 ml (0.25–0.5 tsp)
    - solid extract (10% procyanidins or 1.8% vitexin-4'-rhamnoside): 100–250 mg.
- ***Ammi visnaga* (khella):** an ancient medicinal plant native to the Mediterranean region, khella contains several components effective in dilating the coronary arteries:
  - like the calcium-channel-blocking drugs, khella relaxes blood vessels by blocking the entry of calcium, which causes constriction, into blood vessel cells.
  - khella extracts, standardized for khellin (an active component), typically at 12%, are the preferred form since they deliver a consistent dosage of several active constituents.
  - khella also works well with hawthorn extracts.
  - dosage: dried powdered extract – 12% khellin content, 100 mg t.i.d.

Drug–herb interaction cautions
None.

Physical medicine

- **Aerobic exercise:** a carefully graded, progressive aerobic exercise program. Walking is a good exercise with which to start (30 min, three times a week).

Ascariasis (intestinal roundworms)

DESCRIPTION

Ascaris (roundworms) are large intestinal parasites, reaching 15–40 cm (6–16 in) in length. Infection is spread via food and fingers contaminated by human fecal matter containing mature eggs, particularly in areas where human feces is used as fertilizer. Approximately 25% of the world's population, including 4 million Americans (especially in the southeast of the USA) are infected. In developing areas of the world, where sanitary facilities are lacking, infection in children is almost universal.

When roundworm eggs are ingested, the larvae hatch in the stomach and small intestine, penetrate the wall of the small intestine and travel through the small veins in the lining of the abdominal cavity and the lymph vessels to the heart, and then via the blood to the lungs. From the lungs, they migrate into the throat, are swallowed, and return to the small intestine, where they mature. Within 2–3 months, the female produces enormous numbers of eggs, which are excreted in the feces. The eggs, which can survive in the soil for up to 7 years, become infective after 2–3 weeks. The adult worm may live for a year or more.

FREQUENT SIGNS AND SYMPTOMS

In all age groups:
- Chronic intestinal infection may be asymptomatic if the infection is light.
- Heavy infection may cause abdominal discomfort, with pain, distention or fullness, vomiting, weight loss, weakness, constipation, and diarrhea.
- As the worms pass through the lungs, they cause damage, which may result in bronchitis or pneumonia with fever, cough, shortness of breath, and/or wheezing.

Common symptoms in children may also include:
- irritability
- restlessness at night
- frequent urination
- teeth grinding
- erratic or poor appetite
- frequent fatigue
- colicky abdominal discomfort
- diarrhea (sometimes)
- dry cough and wheezing (rare)
- fever
- twitching in various parts of the body
- convulsions, fits, spasms
- nervousness
- itching of the nose or anus
- anal irritation
- abnormal pallor of the lips, mouth, gums
- worms sometimes seen in bowel movements or in the child's bed; rarely, one may be vomited
- asthma: susceptible individuals have an enhanced tendency to asthma, possibly due to allergic reactions to the *Ascaris* larvae as they pass through the lungs or increased sensitivity to common inhaled allergens caused by exposure to *Ascaris* antigen.

CAUSES

A parasitic worm, *Ascaris*, whose eggs enter the human body through contaminated water, food or soil-contaminated hands.

RISK INCREASES WITH

- Crowded or unsanitary living conditions.
- Use of human feces as fertilizer.
- Environmental toxicity: numerous animal studies suggest that heavy metal toxicity not only increases susceptibility to parasite infection, but also inhibits the body's attempts to limit the infection and allows increased migration of worms throughout the body:
  - studies that looked at the effects of industrial heavy metal emissions (mercury, copper, lead, zinc) on the ability of the guinea pig's immune system to mount a defense during the migration phase of *Ascaris* found an eightfold increase in the number of worm larvae migrating into the lungs.
  - studies of the effects of cadmium and mercury on the immune defenses of roundworm-infected guinea pigs showed an increase of 20% in the number of *Ascaris* larvae reaching the lungs.

PREVENTIVE MEASURES

- Wash hands frequently, and always before eating, with warm water and soap.
- Wash hands carefully after using the toilet.
- Keep nails short and clean.
- Keep fingers away from the mouth.
- Have pets treated for worms. Avoid strange animals.
- Wash all produce. Soak produce in a mild solution of additive-free soap like Ivory or pure castille soap from the health food store. All-natural, biodegradable produce cleansers are also available at most health food stores. Simply spray the produce with the cleanser, gently scrub, then rinse off.
- To prevent infecting others or re-infecting oneself, wash the anus and genitals with warm water and soap at least twice a day until the infection is completely eliminated. Rinse well, preferably under a shower. Don't take tub baths.
- If possible, boil all soiled linen, nightclothes, underwear, towels and washcloths that have been used by anyone with roundworms. Fabrics that cannot be boiled can be soaked in an ammonia solution (1 cup of household ammonia to 5 gallons of cold water).
- After treatment, scrub all toilet seats, bathroom floors and fixtures. Vacuum rugs, tables, curtains, sofa and chairs carefully. Sterilize metal toys or similar objects in a hot oven. All cooking areas and utensils should be thoroughly cleaned.

Expected outcomes

Ascaris infection is almost always curable using the 4-day protocol outlined below. However, to ensure all worms have been eliminated, the entire 4-day program should be repeated twice: 2 weeks later, and then once more after an additional week later.

TREATMENT

Diet

- A diet high in unrefined carbohydrates and raw green vegetables, and moderate in protein, with no meat, dairy, or sugar, provides high resistance to roundworm infections.
- *Ascaris* prefers an environment that is acidic (the result of meat and dairy consumption), sweet (sugar, refined carbohydrates), and constipated (the result of a low-fiber diet).
- An inhospitable diet for roundworms – a whole foods, primarily vegetarian diet (which is alkaline, low in sugar and high in fiber) – is recommended. This health-promoting diet also prevents reinfection by boosting immune function.

Botanical medicines

- Extracts of garlic, onion, pomegranate rind, turmeric (*Curcuma longa*), and various citrus rinds have all been shown to be effective against *Ascaris*.
- Bromelain and papain are useful in dissolving the worms' outer layer that shields them from the body's digestive enzymes.
- Fig powder is helpful due to its laxative effect.
- *Lactobacillus* supplementation may be recommended because the lactic acid this friendly flora produces inhibits the growth of pathogens, decreases any tendency to constipation, and generally promotes healthy bowel activity, which prevents reinfection.
- *Artemesia absinthium* (wormwood), *Inula helenium* (elecampane), and *Picraena excelpa* (quassia) are botanical agents that destroy or expel intestinal worms with the least toxic side effects for the patient.
- Elecampane is recommended as the safest for children.

Therapeutic *Ascaris* elimination protocol

Days 1–3

Eat nothing but 75–150 g (3–5 oz) of pumpkin seeds, plus three to eight cloves of garlic q.d.

- On an empty stomach, the patient should take the following dosages t.i.d.:
  - bromelain (1,200 MCU): 500 mg
  - papain: 500–1,000 mg
  - pancreatin (8 × USP): 500 mg
  - fig powder: 1 tsp.
- Take one botanical therapy t.i.d.:
  Children
  - *Inula helenium* (elecampane): powdered root (1–2 g) or a 1 : 1 fluid extract (1–2 ml)
  Adults
  - *Artemesia absinthium* (wormwood): oil (1–5 drops), infusion (0.5–1 tsp/cup), powdered root (1–2 g), 1 : 1 fluid extract (2–4 ml)
  - *Picraena excelpa* (quassia): powdered wood (1–2 g).

Day 4

Administer a purging dose of licorice root (recommended for children), magnesium citrate, senna or *Cascara sagrada*. Licorice root or coriander may be added to strong laxatives to make them more palatable and/or milder in action if desired.

Before taking the purging dose, soaked raisins may be eaten as the sweetness will help lure any remaining worms out of hiding and enhance their expulsion.

Maintain the recommended preventive diet while continuing the same quantities of pumpkin seeds and garlic.

Two weeks later

Repeat the entire 4-day program, then maintain the recommended preventive diet while continuing the same quantities of pumpkin seeds and garlic.

An additional week later

Repeat the entire 4-day program once more.

Drug—herb interaction cautions

- *Glycyrrhiza glabra* (licorice):
  - plus *digoxin, digitalis*: due to a reduction of potassium in the blood, licorice potentiates the toxicity of cardiac glycosides. Interaction with these cardiac glycoside drugs could lead to arrhythmias and cardiac arrest.
  - plus *stimulant laxatives or diuretics* (thiazides, spironolactone or amiloride): licorice should not be used with these drugs because of the additive increase of potassium loss to potentially dangerous levels.
- **Senna or *Cascara sagrada*:**
  - plus *oral drugs*: may decrease absorption due to decreased bowel transit time.
  - plus *cardiac glycosides*: overuse or misuse can cause potassium loss leading to increased toxicity of cardiac glycosides such as in *Digitalis, Adonis, Convallaria, Urginea, Helleborus, Strophanthus*.
  - plus *diuretics*: use aggravates loss of potassium associated with diuretics.

Asthma

DESCRIPTION

Asthma is an allergic disorder characterized by spasm of the *bronchi* (the airway tubes), swelling of the mucous linings of the lungs, and excessive production of thick, viscous mucus, all of which combine to trigger attacks of wheezing, shortness of breath, coughing and the expectoration of tenacious sputum. Severe attacks can lead to respiratory failure – the inability to breathe.

Asthma has typically been divided into two major categories: extrinsic and intrinsic. *Extrinsic* or atopic asthma is generally considered an allergic condition, with a characteristic rise in levels of IgE – the allergy antibody. *Intrinsic* asthma is associated with bronchial spasm in response to factors such as toxic chemicals, cold air, exercise, infection and emotional upset.

Both categories of asthma trigger the release of inflammation-producing chemicals from specialized white blood cells called mast cells, which are found in various body tissues including the lining of the respiratory passages. The most potent of these asthma-provoking chemicals are the leukotrienes, some of which are 1,000 times more powerful than histamine in stimulating bronchial constriction.

Asthma now afflicts approximately 17.3 million Americans, a number that has more than doubled since the early 1980s, and more than tripled among those aged 5–24 years. Although most common in children under age 10, with affected boys outnumbering girls two-to-one, asthma is no longer a disease outgrown after childhood. A recent study found that in 75% of children with moderate to severe asthma who were followed into their twenties, the disease steadily worsened.

FREQUENT SIGNS AND SYMPTOMS

Mild/moderate attack symptoms
- Chest tightness and shortness of breath
- Wheezing when breathing out
- Rapid, shallow breathing that is easier when sitting up
- Difficulty breathing
- Neck muscles tighten
- Coughing, especially at night, occasionally with thick clear or yellow sputum

Severe attack symptoms
- Bluish skin
- Grunting respiration
- Inability to speak
- Exhaustion
- Mental changes, including restlessness or confusion

CAUSES

The following are all potential contributing factors to the rapid escalation of asthma in the US, especially among young children.

- **Pollution:** increased stress on the immune system due to increased chemical pollution of air, water and food.
- **Earlier weaning and introduction of solid foods to infants:** ideally, an infant should be breastfed for 6–9 months. Weaning earlier than 6 months increases the likelihood of food allergy.
- **Hypochlorhydria:** analysis of asthmatic children has shown that many are hypochlorhydric, i.e., have gastric acid secretions below normal levels, which may predispose these children to the development of food allergies. If not corrected, this may also have a significant negative impact on the success of rotation and/or elimination diets.
- **Food allergy:** food allergens damage the intestinal lining, which allows large molecules that normally are not absorbed to enter the general circulation. This increased antigenic load overwhelms the immune system, increases the level of allergenic compounds that can trigger asthma, and increases the likelihood of developing additional allergies.
- **Food additives:** these chemicals may trigger an immune response in sensitive individuals.
- **Genetic manipulation of plants:** results in food components with greater allergenic tendencies.
- **Pertussis (whooping cough) vaccine:** a British study of 448 children found the relative risk of developing asthma is about 1% in children who receive no immunizations; 3% in those who receive vaccinations other than pertussis, and 11% in those who receive pertussis vaccine. However, in the group not

immunized to pertussis, 16 developed whooping cough compared to only one in the immunized group. These results indicate a greater risk for asthma with the pertussis vaccine versus a greater risk for whooping cough without it.

Common asthmatic attack triggers

- **Environmental triggers:** pollen, house dust, animal dander, stuffed animals, feather pillows, down comforters, cockroaches, molds, smoke, perfumes, household cleaning products, paint or solvents, insecticides, gasoline fumes, natural and cooking gas, strong odors, out-gassing of chemicals from new furnishings or carpets, exposure to occupational chemicals, excessively dry or cold air, exercise, chlorinated pools, viral infections such as colds, flu, bronchitis.

- **Non-steroidal anti-inflammatory drugs (NSAIDs):** asthmatics tend to form higher amounts of leukotrienes, inflammation-producing chemicals that stimulate bronchial constriction and allergy:
  - this abnormality is even more pronounced in patients with "aspirin-induced asthma" in which ingestion of aspirin and other NSAIDs (e.g., indometacin and ibuprofen) results in the production of excessive levels of leukotrienes in sensitive individuals.

- Dietary triggers: yeast (breads, sauces, dried fruits, cheese, mushrooms), cow's milk and dairy products, eggs, soy, wheat, sulfites, pesticide residues on food, and food additives – most notably tartrazine (FD&C yellow dye #5):
  - tartrazine, which is added to most processed foods and can even be found in vitamin preparations and antiasthma prescription drugs (e.g., aminophylline), promotes the tendency to leukotriene formation and is a frequent asthma trigger, especially in children.

RISK INCREASES WITH

- Pertussis vaccination
- Other allergic conditions, such as eczema or hay fever
- Family history of asthma or allergies
- Exposure to air pollutants or other toxic chemicals
- Consumption of processed foods (food additives)
- Smoking or exposure to second-hand smoke
- Use of NSAIDs
- Stressors such as viral infection, exercise, cold air, emotional upset, noxious odors
- High salt intake: strong evidence suggests that increased salt intake increases bronchial reactivity and mortality from asthma

PREVENTIVE MEASURES

Environmental factors

- Install HEPA (high-energy particulate arresting) air filters in the bedroom and other rooms in regular use.
- Cover mattress, box springs, and pillows with allergen-proof cases, tape over the zippers, and wipe down with a wet cloth once a week. Use hypoallergenic or 100% cotton bedding. Wash sheets, blankets, pillowcases, and mattress pads weekly in hot water with additive- and fragrance-free detergent. Purchase new pillows at least once each year; old, sweaty pillows incubate mold.
- Replace wall-to-wall carpeting with hardwood (i.e., real wood; imitation "wood" will out-gas many more chemicals) floors or ceramic tile. Use leather or wood rather than upholstered furniture. If this is not possible, treat carpet and furnishings with a tannic acid spray. Tannic acid, a natural compound found in coffee, tea and cocoa, can help neutralize the dust mite and animal dander proteins responsible for allergic reactions.
- Use a vacuum with a built-in HEPA filter and vacuum frequently.
- Keep pets out of the bedroom. Brush dogs and cats regularly and give them a weekly bath.
- If cockroaches are suspect, sprinkle boric acid – a non-allergenic, relatively safe insecticide – in all potentially infested areas.
- Clean mold-prone areas regularly with a non-toxic solution made from borax and vinegar mixed with water in a spray bottle. Spray on and wipe off.
- Replace all harsh cleaning products with non-toxic products. Avoid soft plastics and plastic wrap for food. Use waxed paper, glass, ceramic or steel containers for food storage and serving.
- Check local pollen and mold counts daily. Information can be obtained on the Internet (e.g., http://www.aaaai.org for the US; http://www.metoffice.com for the UK). Local radio/television stations usually broadcast pollen count forecasts during high-risk periods. When pollen counts are highest, try to stay indoors.
- Shower and change clothes after being outdoors, so pollen will not be transferred to furniture and bedding.

Dietary factors

- Identify and eliminate food allergens and additives.
- Evaluate and, if necessary, reduce salt intake.
- Choose organic produce whenever possible.
- Minimize exposure to pesticides, waxes, fungicides, and fertilizers from produce:
  - avoid animal fat, meat, eggs, cheese, and milk; pesticide residues are concentrated in these foods.

- if organic produce is not readily available, try to buy local in-season produce.
- to remove surface pesticide residues, waxes, fungicides, and fertilizers, soak the produce in a mild solution of additive-free soap like Ivory or pure castile soap from the health food store. All-natural, biodegradable cleansers are also available at most health food stores. Simply spray the produce with the cleanser, gently scrub, then rinse off.
- peel off the skin or remove the outer layer of leaves. The downside here is that many of the nutritional benefits are concentrated in the skin and outer layers.

Expected outcomes

Within 1 month, asthma attacks should decrease in frequency and severity. Within 6 months to 1 year, the problem should be under control.

TREATMENT

Note: In severe cases of asthma, the best treatment is a combined approach, using natural therapies to reduce the allergic threshold and prevent acute attacks, together with drug treatment of acute attacks.

Diet

- **Eliminate food allergens:** food allergies play an important role in asthma, as explained above. Adverse reactions may be immediate or delayed. Immediate-onset sensitivities in children are usually due to (in order of frequency): eggs, fish, shellfish, nuts, and peanuts. Foods most commonly associated with delayed-onset sensitivities include (in order of frequency): milk, chocolate, wheat, citrus, and food colorings.
- **Onions and garlic:** enjoy onions and garlic liberally and frequently, if you are not allergic to them: both inhibit lipoxygenase and cyclo-oxygenases, which generate inflammatory prostaglandins and thromboxanes. Onions also contain other anti-inflammatory agents – the isothiocyanates and the flavonoid, quercetin.
- **Elimination diet:** elimination diets have been successful in identifying allergens and treating asthma. Elimination of common allergens during infancy (the first 2 years) has been shown to reduce allergenic tendencies in children with a strong familial history of asthma.
- **Allergen identification diet:** for 1 week, go on a hypoallergenic diet – for example, consume only lamb, turkey, rice, carrots, pears, and sweet potatoes. Reintroduce one new food every day for 3 days,

monitoring for any adverse reactions. Reintroduce top allergens in pure, unadulterated form, for example, cream of wheat rather than bread.

- **Vegan diet:** in one study, asthma significantly improved or was entirely relieved in 92% of patients following a vegan diet; 71% responded within 4 months, while the remaining 21% needed a full year of diet therapy:
  - the diet in this study excluded all meat, fish, eggs, and dairy products, and also excluded coffee, ordinary tea, chocolate, sugar and salt.
  - for beverages, only spring water (chlorinated tap water was specifically prohibited) and herbal teas were allowed.
  - vegetables used freely were: lettuce, carrots, beets, onions, celery, cabbage, cauliflower, broccoli, nettles, cucumber, radishes, Jerusalem artichokes, and all beans except soy and green peas. Potatoes were allowed in restricted amounts.
  - freely used fruits were: blueberries, cloudberries, raspberries, strawberries, blackcurrants, gooseberries, plums and pears. Apples and citrus fruits were not allowed, and grains were either highly restricted or eliminated.
  - this diet not only eliminates allergens while increasing intake of antioxidants and magnesium, but also avoids arachidonic acid. In the body, arachidonic acid, which is derived from animal products, is used to form inflammatory prostaglandins and leukotrienes that significantly contribute to the allergic reaction in asthma.
- **Increase consumption of cold-water fish:** one possible exception to the avoidance of animal products is cold-water fish (salmon, mackerel, herring, halibut, etc.), as they contain high amounts of anti-inflammatory omega-3 fatty acids.
- **Eliminate food additives:** artificial dyes (particularly tartrazine, an orange food coloring) and common preservatives (benzoates, sulfur dioxide, and, especially, sulfites) are widely used in foods, beverages, and drugs, and have been reported to cause asthma attacks in susceptible individuals:
  - US citizens consume an average of 2–3 mg of sulfites each day; wine and beer drinkers ingest an additional 5–10 mg.
  - a molybdenum deficiency may be responsible for sulfite sensitivity since sulfite oxidase, the enzyme responsible for neutralizing sulfites, requires molybdenum.

Nutritional supplements

Dosages given are for adults; for children, divide the dosage in half if they weigh between 23 and 45 kg

(50 and 100 lb). For children weighing less than 23 kg (50 lb), use one-third the adult dosage.

- **Vitamin B$_5$:** allergies frequently signal inadequate pantothenic acid (B$_5$); dosage: 150 mg q.d.
- **Vitamin B$_6$:** children with asthma have been shown to have a defect in their metabolism of the amino acid tryptophan. Tryptophan is converted to serotonin, a compound that can cause the airways of asthmatics to constrict. Vitamin B$_6$ is required for tryptophan metabolism and, when used in a study that included 76 asthmatic children, produced significant reductions in symptoms and in the dosages of drugs (bronchodilators and corticosteroids) required.
  - in adult asthmatics, blood levels of B$_6$ have been found to be significantly lower than those in healthy controls, and B$_6$ supplementation has produced dramatic decreases in frequency and severity of wheezing and asthmatic attacks, except in patients dependent upon steroids for control of symptoms.
  - while B$_6$ may not help patients dependent upon steroids, it is definitely recommended for those treated with the drug theophylline as this drug significantly depresses levels of the active form of B$_6$.
  - B$_6$ supplementation has also been shown to effectively reduce typical side effects of theophylline (headaches, nausea, irritability, sleep disorders, etc.).
  - dosage: 25–50 mg b.i.d.
- **Vitamin B$_{12}$:** especially effective in treating sulfite-sensitive individuals, B$_{12}$, when given orally before challenge, forms a sulfite–cobalamin complex that blocks sulfite's allergic effect. Weekly IM injections have also produced definite improvement in asthmatic patients including less shortness of breath with exertion, and improved appetite and sleep; dosage: oral B$_{12}$: 1–4 µg; IM injections: 1,000 µg.
- **Magnesium:** a natural bronchodilator, magnesium stabilizes mast cells and relaxes muscles, dilating bronchioles and quickly opening up airways:
  - IV magnesium (2 g of magnesium sulfate every hour, up to a total of 24.6 g) is a well-proven, clinically accepted measure to halt an acute asthma attack.
  - oral magnesium therapy can also raise magnesium stores over a period of about 6 weeks.
  - dietary intake of magnesium, which relaxes bronchial smooth muscle, is directly related to lung function and asthma severity.
  - dosage: 200–400 mg of magnesium citrate or aspartate t.i.d.
- **DHEA:** decreased levels of this adrenal hormone are common among postmenopausal women with asthma. Given its importance to proper immune

function, supplementation may produce positive effects; dosage: 15–50 mg q.d.
- **Antioxidants:** these inhibit leukotriene formation and histamine release from mast cells, increase the integrity of the epithelial lining of the respiratory tract, and protect the lung against free radicals and other oxidizing agents that stimulate bronchial constriction and increase reactivity to other agents. Antioxidants typically work together as a team, so it's best to include a variety of antioxidant nutrients such as the carotenes, vitamins A, C, and E, the mineral cofactors essential for antioxidant defense actions such as zinc, selenium, and copper, and flavonoids, particularly quercetin:
  - *carotenes*: quench free radicals, help detoxify smoke and other air pollutants, and modulate the release of anti-inflammatory prostaglandins and leukotrienes; dosage: 25,000–50,000 IU q.d.
  - *vitamin A*: essential for the health of epithelial cells and mucus membranes in the respiratory system; dosage: 10,000 IU q.d. **Caution:** should not be taken by pregnant women.
  - *vitamin C*: an antihistamine and antioxidant, vitamin C also stimulates white cells to fight infection, directly kills many bacteria and viruses, and regenerates vitamin E after it has been inactivated by disarming free radicals; dosage: 10–30 mg q.d. for every 0.9 kg (2 lb) of body weight, in divided doses.
  - *vitamin E*: protects the cell's fatty membrane and helps neutralize damaging effects of ozone, a major component of smog which worsens asthma; dosage: 200–400 IU q.d. of mixed tocopherols.
  - *zinc*: along with copper, zinc is necessary for the production of one of the body's most important endogenous antioxidants, superoxide dismutase. Zinc also boosts immunity by increasing circulating lymphocytes and antibody production; dosage: 15–45 mg q.d.
  - *selenium*: an antioxidant itself, this trace mineral also activates one of the premier internally produced antioxidants, glutathione, which protects the liver cells responsible for clearing pathogens and toxins from the body; dosage: 200–400 µg q.d.
  - *copper*: a constituent of the important antioxidant enzyme, superoxide dismutase; dosage: 1–2 mg q.d.
  - *quercetin*: a bioflavonoid that works synergistically with vitamin C as an antihistamine; dosage: 400 mg, taken 20 min before each meal.

Botanical medicines
- ***Ginkgo biloba*:** ginkgo contains several unique molecules known collectively as *ginkgolides* that block platelet activating factor (PAF), an important part of

the inflammatory cascade that triggers allergies and asthma:

- in some clinical trials, 12 weeks were needed to produce results.
- dosage: 80 mg of a 24% standardized extract t.i.d.

Ephedra sinica (Ma huang): *Ephedra* and its alkaloid constituents are effective bronchodilators for the treatment of mild to moderate asthma. Peak bronchodilation occurs in 1 hour and lasts about 5 hours:

- *Ephedra* can be combined with the herbs *Glycyrrhiza glabra* and *Lobelia inflata*.
- dosage: optimal dosage of *Ephedra* depends on the alkaloid content of the form used. Each dose should have an ephedrine content of 12.5–25.0 mg and be taken b.i.d.–t.i.d. For the crude herb, this dosage would most likely be 500–1,000 mg t.i.d.
- **caution:** *Ephedra* is contraindicated during pregnancy due to the uterine stimulant action associated with its alkaloids ephedrine and pseudoephedrine in *in vitro* (test tube) and animal studies.

Lobelia inflata (Indian tobacco): lobelia stimulates the adrenal gland to produce hormones that relax bronchial muscles and is also an expectorant; dosage: tincture, 20 drops t.i.d.

Tylophora asthmatica: *Tylophora* has been used extensively in Ayurvedic medicine for treating asthma and other respiratory conditions. Its alkaloids are reported to possess antihistamine and antispasmodic activity as well as inhibiting mast cell release of histamine and other inflammatory compounds:

- *Tylophora* can be combined with the herbal expectorant *Glycyrrhiza glabra*.
- dosage: 200 mg of *Tylophora* leaves or 40 mg of the dry alcoholic extract b.i.d.

Glycyrrhiza glabra (licorice root): licorice is an effective anti-inflammatory and antiallergic agent. Glycyrrhetinic acid, a component in licorice with cortisol-like effects, inhibits prostaglandin and leukotriene manufacture in a manner similar to corticosteroids like prednisone (prednisolone). It is also an expectorant; dosage: choose one of the following forms and take t.i.d.:

- powdered root: 1–2 g
- fluid extract (1 : 1): 2–4 ml
- solid extract (4 : 1): 250–500 mg.

Drug–herb interaction cautions

Ginkgo biloba:

- plus *aspirin*: may induce spontaneous bleeding when combined with chronic use of aspirin. Increased bleeding potential reported after *Ginkgo biloba* usage in a chronic user (2 years) of aspirin.

Glycyrrhiza glabra (licorice):

- plus *digoxin, digitalis*: due to a reduction of potassium in the blood, licorice potentiates the toxicity of cardiac glycosides. Interaction with these cardiac glycoside drugs could lead to arrhythmias and cardiac arrest.
- plus *stimulant laxatives or diuretics* (thiazides, spironolactone or amiloride): licorice should not be used with these drugs because of the additive increase of potassium loss to potentially dangerous levels.

Ephedra sinica (Ma huang):

- plus *monoamine oxidase inhibitors*: ephedrine can induce toxicity with MAO inhibitors due to dangerous elevations in blood pressure from increased vasoconstriction and release of noradrenaline. Ephedrine should be avoided for 2 weeks after stopping MAO inhibitors.
- plus *diabetes drugs*: monitor for hyperglycemia while using *Ephedra* as it may diminish insulin response.
- plus *dexamethasone*: ephedrine increases the clearance and thereby reduces the effect of this corticosteroid.

Atherosclerosis

DESCRIPTION

Atherosclerosis (athero = artery, sclerosis = hardening) is a hardening of the arteries in which plaque deposits containing cholesterol, fatty material, and cellular debris form in the walls of the blood vessels that carry oxygen and other nutrients from the heart to the rest of the body. Atherosclerosis may lead to kidney damage, decreased circulation to the brain and extremities and coronary artery disease.

Plaques form when patches of fatty tissue composed of low density lipoprotein (LDL) collect at artery junctions and, along with other fatty substances, get trapped in and damage the inner lining of the artery. As these fatty deposits accumulate – a process that may begin in early adulthood – they reduce blood vessel elasticity and narrow the passageways, interfering with blood flow. In addition, these plaques can crack or tear, forming clots that can completely block off an artery. If blood flow is severely restricted or blocked in a coronary artery, the heart muscle may suffer severe damage, resulting in a "heart attack". If the blockage occurs in arteries providing blood to the brain, it is called a "stroke".

Atherosclerosis is a significant cause of premature death, affecting 60 million Americans. An estimated 1,100,000 new or recurrent heart attacks occur annually, which translates to the grim statistic that every 20 seconds a person in the US has a heart attack; one-third of these attacks leads to death. Significant atherosclerosis may have developed as early as the 30s. Although up to age 45 atherosclerosis is more common in men, postmenopausal women experience the same incidence. Atherosclerosis is a disease directly related to unhealthy diet and lifestyle, and can therefore not only be stopped but dramatically reversed by changing to health-promoting dietary and lifestyle habits.

FREQUENT SIGNS AND SYMPTOMS

- Blood vessels do not contain nerves, so no pain alarms sound until atherosclerosis reaches advanced stages.
- Symptoms depend upon what part of the body is suffering from decreased blood flow, the extent of the blockage and what damage results:
  - *leg muscle cramps* – if vessels in the legs are damaged.

- *angina pectoris or a heart attack* – if blood vessels to the heart are compromised.
- *stroke or transient ischemic attack* – if blood vessels to the neck and brain are involved.

CAUSES

- **Smoking:** tobacco smoke contains over 4,000 chemicals, more than 50 of which are classified as carcinogens. These chemicals are carried in the bloodstream on LDL cholesterol molecules, and either damage the lining of the arteries directly or damage the LDL molecule, which then damages the artery:
  - smoking also contributes to elevated LDL cholesterol by damaging feedback mechanisms in the liver that control how much LDL is manufactured.
  - not only does smoking elevate LDL cholesterol, but an elevated LDL renders smoking even more damaging because more LDL means more cigarette toxins are carried through the vascular system.
  - smoking also promotes platelet aggregation and elevated fibrinogen levels, both of which increase the risk of blood clots and are considered important risk factors in their own right for heart disease and stroke.
  - smoking contributes to high blood pressure.
- **Passive exposure to smoking:** secondhand smoke actually contains higher concentrations of certain toxic smoke constituents:
  - pathophysiological and biochemical data after short- and long-term exposure to environmental tobacco smoke show changes in the arterial lining, in platelet aggregation, and in diminished exercise capacity similar to those found in active smokers.
  - in the US, more than 37,000 coronary heart disease deaths each year are attributed to secondhand smoke.
- **Disease-promoting diet:** a diet high in refined carbohydrates, sugars, saturated fat, cholesterol, and/or *trans* fats (also called partially hydrogenated fats), and low in fresh vegetables, legumes, fruits, nuts and seeds, and whole grains has been conclusively linked to heart disease, stroke, obesity, diabetes, and cancer. This damaging diet is a root cause of high cholesterol and high

blood pressure:

- refined carbohydrates, sugars, and *trans* fats are the primary ingredients in processed foods.
- saturated fats and cholesterol are derived from animal products.

■ **Physical inactivity:** without regular exercise, negative risk factors including high cholesterol levels, high blood pressure, and obesity tend to rise, while protective factors such as the supply of blood and oxygen to the heart muscle and its functional capacity drop.

■ **Psychological factors:**

- *type A personality*: type A behavior is characterized by an extreme sense of time urgency, competitiveness, impatience, and aggressiveness. An inability to control anger or express it appropriately has been shown to result in higher levels of LDL (bad) cholesterol in relation to high density lipoprotein (HDL) (good) cholesterol. The reverse has also been shown to be true: the greater the ability to control anger, the more healthful the LDL : HDL ratio.
- *excessive worrying*: stress, overwork, and anxiety are all associated with increased risk of heart attack. Worry, particularly about social conditions (political, economic, environmental) over which a person has little, if any, control, has been strongly associated with heart disease.

RISK INCREASES WITH

■ **Smoking:** according to the US Surgeon General, "Cigarette smoking should be considered the most important risk factor for coronary heart disease". Smokers have three to five times the risk of coronary artery disease as non-smokers.

■ **Elevated cholesterol levels:** high levels of LDL, the low density lipoprotein, and low levels of HDL, the high density lipoprotein, greatly increase risk of death as a result of heart disease:

- cholesterol is transported in the blood by lipoproteins: LDL carries fats (primarily cholesterol and triglycerides) from the liver to body cells, while HDL is responsible for returning these fats to the liver.
- the ratio of total cholesterol to HDL should be no higher than 4.2; the ratio of LDL to HDL should be no higher than 2.5.

■ **Elevated lipoprotein(a):** a more damaging form of cholesterol is lipoprotein(a), or Lp(a). Lp(a) resembles LDL but has an additional molecule of an adhesive protein (apolipoprotein(a)) which allows it to stick more easily to artery walls:

- a high level of Lp(a) has been shown to carry a 10 times greater risk of heart disease than an elevated LDL.

■ **High blood pressure:** blood pressure denotes the resistance produced each time the heart beats and sends blood coursing through the arteries. The peak reading is the systolic pressure, while the reading taken between beats when the heart relaxes is the diastolic pressure:

- blood pressure for a healthy adult is 120 (systolic)/ 80 (diastolic).
- even mild hypertension (140–160/90–104) is highly suggestive of atherosclerosis and should be aggressively treated with natural measures.

■ **Diabetes mellitus:** in diabetics, hyperglycemia, a state of excessively high blood sugar levels, is a frequent complication. Excessive blood sugar causes damage to arterial walls:

- a diabetic has a two to three times higher risk of dying prematurely of atherosclerosis than a non-diabetic individual.

■ **Obesity:** leads to insulin insensitivity, resulting in type II diabetes mellitus, high cholesterol levels, and coronary artery disease.

■ **Sedentary lifestyle:** studies have shown that an unfit individual has an eight times greater risk of a heart attack or stroke than a physically fit individual. In addition, researchers estimate that for every hour of exercise, there is a 2-hour increase in longevity.

■ **Low antioxidant status:** antioxidants such as beta-carotene, selenium, vitamin E, and vitamin C work together to protect damage-susceptible fats and cholesterol from free radicals. If damaged, fats and cholesterol form toxic derivatives known as *lipid peroxides* and *oxidized cholesterol*, respectively, which damage artery walls, accelerating the progression of atherosclerosis.

■ **Low levels of essential fatty acids:** population and autopsy studies have demonstrated that people who consume a diet rich in omega-3 oils from either fish or vegetable sources have the least coronary artery disease; conversely, those who consume the least omega-3 oils have the highest degree of coronary artery disease.

■ **Low levels of magnesium and/or potassium:** both minerals are essential to the proper functioning of the entire cardiovascular system. It has been well established that people who die from a heart attack have lower heart magnesium levels than people of the same age who die from other causes. Potassium interacts with magnesium in many body systems, and a diet low in potassium and high in sodium is clearly associated with high blood pressure.

■ **Increased platelet aggregation:** when platelets adhere to each other, they release potent compounds that dramatically promote the formation of atherosclerotic plaque. They may also form a clot that can block small arteries, producing a heart attack or stroke.

- **Increased fibrinogen formation:** fibrinogen, a protein involved in the clotting system, also plays other important roles, several of which promote atherosclerosis, such as acting as a cofactor for platelet aggregation, determining the viscosity of blood, and stimulating the formation of plaque.
- **Elevated levels of homocysteine:** an intermediate compound produced during the conversion of the amino acid methionine to cysteine, homocysteine directly damages the arterial wall, reduces the integrity of the vessel wall, and interferes with the formation of collagen, the main protein in connective tissue:
  - when adequate folic acid, vitamin B_6 and vitamin B_{12} are present, homocysteine is quickly converted into cysteine; however, if these nutrients are relatively deficient, homocysteine will stockpile.
  - elevations in homocysteine are found in approximately 20–40% of patients with heart disease.
- **Elevated blood levels of C-reactive protein:** C-reactive protein is a highly accurate marker of coronary artery disease, even in the absence of classical clinical signs such as high cholesterol, triglycerides and blood pressure:
  - C-reactive protein is not merely a marker, but an active participant in the inflammatory process that leads to atherosclerosis. C-reactive protein triggers the expression of adhesion molecules in arterial cells, thus initiating the inflammation process and causing plaque to stick to vessel walls.
  - a recent 8-year study of 1,086 apparently healthy men showed that those with the highest levels of C-reactive protein had a threefold increase in their risk of a future heart attack and a twofold increase in their risk of a future stroke, compared to men with lower C-reactive protein levels.
- **Disease-promoting diet:** a diet based on animal products and processed foods, with little consumption of fresh vegetables, legumes, fruits, nuts and seeds, and whole grains is low in protective factors – antioxidants, essential fatty acids, magnesium and potassium – and high in damaging factors that elevate cholesterol levels and blood pressure, and increase the risk for obesity and diabetes – saturated fat, *trans* fats (also called partially hydrogenated fats), sugars and refined carbohydrates.
- **Family history of atherosclerosis:** elevations of blood cholesterol and/or triglycerides can be the result of genetic factors; such familial tendencies affect about 1 : 500 people. Atherosclerosis is also directly related to diet and lifestyle, both of which are greatly influenced by learned family behaviors.

- **Type A personality:** a predominantly aggressive (hostile), angry coping style doubles an individual's risk of coronary artery disease.
- **Excessive worrying:** when researchers assessed the impact of worrying (an important component of anxiety), they found that men who worried about social conditions (political, economic, environmental) over which a person has little, if any, control, had a 241% increased risk of developing heart disease.
- **Diagonal earlobe crease:** the earlobe is richly veined, and a decrease in blood flow over a period of time is believed to result in collapse of the vascular bed. Since 1973, over 30 studies have documented this correlation, with the largest to date involving 1,000 patients. In one study, angiograms performed on 205 patients showed an 82% accuracy in predicting heart disease based on the earlobe crease.

PREVENTIVE MEASURES

- Don't smoke.
- Follow the dietary and nutritional supplement guidelines given in the treatment protocol below.
- Exercise regularly – a minimum of 30 min, at least three times a week. A carefully graded, progressive aerobic exercise program is essential. Walking is a good exercise with which to start.
- Learn how to control anger or express it appropriately. The following subjective suggestions will help:
  - be kind to yourself; make time to give and receive love in your life.
  - be an active listener. Allow others to really share their feelings and thoughts uninterrupted. Empathize. Put yourself in their shoes.
  - if you find yourself being interrupted, relax. If you are courteous and let others speak, they will eventually respond in kind (unless they are extremely rude). If they don't, point out to them that they are interrupting the communication process (you can only do this if you have been a good listener).
  - avoid aggressive or passive behavior. Be assertive, but express your thoughts and feelings in a kind way, as you would wish to be treated, to help improve relationships at work and at home.
  - avoid excessive stress as best you can by avoiding excessive work hours, poor nutrition, and inadequate rest.
  - avoid stimulants like caffeine and nicotine that promote the fight-or-flight response and tend to make people more irritable.
  - take time to build your long-term health by performing stress-reduction techniques and deep-breathing exercises.

- focus your energy on those things you can do something about, and let go of the burden of those things over which you have no control.
- be patient and tolerant of others, and yourself. Remember you, and they, are human and will make mistakes, which are always opportunities to learn and grow.

Expected outcomes

Significant overall regression of atherosclerosis of the coronary blood vessels should be measurable within 1 year.

TREATMENT

Diet

- Consume a heart-healthy diet rich in whole, unprocessed, preferably organic foods, especially plant foods (fruits, vegetables, whole grains, beans, nuts and seeds) and cold-water fish:
  - one example of such a diet is the Mediterranean or Cretan diet, as used in the Lyon Heart Study. Compared to the Standard American Diet (SAD), the Cretan diet consists of more wholegrain bread, more root vegetables, more green vegetables, more fish, less meat (beef, lamb, and pork are replaced with poultry), fruit every day, and canola and olive oil instead of butter and cream.
  - compared to the control group, the group following the Cretan diet had a 60% reduction in overall mortality (for more detailed information, Appendix 1).
- Avoid saturated fats, margarine and foods containing *trans* fatty acids; a great deal of research links these fats to heart disease, strokes, and cancer.
- Avoid processed foods because their primary ingredients – sugars, refined carbohydrates, and *trans* fats – elevate cholesterol levels and blood pressure, and increase the risk for obesity and diabetes.
- Increase consumption of omega-3 essential fatty acids by consuming flaxseed oil (1 tbsp q.d.) and/or eating cold-water fish – salmon, mackerel, tuna, herring, halibut (110 g [4 oz] at least three times a week).

Nutritional supplements

- **A high-potency multiple vitamin and mineral supplement:** this should include 400 µg of folic acid, 400 µg of vitamin B_{12}, and 50–100 mg of vitamin B_6. (Folic acid supplementation should always be accompanied by vitamin B_{12} supplementation to prevent folic acid from masking a vitamin B_{12} deficiency.) A daily multiple providing all of the known vitamins and minerals serves as a foundation upon which to build an individualized health-promotion program.

- **Vitamin E:** of all the antioxidants, the fat-soluble antioxidant, vitamin E, may offer the most protection against arteriosclerosis because it is easily incorporated into the low density lipoprotein (LDL) cholesterol molecule where it prevents free radical damage:
  - vitamin E not only reduces LDL *peroxidation* (free radical damage to LDL that results in the formation of toxic derivatives called lipid peroxides) but also improves plasma LDL breakdown, inhibits excessive platelet aggregation, increases high density lipoprotein (HDL) cholesterol levels, and increases the breakdown of fibrin, a clot-forming protein.
  - although dosages as low as 25 IU offer some protection, doses of greater than 400 IU are required to produce clinically significant effects, especially in smokers and people exposed to greater oxidative stress.
  - dosage: 400–800 IU mixed tocopherols q.d.
- **Vitamin C:** a powerful antioxidant, vitamin C is the body's first line of defense, covering all the water-soluble environments in the body both inside and outside cells, and working with its fat-soluble partners, vitamin E and the carotenes, as well as with the antioxidant enzymes glutathione peroxidase, catalase, and superoxide dismutase:
  - vitamin C also regenerates oxidized vitamin E, enabling it to resume its antioxidant defense activities.
  - vitamin C is not only extremely effective in its own right in preventing the oxidation of LDL cholesterol, it also strengthens the collagen structures of the arteries, lowers total cholesterol level and blood pressure, raises HDL cholesterol levels, and inhibits platelet aggregation.
  - dosage: 1,000–4,000 mg q.d.
- **Magnesium:** the beneficial effects of magnesium on the cardiovascular system result from its ability to: dilate the coronary arteries, thus improving delivery of oxygen to the heart; lower peripheral vascular resistance, thus reducing the effort with which the heart must pump; inhibit platelets from aggregating and forming blood clots; improve the heart rate, while preventing arrhythmias; and reduce the size of the infarct (blockage) in a heart attack:
  - the average intake of magnesium by healthy adults in the US ranges between 143 and 266 mg per day, well below the recommended dietary allowance (RDA) of 350 mg for men and 300 mg for women.
  - the diet of most Americans is low in magnesium because they eat primarily processed foods (processing refines out most of the magnesium), meat and dairy products, which contain little magnesium.
  - best dietary sources of magnesium are tofu, legumes, seeds, nuts, whole grains, and green leafy vegetables.

- magnesium bound to aspartate, citrate, or other intermediate of the Krebs cycle (a part of the energy production process in the mitochondria) is more effectively assimilated and utilized.
- dosage: 200–400 mg t.i.d.
- **Glycosaminoglycans (GAGs):** GAGs are structural components essential to maintaining the health of arteries and other blood vessels:
  - a mixture of highly purified bovine-derived GAGs equivalent to those naturally present within the human aorta (including dermatan sulfate, heparan sulfate, hyaluronic acid, chondroitin sulfate, and related hexosaminoglycans) has been shown to inhibit platelet aggregation and to improve the structure, function, and integrity of arteries, as well as improving blood flow.
  - GAGs have been shown to be effective in improving both cerebral (brain) and peripheral (hands and feet) vascular insufficiency, relieving symptoms and increasing blood flow.
  - GAGs should be used for at least 6 months after a stroke.
  - dosage: 50–100 mg q.d.

Botanical medicines

- **Garlic:** garlic oil and garlic preparations standardized for *alliin* (the storage form of allicin, a key active compound in garlic) have demonstrated inhibition of platelet aggregation; dosage: 900 mg q.d. of a dried garlic preparation containing 1.3% alliin.
- **PCO extracts from grape seed and pine bark:** procyanidolic oligomers (PCOs) are naturally bound mixtures of beneficial flavonoids. PCOs exist in many plants and are found in red wine. Commercially available sources of PCO include extracts from grape seeds and the bark of the maritime (Landes) pine:
  - PCOs have been shown to have a 20–50 times more potent antioxidant activity than vitamin E or C.
  - in animal studies, PCO extracts have prevented damage to the lining of the artery, lowered blood cholesterol levels, and shrunk the size of the cholesterol deposit in the artery. PCOs also inhibit platelet aggregation and vascular constriction.
  - dosage: for prevention, 50 mg q.d. of either grape seed or pine bark extract. For therapeutic purposes, increase dosage to 150–300 mg q.d.
- ***Ginkgo biloba* extract (GBE):** GBE (standardized to contain 24% ginkgo flavonglycosides and 6% terpenoids) has been shown to increase blood flow to the brain in more than 40 double-blind studies:
  - GBE has demonstrated effectiveness comparable to Federal Drug Administration approved drugs used in the treatment of cerebral vascular insufficiency and Alzheimer's disease.
  - in addition to increasing blood flow to the brain, and therefore oxygen and glucose utilization by brain cells, GBE also reduces blood viscosity, thus offering additional protection against stroke.
  - a study of post-stroke patients demonstrated that GBE improved blood flow and reduced blood viscosity.
  - dosage: *Ginkgo biloba* extract, 24% ginkgo flavonglycosides, 80 mg t.i.d.

Drug–herb interaction cautions

- **Garlic:**
  - plus *insulin*: animal studies suggest insulin dose may require adjusting because of hypoglycemic effects of whole garlic (in rats) and its constituent allicin (in rabbits).
  - plus *warfarin*: the anticoagulant activity of warfarin is enhanced due to increased fibrinolytic activity and diminished platelet aggregation caused by garlic components allicin, ajoene, trisulfides, and adenosine.
- ***Ginkgo biloba*:**
  - plus *aspirin*: may induce spontaneous bleeding when combined with chronic use of aspirin. Increased bleeding potential reported after *Ginkgo biloba* usage in a chronic user (2 years) of aspirin.

Atopic dermatitis (eczema)

DESCRIPTION

A common chronic allergic skin disorder that affects approximately 2–7% of the population, eczema may begin between the age of 1 month and 1 year, often subsides somewhat by age 3, but may flare up again at any age. Eczema typically manifests on the skin of the hands, scalp, face, back of the neck or skin creases of elbows and knees. Affected skin is very dry, itchy, inflamed and scaly. Scratching and rubbing may lead to darkened, hardened areas of thickened skin with accentuated furrows, most commonly seen on the front of the wrist and elbows and the back of the knees.

FREQUENT SIGNS AND SYMPTOMS

Skin affected by eczema exhibits the following characteristics:
- itching (sometimes severe)
- inflammation (redness)
- dryness, with a decreased capacity to retain moisture
- small blisters with oozing
- thickening and scaling from chronic inflammation, rubbing and scratching
- a tendency to be overgrown by bacteria, especially *Staphylococcus aureus*
- increased susceptibility to potentially severe skin infections from *S. aureus*, herpes simplex, and common wart viruses.

CAUSES

- **Allergy:**
  - eczema signals an immediate allergic reaction.
  - serum IgE (an allergic antibody) levels are elevated in 80% of patients.
  - virtually 100% of eczema patients have positive allergy tests.
  - two-thirds of eczema patients have a family history of eczema.
  - many eczema patients eventually develop hay fever and/or asthma.
  - most eczema patients improve with a diet that eliminates common food allergens: milk, eggs, and peanuts, and, to a lesser extent, fish, soy, wheat, citrus, and chocolate. Any food can, however, be an offending agent.
  - environmental allergens may also trigger eczema: wool clothing; skin lotions and ointments; soaps, detergents, cleansers; plants; tanning agents used for shoe leather; dyes; topical medications.
- **Immune system abnormalities:**
  - mast cell abnormalities: mast cells (specialized immune defense white blood cells) from the skin of people with eczema have abnormalities that cause them to release higher amounts of histamine and other allergenic compounds than mast cells in persons without eczema. Histamine and the other allergenic compounds are what cause the itching of eczema.
  - a defect in the alternate complement pathway (ACP): in many persons with eczema, the ACP, an immune mechanism important for destroying bacteria and foreign particles, does not activate properly. Use of botanical medicines such as burdock root (*Arctium lappa*) and dandelion root (*Taraxacum officinale*) that contain inulin, a polysaccharide that activates the ACP, can result in restoration of the ability to destroy bacteria.
- **Essential fatty acid and prostaglandin metabolism abnormalities:**
  - analysis of fatty acids in blood, red blood cells and white blood cells in patients with eczema demonstrates a tendency for the ratio of omega-3 to omega-6 essential fatty acids (EFAs) to be significantly lower in people with eczema. This imbalance leads to a greater tendency to inflammation and allergies because omega-6 EFAs are used to produce pro-inflammatory prostaglandins (hormone-like compounds), while omega-3 EFAs are used in the production of anti-inflammatory prostaglandins.
- ***Candida albicans*:**
  - overgrowth of the common yeast, *Candida albicans*, in the gastrointestinal tract has been implicated as a causal factor in many allergic conditions, including eczema.
  - elevated levels of anti-Candida antibodies are common in atopic individuals; the higher the level of IgE

antibodies to *Candida* antigens (which signifies a greater overgrowth), the more severe the eczema.

■ **Emotional tension:**

■ emotional stress can provoke and aggravate itching in patients with eczema.

■ eczema patients show higher levels of anxiety, hostility and neurosis than matched controls.

RISK INCREASES WITH

■ A family history of eczema

■ Medical history of other allergic conditions such as hay fever, asthma or sensitivity to certain drugs

■ A diet low in sources of omega-3 essential fatty acids, i.e., cold-water fish (salmon, halibut, herring, mackerel), flaxseed oil, hemp oil, nuts and seeds

■ Stress

■ Clothing made of synthetic fabric or unlined rubber gloves which trap perspiration, or, in some individuals, clothing made of wool

■ Use of harsh detergents and cleaning products

■ Weather extremes, including high humidity, severe cold and severe heat (especially with increased sweating)

PREVENTIVE MEASURES

■ Breast-feeding in infancy offers significant protection against eczema and allergies in general:

■ if breast-fed infants develop eczema, it is usually due to transfer of allergenic antigens in the breast milk. If this occurs, the mother should avoid the common food allergens: milk, eggs, and peanuts, and, to a lesser extent, fish, soy, wheat, citrus, and chocolate.

■ in older or formula-fed infants, milk, eggs and peanuts are the food allergens that most commonly induce eczema, followed by fish, wheat and soybeans. If these children develop eczema, any of these potential food allergens should be avoided.

■ Avoid rough-textured clothing; wear clothing made of natural, non-irritating fibers such as cotton.

■ Use cotton-lined rubber gloves for household cleaning tasks.

■ Use gentle, hypoallergenic detergents and cleaning products.

■ Wash clothing with mild soaps only and rinse thoroughly.

■ Avoid exposure to chemical irritants and any other agents that might cause skin irritation.

■ Avoid greasy lotions since they block sweat ducts.

Expected outcomes

Once susceptibility to any of the causative factors noted above has been identified and corrected, a discovery process that may take 4–6 weeks, significant clinical improvement or complete resolution of eczema should occur within 1–2 weeks.

TREATMENT

Diet

■ Identify and eliminate food allergens as quickly as possible:

■ consumption of allergenic foods damages the lining of the intestinal tract, resulting in a permeable "leaky gut", a condition that allows allergens and other toxins to leak into the general circulation. This puts the immune system in a state of continuous alarm, significantly increasing a trigger-happy response to other foods and the chance of developing additional allergies.

■ trying to deal with multiple food allergies is much more difficult, as the diet becomes more restrictive, but early elimination of allergenic foods appears to stop the development of new allergies.

■ Diagnosis of food allergy is most effectively and least expensively achieved using the "elimination diet and challenge" method – eliminate suspected allergens for a period of at least 10 days followed by careful reintroduction (see the chapter on Food allergy for more information).

■ Start by eliminating all major allergens (milk, eggs, and peanuts account for approximately 81% of all cases of childhood eczema). If this does not resolve the problem, eliminate the less common allergens (fish, soy, wheat, citrus, and chocolate).

■ If laboratory methods are used to identify food allergies in eczema, the most useful method appears to be ELISA IgE and IgG4 (see the chapter on Food allergy for more information).

■ Once an allergy to a particular food has been determined, this should be avoided for at least 1 year. Studies show that in many cases, if patients avoid allergenic foods for a year, their immune response will no longer be triggered by these foods.

■ If not allergic to fish, increase consumption of omega-3 essential fatty acids by eating cold-water fish – salmon, mackerel, tuna, herring, halibut (110 g [4 oz] at least three times a week). For vegetarians or those allergic to fish, flaxseed oil (1 tbsp q.d.), hemp oil and walnuts are good sources of alpha-linolenic acid, an omega-3 precursor. Fish or fish oil supplements, which contain already formed omega-3 fatty acids, are likely to produce greater and more rapid benefit.

- After identifying and removing allergenic foods from your diet, choose a health-promoting diet rich in whole, unprocessed, preferably organic foods, especially plant foods (fruits, vegetables, whole grains, beans, nuts [especially walnuts] and seeds) and cold-water fish (for more detailed information, see Appendix 1).

- If not allergic to onions and/or garlic, enjoy them liberally and frequently. Both contain compounds that inhibit lipoxygenase and cyclo-oxygenases, which generate inflammatory prostaglandins and thromboxanes. Onions also contain other anti-inflammatory agents – the isothiocyanates and the flavonoid, quercetin.

Nutritional supplements

- **Vitamin A:** because of its critical importance in epithelial and mucosal tissues, the fat-soluble nutrient, vitamin A, is beneficial in the treatment of skin and gastrointestinal diseases.
  - the epithelium is a layer of cells forming the epidermis of the skin and the surface layer of mucous and serous membranes. All epithelial surfaces including the skin, vaginal epithelium, and gastrointestinal tract rely upon vitamin A.
  - when vitamin A status is inadequate, keratin is secreted in epithelial tissues, transforming them from their normally pliable, moist condition into stiff dry tissue that is unable to carry out its normal functions, and leading to breaches in epithelial integrity that significantly increase susceptibility to the development of allergy and infection.
  - dosage: 5,000 IU q.d.

- **Vitamin E:** a powerful antioxidant, vitamin E protects fat-soluble components of the body such as cell membranes, brain neurons, and cholesterol from damaging free radicals. In the treatment of eczema, vitamin E plays an important role in protecting vitamin A and increasing its storage; dosage: 400 IU mixed tocopherols q.d.

- **Zinc:** a cofactor in numerous enzymatic reactions, zinc is required to create delta-6 desaturase, the enzyme responsible for converting the omega-6 essential fatty acid, linoleic acid, into gamma-linolenic acid (GLA). The body uses GLA to produce a type of anti-inflammatory (series 1) prostaglandin.
  - when zinc levels are inadequate, linoleic acid is converted into arachidonic acid, which is used to produce pro-inflammatory (series 2) prostaglandins and leukotrienes.
  - low zinc levels are common not only in eczema patients but also in numerous inflammatory

disorders including acne, psoriasis, rheumatoid arthritis, and inflammatory bowel disease.
  - dosage: 45–60 mg q.d. until eczema clears, then decrease to 30 mg q.d.

- **Flavonoids:** the following flavonoids all inhibit allergenic mechanisms (choose one):
  - *quercetin*: a potent antioxidant and antihistamine, quercetin not only inhibits histamine release, it inhibits the formation of histamine and other allergenic compounds; dosage: 400 mg 20 min before meals.
  - *grape seed extract*: dosage: 95% procyanidolic oligomers content, 50–100 mg t.i.d.
  - *green tea extract*: dosage: 50% polyphenol content, 200–300 mg t.i.d.

- ***Ginkgo biloba* extract** (24% ginkgo flavonglycosides and 6% terpenoid): in addition to flavonoids, *Ginkgo biloba* contains several unique terpene molecules collectively called *ginkgolides* that block the effects of platelet activating factor (PAF), a key chemical mediator in eczema; dosage: 80 mg t.i.d.

- **Omega-3 essential fatty acids:** levels of omega-3 essential fatty acids, which are used in the production of anti-inflammatory prostaglandins, are often significantly reduced in people with eczema:
  - dosage: EPA and DHA, 540 and 360 mg q.d. or flaxseed oil, 1 tbsp q.d. If no response after 3 months, try evening primrose oil, 3,000 mg q.d.

Botanical medicines

- ***Glycyrrhiza glabra* (licorice):** antiallergy and anti-inflammatory effects due to glycyrrhetinic acid, a component in licorice that inhibits inflammatory prostaglandin and leukotriene manufacture:
  - glycyrrhetinic acid works, in a manner similar to cortisone, by blocking production of the enzyme phospholipase A2. Phospholipase A2 mobilizes arachidonic acid (AA), which is used to produce pro-inflammatory (series 2) prostaglandins and leukotrienes.
  - dosage: choose one of the following forms and take the recommended dosage t.i.d.:
    - powdered root: 1–2 g
    - fluid extract (1 : 1): 2–4 ml
    - solid (dry, powdered) extract (4 : 1): 250–500 mg.

- ***Arctium lappa* (burdock root) or *Taraxacum officinale* (dandelion root):** both herbs contain inulin, a polysaccharide that activates the alternate complement pathway (ACP). The ACP, an important immune mechanism for destroying bacteria and foreign particles, does not activate properly in many persons with eczema:

■ dosage: for either herb, choose one of the following forms and take the recommended dosage t.i.d.:
- ● dried root: 2–8 g by infusion or decoction
- ● fluid extract (1 : 1): 4–8 ml (1–2 tsp)
- ● juice of fresh root: 4–8 ml (1–2 tsp)
- ● powdered solid extract (4 : 1): 250–500 mg.

Drug–herb interaction cautions

■ *Glycyrrhiza glabra* **(licorice):**

■ plus *digoxin, digitalis*: due to a reduction of potassium in the blood, licorice potentiates the toxicity of cardiac glycosides. Interaction with these cardiac glycoside drugs could lead to arrhythmias and cardiac arrest.

■ plus *stimulant laxatives or diuretics* (thiazides, spironolactone, or amiloride): licorice should not be used with these drugs because of the additive increase of potassium loss to potentially dangerous levels.

■ *Arctium lappa* **(burdock root):**

■ plus *insulin*: due to burdock's hypoglycemic effect (in rats), insulin dosage may need to be adjusted.

■ *Taraxacum officinale* **(dandelion root):**

■ plus *lithium*: enhanced sodium excretion resulting from the diuretic effect of the roots and leaves (in rats) may cause sodium depletion, which might then worsen lithium toxicity.

Topical medicines

■ *Glycyrrhiza glabra* **(licorice):** commercial topical preparations featuring pure glycyrrhetinic acid have been shown to exert an effect similar to that of topical hydrocortisone in the treatment of eczema, contact dermatitis (e.g., poison oak), allergic dermatitis, and psoriasis.

■ **Lotions:** local application of soothing lotions containing chamomile, witch hazel or zinc oxide can also help reduce inflammation and itching in patients with eczema.

■ **Caution:** avoid heavy, greasy creams that may interfere with perspiration.

Attention deficit disorders

DESCRIPTION

A pattern of behavior in children characterized by short attention spans and impulsivity, with or without hyperactivity, attention deficit disorder (ADD) is implicated in learning disorders and estimated to affect 5–10% of school-aged children with incidence substantially greater in boys than girls (10:1). Over two million American school-aged boys take the drug methyl-phenidate (Ritalin) for ADD. Onset is usually by 3 years of age, but diagnosis is generally not made until later when the child is in school.

Three separate attention deficit disorders exist:

- *hyperactivity* (attention deficit disorder with hyperactivity) – signs of inattention, impulsiveness, and hyperactivity inappropriate for the child's age
- *learning disability* (attention deficit disorder without hyperactivity) – developmentally inappropriate brief attention span and poor concentration for the child's age
- *ADD, residual type* (in individuals 18 years old or older) – a continuation of the process of ADD into adulthood.

FREQUENT SIGNS AND SYMPTOMS

Characteristics of ADD with hyperactivity in order of frequency

- Hyperactivity (squirms in seat, fidgets with hands or feet, unable to stay seated when required to do so, difficulty waiting turn in lines and games, difficulty playing quietly)
- Perceptual motor impairment
- Emotional instability
- General coordination deficit
- Disorders of attention (short attention span, easily distracted, lack of perseverance, failure to finish things, shifts from one uncompleted project to another, not listening, poor concentration)
- Impulsiveness (action before thought, abrupt shifts in activity, poor organizing, jumping up in class, talks excessively, blurts out answers before a question is finished, interrupts or intrudes on others, often engages in dangerous activities without considering consequences)
- Disorders of memory and thinking (difficulty following instructions, doesn't appear to listen, frequently loses items necessary for tasks)

- Specific learning disabilities
- Disorders of speech and hearing
- Equivocal neurological signs and electroencephalographic irregularities

Characteristics of ADD without hyperactivity

- Frequent ear infections (otitis media)
- Moderate to severe hearing loss
- Impaired speech and language development
- Lowered general intelligence scores
- Learning difficulties

CAUSES

Although ADD with hyperactivity and ADD without hyperactivity (learning disabilities) are discussed separately, the factors discussed under one may be equally relevant to, and should be considered in treatment of, the other.

ADD with hyperactivity

- **Food additives:**
  - some 5,000 additives are used in the US including anticaking agents (e.g., calcium silicate), antioxidants (e.g., BHT, BHA), bleaching agents (e.g., benzoyl peroxide), colorings (e.g., artificial azo dye derivatives, particularly the yellow dye tartrazine), flavorings (emulsifiers, mineral salts), preservatives (e.g., benzoates, nitrates, sulfites), thickeners, and vegetable gums.
  - each person in the US is estimated to consume 3.5–4.5 kg (8–10 lb) of food additives per year with daily per capita consumption averaging 13–15 g. For the US population, total annual consumption of artificial food colors alone is approximately 45 million kg (100 million lb).
  - based on his experience with over 1,200 cases in which food additives were linked to learning and behavior disorders, Benjamin Feingold MD has proposed that food additives are a major cause in hyperactivity. According to Feingold, many hyperactive children – perhaps 40–50% – are sensitive to artificial food colors, flavors, and preservatives and to naturally occurring salicylates and phenolic compounds.

- although Feingold's hypothesis has been hotly debated, the published studies yield some clear conclusions. Virtually every study has demonstrated that some hyperactive children consistently react with behavioral problems when challenged by specific food additives, and their responses are reproducible under double-blind conditions.
- studies evaluating Feingold's hypothesis in the US (funded by the Nutrition Foundation, an organization supported by the major food manufacturers – Coca Cola, Nabisco, General Foods, etc. – which would suffer economically if food additives were found harmful) have been largely negative, while studies in Australia and Canada have been supportive. The use of artificial food additives has been significantly restricted in other countries because of the possibility of harmful effects.

Sucrose (sugar) consumption:

- destructive–aggressive and restless behavior has been found to significantly correlate with the amount of sucrose consumed.
- a high percentage – 74% of 261 hyperactive children in a recent study – has been shown to have abnormal glucose tolerance curves exhibiting hypoglycemia, which would promote hyperactivity via increased adrenaline secretion.
- refined carbohydrate consumption appears to be the major factor in promoting reactive hypoglycemia, i.e., hypoglycemia resulting from a rapid elevation in blood sugar for 1–2 hours followed by a severe drop in blood sugar levels.

Food allergies:

- while artificial colorings and preservatives have been the most common substances causing hyperactivity in studies, no child has been found to be sensitive to these alone. Food allergies or sensitivities can also cause psychological symptoms. A number of studies have demonstrated that to effectively heal ADD, both food additives and allergens must be eliminated from the diet.
- in a double-blind study of 26 hyperactive children, 19 responded well when both food additives and allergens were eliminated, and in a larger study of 185 children with hyperkinetic syndrome, 116 improved. In a retrospective study, 86% of hyperactive children were found to have elevated levels of eosinophils, white blood cells that are linked to allergies.

Learning disabilities (ADD without hyperactivity)
Three factors appear to be particularly relevant to learning disabilities.

Otitis media (ear infections):

- current and recurrent ear infections have been reported to be twice as common in learning-disabled children as non-learning-disabled children.
- children with moderate to severe hearing loss tend to have impaired speech and language development, lowered general intelligence scores, and learning disabilities.

Nutrient deficiency:

- low levels of nutrients in the diet prevent the brain from functioning properly, and poor nutritional status may be most harmful earlier in life, during physical, mental and social development. Even a subclinical deficiency of virtually any nutrient can result in hampered nerve cell function and impaired mental performance.
- iron deficiency, the most common nutrient deficiency in American children, is associated with markedly decreased attentiveness; less complex or purposeful, narrower attention span; decreased persistence; and decreased voluntary activity – all of which are usually responsive to supplementation.
- several clinical studies have demonstrated that nutritional supplementation can significantly improve mental function in school-age children.
- nutrients especially important to proper brain and nervous system function include thiamin, niacin, vitamin B_6, vitamin B_{12}, copper, iodine, iron, magnesium, manganese, potassium, and zinc.

Heavy metals:

- numerous studies have demonstrated a strong relationship between childhood learning disabilities (and other disorders including criminal behavior) and body stores of heavy metals, particularly lead.
- learning disabilities are frequently characterized by a pattern of high levels of mercury, cadmium, lead, copper, and manganese as determined by hair analysis.

RISK INCREASES WITH

- **Ear infections:** frequent ear infections and antibiotic use are associated with greater likelihood of developing ADD.
- **A nutrient-poor diet** composed largely of additive and sugar-laden (processed) foods.
- **Exposure to heavy metals:** common sources – in addition to environmental contamination of air, water and food crops due to industrial processes and leaded gasoline – include lead from pesticide sprays, cooking utensils, the solder in tin cans; cadmium and lead from cigarette smoke; mercury from dental fillings,

contaminated fish, and cosmetics; and aluminum from antacids, antiperspirants, cookware and aluminum foil.
- **History:** a family history of ADD.

PREVENTIVE MEASURES

- **Avoid processed foods:** the debilitating load of sugars, refined carbohydrates, *trans* fats and food additives that these foods contain contributes to ADD in children – and to elevated cholesterol levels, blood pressure, and a significantly increased risk for obesity and diabetes in adults.
- **Provide a health-promoting diet** rich in whole, unprocessed, preferably organic foods, especially plant foods (fruits, vegetables, whole grains, beans, nuts and seeds), and cold-water fish.
- **Eat organic produce:** both for maximum nutrient density and minimal pesticides, herbicides, fungicides and waxes, choose organic produce whenever possible. If organic produce is not readily available, try to buy local in-season produce. Soak the produce in a mild solution of additive-free soap or pure castille soap from the health food store. All-natural, biodegradable cleansers are also available at most health food stores. Simply spray the produce with the cleanser, gently scrub, then rinse off.
- **Minimize exposure to heavy metals:** this is another reason to choose organic produce. Don't smoke or allow your child to be around smokers. Avoid being outside when smog levels are high. If pesticide use is necessary, sprinkle boric acid – a non-allergenic, relatively safe insecticide – in all potentially infested areas. Use waxed paper, glass, ceramic or steel containers for storage and serving. Avoid canned foods; purchase fresh or frozen foods or dried beans.

Expected outcomes

Identification and elimination of clear causative factors, such as food allergies or sensitivities to food additives, will often bring about dramatic improvements within the first 2 weeks of treatment in many cases. However, in cases where food allergies/sensitivities do not appear to be the primary factors, improvements will be more subtle and gradual.

TREATMENT

Screening for heavy metal toxicity

Hair mineral analysis and EDTA challenge should be used to screen for heavy metal toxicity as these tests illustrate long-term burden versus blood measurements;

the latter reflect only recent exposure and do not accurately evaluate heavy metal concentration in the brain.

Diet
- Eliminate all refined sugars and as many food additives as possible by providing a diet composed from whole, unprocessed, preferably organic foods prepared at home. When in control of food preparation, consumption can be monitored accurately.
- To identify and eliminate food allergens, the most sensible and least expensive method is a 4-week program of the oligoantigenic diet (*oligo* = from the Greek *oligos* meaning little, plus *antigenic* = allergy-provoking – in other words, a diet containing the least amount of potentially allergenic foods).
- The oligoantigenic diet consists of lamb, chicken, potatoes, rice, banana, apple, cabbage-family vegetables, a multiple vitamin, and 3 g q.d. of calcium gluconate (for detailed information see the chapter on Food allergy).
- After 4 weeks on the oligoantigenic diet, reintroduce suspected problem foods (full servings at least once a day, one food introduced per week). If symptoms recur or worsen upon reintroduction/challenge, the food should be removed from the diet.
- If no improvement occurs on the oligoantigenic diet, the child may be reacting to something else in the diet or environment, and further testing for allergens or heavy metals may be indicated.
- To help chelate heavy metals, increase consumption of foods high in sulfur such as garlic, onions, and eggs, provided your child is not allergic to these foods. In addition, water-soluble fibers (e.g., guar gum, oat bran, pectin, and psyllium seed) bind toxins in the gut and help promote their excretion.

Nutritional supplements
- A high-potency children's general multivitamin and mineral supplement – with special care used to ensure the child is not allergic to any of the product's constituents.
- Should a child be found to have heavy metal toxicity, the following minerals and vitamins are of particular importance in combating heavy metal poisoning: calcium, magnesium, zinc, iron, copper, and chromium; vitamin C and B-complex vitamins. The sulfur-containing amino acids (methionine, cysteine, and taurine) may also be prescribed.

Botanical medicines
- **Silymarin:** a special extract from *Silybum marianum* (milk thistle), silymarin contains a group of flavonoid compounds that exert powerful beneficial effects in

protecting the liver from damage and enhancing detoxification processes:

- silymarin is an antioxidant many times more potent than vitamin E and vitamin C.
- silymarin prevents the depletion of glutathione, perhaps the most important detoxification enzyme in the liver. Glutathione has primary responsibility for the elimination of fat-soluble toxins, a group that includes not only heavy metals, but also many of the toxins from pesticides, gasoline and cigarette smoke. The higher its glutathione levels, the greater the liver's capacity to detoxify harmful chemicals.
- dosage: 70–210 mg t.i.d.

Drug–herb interaction cautions
None.

Physical medicine
- Help the child at home by providing a structured environment, well-defined behavior limits and consistent use of parenting techniques. Professional counseling for parents and child may be helpful.
- Behavior and cognitive therapies involve the child with self-monitoring, role playing and self-recording, focusing on strategies that alter the undesired behavior.
- Stay in close contact with the child's teacher. Arrange for extra lessons or tutoring if needed.

Autism

DESCRIPTION

A biochemical and/or genetic disorder that causes an organic defect in brain development, autism occurs in early childhood (first diagnosis is typically no later than 30 months), and results in a neurological disorder that disrupts normal brain function, manifesting in the areas of social interaction and communication skills. Autistic children are usually retarded in their intellectual development, have significant difficulty with both verbal and non-verbal communication, and do not develop social relationships. Compulsive, and in some cases, aggressive and/or self-injurious behavior may be present.

More than a half a million people in the US have some form of autism, which is the third most common developmental disorder and occurs in as many as 1 in 500 births. (In comparison, Down's syndrome occurs in 1–2 of every 1,000 births.) Eighty percent of children born with autism are low birth weight males; the lower the birth weight, the higher the risk of autism.

FREQUENT SIGNS AND SYMPTOMS

- Low birth weight
- Profound failure to develop social relationships
- Language disorder with impaired understanding, involuntary parrot-like repetition of a word or sentence just spoken by another person, and reversal of pronouns
- Rituals and compulsive actions
- General retardation in intellectual development (in most cases)

CAUSES

- **A defect in serotonin metabolism in the brain:** the basic defect appears to be a decrease in central nervous system serotonin activity despite elevated free tryptophan levels in the serum (tryptophan is the amino acid from which the body makes serotonin).
- **Biochemical mechanisms:** the following biochemical mechanisms are the most plausible theories to explain the decrease in brain serotonin activity seen in autism:
  - reduced activity of tryptophan hydroxylase or L-aromatic amino acid decarboxylase results in impaired serotonin synthesis that, via feedback control, leads to increased levels of free tryptophan in the serum.
  - increased activity of the enzyme tryptophan oxygenase results in the production of high levels of kynurenine (a product of the metabolism of L-tryptophan, elevated in cases of vitamin B_6 deficiency), reduces the tryptophan available for serotonin synthesis, and inhibits tryptophan transport across the blood–brain barrier. A further increase in tryptophan oxygenase activity is triggered when tryptophan levels rise, setting up a vicious cycle that continues the problem.
- **Trigger mechanisms:** researchers are uncertain as to what may initially trigger the biochemical mechanisms that then result in defective serotonin metabolism. Although genetic disorders are definitely a root cause, studies suggest the following environmental factors may contribute: infant vaccinations, food allergies, viral infections, fetal alcohol syndrome, lead poisoning, parasite infestation, yeast infections, trauma during birth delivery.
- **Food allergies and intestinal permeability:** gluten (a protein in wheat and other grains) and milk are thought to be major food allergens in autistic patients. Children with autism frequently suffer from metabolic defects in the enzymes that break down certain opiate-like peptides in milk and wheat. These peptides then gain entry into the brain and significantly disrupt brain chemistry.
- ***Candida albicans*:** some evidence suggests that an overgrowth of the yeast, *Candida albicans*, may exacerbate behavior problems in autistic children. The by-products of this yeast's metabolism are toxins that damage the intestinal wall and thus can leak into the general circulation, impairing central nervous system and immune system function:
  - behaviors related to *Candida* overgrowth may include confusion, hyperactivity, short attention span, lethargy, irritability, and aggression.

- health problems associated with *Candida* can include headaches, constipation, diarrhea, flatulence, distended stomach, and cravings for carbohydrates, fruits and sweets. Skin rashes, unpleasant odor of hair and feet, and an acetone smell from the mouth may also be present.

RISK INCREASES WITH

- Low birth weight
- Male sex
- Fetal alcohol syndrome
- Lead poisoning
- Parasite infestation
- Yeast infections
- Trauma during birth delivery
- Food allergies
- Infant vaccinations
- Viral infections

PREVENTIVE MEASURES

Pregnancy
- Don't consume alcohol.
- Avoid known food allergens.
- Seek prompt treatment of any infection.
- Check water supplies for heavy metals.

Infant care
- Parents should become well informed about the pros and cons of infant vaccinations and make educated decisions as to which vaccinations their child receives.
- In allergy-induced autism, symptoms become apparent during early infant life. Should a child exhibit excessive thirst, excessive sweating (especially at night), low blood sugar, diarrhea, bloating, rhinitis, inability to control body temperature, red face and/or ears, and dark circles under the eyes, act aggressively to identify and remove potential allergens.
- Some children have autism that has been triggered by intolerance to foods and/or chemicals with the main offenders being wheat, dairy products, corn, sugar, and citrus fruits. Allergies may, however, be a reaction to virtually any substance.

Expected outcomes

Sadly, the prognosis for the autistic child is currently poor; typically, only one in 20 will show any improvement by adulthood. The likelihood of improvement appears to be related to the results of IQ testing. As testing is difficult in autistic children, an experienced examiner is essential for an accurate assessment.

Typically, about half of those children with an IQ over 50 can do moderately well, and some can attain normal adjustment, especially with appropriate behavioral therapy, psychotherapy, and special schooling. In those children with IQ scores under 50, temporal lobe epilepsy usually manifests eventually.

TREATMENT

No effective medical treatments currently exist for autism. Phenothiazines are used to control severe forms of aggressive and self-destructive behavior but do not affect the underlying defect in serotonin metabolism, so do not correct the mental disorder. Natural therapies (including nutrient supplementation, allergy elimination, and a diet geared towards enhancing bowel detoxification of potential central nervous system toxins), which support normal serotonin metabolism and help minimize levels of central nervous system toxins, have been shown in a number of studies to greatly help a significant portion of children with autism.

Diet
- Identify and eliminate allergens from the diet.
- Milk and wheat are highly suspect since both contain highly allergenic proteins:
  - in a study of 19 autistic children who were given diets that eliminated milk and/or gluten (a protein found in wheat and other grains) for 1 year, a decrease was seen in the excretion of peptides (the building blocks of proteins) in the urine. This decrease was accompanied by several behavioral improvements: an increase in social contact, an end to self-mutilation like head-banging, and a decrease in "dreamy state" periods.
- Foods rich in factors that help improve the liver's detoxification ability include:
  - high-sulfur-content foods such as garlic, legumes, onions, and eggs
  - good sources of soluble fibers such as pears, oat bran, apples, and legumes
  - cabbage-family vegetables, especially broccoli, Brussels sprouts, and cabbage
  - artichokes, beets, carrots, dandelion, and herbs and spices including turmeric, cinnamon, and licorice.

Nutritional supplements
Doses given below are suitable for children between the ages of 2 and 6 years and should be tailored to the size as well as the age of the patient:
- **Folic acid, vitamin B$_{12}$, and vitamin C:** if the defect in serotonin metabolism is due to a decrease in activity

of the enzyme tryptophan hydroxylase, supplementation with these three nutrients may help. Folic acid, vitamin B_{12} and vitamin C work together to increase levels of an enzyme called tetrahydrobiopterin [BH4] upon which the tryptophan hydroxylase enzyme depends. Increasing central nervous system levels of BH4 has helped patients with affective disorders and Parkinson's disease; dosages:

- vitamin C: 1 g q.d.
- folic acid: 500 µg q.d.
- vitamin B_{12}: 500 µg q.d.

■ **Pyridoxal phosphate, pyridoxine (vitamin B_6) and magnesium:** if the defect in serotonin metabolism is due to abnormal decarboxylation or kynurenine metabolism, then supplementation with vitamin B_6 may be of significant help. Vitamin B_6 (which is synthesized into its metabolically active coenzyme form, pyridoxal phosphate, in the liver) is associated with numerous enzymes necessary for the production of serotonin and other neurotransmitters including dopamine, noradrenaline and gamma-amino-butyric acid (GABA). Magnesium is required for the synthesis of pyridoxal phosphate; dosages:

- pyridoxal phosphate: 5–20 mg q.d.
- pyridoxine: 25–100 mg q.d.
- magnesium: 75–100 mg q.d.

Botanical medicines

■ **Silymarin:** a special extract from *Silybum marianum* (milk thistle), silymarin contains a group of flavonoid compounds that exert powerful beneficial effects in protecting the liver from damage and enhancing detoxification processes:

- silymarin is an antioxidant many times more potent than vitamin E and vitamin C.
- silymarin prevents the depletion of glutathione, a powerful antioxidant essential to numerous detoxification processes in the liver.
- glutathione has the primary responsibility for eliminating fat-soluble toxins. The higher its glutathione levels, the greater the liver's capacity to detoxify harmful chemicals.
- dosage: 70–210 mg t.i.d.

Drug–herb interaction cautions
None.

Counseling
Autism requires specialized behavioral and psychological attention. Referral to a counselor experienced in working with autistic children is warranted.

Bacterial sinusitis

DESCRIPTION

An inflammation of the sinuses (air-filled cavities) adjacent to the nose, sinusitis commonly affects the ethmoidal sinuses (located between the eyes), and the maxillary sinuses (located in the cheekbones). Any factor that causes swelling of the mucous membranes that line the sinuses may result in obstruction of drainage. Fluid is then trapped, becoming a source of food for bacteria, which multiply causing an infection. Pain, tenderness, redness and swelling over the involved sinus, often along with nasal congestion and thick discharge, signal sinusitis.

The most common predisposing factor to acute bacterial sinusitis is viral upper respiratory infection – the common cold. And, like the common cold, sinusitis is contagious. When sinusitis primarily affects the maxillary (cheek) sinuses, underlying dental infection is the cause in about one-quarter of cases. When sinusitis is chronic, food allergies, hay fever (allergic rhinitis), and low immune function are frequently causal factors.

FREQUENT SIGNS AND SYMPTOMS

Early stage acute sinusitis
- Nasal congestion with thick green-yellow discharge (sometimes tinged with blood)
- Feeling of pressure inside the head
- Eye pain
- Frontal headache, often worse in the morning or when leaning forward

Late stage acute sinusitis
- Pain, tenderness, redness, and swelling over the involved sinus
- Fever, chills, and frontal headache
- Cheek pain that may resemble a toothache
- Complete blockage of the sinus openings, resulting in no nasal discharge and increased pain

Chronic sinusitis
- Post-nasal drip
- Musty odor
- Non-productive cough

CAUSES

- **Viral upper respiratory infection** (the common cold)
- **Underlying dental infection**
- **Food and environmental allergies:** sinusitis affects between 25 and 75% of people with environmental or food allergies.
- **Low immune function due to:**
  - excessive consumption of refined carbohydrates and sugars: consuming 75 g (3 oz) of sugar in one sitting in any form (sucrose, honey, fruit juice) depresses white (immune) cell activity by 50% for 1–5 hours.
  - nutrient deficiency: an overwhelming number of studies demonstrate that even a subclinical deficiency of any nutrient can impair immune function.
  - stress: the mind and emotions significantly impact immune function.
  - inadequate rest: a minimum of 7 hours sleep per night is recommended.
  - obesity: the white blood cells of overweight individuals have been shown in experimental studies to be less able to destroy bacteria.
  - alcohol consumption profoundly depresses the rate at which white blood cells move into areas of infection; the more alcohol consumed, the greater the impairment of white blood cell mobility.
- ***Helicobacter pylori* infection:** when asthma and eczema patients with peptic ulcer symptoms were treated (using antibiotic therapy) for *H. pylori* infection, elimination of this ulcer-causing bacterium also resolved allergy symptoms, including chronic sinusitis. If you have chronic sinusitis, your physician may suggest screening for *H. pylori*.

RISK INCREASES WITH

- Common cold or other upper respiratory infection
- Irritation of the nasal passages from cigarette smoke, chemicals in the environment that irritate the respiratory tract, harsh sneezes with the mouth closed, chilling, swimming (especially jumping into the water without holding the nose), and fatigue

- Exposure to others in public places; swimming in contaminated water
- Illness or drugs that have lowered immune resistance
- Frequent consumption of refined carbohydrates and sugars
- Smoking
- Alcohol consumption
- *Helicobacter pylori* infection
- Dental infection
- Food or environmental allergies

PREVENTIVE MEASURES

- **Minimize** consumption of refined carbohydrates, sugars and alcohol.
- **An immune supportive diet:** after identifying and removing any allergenic foods from your diet, consume a nutrient-dense diet rich in whole, unprocessed, preferably organic foods, especially plant foods (fruits, vegetables, whole grains, beans, nuts and seeds), and cold-water fish (for more detailed information, see Appendix 1).
- **A high-potency multiple vitamin and mineral supplement:** a daily multiple providing all of the known vitamins and minerals serves as a foundation upon which to build an individualized health-promotion program. Any good multiple should include 400 µg of folic acid, 400 µg of vitamin B_{12}, and 50–100 mg of vitamin B_6. (Folic acid supplementation should always be accompanied by vitamin B_{12} supplementation to prevent folic acid from masking a vitamin B_{12} deficiency.)
- **Maintain good oral health:** brush and floss teeth after meals and have regular dental checkups.
- **Minimize respiratory tract irritants:** everyone should minimize exposure to noxious chemicals, especially cigarette smoke. Studies have shown that people who live in households where one or more members smoke and/or in well-insulated homes with wood stoves have more upper respiratory infections than average. Individuals with chronic sinusitis should consider the use of air-filtering vacuum cleaners and installation of a HEPA air filtration system in their home and workplace. Particularly sensitive people may need to remove carpeting, feather bedding and pets – at least from bedrooms. Live plants may also help purify the air.
- **Nose blowing:** blow the nose gently with both nostrils open. **Do not** hold one nostril closed and blow with force; this can send mucus back up into the sinus cavities.

Expected outcomes

Even chronic sinusitis should be resolved within 2–3 weeks of instituting the recommended preventive and treatment measures.

TREATMENT

Diet

- Limit consumption of simple sugars (primarily found in refined carbohydrates but also including fruit sugars) to less than 50 g q.d.
- Drink extra fluids to help thin secretions. Choose water, sparkling water, herb teas, diluted vegetable juices, and soups; avoid fruit juices, sodas, and other sweetened fluids.

Nutritional supplements

- **Vitamin C:** directly antiviral and antibacterial, vitamin C's main claim to fame is its many different immune-enhancing effects including white blood cell response and function, increasing levels of interferon (a special chemical factor that fights viral infection and cancer), and increasing secretion of hormones from the thymus gland (the major gland of the immune system); dosage: 500 mg every 2 hours.
- **Bioflavonoids:** a group of plant pigments largely responsible for the colors of fruits and flowers, flavonoids are powerful antioxidants in their own right, and, when taken with vitamin C, significantly enhance its absorption and effectiveness; dosage: 1,000 mg q.d.
- **Vitamin A:** known as the "anti-infective vitamin", vitamin A plays an essential role in immune function by:
  - maintaining the surfaces of the skin, respiratory tract, and gastrointestinal tract and their secretions – all of which constitute a barrier that is the body's first line of defense against micro-organisms.
  - stimulating and/or enhancing numerous immune processes including white blood cell function and antibody response.
  - direct anti-viral activity.
  - preventing immune suppression resulting from stress-induced adrenal hormones, severe burns, and surgery.
  - some of these latter effects are likely the result of the ability of vitamin A to prevent stress-induced shrinkage of the thymus gland and to promote thymus growth.
  - dosage: 5,000 IU q.d.
- **Beta-carotene:** also called "pro-vitamin A" since it can be converted into vitamin A, beta-carotene is a more powerful antioxidant than vitamin A and exerts

additional immune-stimulating effects, including enhancing thymus function. Specifically, beta-carotene has been shown to increase the production of helper/inducer T cells by 30% after 7 days and all T cells after 14 days; dosage: 25,000 IU q.d.

■ **Zinc:** the most critical mineral for immune function, zinc promotes the destruction of foreign particles and micro-organisms, protects against free radical damage, acts synergistically with vitamin A, is required for proper white cell function, and is necessary for the activation of serum thymic factor – a thymus hormone with profound immune-enhancing actions. Zinc also inhibits replication of several viruses, including those of the common cold; dosage: 20–30 mg q.d.

■ **Thymus extract:** substantial clinical data demonstrate that thymus extracts restore and enhance immune system function via improving thymus function:
  ■ in double-blind studies, thymus extracts have been shown not only to treat current respiratory tract infections but also, over the course of a year, to reduce significantly the number of respiratory infections and improve numerous immune parameters.
  ■ specifically, thymus extract has been shown to normalize the ratio of T helper cells to suppressor cells, whether the ratio is low (as in AIDS or cancer) or high (as in allergies or rheumatoid arthritis).
  ■ dosage: consume the equivalent of 120 mg pure polypeptides with molecular weights less than 10,000, or roughly 500 mg of the crude polypeptide fraction.

Botanical medicines

■ **Bromelain:** good to excellent results have been obtained in bromelain-treated patients with acute sinusitis. Bromelain is a group of sulfur-containing proteolytic (protein-digesting) enzymes obtained from the pineapple plant; dosage: (1,200–1,800 MCU) 250–500 mg between meals.

■ *Echinacea* **species:** the two most widely used species are *Echinacea angustifolia* and *Echinacea purpurea*, both of which exert numerous immune-enhancing effects.
  ■ one of *Echinacea*'s most important immune-stimulating components is *inulin*, a large polysaccharide that activates the alternative complement pathway, part of the immune system's first line of defense, and increases the production of immune chemicals that activate macrophages. The result is increased activity of many key immune parameters: production of T cells, macrophage phagocytosis, antibody binding, natural killer cell activity, and levels of circulating neutrophils.
  ■ in addition to immune support, *Echinacea* is directly antiviral and helps prevent bacterial infection by inhibiting the bacterial enzyme hyaluronidase. Bacteria secrete hyaluronidase to break through the body's first line of defense – its protective membranes such as the skin or mucous membranes – so the bacteria can enter the body.
  ■ dosage: choose one of the following forms and take the recommended dosage t.i.d.:
    ● dried root or as tea: 0.5–1 g
    ● freeze-dried plant: 325–650 mg
    ● juice of aerial portion of *E. purpurea* stabilized in 22% ethanol: 2–3 ml
    ● tincture (1 : 5): 2–4 ml
    ● fluid extract (1 : 1): 2–4 ml
    ● solid (dry powdered) extract (6.5 : 1 or 3.5% echinacoside): 150–300 mg.

■ *Hydrastis canadensis* **(goldenseal):** goldenseal is a remarkably safe and effective natural antibiotic. Its most active alkaloid constituent, berberine sulfate, exhibits a broad range of antibiotic action against a wide variety of bacteria (including streptococci and staphylococcus), fungi (including Candida), and protozoa. Its action against some of these pathogens is actually stronger than that of commonly used antibiotics, but, unlike antibiotic drugs, goldenseal does not destroy the protective bacteria (lactobacilli) in our intestines:
  ■ berberine is a more effective antimicrobial agent in an alkaline environment. Alkalinity can be increased by consuming less animal products and more plant foods, especially fruits. Although most fruits are acidic, digestion uses up their acid components leaving behind an alkaline residue.
  ■ dosage: choose one of the following forms and take the recommended dosage t.i.d. (the dosage should be based on berberine content, and standardized extracts are recommended):
    ● dried root or as infusion (tea): 2–4 g
    ● tincture (1 : 5): 6–12 ml (1.5–3 tsp)
    ● fluid extract (1 : 1): 2–4 ml (0.5–1 tsp)
    ● solid (dry powdered) extract (4 : 1 or 8–12% alkaloid content): 250–500 mg.

Drug–herb interaction cautions
None.

To help re-establish drainage, the following topical and physical medicine treatments may be used.

Topical medicines
■ **Nasal saline flush:** dissolve 0.25 tsp of salt and 0.12 tsp of baking soda in 120 ml (4 US fl oz) of water. Spray the mixture inside the nose with a bulb syringe, then use the syringe to suction out the loosened mucus.

- **Swab nasal passages with oil of bitter orange:** oil of bitter orange (4% dilution) has been shown to have strong antibacterial and antifungal activity. It is essential to use the genuine versions, Neroli Bigarade or Pettigrain Bigarade, of this much adulterated and simulated oil. Neroli Portugal, the oil distilled from the flowers of the sweet orange tree, is of a lesser quality.
- **Sinus compress:** apply a compress of menthol or eucalyptus over the sinuses (take care to avoid irritation). To prepare a compress, disperse two drops of essential oil in a cup of warm water, dip a clean cotton cloth or washcloth in the mixture, wring it out slightly so it is no longer dripping, apply to the affected area, and leave it in place for 10–15 min.
- **Vapor inhalation treatment:** add 4–5 drops of essential oil of eucalyptus and/or rosemary to a sink-full or large pot of hot, steaming water. Drape a large towel over your head, forming a tent. Lean over the pot and inhale the steam for at least 5 min.

Physical medicine
- Local applications of hot packs (discontinue if pain increases without drainage).

Benign prostatic hyperplasia

DESCRIPTION

The prostate, a donut-shaped gland about the size of a walnut that lies below the bladder and surrounds the urethra in males, secretes a fluid that increases sperm motility and lubricates the urethra to prevent infection. As men age, benign (non-malignant) prostate enlargement (hyperplasia) (BPH) is extremely common, affecting 5–10% of men at age 30 and over 90% of men over age 85. If the enlarged prostate pinches off the flow of urine from the bladder, problems associated with bladder obstruction occur, such as increased urinary frequency, nighttime awakening to empty the bladder, and a reduction in the force and speed of urinary flow.

If experiencing any symptoms associated with BPH, self-diagnosis is definitely not recommended. For the most accurate diagnosis, a digital prostate examination will likely be performed and/or an ultrasound along with a blood test for prostate-specific antigen. The digital examination simply involves a doctor inserting a gloved finger into the rectum and feeling the lower part of the prostate for any abnormality. The classic enlarged prostate due to BPH is softer (boggy) and may be two to three times larger than normal, but is not tender, as is the case in prostatitis. In prostate cancer, the prostate typically feels much harder than normal, and its border is not well defined like that of a normal prostate.

A definitive diagnosis of BPH can be made with the aid of ultrasound measurements, but because symptoms of BPH and prostate cancer can be similar, a blood test is also used to differentiate the two. The blood test measures levels of a protein produced in the prostate: prostate specific antigen (PSA). Normal value for PSA is less than 4 ng/ml. A level above 10 ng/ml is highly indicative of prostate cancer, while mid-range elevations in PSA can be caused by BPH. In some instances, however, prostate cancer may be present without elevations in PSA levels, so, in a man over 50 with an immediate relative who has had prostate cancer, a yearly digital prostate examination as well as a PSA test is recommended.

FREQUENT SIGNS AND SYMPTOMS

- Increased, progressive urinary frequency, especially at night
- Weak urinary stream
- Straining and dribbling on urination
- Feeling that the bladder cannot be completely emptied
- Excessive sensitivity to the presence of any residual urine in the bladder
- Urine of abnormal color
- Impotence (sometimes)
- Burning on urination

CAUSES

- **Hormonal changes associated with aging:** as men age, hormonal changes, including an increase in prolactin and estrogen levels, occur, resulting in an increased concentration of testosterone in the prostate and increased conversion of this hormone to a more potent form called dihydrotestosterone (DHT). Increases in DHT levels are primarily due to two factors: (1) an increase in the activity of the enzyme 5-alpha-reductase, which converts testosterone to DHT, and (2) a decrease in DHT removal due to the increase in estrogen, which inhibits the elimination of DHT from the prostate.

RISK INCREASES WITH

- **Aging**
- **Inadequate zinc intake:** zinc is critical to many aspects of hormone metabolism. Intestinal uptake of zinc is impaired by estrogens, but enhanced by androgens. Zinc inhibits the activity of 5-alpha-reductase (the enzyme that converts testosterone to DHT), and the pituitary gland's secretion of prolactin. Prolactin increases the prostate's uptake of testosterone, leading to an increase in the formation of DHT.
- **Beer:** the hops in beer cause an increase in prolactin secretion.

Natural Medicine Instructions for Patients

- **Stress:** this increases prolactin secretion.
- **Low-protein diet:** a 10% protein, 70% carbohydrate, 20% fat diet stimulates 5-alpha-reductase, the enzyme that converts testosterone to DHT.
- **Alcohol consumption:** while only beer raises prolactin levels, consumption of 740 ml (25 US fl oz) or more per month of any form of alcohol, especially beer, wine and sake, is directly correlated with a diagnosis of BPH.
- **Essential fatty acid deficiency:** the prostatic and seminal lipid (fat) levels and ratios are often abnormal in patients with BPH. Supplementation with essential fatty acids has resulted in significant improvement for many BPH patients.
- **High cholesterol:** cholesterol damaged by free radicals is particularly toxic and carcinogenic to the prostate. Damaged forms of cholesterol are thought to play a role in stimulating prostate cell formation in BPH.
- **Smoking or exposure to cigarette smoke:** cigarette smoke is a major source of cadmium, which is a known antagonist of zinc and increases the activity of 5-alpha-reductase.

PREVENTIVE MEASURES

- **Limit alcohol consumption:** intake of 740 ml (25 US fl oz) or more of alcohol per month is directly correlated with a diagnosis of BPH.
- **Pesticides:** avoid environmental exposure to pesticides and choose organically grown produce whenever possible; many pesticides increase the activity of 5-alpha-reductase.
- **Increase consumption of soy and soy foods:** soy contains the flavonoids genistein and daidzein which attach to estrogen receptors, thus preventing estrogen's attachment. In addition, genistein and daidzein inhibit 5-alpha-reductase.
- **Diet:** increase consumption of deep sea, cold-water fish (salmon, herring, mackerel, tuna), and also nuts and seeds, especially flaxseed and walnuts; these foods are the best sources of omega-3 essential fatty acids.
- **Smoking:** don't smoke and avoid exposure to second-hand smoke.
- **Maintain healthful cholesterol levels:** total blood cholesterol level should be less than 200 mg/dl; the level of low density lipoprotein (LDL) cholesterol should be less than 130 mg/dl, and the high density lipoprotein (HDL) cholesterol level should be greater than 35 mg/dl, i.e., the ratio of LDL to HDL should be no higher than 2.5.

Expected outcomes

The chance of significant improvement within the customary 4–6-week period of use with any of the botanical treatments appears to be determined by the degree of obstruction, as indicated by residual urine content:

- For levels below 50 ml, results are usually excellent.
- For levels between 50 and 100 ml, results are usually quite good.
- For residual levels between 100 and 150 ml, it may take longer to produce improvement.
- For residual urine content greater than 150 ml, botanical medicines are not likely to produce significant improvement.
- Severe BPH, resulting in significant urinary retention, may require catheterization for relief.
- A sufficiently advanced case may not respond to therapy rapidly enough and may require short-term use of an alpha-1 antagonist drug (e.g., Hytrin or Cardura) or surgical intervention.

TREATMENT

Diet

- A high-protein diet (44% protein, 35% carbohydrate, 21% fat) inhibits 5-alpha-reductase (the enzyme that converts testosterone to DHT).
- To reduce pesticide exposure, choose organically grown foods whenever possible. Increase intake of cold-water fish, flaxseed oil, and walnuts – foods that are excellent sources of essential fatty acids.
- Nuts and seeds, particularly pumpkin seeds, are rich in zinc, so should also be frequently consumed; 85–150 g (3–5 oz) of pumpkin seeds daily is suggested.
- To maintain or achieve healthful cholesterol levels, limit consumption of animal-derived foods and make plant foods – fresh fruits, vegetables, whole grains, legumes, nuts and seeds – the primary dietary constituents.
- Soy products should also be a dietary staple:
  - soybeans, an excellent source of high quality protein, are especially rich in compounds, such as beta-sitosterol, that resemble cholesterol in structure and have well-documented cholesterol-lowering effects.
  - soy's phytosterols have also been shown to significantly relieve BPH. In the latest double-blind study, a group of 200 men received either beta-sitosterol or placebo. No changes were observed in the placebo group, but in those receiving beta-sitosterol (20 mg t.i.d.), maximum urine flow rate increased from a baseline of 9.9 ml/sec to 15.2 ml/sec, and the amount of urine left in the bladder after

urination decreased from 65.8 to 30.4 ml. A 100 g (3.5 oz) serving of soybeans, tofu or other soy food provides approximately 90 mg of beta-sitosterol.

■ increased consumption of soy is associated with decreased risk of prostate cancer, largely due to the action of two soy phytoestrogens, genistein and daidzein. These compounds bind to estrogen receptors, thus preventing estrogen attachment, and also inhibit 5-alpha-reductase.

Nutritional supplements

■ **Zinc:** zinc inhibits 5-alpha-reductase activity (the enzyme that converts testosterone to DHT), and prolactin secretion. Prolactin increases the prostate's uptake of testosterone, leading to an increase in the formation of DHT; dosage: 45–60 mg q.d.

■ **Flaxseed oil:** a good source of essential fatty acids. Be sure to purchase flaxseed oil in a dark, opaque container, store in the refrigerator, and do not heat; dosage: 1 tbsp q.d.

■ **Amino acid mixture:** a combination of the amino acids glycine, glutamic acid and alanine has been shown in controlled studies to provide significant symptomatic relief for men with BPH. The mechanism of action is thought to be related to these amino acids acting as inhibitory neurotransmitters and reducing the feelings of a full bladder; dosage: 200 mg q.d. of each of the three amino acids glycine, glutamic acid, and alanine.

Botanical medicines

Careful review of the published medical literature suggests the relative effectiveness of the botanicals used for BPH are as follows: Saw palmetto, Cernilton, Pygeum, Urtica. Each plant, however, has a slightly different mechanism of action, so in some situations, Urtica, though rated lowest, may produce the best results.

■ ***Serenoa repens* (Saw palmetto):** in numerous clinical studies, the fat-soluble extract of the fruit of the saw palmetto tree has significantly diminished all major symptoms of BPH, especially nocturia (nighttime awakenings to urinate), in roughly 90% of men with BPH.

■ mechanisms of action include inhibition of DHT binding to cellular receptors, inhibition of 5-alpha-reductase, and interference with prostate estrogen receptors.

■ most patients achieve some relief of symptoms within the first 30 days of saw palmetto extract treatment versus the drug finasteride (Proscar), which typically takes up to a year to produce significant benefits. In addition, saw palmetto extract has no demonstrable effect on serum prostate specific antigen (PSA) levels.

■ dosage: saw palmetto extract standardized to contain 85–95% fatty acids and sterols: 160 mg b.i.d.

■ **Cernilton:** an extract of flower pollen, cernilton's overall success rate in patients with BPH is about 70%. Responsive patients typically have significant reductions in residual urine volume, plus reductions in nocturia and daytime frequency of around 70%; dosage: 63–126 mg b.i.d./t.i.d.

■ ***Pygeum africanum*:** the bark of this evergreen tree contains fat-soluble sterols and fatty acids with demonstrated effectiveness in reducing both the symptoms and clinical signs of BPH:

■ although less effective when compared to saw palmetto extract, pygeum has produced some beneficial effects on prostate secretion that saw palmetto has not. The two extracts, with their somewhat overlapping mechanisms of action, can be used in combination.

■ dosage: *Pygeum* extract standardized to contain 14% triterpenes including beta-sitosterol and 0.5% *n*-docosanol: 50–100 mg b.i.d.

■ ***Urtica dioica* (Stinging nettle):** although less research has been done with stinging nettle, it has been shown to produce beneficial effects in two double-blind studies. Although not as effective as saw palmetto, urtica appears to act similarly, by interfering with the binding of DHT to cytosolic and nuclear receptors; dosage: *Urtica dioica* extract: 300–600 mg q.d.

Drug–herb interaction cautions

None.

Canker sores

DESCRIPTION

Recurrent oral canker sores (aphthous stomatitis) are a common condition affecting about 20% of the US population. Outbreaks vary from a single lesion, two or three times a year, to an uninterrupted succession of multiple lesions. While neither cancerous nor herpes infections (with which they are often confused), these small, shallow mouth ulcers are painful and quite bothersome. They appear either singly or in clusters on the lips, gums, inner cheeks, tongue, palate and/or throat. Ulcerations typically heal without scarring within 7–21 days.

FREQUENT SIGNS AND SYMPTOMS

- Ulcers are sometimes preceded by a feeling of tingling or burning for 24 hours.
- Ulcers are small, shallow, very painful, and covered by a grey membrane. Borders are surrounded by an intense red halo.
- Ulcers may appear anywhere in the oral cavity: lips, gums, inner cheeks, tongue, palate and/or throat.
- Typically only two or three ulcers appear during an attack, but episodes with 10–15 ulcers are not uncommon.
- Ulcers may be so painful during the first 2–3 days that they interfere with eating or speaking.

CAUSES

- **Food sensitivities or allergies** (especially to milk and gluten): microscopic evaluation of lesions plus elevated levels of allergy-induced white blood cells and antibodies confirm a causal link between recurrent canker sores and allergens in many cases. Gluten, a protein found in grains, is often the culprit. Patients with celiac disease, a condition characterized by diarrhea and malabsorption due to gluten sensitivity, have a high frequency of recurrent canker sores.
- **Environmental allergens:** preservatives such as benzoic acid, methylparaben, dichromate, and sorbic acid commonly induce canker sores.
- **Nutrient deficiency:** due to the rapid rate of turnover in the cells that line the surfaces of the mouth and throat, the oral lining is often the first place where the effects of a nutrient deficiency become visible. A number of nutrient deficiencies can lead to canker sores. Several studies have clearly demonstrated a causal association between thiamin deficiency and recurrent canker sores. Other studies show nutrient deficiencies – including not only thiamin, but also iron, folate, vitamin B_{12}, riboflavin, and pyridoxine – are much more common in recurrent canker sore sufferers than in the general population.
- **Stress:** often a precipitating factor in recurrent canker sores, stress may disrupt normal immune function and/or result in damage to the integrity of the mucosal lining.
- **Trauma:** injury to the mucosal lining caused by rough dentures, excessively hot food, toothbrushing or dental work, or irritation from frequent or prolonged consumption of highly acidic (vinegar, pickles) or salty (salted nuts, popcorn, potato chips) foods.

RISK INCREASES WITH

- Recent dental treatment
- Emotional or physical stress, anxiety or premenstrual tension
- Frequent consumption of processed foods containing numerous preservatives

PREVENTIVE MEASURES

- Brush teeth thoroughly, but not abrasively, at least twice a day and floss regularly to keep the mouth clean and healthy.
- Check dentures and mouth guards for proper fit and smoothness.
- Avoid consumption of excessively hot, acidic or salty foods.

Expected outcomes

Eliminating food allergens, sources of gluten, and nutritional deficiencies results in complete cure within 1 month in most cases.

TREATMENT

Diet
- **Evaluate for potential allergens and gluten sensitivity** and, if indicated, remove all allergens and gluten sources (grains) from the diet. The best method of diagnosing sensitivity to gluten is to measure the level of antibodies against gluten in the blood, a test called the *alpha-1-gliadin antibody assay*.
- **Consume a nutrient-dense diet** rich in whole, unprocessed, preferably organic foods, especially plant foods (fruits, vegetables, beans, seeds and nuts), and cold-water fish, and low in animal products (for more detailed information, see Appendix 1).

Nutritional supplements
- **A high-potency multiple vitamin and mineral supplement:** this should provide all of the known vitamins and minerals (see the guidelines provided in Appendix 2).
- **Vitamin C:** necessary for the production of healthy collagen used to form connective tissue, repair wounds, improve gum and mucosal health, and reduce bruising; dosage: 1,000 mg q.d.
- **Quercetin:** a bioflavonoid known to inhibit mast cells from releasing inflammatory compounds and causing symptoms of allergy. The antiallergy drug, sodium cromoglicate, which has been shown to increase the number of canker sore-free days, is similar in structure and function; dosage: 400 mg, 20 min before meals.

Botanical medicines
- **Deglycyrrhizinated licorice (DGL):** a special licorice extract with anti-inflammatory, antiallergic activity, DGL accelerates the growth and regeneration of mucosal cells. In a study of 20 patients with canker sores given DGL as a mouthwash, 15 of the 20 experienced 75% improvement within 1 day, and complete healing of the ulcers by the third day. Tablets, being a more concentrated form, may produce even better results; dosage: one to two 380 mg chewable tablets 20 min before meals.

Drug–herb interaction cautions
None.

Physical medicine
- Learn how to cope effectively with stress. Use stress-management techniques such as abdominal breathing, progressive relaxation, meditation or guided imagery.

Carpal tunnel syndrome

DESCRIPTION

Carpal tunnel syndrome (CTS) is a common, painful nerve disorder caused by compression of the median nerve that passes between the bones and ligaments of the wrist, resulting in numbness, tingling, and burning pain in the first three fingers of the hand. Symptoms may be occasional or constant and typically occur most frequently at night. CTS is often found in people who perform repetitive strenuous work with their hands (e.g., carpenters), but may also occur with light, repetitive work (e.g., typists, keyboard operators). Although injury to the wrist may precipitate CTS, it usually occurs with no history of significant trauma. More prevalent among women, particularly between the ages of 40 and 60, CTS occurs most frequently in pregnant women, women taking oral contraceptives, menopausal women, and patients on hemodialysis as a result of kidney failure. These individuals tend to have a greater need for vitamin B_6; B_6 supplementation has been shown to be helpful in many cases, even when no apparent deficiency exists.

FREQUENT SIGNS AND SYMPTOMS

- Numbness, tingling and/or pain in the first three fingers of the hand, particularly at night
- Sharp pains that shoot from the wrist up the arm, especially at night
- Burning sensation in the fingers
- Burning, tingling or aching that may radiate to the forearm and shoulder
- Morning stiffness or cramping of hands
- Thumb weakness
- Pain when gripping
- Frequent dropping of objects
- Inability to make a fist
- Appearance or worsening of symptoms caused by flexing the wrist for 60 sec and relieved by extending the wrist

CAUSES

- **Nerve pressure:** pressure on the nerves at the wrist caused by swollen, inflamed or scarred tissue. Sources of pressure include:
  - inflammation of the tendon sheaths, frequently from rheumatoid arthritis.
  - sprain or dislocation of the wrist or fracture of the forearm.
  - hypothyroidism, which produces an edema known as myxedema. This accumulation of fluid causes swelling, placing pressure on the nerve as it passes through the carpal tunnel.
- **Inadequate vitamin B_6:** the increased frequency of CTS since its initial description by George Phalen MD in 1950 parallels the increased presence of compounds that interfere with vitamin B_6 in the body, particularly tartrazine (FD&C yellow dye #5).
- **High protein intake:** this can lead to a relative shortage of vitamin B_6 since B_6 is involved in protein metabolism.

RISK INCREASES WITH

- Work that requires repetitive hand or wrist action
- Fracture to the forearm or sprain or dislocation of the wrist
- Chronic inflammatory conditions such as diabetes mellitus, Raynaud's disease, rheumatoid arthritis, gout, ganglion cyst
- Conditions that increase the need for vitamin B_6 such as pregnancy, menopause, use of oral contraceptives, hemodialysis, hypothyroidism

PREVENTIVE MEASURES

- Avoid processed foods containing the additive, tartrazine (FD&C yellow dye #5).
- Ensure adequate levels of vitamin B_6 by consuming foods rich in this nutrient (see Diet recommendations below) as well as a high-potency multiple vitamin and mineral supplement including 400 µg of folic acid,

400 µg of vitamin B_{12}, and 50–100 mg of vitamin B_6. (Folic acid supplementation should always be accompanied by vitamin B_{12} supplementation to prevent folic acid from masking a vitamin B_{12} deficiency.) A daily multiple providing all of the known vitamins and minerals serves as a foundation upon which to build an individualized health-promotion program.

- If possible, avoid activities that cause trauma to the median nerve by repeated flexion and extension of the wrist.
- Take a 5-min break at least once an hour when doing repetitive hand work.
- Wear a wrist brace during repetitive hand work.

Expected outcomes

Symptoms may begin to lessen within 2 weeks of initiating treatment, but full benefits may take as long as 3 months.

TREATMENT

Diet

- Avoid processed foods containing the additive, tartrazine (FD&C yellow dye #5).
- Ensure adequate levels of vitamin B_6 by consuming foods rich in this nutrient: seafood, walnuts and other nuts, sesame seeds, wheat germ, legumes, leafy green vegetables, avocado, watercress, Brussels sprouts, cauliflower, cabbage, bananas, cantaloupe, molasses, and milk.
- Limit daily protein intake to a maximum of 0.75 g/kg of body weight.

Nutritional supplements

- **Vitamin B_6 (pyridoxine):** John Ellis MD and Karl Folkers PhD at the University of Texas have successfully treated hundreds of patients suffering from CTS with vitamin B_6, even those with no apparent vitamin B_6 deficiency; dosage: 25 mg t.i.d.

- **Vitamin B_2 (riboflavin):** vitamin B_2 functions in the conversion of vitamin B_6 into its more active form, pyridoxal-5-phosphate; dosage: 10 mg q.d.

Botanical medicines

- **Bromelain:** bromelain, an enzyme found in pineapple, has demonstrated effectiveness in reducing swelling, bruising, healing time, and pain following various injuries and surgeries, and is a well-documented anti-inflammatory in virtually all inflammatory conditions. If surgery for CTS is absolutely necessary, bromelain should definitely be taken for 3 days prior to surgery and for at least 2 weeks after surgery:
  - dosage: bromelain standardized to include 1,200–1,800 MCU/gdu, 250–750 mg b.i.d. between meals.

Drug–herb interaction cautions

None.

Topical medicine

- **Contrast hydrotherapy:** alternating immersion in first hot and then cold water provides a simple, efficient way to increase circulation to an area of inflammation, thereby increasing local nutrition, eliminating waste, decreasing pain, and reducing swelling. Immerse the hand and forearm in hot water for 3 min, then in cold water for 30 sec. Repeat the process three to five times; perform daily.

Physical medicine

- **Acupuncture:** in a study of 36 CTS patients, 14 of whom had been previously treated unsuccessfully with surgery, 35 responded positively to acupuncture.
- **Stretching:** researchers have suggested that stretching exercises might reduce the need for surgery by 50%. Flex the wrists and fists, with the arms extended, for 5 min before work starts and during every break. This sustained stretching helps prepare the carpal tunnel nerve for repetitive actions.

Celiac disease

DESCRIPTION

Also called *non-tropical sprue*, *gluten-sensitive enteropathy* or *celiac sprue*, celiac disease is an allergic response to gluten (a protein found primarily in wheat, barley and rye grains) and its smaller derivative, *gliadin*, which damages the small intestine resulting in diarrhea, weight loss and multiple vitamin and mineral deficiencies. Symptoms typically appear either during the first 3 years of life when cereals are introduced into the diet, or during the third decade of life. In adults, symptoms may develop gradually over months or even years.

FREQUENT SIGNS AND SYMPTOMS

- Weight loss or slowed weight gain in an infant following the introduction of cereal to the diet
- Bulky, pale, frothy, foul-smelling, greasy stools with increased fecal fat
- Swollen and/or painful abdomen
- General undernourished appearance
- Anemia or vitamin deficiency, with fatigue, paleness, skin rash, or bone pain
- Poor appetite, vague tiredness, breathlessness
- Mouth ulcers
- Swollen legs, mildly bowed legs in children
- Increased blood levels of antibodies for alpha-gliadin: blood tests for anti-alpha-gliadin antibodies have a diagnostic sensitivity for celiac disease of 100%
- Diagnosis confirmed by biopsy of the small intestine: usually unnecessary due to the sensitivity of the blood test for anti-alpha-gliadin antibodies
- Schizophrenia: partially digested wheat gluten has demonstrated opiate-like activity, which may explain the association between wheat consumption and schizophrenia that has been substantiated in epidemiological, clinical and experimental studies
- Lactose intolerance: celiac disease often leads to lactose deficiency, causing lactose intolerance and increased intestinal permeability, and frequently resulting in multiple food allergies
- Associated conditions: thyroid abnormalities, insulin-dependent diabetes mellitus, psychiatric disturbances (including schizophrenia), and hives have also been linked to gluten intolerance. Celiac patients also have an increased risk for malignant cancers that may be due to decreased absorption of vitamins and minerals, particularly vitamin A and carotenoids, or to a gliadin-activated suppression of immune function. Alpha-gliadin has demonstrated suppressive effects on immune function in celiac patients but has no effect on the immune function of healthy controls or patients with Crohn's disease.

CAUSES

- **Genetic factors:** people with specific genetic markers known as HLA-B$_8$ and DR$_{w3}$ that appear on the surface of cells (like the genetic markers of blood type) are significantly more likely to have celiac disease than persons without these markers. The HLA-B$_8$ marker is found in 85–90% of celiac patients versus 20–25% of normal subjects. The frequency of HLA-B$_8$ is low in Asia, an area in which farming has a much longer history than in northern and central Europe and the northwest Indian subcontinent, where HLA-B$_8$ incidence is much higher and wheat cultivation, which began around 1000 BC, is a relatively recent development. Celiac disease is virtually unknown in Asia, but is estimated to occur in 1 : 300 people in southwest Ireland, and in 1 : 2,500 people in the US, a much more genetically diverse population.
- **Gluten:** the major protein component of wheat, gluten, is composed of *gliadins* and *glutenins*. Only the gliadin portion has been demonstrated to activate celiac disease. Among the different cereal grains, which are all members of the family *Gramineae*, the more closely a grain is related to wheat, the greater its ability to activate celiac disease. Rice and corn, the grains the farthest removed from wheat, do not appear to activate celiac disease.
- **Protein digestion abnormality:** gliadin that has been completely broken down by digestion does not activate celiac disease in susceptible individuals. This suggests that celiac disease may arise from a deficiency either of enzymes that break down gliadin or of some other factor involved in protein digestion.

- **Immune system abnormality:** the damage to the intestinal tract seen in celiac disease is not due to some toxic property of gliadin, but results when the immune system, in the process of trying to neutralize gliadin, destroys surrounding intestinal tissue.
- **Early introduction of cow's milk:** cow's milk contains a number of highly allergenic proteins. A major portion of the immune system – the gut-associated lymphoid tissue (GALT) – clusters around the intestines. Particularly during the first 4–6 months of life, when the intestinal system is not yet fully developed, allergenic protein can leak across the intestinal wall, triggering an immune response from the GALT and the development of food allergies.

RISK INCREASES WITH

- Not having been breast-fed as an infant
- Early introduction of cereal grains and/or cow's milk into the diet
- Northern and central European or northwest Indian ancestry
- Family history of celiac disease
- Lactose intolerance
- Other allergies

PREVENTIVE MEASURES

- Breast-feeding for a minimum of 6 months.
- Delay introduction of cow's milk and high-gluten cereal grains (wheat, barley, rye) into the diet of high-risk individuals for at least the first year of life.
- Once these potentially problematic foods have been introduced, rotate foods in the child's diet so that high-gluten cereal grains and cow's milk are consumed no more frequently than every fourth day.

Expected outcomes

Significant improvement will usually be apparent within a few days or weeks. Thirty percent of celiac patients respond within 3 days; another 50% within 1 month, and 10% after 2 months. Ten percent, however, only respond after 24–36 months of gluten avoidance. Milk and milk products should also be eliminated until intestinal structure and function return to normal.

If improvement does not occur after following a gluten-free diet for 2 months, consider the following:
- Diagnosis may be incorrect.
- Gliadin may still be being consumed from hidden sources in the diet. Gliadin is found in some brands of soy sauce, modified food starch, ice cream, soup, beer, wine, vodka, whiskey, malt, and other foods.

- Complications of celiac disease, such as an underlying nutrient deficiency, may prevent healing. Zinc deficiency in particular will prevent healing as zinc is a necessary cofactor for growth and repair.

TREATMENT

Diet

- Follow a gluten-free diet. Eliminate any wheat, rye, barley, triticale, or oats. Buckwheat and millet are often excluded as well. Although buckwheat is not in the grass family, and millet is more closely related to rice and corn, both do contain proteins similar to alpha-gliadin.
- Eliminate milk and milk products until intestinal structure and function return to normal.
- Rotate other foods to minimize the potential for developing allergies.

Resources for gluten-free recipes and further education

American Celiac Society
45 Gifford Avenue
Jersey City, NJ 07304

American Digestive Disease Society
7720 Wisconsin Avenue
Bethesda, MD 20014

Gluten Intolerance Group of North America
5110 10th Avenue SW, Suite A
Seattle, WA 98166-1820
206-246-6652 (Voice)
206-246-6531 (FAX)

Coeliac UK
PO Box 220
High Wycombe
Bucks HP11 2HY, UK

Digestive Disorders Foundation
3 St Andrew's Place
London NW1, UK

Websites

- Gluten Intolerance Group of North America: http://www.gluten.net/
- American Autoimmune Related Diseases Association, Inc.: http://www.aarda.org/
- Celiac Sprue Association/United States of America, Inc.: http://www.csaceliacs.org/
- Coeliac UK: http://www.coeliac.co.uk/
- Digestive Disorders Foundation: http://www.digestivedisorders.org.uk/

Nutritional supplements

- **A high-potency multiple vitamin and mineral supplement:** this should include 400 µg of folic acid, 400 µg of vitamin B_{12}, and 50–100 mg of vitamin B_6. (Folic acid supplementation should always be accompanied by vitamin B_{12} supplementation to prevent folic acid from masking a vitamin B_{12} deficiency.) In addition to treating any underlying deficiency, a daily multiple providing all of the known vitamins and minerals provides the cofactors for growth and repair. Celiac disease will often not clear up if there is an underlying nutrient (e.g., zinc) deficiency.

- **Pancreatic enzymes:** a deficiency of pancreatic enzymes is found in 8–30% of celiac patients. A double-blind study found that pancreatic enzyme supplementation enhanced the clinical benefits of a gluten-free diet during the first 30 days but did not provide greater benefit than placebo after 60 days:
  - dosage: pancreatic enzyme capsules each containing: lipase 5,000 IU, amylase 2,900 IU, and protease 330 IU. Two capsules with each meal for 30 days.

Cellulite

DESCRIPTION

A cosmetic defect rather than a disease, cellulite – a pitting, bulging deformation of the skin surface resulting from weakened underlying connective tissue structures – is nevertheless a cause for great distress among millions of European and American women. Because of structural differences in the subcutaneous layer immediately below the surface of the skin in men and women, cellulite is rarely found in men and, if present, is a highly probable sign of androgen (male hormone) deficiency. Women, however, unless slim and athletic, are nine times more likely to develop cellulite, and their susceptibility increases with age.

FREQUENT SIGNS AND SYMPTOMS

- The "mattress phenomenon": pitting, bulging and deformation of the skin surface, most typically on the thighs and buttocks, but also, to a lesser extent, on the lower part of the abdomen, the nape of the neck, and the upper parts of the arms.
- Possible feelings of tightness and heaviness in affected areas, particularly the legs.
- Tenderness of the skin when pinched, pressed upon, or vigorously massaged.
- Varicose veins are often found in conjunction with cellulite, and both conditions share a common cause: a loss of integrity in supporting connective tissue.

CAUSES

Women's subcutaneous tissue structure
- Subcutaneous tissue lies just below the surface of the skin and binds the skin loosely to underlying tissue or bones. On the thighs, a primary area for cellulite, subcutaneous tissue is composed of three layers of fat with two layers of connective tissue between them.
- In women, the uppermost subcutaneous layer consists of large vertically standing fat cell chambers, separated by walls of connective tissue that are anchored to the overlying connective tissue of the skin. In men,

this uppermost layer of subcutaneous tissue is much thinner and, instead of connective tissue walls separating vertical fat cells, has a network of crisscrossing connective tissue holding the fat in place. In addition, the corium, the connective tissue structure immediately below the epidermis (the visible skin) and between it and the subcutaneous tissue, is thicker and stronger in men than in women.

The breaking down or thinning of connective tissue structures
- As women age, their corium layer becomes progressively thinner and looser. This thinning allows fat cells from the subcutaneous layer immediately below to migrate into the corium. The connective tissue walls between the fat cell chambers also become thinner, allowing the fat cell chambers to enlarge excessively. The resulting alternating depressions and protrusions in the subcutaneous layer appear as cellulite in the epidermis.

RISK INCREASES WITH

- Obesity
- Age: cellulite is very common after menopause
- Sedentary lifestyle

PREVENTIVE MEASURES

Maintain a slim subcutaneous fat layer by:
- maintaining normal body weight throughout life
- regular exercise.

Expected outcomes
At least 3 months of treatment is required before improvement in the skin's appearance is noted.

TREATMENT

Diet
- A health-promoting diet, along with regular exercise, will normalize weight and reduce stress on connective

tissue structures by reducing the size of fat cells. Consume a nutrient-dense diet rich in whole, unprocessed, preferably organic foods, especially plant foods (fruits, vegetables, beans, seeds and nuts), and cold-water fish, and low in animal products, refined carbohydrates and fats (for more detailed information, see Appendix 1).

■ Weight reduction should be gradual, especially in women over the age of 40 years. A rapid loss of weight in individuals whose skin and connective tissues are already undergoing changes from aging will often make cellulite more apparent.

Nutritional supplements

■ **A high-potency multiple vitamin and mineral supplement:** a daily multiple providing all of the known vitamins and minerals serves as a foundation upon which to build an individualized health-promotion program. Any good multiple should include $400\,\mu g$ of folic acid, $400\,\mu g$ of vitamin B_{12}, and $50{-}100\,mg$ of vitamin B_6. (Folic acid supplementation should always be accompanied by vitamin B_{12} supplementation to prevent folic acid from masking a vitamin B_{12} deficiency.)

Botanical medicines

The following botanical medicines increase the integrity of connective tissue structures.

■ *Centella asiatica* **(gotu kola) extract:** in the treatment of cellulite and varicose veins, an extract of *Centella* has demonstrated very good results in several studies in approximately 80% of patients over a period of 3 months:
  ▪ centella enhances connective tissue strength by stimulating the manufacture of important structural components of connective tissue known as glycosaminoglycans (GAGs).
  ▪ GAGs are the major components of the ground substance in which collagen (the main protein of connective tissue and bone) fibers are embedded.
  ▪ dosage: 30 mg of triterpenes t.i.d.

■ *Aesculus hippocastanum* **(horse chestnut) extract:** the key compound in horse chestnut extracts, *escin*, has anti-inflammatory and anti-swelling effects useful in the treatment of cellulite and varicose veins:
  ▪ one of escin's key actions is that it decreases capillary permeability by reducing the number and size of the small pores in capillary walls.
  ▪ dosage: 10–20 mg of escin t.i.d.

Drug–herb interaction cautions

■ *Aesculus hippocastanum* **(horse chestnut):**
  ▪ plus *aspirin or anticoagulants*: it has been speculated that horse chestnut should not be taken with aspirin or anticoagulants because the antithrombin activity of its hydroxycoumarin component, *aesculin*, might cause increased bleeding time.

Topical medicine

Salve, ointment, etc., apply twice per day.

■ **Escin:** applied topically, escin is also beneficial in the treatment of bruises because of its ability to decrease capillary fragility and swelling (use a salve containing 0.5–1.5% escin).

■ *Cola vera* **extract (14% caffeine):** cola is a rich source of caffeine and related compounds which potentiate fat breakdown. Topical application is preferable since effects are primarily local (use a salve containing 0.5–1.5% *Cola vera* extract).

■ *Fucus vesiculosus* **(bladderwrack):** a seaweed with soothing, softening and toning effects that has been used in the treatment of obesity since the 17th century, bladderwrack's high iodine content is thought to stimulate thyroid function (use a salve containing 0.25–0.75% *Fucus vesiculosus*).

Physical medicine

Reduce subcutaneous fat and improve circulation of blood and lymph in affected areas through exercise and massage.

■ **Exercise:** 20–30 min of aerobic exercise a minimum of 5 days per week.

■ **Massage:** regular self-massage of the affected area with hand or brush. The direction of any massage should always be towards the heart.

Cervical dysplasia

DESCRIPTION

Cervical dysplasia, abnormal cell growth on the surface of the cervix, is typically a precancerous condition, but if left untreated, can progress to cervical cancer. The cervix is a small cylindrical organ that comprises the lower part and neck of the uterus, and contains a central canal for the passage of menstrual blood and sperm, and for childbirth. Both the canal and outer surface of the cervix are lined with two types of cell: mucus-producing cells and protective (*squamous*) cells. Cervical dysplasia refers to abnormal changes in these cells, which although they produce no symptoms, can be detected by routine Papanicolaou (Pap) smears long before abnormality has progressed to cancer.

Cancer of the cervix is currently one of the most common cancers affecting women and is the second most common malignant cancer found in women between the ages of 15 and 34, although it can occur at any age. After menarche (the onset of menstruation), all women should have an annual Pap smear (which takes a sampling of cells from the surface of the cervix) to ensure early detection and, thus, successful treatment if cervical dysplasia is present.

Treatment of cervical dysplasia depends upon its severity. Most doctors use a numerical rating system in which "I" represents normal and "V" represents cancer, although the cervical intraepithelial neoplasia (CIN) and Bethesda scales are also used (see table below). If the Pap smear indicates Class II or III, the treatment recommendations below can be used *with careful monitoring*: a Pap smear should be taken every 1–3 months, depending upon dysplasia severity, until results are normal.

FREQUENT SIGNS AND SYMPTOMS

- Usually no signs or symptoms
- Diagnosis results from routine Pap smear evaluation

CAUSES

- **Viruses:** because early age at first intercourse and/or multiple sexual contacts are associated with increased risk of cervical dysplasia/cancer, it has been suggested that cervical cancer is a venereal disease, in the sense that the implicated infectious agents appear to be sexually transmitted. Viruses are the most likely candidates for the infectious agents:
  - two classes of virus are currently suspected as causative agents in cervical dysplasia and cervical cancer: herpes simplex type II (HSV-II) and the human papillomavirus (HPV).
  - HSV-II is the sexually transmitted type of herpes, and outbreaks typically occur on the genitals.
  - HPV is the virus that causes venereal warts. Over 45 strains of HPV have been identified, but one strain, HPV16, has been found in 90% of all cervical cancers and 50–70% of all cases of cervical dysplasia.
  - although these viruses are known to be related to cervical dysplasia, whether they indicate decreased immunity or some other defense mechanism, or are themselves the causative agents has not yet been determined.
- **Smoking:** smokers have at least a two to three times greater risk of cervical dysplasia compared to non-smokers (one study showed the risk to be as much as 17 times greater in women smokers aged 20–29 years). Several hypotheses have been suggested to explain the association:
  - smoking may depress immune functions, enabling a sexually transmitted agent to promote abnormal cellular development.
  - smoking induces vitamin C deficiency. Vitamin C is necessary for normal epithelial integrity, wound

Classification systems for Pap smears

Numerical class	Dysplasia	CIN	Bethesda system
I	Benign	Benign	Normal
II	Benign with inflammation	Benign with inflammation	Normal
III	Mild dysplasia	CIN I	Low-grade SIL
III	Moderate dysplasia	CIN II	Low-grade SIL
III	Severe dysplasia	CIN III	High-grade SIL
IV	Carcinoma *in situ*	CIN III	High-grade SIL
V	Invasive cancer	Invasive cancer	Invasive cancer

CIN, cervical intraepithelial neoplasia; SIL, squamous epithelial lesion.

healing, and immune function, and is an anti-oxidant that inhibits carcinogen formation.
- ▪ vaginal or endometrial cells may concentrate carcinogenic compounds derived from cigarette smoke.
- ▪ unrecognized associations may exist between smoking and sexual behavior.
- **Oral contraceptives:** birth control pills increase the adverse effects of cigarette smoking and decrease levels of numerous important nutrients including vitamins C, B$_6$, and B$_{12}$, folic acid, riboflavin, and zinc.
- **Nutrient deficiencies:** 67% of patients with cervical cancer have nutritional deficiencies. In particular, deficiencies of beta-carotene and vitamin A, folic acid, vitamin B$_6$, vitamin C, and selenium play a significant role in the onset of cervical dysplasia/cancer.

RISK INCREASES WITH

Cervical dysplasia is associated with the same risk factors as cervical cancer.
- **Early age (younger than 18) at first intercourse:** risk for cervical dysplasia/cancer is 2.76 times higher in women who became sexually active before the age of 18.
- **Multiple (2–5) sexual partners:** risk for cervical dysplasia/cancer is 3.46 times higher in women with multiple sexual partners.
- **Pregnancy:** multiple pregnancies and pregnancy before age 20.
- **Viruses:** herpes simplex type II and human papillomaviruses.
- **Immune suppression:** repeated infections signal immune suppression. A suppressed immune system is less effective in eliminating abnormal cells and in protecting the body against viruses.
- **Smoking (more than 10 cigarettes a day):** incidence of cervical dysplasia/cancer in smokers is two to three times greater than in non-smokers.
- **Oral contraceptive use (5–8 years):** birth control pills are thought to block folic acid uptake within cells, thus causing a cellular folic acid deficiency that results in abnormal changes in cells lining the cervix.
- **Deficient dietary vitamin C (less than 30 mg q.d.):** women with low levels of vitamin C are 6.7 times more likely to develop cervical dysplasia than women with sufficient vitamin C levels.
- **Deficient dietary beta-carotene (less than 5,000 IU q.d.):** a strong inverse relationship exists between beta-carotene intake and the risk of cervical dysplasia/cancer. The more severe the dysplasia, the lower the level of beta-carotene. Women with low serum beta-carotene levels have a three times greater

risk for severe dysplasia than women with normal beta-carotene levels.
- **Low intake of folic acid:** folic acid deficiency is typically characterized by abnormal red and white blood cells, but similar changes occur in the cells of the cervix weeks or even months earlier. Many abnormal Pap smears may actually reflect folate deficiency rather than true dysplasia:
  - ▪ folic acid deficiency is the most common vitamin deficiency in the world and is extremely common in women taking birth control pills. It is thought that birth control pills block the effects of folic acid by stimulating a molecule that inhibits folic acid uptake by cells, so serum levels of folic acid may be normal or even increased in patients with cervical dysplasia while the level within the cells of the cervix is low.
  - ▪ low levels of folic acid in red blood cells enhance the effects of other risk factors for cervical dysplasia, especially human papillomavirus (HPV) infection. Conversely, when folic acid status within the cells of the cervix is high, HPV does not infect the cells.
- **Low levels of vitamin B$_6$:** vitamin B$_6$ status is depressed in one-third of patients with cervical cancer. Vitamin B$_6$ is necessary for the proper metabolism of estrogens and for immune response. Estrogens promote cell division and proliferation, so a buildup of estrogen increases the likelihood of abnormal cell division. The immune system is responsible for the identification and elimination of abnormal cells.
- **Low serum levels of selenium:** serum levels and dietary intake of selenium are significantly lower in patients with cervical dysplasia. Selenium is an essential cofactor of glutathione peroxidase, an internally produced antioxidant critical for the detoxification of carcinogenic compounds:
  - ▪ selenium is found in highest amounts in fish, vegetables, and whole grains. In areas where the soil is selenium-poor, the plant content of selenium is low, which translates to lower dietary selenium intake in these areas and a higher risk for cervical dysplasia.
- **High fat intake:** high consumption of fats, particularly animal fats, has been associated with an increased risk for cervical cancer. The more fat, the more estrone (the most potent form of estrogen) a woman's body makes.

PREVENTIVE MEASURES

- ▪ Don't smoke.
- ▪ If using oral contraceptives, switch to a different form of birth control.

- A high-potency multiple vitamin and mineral supplement including 400 µg of folic acid, 400 µg of vitamin B_{12}, and 50–100 mg of vitamin B_6. (Folic acid supplementation should always be accompanied by vitamin B_{12} supplementation to prevent folic acid from masking a vitamin B_{12} deficiency.) A daily multiple providing all of the known vitamins and minerals serves as a foundation upon which to build an individualized health-promotion program.
- Consume a nutrient-dense diet rich in whole, unprocessed, preferably organic foods, especially plant foods (fruits, vegetables, beans [especially soy beans], seeds and nuts), and cold-water fish, and low in animal products (for more detailed information, see Appendix 1).

Expected outcomes

With early diagnosis and treatment, the outcome is excellent. Spontaneous regression occurs in a significant number of patients within 3–5 months.

TREATMENT

Diet

- **Saturated fats:** decrease consumption of meat and dairy products, which are high in saturated fats. Extensive research links a diet high in saturated fat and cholesterol to numerous cancers, including cervical cancer.
- **Animal protein:** limit intake of animal protein sources to 110–175 g (4–6 oz) per day and choose fish, skinless poultry, and lean cuts of meat.
- **Increase consumption of soy foods:** soy foods are not only excellent sources of protein free of saturated fat, they also contain *phytoestrogens* (plant estrogens) that bind to estrogen receptors. Since their estrogenic effect is only 2% as strong as human estrogen, when phytoestrogens occupy estrogen-receptor sites, the end result is a decrease in estrogenic effects.
- **Increase consumption of plant foods** (vegetables, fruits, legumes, whole grains, nuts and seeds): a diet rich in fruits and vegetables correlates with significantly lower incidence of cervical cancer, probably due to its higher levels of fiber, beta-carotene, folic acid, vitamin C, vitamin B_6, and selenium.
- **Reduce sugar intake:** high sugar intake impairs estrogen metabolism and is associated with high estrogen levels, which have been linked to premenstrual syndrome, breast cancer, and low sperm counts. In addition, sugar is the preferred fuel for cancerous cells.
- **Organic foods:** consume organically grown foods in preference to foods sprayed with pesticides and

herbicides. Many pesticides contain chemicals known to mimic estrogen in the body and are thought to be a major factor in a growing number of estrogen-related health problems.

Nutritional supplements

- **Folic acid:** supplementation with folic acid (10 mg q.d.) has resulted in improvement or normalization of Pap smears in patients with cervical dysplasia in placebo-controlled and clinical studies. The regression-to-normal rates ranged from 20% in one study to 100% in another (regression rates for untreated cervical dysplasia are typically 1.3% for mild and 0% for moderate dysplasia):
  - as noted above, folic acid deficiency, which is extremely common, causes abnormal changes in the cells of the cervix, and many abnormal Pap smears may actually indicate folate deficiency rather than true dysplasia.
  - dosage: 10 mg q.d. for 3 months, then 2.5 mg q.d. until normalization of the Pap smear.
- **Vitamin B_{12}:** B_{12} supplementation should always accompany folate supplementation to prevent folic acid from masking a vitamin B_{12} deficiency; dosage: 1 mg q.d.
- **Vitamin B_6:** necessary for normalization of estrogen metabolism and immune response; dosage: 25 mg t.i.d.
- **Beta-carotene:** also known as pro-vitamin A since it can be converted to vitamin A in the body, beta-carotene is a powerful antioxidant essential to epithelial health:
  - a strong inverse correlation has been shown between serum levels of beta-carotene and cervical dysplasia/cancer. Studies have also found that the higher the intake of beta-carotene, the lower the risk for cervical dysplasia/cancer.
  - dosage: 25,000–50,000 IU q.d.
- **Vitamin C:** an essential antioxidant found in all body compartments composed of water, vitamin C strengthens and maintains normal epithelial integrity, improves wound healing, enhances immune function, and inhibits carcinogen formation. In addition, vitamin C regenerates vitamin E after it has used up its antioxidant potential:
  - inadequate intake of vitamin C has been identified as an independent risk factor for the development of cervical dysplasia and carcinoma *in situ*.
  - dosage: 500–1,000 mg t.i.d.
- **Vitamin E:** while vitamin C protects the body's water-soluble areas, vitamin E is the primary antioxidant in the fat-soluble compartments such as cell membranes and fatty molecules like cholesterol:
  - vitamin E also significantly enhances both types of immune defense: non-specific or cell-mediated

immunity and specific or humoral immunity. Cell-mediated immunity is the body's primary mode of protection against cancer.

  ■ dosage: 200–400 IU q.d.
- **Selenium:** as a cofactor necessary for the production of glutathione peroxidase, selenium helps to prevent cancer. Serum and dietary selenium levels are significantly lower in patients with cervical dysplasia; dosage: 200–400 μg q.d.

Topical medicine

- **Vaginal depletion pack:** this promotes drainage from damaged tissues. Essentially, a vaginal depletion pack is a cotton tampon containing a formula composed of several botanical medicines and minerals that promotes a cleansing drainage and tissue healing. If this procedure is suggested, a vaginal depletion pack will be prepared and inserted by a physician, who will provide full instructions at that time. After insertion, the pack is left in for 24 hours, then removed by pulling on the string. A chlorophyll douche should be performed after the vaginal depletion pack has been removed.

Chlamydial infections

21

DESCRIPTION

Chlamydia are a large group of sexually transmitted intracellular parasitic bacteria that infect mucosal surfaces causing inflammation of the *urethra* (the tube that allows urine from the bladder to be excreted from the body), vagina, cervix, uterus, fallopian tubes, anus, and ovaries. *Chlamydia* infection may also be transmitted to the eyes or lungs of a newborn infant and is thought to be responsible for half of the pneumonias in infants.

For genital infections, the incubation period is 7–28 days, and the primary site of infection is the urethra in men and the cervix in women. *Chlamydia* is highly infectious; if found by microscopic examination or culture of discharge in any person who is sexually active, all sexual partners must be treated. In newborns, *conjunctivitis* (eye infection) due to *Chlamydia* is transmitted via genital infection in the mother. The incubation period in newborns is 3–14 days. Although blindness does not occur, chronic cases can lead to permanent changes in the *conjunctiva* (the mucous membrane on the surface of the eye and inside of the eyelid) or cornea. An infant with a chlamydial infection is quite infectious, so careful hygiene is essential.

About four million cases of genital chlamydial infection are reported annually in the United States. Worldwide, more than 50 million new cases are reported each year, making chlamydial infection the most common sexually transmitted disease (STD) in developed countries. Since genital chlamydial infection often produces no symptoms, the actual incidence may be much higher.

FREQUENT SIGNS AND SYMPTOMS

Sexually active individuals
- Often no symptoms, especially in the early stages
- Vaginal discharge in females
- Urethral discharge in males
- Anal swelling, pain or discharge
- Reddening of the vagina or tip of the penis
- Abdominal pain
- Fever
- Discomfort on urinating
- Genital discomfort or pain

Infants
- **Pneumonia:** fluid in the lungs and a protracted staccato cough

Infants and children
- **Conjunctivitis:** redness, irritation, and pus-containing discharge from the eyes

CAUSES

Chlamydia trachomatis bacteria spread by:
- vaginal sexual intercourse
- rectal sexual intercourse
- oral–genital contact
- vaginal infection of a newborn during delivery.

RISK INCREASES WITH

- Lowered immune function
- Chronic diseases associated with chlamydial infection include diabetes mellitus, rheumatoid arthritis in some patients, Reiter's syndrome, and coronary artery disease
- Unprotected sexual activity, particularly in young women
- Low levels of vaginal lactobacilli
- Hot weather, non-ventilating clothing (especially underwear), or any other condition that increases genital moisture, warmth and darkness, all of which foster the growth of pathogenic bacteria

PREVENTIVE MEASURES

- Use condoms during sexual activity.
- Wear cotton underpants or pantyhose with a cotton crotch. Avoid underclothes made from non-ventilating material such as nylon.
- Avoid pants that are tight in the crotch or thighs.
- Don't sit around in a wet bathing suit or other wet clothing.
- After urination or bowel movements, cleanse by wiping or washing from front to back (vagina to anus).

- Change tampons frequently.
- Avoid douches.
- Consume a 225 g (8 oz) serving of plain yogurt containing live lactobacillus cultures at least three times a week.

Expected outcomes

A positive response to treatment should occur within no more than 1 week, although 3 weeks should be allowed for complete recovery. Sexual relations should be delayed until treatment is completed, and symptoms are gone. Since ineffective treatment of *Chlamydia trachomatis* can lead to tubal fibrosis and infertility, if there is significant pelvic inflammation or if testing shows continued infection, antibiotics should be used in addition to the therapies suggested below.

TREATMENT

Diet
- Optimal immune function requires a nutrient-dense diet that is:
  - rich in whole, unprocessed, preferably organic foods, especially plant foods (fruits, vegetables, beans, seeds and nuts), and cold-water fish
  - low in high-fat meat and dairy products, saturated fats, and sugars
  - contains adequate amounts of protein.

For more detailed information, see Appendix 1.

Nutritional supplements
- **Vitamin C:** vitamin C is both antiviral and antibacterial, but its main effects are the result of its immune-enhancing effects, including enhancing white blood cell response and function, increasing levels of *interferon* (a special chemical factor that fights viral infection and cancer), increasing the secretion of *thymic hormones* (the thymus is the master gland of the immune system), and improving the integrity of the linings of mucous membranes; dosage: 1,000 mg q.i.d.
- **Vitamin E:** vitamin E boosts both arms of immunity: non-specific or cell-mediated immunity and antibody-related or humoral immunity; dosage: 400 IU mixed tocopherols q.d.
- **Beta-carotene:** oral beta-carotene (approximately 300,000 IU q.d.) has been shown to increase the number of helper/inducer T cells by 30% after 7 days and all T cells after 14 days. T-cells are white cells produced in the thymus that play a critical role in immune function; dosage: 200,000 IU q.d.

- **Zinc:** zinc plays a vital role in many immune system reactions: it promotes the destruction of foreign particles and micro-organisms, protects against free radical damage, acts synergistically with vitamin A, is required for proper white blood cell function, and is necessary for the activation of *serum thymic factor* – a thymus hormone with profound immune-enhancing properties. Even in elderly subjects, zinc supplementation has been shown to result in increased numbers of T cells and enhanced cell-mediated immune responses. Zinc also inhibits the growth of several viruses, including the common cold and herpes simplex virus; dosage: 30 mg q.d.; picolinate form is recommended.

Botanical medicines
- **Hydrastis canadensis (goldenseal):** berberine, an active component of goldenseal, has been shown to be very effective in the treatment of *ocular* (eye) *Chlamydia trachomatis* infections and should be equally effective against genital *C. trachomatis* infections; dosage: choose any one of the following forms and take the recommended dosage t.i.d.:
  - dried root: 2–3 g
  - tincture (1 : 5): 6–12 ml
  - fluid extract (1 : 1): 1–2 g
  - solid extract (4 : 1): 250 mg

Drug–herb interaction cautions
None.

Topical medicine
- **Vaginal depletion pack:** this treatment, administered in the physician's office, consists of the application of a tampon saturated with a formula containing several antibacterial botanical agents, including goldenseal. The tampon is left in place for 24 hours and then removed by simply pulling on the string. An additional 24 hours later, a mild vinegar or Betadine (see below) douche is performed. The procedure can be repeated weekly until desired results are obtained. Typically, an increase in drainage occurs while the vaginal pack is in place and during the following 24–48 hours. Light sanitary pads may be worn during this time but should be changed frequently to keep the genital area as clean and dry as possible.
- **Povidone-iodine:** betadine, or other source of povidone-iodine, has been shown to be an effective antichlamydial agent. It can be used in a douche containing 2 tbsp of Betadine to 950 ml (2 US pints) of water.

Chronic candidiasis

DESCRIPTION

An overgrowth of the normally benign yeast (or fungus) *Candida albicans*, chronic candidiasis (also called the yeast syndrome) results in a wide variety of symptoms in virtually every system of the body, the most susceptible being the gastrointestinal, genitourinary, endocrine (hormonal), nervous, and immune systems. Normally, *C. albicans* lives harmoniously in the inner warm creases and crevices of the digestive tract and, in women, also in the vaginal tract. However, when conditions in the body allow this yeast to overgrow, when immune system mechanisms are depleted, or when the normal lining of the intestinal tract is damaged, then yeast cells, particles of yeast cells, and various toxic by-products of yeast metabolism can enter the general circulation and significantly disrupt body processes. Due to the effects of estrogen, birth control pills, and a higher number of prescriptions for antibiotics, women are eight times more likely to experience candidiasis than men. The typical patient with chronic candidiasis is a female between the ages of 15 and 50 years.

FREQUENT SIGNS AND SYMPTOMS

Since virtually any system can be affected, chronic candidiasis can trigger a multitude of symptoms. Patients often say they "feel sick all over". Fatigue, allergies, immune system malfunction, depression, chemical sensitivities, and digestive disturbances are just some of the symptoms patients with yeast syndrome can experience.

The more symptoms listed below that are present, the higher the likelihood of yeast overgrowth.

General symptoms
- Chronic fatigue or lethargy
- Feeling of being drained
- Loss of energy
- General malaise
- Headache
- Decreased libido
- Numbness, burning or tingling
- Muscle aches, weakness or paralysis
- Dizziness, loss of balance

- Pain and swelling in joints
- Craving for foods rich in carbohydrates or yeast, e.g., sugar-laden foods, bread, alcoholic beverages

Gastrointestinal system symptoms
- Thrush
- Abdominal pain
- Bloating, belching, gas (flatulence)
- Intestinal cramps
- Rectal itching
- Indigestion
- Heartburn
- Altered bowel function – constipation, diarrhea
- Irritable bowel syndrome
- Mucus in stools
- Hemorrhoids
- Bad breath

Genitourinary system symptoms
- Persistent vaginal itch or burning
- Vaginal yeast infection
- Frequent bladder infections
- Urinary urgency or frequency
- Burning on urination
- Endometriosis
- Impotence

Endocrine system symptoms
- Primarily menstrual complaints:
  - premenstrual syndrome
  - cramps and/or other menstrual irregularities.

Nervous system symptoms
- Depression
- Frequent mood swings
- Irritability
- Inability to concentrate
- Feeling "spacey" or "unreal"
- Poor memory
- Spots in front of the eyes
- Erratic vision

Immune system symptoms
- Allergies

- Sensitivity to foods, environmental allergens, chemicals:
  - symptoms provoked by exposure to perfumes, insecticides, cleaning products, tobacco smoke, fabric odors, etc.
  - symptoms worse on damp muggy days or in moldy places
- Low immune function (susceptibility to infection)
- Burning or tearing of eyes
- Recurrent infections or fluid in ears
- Ear pain or deafness

Respiratory symptoms
- Nasal congestion or discharge
- Postnasal drip
- Nasal itching
- Sore or dry throat
- Cough
- Pain or tightness in chest
- Wheezing or shortness of breath

Dermatological symptoms
- Eczema
- Psoriasis
- Athlete's foot, "jock itch", ringworm or other chronic infections of the skin or nails
- Candidiasis of the skin:
  - bright red itchy plaques with poorly defined borders
  - severe itching
  - skin appears moist and crusted
  - typically affects skin of the scrotum, vagina and vaginal lips, underarms, spaces between fingers and toes, inner thighs, under breasts, over the base of the spine (sacrum).

Past history
- Chronic vaginal yeast infections or vaginitis (inflammation of the vagina)
- Chronic prostatitis (inflammation of the prostate)
- Chronic antibiotic use for infections or acne:
  - use of tetracycline or other antibiotics for acne for 1 month or longer
  - use of "broad-spectrum" antibiotics for respiratory, urinary, or other infections for 2 months or longer, or in short courses four or more times in a 1-year period
- Use of oral birth control pills
- Oral steroid hormone usage:
  - prednisone (prednisolone) or other cortisone-type drugs.

Laboratory tests
- Stool cultures positive for Candida
- Higher than normal levels of Candida antibodies or antigens in the blood

CAUSES

Chronic candidiasis is typically due to multiple factors that predispose an individual to yeast overgrowth including:
- **Antibiotics:**
  - prolonged antibiotic use is believed to be the most important factor in the development of chronic candidiasis. Antibiotics suppress the immune system and kill the normal intestinal bacteria that prevent yeast overgrowth.
  - drugs such as nystatin, ketoconazole, and fluconazole, as well as various natural anti-Candida agents, rarely produce significant long-term results because they do not address the underlying factors that promote Candida overgrowth.
  - use of natural anti-Candida therapies such as timed-release caprylic acid preparations, enteric-coated volatile oil preparations, or fresh garlic preparations (see below) can be helpful. These therapies do not eliminate health-promoting intestinal bacteria. If a follow up stool culture and Candida antigen test show Candida has been eliminated but symptoms are still present, it is likely that Candida is not the culprit.
  - similar symptoms to those attributed to Candida can be caused by small intestine bacterial overgrowth, in which case pancreatic enzymes and berberine-containing botanicals such as *Hydrastis canadensis* (goldenseal) can be helpful.
- **Dietary factors:**
  - sugar is the chief nutrient for *Candida albicans*. Avoiding sugar – which may appear on labels as fructose, maltose, dextrose, polydextrose, corn syrup, molasses, sorbitol, maltodextrin, honey, or maple syrup – is absolutely essential. Fruit juice, which concentrates fruit sugars, should also be avoided.
  - milk and dairy products should be restricted or eliminated for several reasons. Milk's high content of lactose (milk sugar) promotes Candida overgrowth. Milk is one of the most common food allergens. Milk may contain trace levels of antibiotics, which can further disrupt gastrointestinal bacterial flora and promote Candida overgrowth.
  - mold and yeast-containing foods including alcoholic beverages, cheeses, dried fruits, and peanuts should be eliminated from the diet until the situation is under control.
- **Food allergies:**
  - food allergies are commonly found in patients with yeast syndrome.
  - ELISA tests, which determine both IgE- and IgG-mediated food allergies are often helpful (see the chapter on Food allergy for more information).

- **Decreased digestive secretions:**
  - gastric hydrochloric acid, pancreatic enzymes, and bile all inhibit the overgrowth of Candida and prevent its penetration into the absorptive surfaces of the small intestine. Decreased secretion of any of these digestive components can lead to yeast overgrowth.
  - antiulcer drugs such as Tagamet (cimetidine) and Zantac (ranitidine), which shut down hydrochloric acid production, actually develop Candida overgrowth in the stomach.
  - proteases (enzymes that break down protein) are also largely responsible for keeping the small intestine free from parasites including, not only yeast but also bacteria, protozoa, and intestinal worms. A lack of proteases or other digestive secretions greatly increases risk for an intestinal infection, including chronic candidiasis.
- **Impaired immunity:**
  - patients with chronic candidiasis typically suffer from other chronic infections such as repeated viral infections (including the common cold), outbreaks of cold sores or genital herpes, and prostatic (men) or vaginal (women) infections.
  - a triggering event such as antibiotic or corticosteroid use, a nutrient deficiency, food allergy, stress or high-sugar diet can suppress the immune system, allowing *Candida albicans* to overgrow and become entrenched in the lining of the gastrointestinal tract where it competes for, and robs the body of, nutrients rendering the body more susceptible to further infection.
  - *Candida albicans* is referred to as a "polyantigenic" organism because it secretes so many toxins and antigens (compounds the body sees as foreign invaders and against which it develops antibodies). More than 79 distinct *C. albicans* antigens greatly tax the immune system, draining many of its resources.
- **Impaired liver function:**
  - experimental animal studies have repeatedly demonstrated that impaired liver function suppresses the immune system. In mice studies, when the liver is even slightly damaged, Candida runs rampant through the body.
  - indications of an excessively taxed liver include:
    - being more than 9 kg (20 lb) overweight
    - diabetes
    - gallstones
    - history of heavy alcohol use
    - psoriasis
    - natural and synthetic steroid hormone use: anabolic steroids, estrogens, oral contraceptives

  - high exposure to certain chemicals or drugs: cleaning solvents, pesticides, antibiotics, diuretics, non-steroidal anti-inflammatory drugs (aspirin, ibuprofen), thyroid hormone
  - history of viral hepatitis.

RISK INCREASES WITH

- Antibiotic use
- Corticosteroid use
- Oral contraceptive use
- Thyroid hormone use
- Antiulcer drug use (Tagamet, Zantac)
- Frequent use of non-steroidal anti-inflammatory drugs (aspirin, ibuprofen)
- Diuretic use
- High exposure to chemicals such as cleaning solvents, pesticides
- Food allergies
- High-sugar diet
- Heavy alcohol use (alcohol damages the liver, increases intestinal permeability, and raises blood sugar levels)
- Nutrient deficiency
- Inadequate digestive secretions (hydrochloric acid, pancreatic enzymes, bile)
- Stress
- AIDS (suppressed immune system)
- Diabetes (high blood sugar)
- Gallstones (inadequate bile secretion)
- Use of drugs that suppress the immune system
- Frequent infections (colds, cold sores, genital herpes, prostatic or vaginal infections)

PREVENTIVE MEASURES

- Do not use antibiotics, steroids, immune-suppressing drugs, and birth control pills (unless there is absolute medical necessity).
- Identify any lack of digestive secretions and supplement with necessary digestive factors (discussed below).
- Identify and treat food allergies (for more information see the chapter on Food allergy).
- Avoid exposure to chemicals. Consume organically grown food whenever possible. Use environmentally friendly cleaning products.
- Consume a health-promoting diet rich in whole, unprocessed, preferably organic foods, especially plant foods (fruits, vegetables, whole grains, beans, nuts [especially walnuts], and seeds), and cold-water fish (for more detailed information, see Appendix 1).

- Make fresh garlic a frequent addition to your diet. The active component in fresh garlic, allicin, is an effective antifungal agent.
- Limit consumption of refined and simple sugars and alcohol.
- Get adequate rest and sleep to ensure good immune function.

Expected outcomes
Candidiasis treatment usually produces positive changes within 2 weeks.

TREATMENT

Diet
- **Eliminate refined and simple sugars:** sugar, the chief nutrient for *Candida albicans*, may appear on labels as fructose, maltose, dextrose, polydextrose, corn syrup, molasses, sorbital, maltodextrin, honey, or maple syrup. Fruit juice, which concentrates fruit sugars, should also be avoided. Consume no more than one serving of a whole fruit per day.
- **Eliminate alcohol:** alcohol damages the liver, raises blood sugar levels, and increases intestinal permeability, allowing Candida access to the rest of the body.
- **Eliminate milk and dairy products:**
  - milk's high content of lactose (milk sugar) promotes Candida overgrowth.
  - milk is one of the most common food allergens.
  - milk may contain trace levels of antibiotics.
- Eliminate mold and yeast-containing foods including alcoholic beverages, cheeses, dried fruits, and peanuts.
- Eliminate all known or suspected food allergens.
- Follow the dietary recommendations given above in Preventive measures.

Nutritional supplements
- **A high-potency multiple vitamin and mineral supplement:** a daily multiple containing all of the known vitamins and minerals provides a foundation of nutritional support. Any good multiple should include 400 µg of folic acid, 400 µg of vitamin B_{12}, and 50–100 mg of vitamin B_6. (Folic acid supplementation should always be accompanied by vitamin B_{12} supplementation to prevent folic acid from masking a vitamin B_{12} deficiency.)
- **Take additional antioxidants:** look for an antioxidant formula containing carotenes (25,000 IU), vitamin E (200 IU), vitamin C (500–1,000 mg), zinc (15 mg), and selenium (200 µg).
- **Flaxseed oil:** purchase organic flaxseed oil bottled in an opaque container, store it in the refrigerator, and do not heat; dosage: 1 tbsp q.d.

- **Thymus extract:** perhaps the most effective way to re-establish a healthy immune system is to improve the functioning of the thymus. The master gland of the immune system, the thymus is responsible for the production of T cells and thymic hormones, which facilitate numerous immune functions; dosage: thymus extract: 750 mg of crude polypeptide fractions daily.
- **Water-soluble fiber:** water-soluble fiber such as guar gum, psyllium seed, or pectin will promote detoxification and elimination; dosage: 3–5 g taken at night.
- **Probiotics:** friendly intestinal flora are needed to repopulate the intestines, both for their numerous beneficial effects on gut health and also to compete with, and thereby prevent overgrowth of, *Candida albicans*; dosage: 1–10 billion viable *Lactobacillus acidophilus* and *Bifidobacterium bifidum* cells q.d.
- **Lipotropic factors:** the nutrients choline, betaine, and methionine are *lipotropic* agents, i.e., they promote the flow of fat and bile to and from the liver, which improves liver function and fat metabolism. Lipotropic formulas appear to increase levels of two important liver substances: SAM (*S*-adenosylmethionine), the major lipotropic compound in the liver, and glutathione, a powerful antioxidant that is one of the major detoxifying compounds in the liver; dosage: 1,000 mg of choline and 1,000 mg of either methionine and/or cysteine q.d.
- **Caprylic acid:** a naturally occurring fatty acid, caprylic acid has been shown to be an effective antifungal against *Candida albicans*. Take a timed-release or enteric-coated caprylic acid formulation to ensure its gradual release throughout the entire intestinal tract; dosage: 1,000–2,000 mg taken with meals.

Botanical medicines
- **Silymarin:** a special extract of milk thistle (*Silybum marianum*), silymarin is a group of flavonoid (plant pigments with impressive antioxidant effects) compounds that protect the liver from damage and enhance detoxification processes; dosage: standardized extract of silymarin, 70–210 mg t.i.d.
- **Berberine-containing plants:** these include goldenseal (*Hydrastis canadensis*), barberry (*Berberis vulgaris*), Oregon grape (*Berberis aquifolium*), and goldthread (*Coptis chinensis*):
  - berberine, an alkaloid, has a broad spectrum of antibiotic activity against disease-causing bacteria, protozoa and fungi, particularly *Candida albicans*. Since berberine inhibits both pathogenic bacteria and Candida, it prevents the yeast overgrowth that is a common side effect of antibiotic use.
  - berberine has shown remarkable antidiarrheal activity, even in severe cases, and may relieve the diarrhea common in patients with chronic candidiasis.

- the use of berberine or berberine-containing plants is not recommended during pregnancy due to possible uterine-stimulant action, and higher doses than those recommended here may interfere with B vitamin metabolism.
- dosage: use a standardized extract of any of the berberine-containing plants. Choose one of the following forms and take the recommended dosage t.i.d.:
  - dried root or as infusion (tea): 2–4 g
  - tincture (1 : 5): 6–12 ml (1.5–3 tsp)
  - fluid extract (1 : 1): 2–4 ml (0.5–1 tsp)
  - solid (dry powdered) extract (4 : 1 or 8–12% alkaloid content): 250–500 mg.

■ *Allium sativum* **(garlic):** in both animal and *in vitro* (test tube) studies, garlic has demonstrated more potent inhibition of *Candida albicans* than nystatin, gentian violet, and six other reported antifungal agents. The active component, allicin, gives garlic its pungent odor:

- dosage: treatment of candidiasis requires a daily dose of at least 10 mg allicin or a total allicin potential of 4,000 mg, an amount equal to approximately one clove of fresh garlic. To receive the benefits of allicin without the odor, use an enteric-coated tablet preparation.

■ **Enteric-coated volatile oils:** volatile oils from oregano, thyme, peppermint, and rosemary are all effective antifungal agents. Oregano oil has been shown to be more than 100 times more potent than caprylic acid against Candida. As volatile oils are quickly absorbed, an enteric-coated formulation is recommended to prevent possible heartburn and ensure delivery to the small and large intestine:

- **caution:** do not use during pregnancy due to possible stimulation of menses, abortive effects.
- dosage: 0.2–0.4 ml b.i.d. between meals.

Drug–herb interaction cautions

■ **Garlic:**

- plus *insulin*: animal studies suggest insulin dose may require adjusting due to hypoglycemic effects of whole garlic (in rats) and its constituent allicin (in rabbits).
- plus *warfarin*: the anticoagulant activity of warfarin is enhanced due to increased fibrinolytic activity and diminished platelet aggregation caused by garlic components allicin, ajoene, trisulfides, and adenosine.

■ **Psyllium:**

- plus *oral drugs* (e.g., lithium salts): possible reduced absorption unless drug is taken 1 hour before psyllium
- plus *insulin*: insulin dosage may need reduction due to slowing of dietary carbohydrate absorption.

Chronic fatigue syndrome

DESCRIPTION

Chronic fatigue syndrome (CFS) is characterized primarily by the abrupt onset of profound fatigue that does not resolve with bed rest and is severe enough to reduce daily activity by 50% or more for at least 6 months. Fatigue is accompanied by varying combinations of symptoms including sore throat, low-grade fever, lymph node swelling, headache, muscle and joint pain, intestinal discomfort, emotional distress and/or depression, sleep disturbances, and loss of concentration. Chronic fatigue can be caused by a variety of chronic physical and psychological conditions, which should be ruled out. In the United States, the frequency of individuals suffering from CFS is thought to be about 11.5%.

FREQUENT SIGNS AND SYMPTOMS

Symptom/sign	Frequency (%)
Fatigue	100
Low-grade fever	60–95
Muscle pain	20–95
Excessive sleep or insomnia	15–90
Impaired mental function	50–85
Depression	70–85
Headache	35–85
Allergies	55–80
Sore throat	50–75
Anxiety	50–70
Muscle weakness	40–70
After-exercise fatigue	50–60
Premenstrual syndrome (women)	50–60
Stiffness	50–60
Visual blurring	50–60
Nausea	50–60
Dizziness	30–50
Joint pain	40–50
Dry eyes and mouth	30–40
Diarrhea	30–40
Cough	30–40
Decreased appetite	30–40
Night sweats	30–40
Painful lymph nodes	30–40

CAUSES

- **Epstein–Barr virus (EBV):** many research studies have attempted to identify an infectious agent as the cause of CFS, and EBV has emerged as the leading, yet controversial, candidate:
  - EBV is a member of the herpes group of viruses, which includes herpes simplex types I and II, varicella zoster virus, cytomegalovirus, and pseudorabies virus. After the initial infection, all of these viruses establish a lifelong latent infection that is usually kept in check by a healthy immune system. When the immune system is compromised, however, these viruses can become active, replicate and spread. This viral reactivation and recurrence of infection can itself compromise and/or disrupt immunity, increasing susceptibility to other diseases.
  - elevated EBV antibody levels are observed in a significant number of diseases characterized by disorders in immune function. Elevated antibody levels to not only EBV but to the herpes-group viruses, measles, and other viruses have been observed in patients suspected of having CFS.
  - EBV infection is the rule rather than the exception among humans. By the end of early adulthood, virtually all of us demonstrate detectable antibodies to the Epstein–Barr virus in our blood, indicating past infection. When the initial infection occurs in childhood, it usually produces no symptoms, but when it occurs in adolescence or early adulthood, symptoms of infectious mononucleosis develop in approximately 50% of cases.
- **Other infectious agents:** a number of other viruses have been investigated as possible causes of CFS, although the underlying issue – the inability of the individual's immune system to deal with viruses effectively – is not addressed by this focus. The following organisms have been proposed as causative agents in CFS:
  - Epstein–Barr virus
  - human herpes virus-6
  - Inoue–Melnich virus
  - *Brucella*
  - *Borrelia burgdorferi*
  - *Giardia lamblia*

- cytomegalovirus
- enterovirus
- retrovirus
- **Immune system abnormalities:** a disturbed immune system plays a central role in CFS. A variety of immune system abnormalities have been reported in CFS patients:
  - *low natural killer (NK) cell activity*: the most consistent abnormality is a decrease in number or activity of NK cells, immune cells responsible for destroying cells that have become cancerous or infected with viruses.
  - *lack of lymphocyte response*: another consistent finding is a reduced ability of lymphocytes (a type of white blood cell critical in the battle against viruses) to respond to stimuli.
  - *interferon abnormalities*: one of the reasons for the lack of lymphocyte response may be reduced activity or decreased production of interferon, a key compound produced by the body to fight viruses. Both low and high levels of interferon have been reported in CFS, but levels are more often depressed. When interferon levels are low, reactivation of latent viral infection is likely. When interferon levels are high, as is the case when interferon is used as a therapy for cancer and viral hepatitis, the side effects produced are similar to the symptoms of CFS.
  - *immunological abnormalities* that have been reported for CFS:
    - elevated levels of antibodies to viral proteins
    - decreased natural killer cell activity
    - low or elevated antibody levels
    - decreased levels of circulating immune complexes
    - increased cytokine (e.g., interleukin-2) levels
    - increased or decreased interferon levels
    - altered helper/suppressor T cell ratio
    - fibromyalgia (FM): the only difference in diagnostic criteria for FM and CFS is the requirement of musculoskeletal pain in FM and fatigue in CFS. If a rheumatologist or orthopedic specialist is consulted, the patient is more likely to be diagnosed with FM (see the chapter on Fibromyalgia for more information).
    - multiple chemical sensitivities (MCS): one group of researchers carefully compared the symptoms of 90 patients who had been diagnosed as having CFS, MCS, or FM (30 in each category). Eighty percent of both the FM and MCS patients met the CFS criteria of fatigue lasting more than 6 months and causing a 50% reduction in activity. More than 50% of the CFS and FM patients reported adverse reactions to various chemicals.

- **Other causes:** chronic fatigue can be caused by a variety of physical and psychological factors other than CFS. Virtually any chronic disease or chronic use of any drug can disrupt bodily processes causing fatigue. In the following list, which ranks major causes of chronic fatigue in decreasing order of frequency, CFS ranks well below numerous other factors. The most notable factors, which must be addressed if CFS is to be treated effectively, are briefly explained:
  - pre-existing physical condition
  - depression – in the absence of a pre-existing clinical condition, depression is generally regarded as the most common cause of chronic fatigue
  - diabetes
  - heart disease
  - lung disease
  - rheumatoid arthritis
  - chronic inflammation
  - chronic pain
  - cancer
  - liver disease
  - multiple sclerosis
  - prescription drugs
  - antihypertensive drugs
  - anti-inflammatory agents
  - birth control pills
  - antihistamines
  - corticosteroids
  - tranquilizers and sedatives
  - stress – when an individual is stressed, his/her adrenal glands secrete hormones such as cortisol and other corticosteroids. These hormones stimulate the conversion of protein to energy and promote the retention of sodium to keep blood pressure elevated, thus preparing the body to deal effectively with a crisis or for strenuous tasks. To shunt available energy to meet the stress-generated need, bodily systems whose tasks relate to long-term health, such as tissue repair and immune defense, are downregulated. If the body is constantly in an alarm state responding to perceived stress, exhaustion will eventually manifest as a total collapse of body functions or as a collapse of specific organs:
    - two of the major causes of exhaustion are losses of potassium ions and depletion of adrenal glucocorticoid hormones such as cortisol. When cells lose potassium, they function less effectively and eventually die. When adrenal glucocorticoid stores are depleted, hypoglycemia (low blood sugar) results, and cells do not receive enough glucose and other nutrients to function properly.

- exhaustion is also due to a weakening of the organs. Prolonged stress places a tremendous load on many organ systems, especially the heart, blood vessels, adrenals and immune system.
- *low adrenal function*: debilitating fatigue is one of the major symptoms of low adrenal function, also characterized by a stressful event, followed by feverishness, joint pain, muscle ache, swollen lymph glands, fatigue, worsening of allergic responses, and disturbances of mood and sleep.
- *impaired liver function and/or environmental illness*: exposure to food additives, solvents (cleaning materials, formaldehyde, toluene, benzene, etc.), pesticides, herbicides, heavy metals (lead, mercury, cadmium, arsenic, nickel, and aluminum), and other toxins can greatly stress the liver, leading to a reduction in its ability to detoxify:
  - symptoms of impaired detoxification include depression, general malaise, headaches, digestive disturbances, allergies and chemical sensitivities, premenstrual syndrome, and constipation.
  - in a multi-clinic research study, when chronically ill patients diagnosed with CFS were placed on a hypoallergenic diet and provided with a dietary supplement rich in nutrients that support liver detoxification, the patients reported a 52% reduction in symptoms after 10 weeks. Symptom improvement was mirrored by normalization of liver detoxification mechanisms.
- *impaired immune function*: fatigue is the body's response to infection because immune cell production occurs during sleep.
- *chronic fatigue syndrome*
- *chronic Candida infection*: normally, the benign yeast *Candida albicans* lives harmoniously in the inner warm creases and crevices of the digestive tract and, in women, also in the vaginal tract. However, when conditions, such as antibiotic use, allow this yeast to overgrow, when immune system mechanisms are depleted, or when the normal lining of the intestinal tract is damaged, then yeast cells, particles of yeast cells, and various toxic by-products of yeast metabolism enter the general circulation and significantly disrupt body processes. Fatigue, allergies, immune system malfunction, depression, chemical sensitivities, and digestive disturbances are just some of the symptoms patients with yeast syndrome can experience.
- *other chronic infections*
- *food allergies*: chronic fatigue, muscle and joint aches, drowsiness, difficulty in concentration, nervousness and depression are key features of the toxemia resulting from food allergy. Between 55 and 85% of individuals with CFS have allergies.

- *hypothyroidism*: since hormones produced by the thyroid gland affect every cell of the body, a deficiency will cause numerous problems. Depression, weakness and fatigue are usually the first symptoms. Hypothyroidism is often undiagnosed because standard blood measurements of thyroid hormone are not sensitive enough to diagnose the most common, yet milder forms (for more information see the chapter on Hypothyroidism).
- *hypoglycemia*: faulty carbohydrate metabolism induced by a diet too high in refined carbohydrates results in low blood glucose (sugar) levels. Hypoglycemia is associated not only with fatigue, but depression, which is the most common cause of chronic fatigue.
- *anemia and nutritional deficiencies*
- *sleep disturbances*
- *negative or defeatist attitude*: many people with CFS are told that it is "something they will have to live with". This is not true! It is possible to get better. In addition to correcting the underlying physiological causes of CFS, a positive mental attitude is critical to good health and energy levels. Mental states have a direct impact on the production of neurotransmitters that translate our thoughts into physiological changes throughout the body. These neurotransmitters are found, not just in the brain, but also in the immune system, endocrine system, heart, lungs, intestines – everywhere.

RISK INCREASES WITH

- Depression
- Stress/low adrenal function
- Impaired detoxification (liver function)
- Impaired immune function and/or chronic infection, e.g., chronic Candida infection.
- Food allergies/excessive gut permeability
- Hypothyroidism
- Frequent consumption of sugar and/or caffeine: sugar is a major contributor to hypoglycemia, and caffeine stresses the adrenal glands.
- Disease-promoting diet: energy level is directly related to the quality of the foods routinely ingested. A diet based on processed foods, with little consumption of fresh vegetables, legumes, fruits, nuts and seeds, whole grains, and cold-water fish is low in the factors necessary for cellular energy metabolism – antioxidants, vitamin and mineral cofactors, essential fatty acids, magnesium and potassium – and high in factors that disrupt the body's production and use of energy – refined

carbohydrates, *trans* fats (also called partially hydrogenated oils), and chemical additives.

■ Nutrient deficiency: a deficiency of virtually any nutrient can produce symptoms of fatigue and render the body more susceptible to infection.

PREVENTIVE MEASURES

■ **A positive mental attitude:** seek guidance from a physician, or religious or professional counselor to establish a regular pattern of mental, emotional, and spiritual affirmations.

■ **Regular exercise:** a minimum of 30 min, at least three times a week.

■ **Identify** and eliminate food allergens.

■ **Eat** whole, organically grown foods and use environmentally friendly, hypoallergenic cleaning products.

■ **Restrict** intake of refined sugar, alcohol, and caffeine.

■ **Use** antibiotics and other prescription and over-the-counter drugs only when absolutely necessary.

■ **A health-promoting diet:** after identifying and removing allergenic foods from your diet, choose a balanced diet composed of whole, unprocessed, preferably organic foods, especially plant foods (fruits, vegetables, whole grains, beans, nuts [especially walnuts] and seeds), and cold-water fish (for more detailed information, see Appendix 1).

■ **A high-potency multiple vitamin and mineral supplement:** a daily multiple providing all of the known vitamins and minerals serves as a foundation upon which to build an individualized health-promotion program. Any good multiple should include 400 µg of folic acid, 400 µg of vitamin B_{12}, and 50–100 mg of vitamin B_6. (Folic acid supplementation should always be accompanied by vitamin B_{12} supplementation to prevent folic acid from masking a vitamin B_{12} deficiency.)

Expected outcomes

Chronic fatigue syndrome has a broad spectrum of severity. The treatment response is fairly unpredictable even in minor cases due to the fact that an individual's response to CFS has a significant subjective as well as physiological component. A specific treatment approach should be given a trial of at least 3 months before abandoning it, unless it significantly exacerbates the situation.

TREATMENT

Diet

■ Identify and eliminate food allergens (for more information, see the chapter on Food allergies).

■ Increase consumption of water while eliminating consumption of caffeine-containing drinks and alcohol.

■ Adopt a diet of whole, organically grown foods (for more information, see Appendix 1).

■ Control hypoglycemia by eliminating sugar and other refined foods, and consuming regular small meals and snacks.

■ To speed up detoxification, consider a several-week course of a medical food product (e.g., UltraClear, a powdered meal-replacement formula produced by Metagenics, Inc.).

Nutritional supplements

■ **A high-potency multiple vitamin and mineral supplement:** this should include 400 µg of folic acid, 400 µg of vitamin B_{12}, and 50–100 mg of vitamin B_6. (Folic acid supplementation should always be accompanied by vitamin B_{12} supplementation to prevent folic acid from masking a vitamin B_{12} deficiency.)

■ **Vitamin E:** vitamin E is found primarily in the lipid membrane of cells, which it protects from free radical damage. Since a healthy cell membrane is essential for the passage of both nutrients in and wastes out of cells, an inadequate supply of vitamin E can significantly disrupt cellular metabolism. Signs of vitamin E insufficiency include susceptibility to infections, fatigue, weakness, poor coordination, and difficulty digesting fatty foods; dosage: 200–400 IU mixed tocopherols q.d.

■ **Vitamin C:** a potent antioxidant, vitamin C also regenerates vitamin E and enhances immune function. Fatigue is one of the first signs of vitamin C deficiency; dosage: 500–1,000 mg t.i.d.

■ **Thymus extract:** provides support for the thymus, the master gland of the immune system; dosage: 750 mg of the crude polypeptide fraction q.d. or b.i.d.

■ **Magnesium bound to citrate or aspartate:** magnesium is more easily absorbed and utilized when bound to citrate or aspartate, both of which are involved along with magnesium in the Krebs cycle, the final common pathway in which glucose, fatty acids, and amino acids are converted into the energy currency of the body, ATP (adenosine triphosphate); dosage: 200–300 mg t.i.d.

■ **Pantothenic acid (vitamin B_5):** pantothenic acid is involved in the production of adrenal hormones, red blood cells, and the metabolism of fatty acids, proteins and carbohydrates in energy production; dosage: 250 mg q.d.

Botanical medicines

■ *Eleutherococcus senticosus* **(Siberian ginseng):** in addition to supporting adrenal function, and increasing resistance to stress, Siberian ginseng has also been found to produce improvements in immune function, including a significant increase in T-helper cells and an increase in natural killer cell activity; dosage: choose one of the following forms and take the recommended dosage t.i.d.:

- dried root: 2–4 g
- tincture (1 : 5): 10–20 ml
- fluid extract (1 : 1): 2–4 ml
- solid (dry powdered) extract (20 : 1 or standardized to contain greater than 1% eleutheroside E): 100–200 mg.

- **Glycyrrhiza glabra (licorice):** its antiviral and adrenal supportive properties make licorice root an ideal botanical for CFS. If ingested at a dosage of 3 g q.d. for more than 6 weeks, licorice may cause sodium and water retention, resulting in high blood pressure. Blood pressure should therefore be monitored, although patients who normally consume high-potassium foods and restrict sodium intake (which will occur naturally on the health-promoting diet), have been reported to be free of the blood pressure-raising effects of licorice; dosage: choose one of the following forms and take the recommended dosage t.i.d.:
  - powdered root: 1–2 g
  - fluid extract (1 : 1): 2–4 ml
  - solid (dry powdered) extract (4 : 1): 250–500 mg.

Drug–herb interaction cautions
- **Eleutherococcus senticosus (Siberian ginseng):**
  - plus *hexobarbital*: when injected into the peritoneal cavity in mice, Siberian ginseng increases the effect of hexobarbital due to inhibition of its metabolic breakdown.
  - plus *insulin*: when injected into the peritoneal cavity in mice, Siberian ginseng extract has hypoglycemic effects, so insulin dosage may need adjustment.
- **Glycyrrhiza glabra (licorice):**
  - plus *digoxin, digitalis*: due to a reduction of potassium in the blood, licorice potentiates the toxicity of cardiac glycosides. Interaction with these cardioglycoside drugs could lead to arrhythmias and cardiac arrest.
  - plus *stimulant laxatives or diuretics* (thiazides, spironolactone or amiloride): licorice should not be used with these drugs because of the additive increase of potassium loss to potentially dangerous levels.

Physical medicine
- **Regular exercise:** for CFS patients, light to moderate regular exercise has been shown to significantly enhance immune response, leading to an increase of up to 100% in natural killer cell activity. A program including strength training (weight lifting) using light weights, and aerobic activities such as T'ai Chi, yoga, walking, swimming, and dancing will stimulate the immune system, and improve mood and energy utilization.

Congestive heart failure

DESCRIPTION

Congestive heart failure (CHF) refers to an inability of the heart to effectively pump blood throughout the body. There are two types of CHF: *systolic* and *diastolic*. In systolic CHF, blood coming into the heart from the lungs surges back, causing fluid accumulation in the lungs. In diastolic CHF, damage to the heart muscle results in a lessening of its pumping ability, leading to fluid accumulation in the feet, ankles, legs, and abdomen.

Both types of CHF cause a reduction in the heart's output, which leads to a reduction in blood flow to the kidneys. When the kidneys receive less blood, this signals the body to retain fluid, which it does by activating a blood volume management system (the *renin–angiotensin* system). This system increases the amount of force with which the heart's chambers must contract, the resistance of veins to the inflow of blood, and the level of a hormone that causes blood vessels to constrict (*vasopressin*), all of which not only further increase fluid retention, but force an already overtaxed heart muscle to work even harder.

The American Heart Association estimates that 4.7 million Americans have CHF, the leading cause for hospitalization in people over 65. African–Americans are twice as likely to acquire CHF as Caucasians, and mortality from CHF is also twice as great in this group.

FREQUENT SIGNS AND SYMPTOMS

- Shortness of breath, especially with exertion or when lying flat in bed
- A chronic, non-productive cough
- Fatigue, weakness or faintness
- Fluid retention, causing swelling in the ankles, legs, and abdomen (edema)
- Rapid, irregular heartbeat
- Low blood pressure
- Distended neck veins
- Irregularity in the normal rhythm of the heartbeat (arrhythmia)
- Rapid heart beat, over 90 bpm (tachycardia)

CAUSES

CHF is the result of damage to the heart muscle (cardiomyopathy). An understanding of the underlying process responsible for the damage in each individual is important for both treatment and prognosis. There are three basic types of damage to the heart muscle: damage that causes the heart muscle to enlarge and thicken (hypertrophic), damage that causes the heart muscle to become thin and stretched (dilated), and damage that leaves scar tissue that restricts the heart's ability to contract (restricted). Each of these types of damage has different causes:

- **The heart muscle becomes enlarged and thickened as a result of:**
  - high blood pressure: the most common underlying cause of CHF
  - coronary artery disease
  - disorder of a heart valve.
- **The heart muscle becomes thin and stretched as a result of:**
  - alcoholism
  - endocrine diseases such as hyperthyroidism
  - genetic diseases such as congenital heart disease.
- **Damage to the heart muscle that leaves scar tissue that restricts its movement can be caused by:**
  - previous heart attack
  - prior heart surgery
  - chronic lung disease such as emphysema
  - severe anemia
  - rheumatic heart disease
  - infections complicating underlying heart disease
  - heart tumor (rare).

RISK INCREASES WITH

- High blood pressure: according to a recent report from The Framingham Study, high blood pressure increases the risk of developing CHF about twice for men and three times for women
- High cholesterol
- Previous heart attack

Natural Medicine Instructions for Patients

- Diabetes mellitus: incidence of CHF is three to eight times greater in diabetics than in the non-diabetic population
- Smoking
- Infection
- High fever
- Emotional stress
- Pregnancy
- Anemia
- High salt intake
- High environmental temperature
- Alcohol consumption
- Kidney failure
- Liver failure
- Drugs:
  - beta-adrenergic blockers
  - antiarrhythmic drugs
  - drugs that cause sodium retention such as steroids, non-steroidal anti-inflammatory drugs (e.g., aspirin, ibuprofen)
  - diuretics (e.g., Lasix) deplete the body not only of fluid but of nutrients critical for proper heart function, including thiamin, potassium, and magnesium (discussed below). For example, in 1980, it was shown that after only 4 weeks of furosemide (Lasix) use, levels of thiamin (vitamin B_1) and thiamin-dependent enzymes drop significantly.
- Nutrient deficiency: especially of magnesium, thiamin, coenzyme Q_{10}, and carnitine (discussed below)
- Disease-promoting diet: a diet composed of meat and dairy products and processed foods, with little consumption of fresh vegetables, legumes, fruits, cold-water fish, whole grains and nuts and seeds. This diet is:
  - *low in heart-protective factors*: antioxidants, essential fatty acids, magnesium, potassium, B vitamins
  - *high in damaging factors*: salt, saturated fat, *trans* fats (also called partially hydrogenated oils), sugars, refined carbohydrates, and chemical additives. These factors elevate blood pressure and cholesterol levels, and increase the risk for diabetes and obesity.

PREVENTIVE MEASURES

- Don't drink alcohol. Alcohol depresses the functioning of the heart muscle.
- Don't smoke.
- Lose weight if necessary.
- Consume a nutrient-dense diet rich in whole, unprocessed, preferably organic foods, especially plant foods (fruits, vegetables, beans, seeds and nuts), and cold-water fish, and low in animal products and refined foods (for more detailed information, see Appendix 1).
- A high-potency multiple vitamin and mineral supplement including 400 μg of folic acid, 400 μg of vitamin B_{12}, and 50–100 mg of vitamin B_6. (Folic acid supplementation should always be accompanied by vitamin B_{12} supplementation to prevent folic acid from masking a vitamin B_{12} deficiency.) A daily multiple providing all of the known vitamins and minerals serves as a foundation upon which to build an individualized health-promotion program.

Expected outcomes

Fluid retention should be significantly lessened within 1 week. Energy levels should be substantially improved within 1 month. Treatment should be continued indefinitely to maintain improvements. The use of natural therapies either as primary therapy for mild to moderate CHF, or as adjunctive therapy for moderate to severe CHF, is definitely indicated. Using only conventional (drug) treatment: 20% of CHF patients die within 1 year of diagnosis, and 50% die within 5 years.

TREATMENT

In the initial stages of CHF, when shortness of breath is common with exertion, but no symptoms are present at rest, natural measures designed to address the underlying cause (e.g., high blood pressure) or improve the functioning of the heart muscle are often quite effective. In later stages, when even minor exertion results in shortness of breath and fatigue, medical treatment involving the use of diuretics and angiotensin-converting enzyme (ACE) inhibitors and/or digitalis glycosides is indicated in most cases. In these more severe cases, the measures described here should be used as adjunctive therapy.

Diet

- **Reduce excess weight**
- **Strictly limit** salt intake to below 1.8 g daily.
- **Do not consume alcohol**
- **Increase consumption of plant foods:** plant foods are rich in potassium, a critically important dietary *electrolyte* (a mineral salt that can conduct electricity when dissolved in water). Potassium is necessary for water balance and distribution, blood pressure, muscle and nerve cell function, heart function, kidney and adrenal function. During nerve transmission and muscle contraction, potassium exits the cell and sodium enters, causing a nerve impulse or muscle contraction. Potassium is also essential for the conversion

of blood sugar into glycogen (the form in which sugar is stored in the muscles and liver). Because exercising muscles, including the heart, use glycogen for energy, a potassium deficiency causes great fatigue and weakness.

- **Increase consumption of celery, garlic and onions:**
  - celery contains a compound (3-*n*-butyl phthalide) shown in studies to lower blood pressure and cholesterol levels. Consumption of four stalks of celery each day should provide an effective dosage.
  - garlic and onions have also been shown to reduce high blood pressure.
- **Reduce saturated fats:** reduce the intake of saturated fats, found primarily in meat and dairy products. Eliminate margarine and foods containing *trans* fatty acids (also called hydrogenated fats). Considerable research links all these fats to heart disease.
- **Avoid processed foods:** their primary ingredients – sugars, refined carbohydrates, and *trans* fats – elevate cholesterol levels and blood pressure, and increase the risk for obesity and diabetes as well as CHF.
- **Increase consumption of omega-3 essential fatty acids:** over 60 studies have demonstrated that both fish oil and flaxseed oil are very effective in lowering blood pressure. Flaxseed oil should be refrigerated and not heated. Use flaxseed oil (1 tbsp q.d.) in salad dressing, add it to smoothies or mix it into already cooked food. At least three times each week, replace meat and/or dairy protein with cold-water fish – salmon, mackerel, tuna, herring, halibut (110 g [4 oz] at least three times a week).

Nutritional supplements

CHF is characterized by fatigue, which is frequently due to a deficiency of one or more of the following nutrients:

- **Magnesium:** low magnesium levels (particularly white blood cell magnesium) are a common finding in patients with CHF:
  - low magnesium levels correlate directly with lower survival rates – not surprising, as magnesium deficiency is associated with abnormal heart rhythms (cardiac arrhythmias), a poorer cardiovascular prognosis, inadequate circulation of blood to the heart, and a higher likelihood that a heart attack will be fatal.
  - magnesium is a critical nutrient for the production of ATP, the energy currency of the body.
  - conventional drug therapy for CHF (i.e., digitalis, diuretics, and vasodilators including beta-blockers, calcium channel blockers, etc.) causes magnesium depletion. Even in CHF patients receiving conventional drug therapy whose serum magnesium levels are normal, magnesium supplementation has been shown to produce substantial positive effects.

- a recent study of CHF patients at the Arizona Heart Institute found that those who received oral magnesium oxide showed significant improvement in heart rate, mean arterial pressure, and exercise tolerance.
- magnesium is more easily absorbed and utilized when bound to citrate or aspartate, both of which are involved along with magnesium in the Krebs cycle, the final common pathway in which sugars, proteins and fats are converted into ATP, the energy currency of the body.
- dosage: 200–400 mg of magnesium citrate t.i.d.
- **Thiamin (vitamin B$_1$):** thiamin deficiency can result in a buildup of fluid in the lower limbs, and heart failure:
  - a growing body of evidence shows that a significant percentage of the geriatric population are deficient in thiamin and other B vitamins, which are essential to both heart and brain function.
  - furosemide (Lasix), a diuretic drug prescribed for CHF, induces thiamin deficiency after only 4 weeks of use.
  - several studies have shown that daily doses of thiamin (80–240 mg q.d.) increases the amount of blood the heart is able to pump out with each contraction (left ventricular ejection fraction) by 13–22%. In CHF patients, an increase in ejection fraction is associated with a greater survival rate.
  - dosage: 200–250 mg of thiamin q.d.
- **Carnitine:** normal heart function is critically dependent on adequate concentrations of carnitine and coenzyme Q$_{10}$ (discussed below). These compounds are essential in the transport of fatty acids into the heart muscle and mitochondria (the energy production factories in each cell), where they are used to produce energy:
  - while the normal heart stores more carnitine and CoQ$_{10}$ than it needs, if the heart does not have a good supply of oxygen (as is the case in CHF), carnitine and CoQ$_{10}$ levels quickly decrease.
  - several double-blind clinical studies have shown carnitine supplementation improves heart function in patients with CHF. Significant improvement has occurred after only 1 month of treatment, and the longer carnitine was used, the more dramatic the improvement. After 6 months, the CHF patients receiving carnitine demonstrated a 25.9% increase in maximum exercise time and a 13.6% increase in the amount of blood the heart is able to pump out with each contraction (ejection fraction).
  - dosage: 500 mg of L-carnitine t.i.d.
- **Coenzyme Q$_{10}$:** in numerous clinical trials, CoQ$_{10}$ has been an extremely effective adjunct therapy in

improving heart function in patients with CHF:

- in one of the early studies, 17 patients with mild CHF received 30 mg q.d. of CoQ_{10}. All patients improved, and nine (53%) no longer had any symptoms of CHF after 4 weeks.
- in the most recent (1994) and largest study to date, 2,664 patients with mild to moderately severe CHF (New York Heart Association classes II and III) were enrolled in an open study in Italy. After 3 months of CoQ_{10} treatment (most patients received 100 mg q.d.), improvements included reductions in:
  - purplish skin discoloration due to poorly oxygenated blood (cyanosis) – 78.1%
  - fluid retention – 78.6%
  - congestion in the lungs – 77.8%
  - liver enlargement – 49.3%
  - congestion in the veins – 71.8%
  - shortness of breath – 52.7%
  - heart palpitations – 75.4%
  - sweating – 79.8%
  - a feeling that the heart is beating in an abnormal rhythm (subjective arrhythmia) – 63.4%
  - insomnia – 66.2%
  - dizziness (vertigo) – 73.1%
  - nighttime urination (nocturia) – 53.6%

- **Arginine:** the body uses the amino acid arginine to make the natural vein dilator nitric oxide:
  - vein dilation is beneficial in patients with CHF who are typically found to be less able to achieve good blood flow to their extremities (lower limbs and arms), even during exercise.
  - orally administered arginine has been shown in a randomized, double-blind, placebo-controlled study (the gold standard for medical studies) of CHF patients to increase flow to lower limbs and arms by 29%, increase 6-minute walking distance by 8%, and increase the ease with which arteries dilate (arterial compliance) by 19%.
  - dosage: 5.6–12.6 g q.d.

Botanical medicines

- ***Crataegus oxyacantha* (hawthorn):** *Crataegus'* effectiveness in improving heart function in CHF has been repeatedly demonstrated in many double-blind studies:
  - CHF patients receiving *Crataegus* extract have shown an increase in exercise capacity along with reductions in blood pressure and heart rate; no improvements were seen in the CHF patients given a placebo.
  - hawthorn extract (1.8% vitexin-4'-rhamnoside or 10% procyanidin content): 100–200 mg t.i.d.

Drug–herb interaction cautions

None; in fact, in more severe CHF, *Crataegus* extract has been shown to be excellent adjunct therapy.

- *Crataegus* extract contains components (polymeric procyanidins) that enhance the activity of cardiotonic drugs (e.g., digitalis), and cardiac glycosides (e.g., digitoxin and digoxin).
- *Crataegus* extract reduces the toxicity of digitoxin and digoxin by dilating coronary arteries and normalizing heart beat rhythm.

Cystitis

DESCRIPTION

Cystitis, a urinary tract or bladder infection, is most frequently (85% of the time) caused by normal intestinal bacteria, but may be caused by viruses (herpes simplex type II), fungi (*Candida albicans*), and a variety of parasites (worms and protozoa). Lower urinary tract infections occur in the urethra or bladder and, because of differences in male and female anatomy, are more common in women than in men. In women, the urethra is shorter and closer to the anus, a common source of bacteria, which can migrate across the perineum (the narrow band of flesh between the anus and the vagina) to the urethra. The male urethra is much longer, with antimicrobial secretions from the prostate gland providing an additional defense against bacterial invasion.

Urine, as secreted by the kidneys, is sterile until it reaches the urethra, which transports it from the bladder to the urethral opening. Bacteria can reach the urinary tract by ascending from the urethra, or, much less commonly, through the bloodstream.

The body has several defenses against bacterial growth in the urinary tract: urine flow tends to wash away bacteria; the surface of the bladder has antimicrobial properties; the normal pH of the urine inhibits the growth of many bacteria; in men, the prostatic fluid contains many antimicrobial substances; and the immune system quickly mobilizes white cells to control bacteria.

Despite these protective mechanisms, bladder infections in women are surprisingly common: 10–20% of all women have urinary tract discomfort at least once a year; 37% of women with no history of bladder infection will have one within 10 years; and 2–4% of apparently healthy women have elevated levels of bacteria in their urine, indicating an unrecognized urinary tract infection. Women with recurrent bladder infections typically have an episode at least once a year, and as 55% of urinary tract infections eventually involve the upper urinary tract (the kidneys), prompt treatment and learning how to prevent future infections is important.

FREQUENT SIGNS AND SYMPTOMS

- A frequent, urgent desire to urinate
- Burning pain on urination
- Increased urinary frequency, especially at night (nocturia)
- Cloudy, foul-smelling or dark urine
- Blood in the urine
- Painful sexual intercourse
- Pain above the pelvic bone and/or in the lower back
- Bed-wetting in a child
- Fever, irritability in an infant
- Urinalysis may show a significant number of bacteria and white blood cells; only 60% of women with the typical symptoms of cystitis actually have significant levels of bacteria in their urine.

CAUSES

- Bacteria that enter the urinary tract from skin around the genitals and anal area:
  - *Escherichia coli*: although other bacteria can be involved, *E. coli*, a bacterium normally found in the digestive tract and present on the skin around the rectal area, is the culprit in 90% of urinary tract infections when bacteria are identified.
- Bacteria that reach the bladder through the bloodstream.

RISK INCREASES WITH

- **Structural abnormalities** of the urinary tract that block the free flow of urine, as caused by:
  - congenital abnormality
  - kidney stones
  - prior infections of sexually transmitted disease
  - prostate enlargement in older men.
- **Sexual intercourse:** in women, the urethra may be bruised during intercourse; nuns have one-tenth the incidence of cystitis.
- **Mechanical trauma or irritation of the urethra:** for example in childhood sexual abuse.

- **Pregnancy:** cystitis occurs twice as frequently during pregnancy as a result of compression of pelvic organs and a lowering of immunity.
- **Homosexual activity** in males.
- **Use of a urinary catheter** to empty the bladder, such as following childbirth or surgery.
- **Holding urine for too long** a period of time.
- **Infection** in other parts of the genitourinary system.
- **Stress**
- **Illness**, which results in lowered resistance.
- **Excessive sugar consumption:**
  - consumption of 75 g (3 oz) of any form of sugar (glucose, fructose, sucrose, honey, fruit juice), significantly suppresses neutrophil activity for up to 5 hours.
  - neutrophils constitute 60–70% of circulating white blood cells, which engulf and destroy bacteria.
- **Diabetes mellitus:** the spillage of glucose into the urine creates a hospitable medium for bacterial growth.
- **Excess alcohol consumption:**
  - alcohol consumption often results in a rapid increase, followed by a rapid drop, in blood sugar levels.
  - alcohol increases intestinal permeability to bacteria and other toxins, and to potentially allergenic food proteins.
- **Food allergies:**
  - interstitial cystitis has been linked to food allergy.
  - food allergens damage the intestinal lining, increasing the likelihood of bacteria gaining access to the bloodstream.
- **Nutritional deficiencies:** a deficiency of virtually any nutrient can affect immune function.
- **Improper bladder emptying:** from neurological diseases such as paraplegia, valve leakage between the bladder and urethra, and in-dwelling urinary catheters left unchanged for too long a period of time.
- **Wearing** poorly ventilated undergarments.
- **Sitting in bathwater** containing bath salts or bubble bath.
- **Loss of normal suspension of female organs:** resulting from pregnancies and/or surgery.

PREVENTIVE MEASURES

- Drink a glass of water before sexual intercourse and urinate within 15 min after intercourse.
- Use a water-soluble lubricant such as K-Y lubricating jelly during intercourse.
- Use female-superior or lateral positions in sexual intercourse to protect the urethra.
- If using a diaphragm, wash, rinse and carefully dry after each use.

- Take showers rather than tub baths.
- Do not douche, and avoid feminine hygiene sprays or deodorants.
- Cleanse the anal area thoroughly after bowel movements, always wiping from the front to the rear to avoid spreading fecal bacteria to the genital area.
- Wear underwear and pantyhose with cotton crotches. Wear loose-fitting pants.
- Don't postpone urination.
- Avoid caffeine, alcohol and spicy foods, which may irritate the bladder.
- Drink 8–10 glasses of pure water, herbal teas, or fresh fruit and vegetable juices diluted with at least an equal amount of water.
- Avoid soft drinks, concentrated fruit drinks, candy, pastries and other sugar-laden refined foods. Sugar suppresses immune function.

Expected outcomes

Cystitis is usually curable within 1–2 weeks. If an original urine culture indicates the presence of bacteria, it is appropriate to follow up with another culture 7–14 days after treatment is started.

TREATMENT

Diet

- Drink large quantities of fluids (at least 2 L [4 US pints] q.d.), including at least 0.5 L (1 US pint) of *unsweetened* cranberry juice or 0.25 L (8 US fl oz) of blueberry juice per day:
  - in order for bacteria to infect, they must first adhere to the mucosal lining of the urethra and bladder. Components found in cranberry and blueberry juice reduce the ability of *E. coli* to adhere.
  - cranberry extracts are also available in pill form, but if these are used, care should be taken to consume at least 2 L (4 US pints) of fluid per day. Increasing urine flow is essential in flushing bacteria out of the urinary tract.
- In addition to unsweetened cranberry or blueberry juice, liquids consumed should be pure water, herbal teas, and fresh fruit and vegetable juices diluted with at least an equal amount of water.
- Avoid all simple sugars, refined carbohydrates, undiluted fruit juice.
- Identify and eliminate food allergens from the diet:
  - this is especially important in cases of chronic interstitial cystitis, a persistent form of cystitis not due to bacterial infection.
  - food allergies have been shown to produce cystitis in some patients.

Natural Medicine Instructions for Patients

repeated consumption of food allergens could be responsible for the damage to connective tissue lining the bladder wall that is seen in chronic interstitial cystitis.

Nutritional supplements
- **Citrate:** citrate, taken in the form of mineral supplements in which the mineral is bound to citrate, alkalinizes the urine, providing an inhospitable environment for bacteria:
  - treatment with potassium and/or sodium citrate is often started immediately before the results of a urine culture are available as they often provide complete relief of symptoms.
  - many of the herbs used to treat urinary tract infections, such as goldenseal and uva ursi, contain antibacterial components that work most effectively in an alkaline environment.
  - dosage can be based on the level of elemental mineral such as potassium, magnesium, or calcium.
  - dosage: 125–250 mg t.i.d.–q.i.d.
- **Vitamin C:** vitamin C is directly antibacterial, improves the integrity of the mucous lining of the urethra and bladder, and significantly enhances the activity of white blood cells, the immune cells responsible for destroying bacteria; dosage: 500 mg every 2 hours.
- **Bioflavonoids:** plant pigments largely responsible for the colors of fruits and flowers, bioflavonoids provide protection against a wide variety of oxidants and free radicals and have a wide range of health-promoting actions. In the treatment of cystitis, the most important benefits are:
  - bioflavonoids' protective effects on collagen. Collagen, the most abundant protein in the body, is the "ground substance" of all types of tissue. Bioflavonoids inhibit the destruction of collagen by enzymes secreted by white blood cells to destroy bacteria.
  - bioflavonoids prevent the release and synthesis of compounds that promote inflammation.
  - dosage: 1,000 mg q.d.
- **Vitamin A:** once known as the "anti-infective vitamin", vitamin A is critically important for the health of mucosal tissues including those lining the urinary tract:
  - when vitamin A status is inadequate, tissues become stiff and dry, leading to breaches in mucosal integrity that significantly increase susceptibility to infection.
  - dosage: 50,000 IU q.d. for up to 2 days in infants and up to 1 week in adults, or beta-carotene 200,000 IU q.d.
  - **caution:** do not use vitamin A without effective birth control if you are a sexually active woman of childbearing age: at high doses, vitamin A has been linked to birth defects.
- **Zinc:** among its many vital roles in immune system reactions, those most important in the treatment of cystitis are:
  - zinc promotes destruction of bacteria.
  - zinc acts synergistically with vitamin A.
  - zinc is required for proper white blood cell function.
  - dosage: 30 mg q.d.

Botanical medicines
Neither uva ursi nor goldenseal is recommended during pregnancy. Alkaloid components in both herbs may stimulate uterine contraction. If you are not pregnant, choose either one.
- ***Arctostaphylos uva ursi* (uva ursi):** also known as upland cranberry, uva ursi contains an antiseptic component, *arbutin*, which is converted to a related compound (*hydroquinone*) with specific urinary tract antiseptic actions:
  - hydroquinone is most effective in a more alkaline urine.
  - uva ursi is especially effective against *E. coli* and also has diuretic properties.
  - regular use of uva ursi, which appears to be even more effective than cranberry, may prevent recurrent bladder infections.
  - **do not** take more uva ursi than the dose recommended below. As little as 15 g (0.5 oz) of dried leaves has been found to produce side effects (usually nausea) in susceptible individuals. Signs of extreme toxicity include: ringing in the ears, nausea, vomiting, sense of suffocation, and shortness of breath.
  - chose one of the following forms and take the recommended dosage t.i.d. with a large glass of water:
    - dried leaves or as tea: 1.5–4.0 g (1–2 tsp)
    - freeze-dried leaves: 500–1,000 mg
    - tincture (1 : 5): 4–6 ml (1–1.5 tsp)
    - fluid extract (1 : 1): 0.5–2.0 ml (0.25–0.5 tsp)
    - powdered solid extract (10% arbutin): 250–500 mg.
- ***Hydrastis canadensis* (goldenseal):** goldenseal has a long history of use in the treatment of infection, and its significant antimicrobial properties are well documented in the scientific literature:
  - of particular importance in cystitis is goldenseal's activity against many common causes of bladder infections, including *E. coli* and Proteus species.
  - the principal antibiotic substance in goldenseal, berberine, works best in a more alkaline urine.
  - chose one of the following forms and take the recommended dosage t.i.d. with a large glass of

water:
- dried root (or as tea): 1–2 g
- freeze-dried root: 500–1,000 mg
- tincture (1 : 5): 4–6 ml (1–1.5 tsp)
- fluid extract (1 : 1): 0.5–2.0 ml (0.25–0.5 tsp)
- powdered solid extract (8% alkaloid): 250–500 mg.

Drug–herb interaction cautions

None.

Topical medicines

■ *Lactobacillus acidophilus*: although antibiotics are typically prescribed, a natural approach is preferable for most bladder infections. Antibiotic therapy actually promotes recurrent bladder infection by killing the protective bacteria in the vagina and by giving rise to antibiotic-resistant strains of *E. coli*. One of the body's most important defenses against bacterial colonization of the bladder is a shield of bacteria that line and protect the external portion of the urethra. When antibiotics are used, this normal protective shield is stripped away or replaced by less effective organisms.

■ **Friendly bacteria:** if antibiotics have been used or if a woman suffers from recurrent cystitis, friendly bacteria should be reintroduced into the vagina. Use a *Lactobacillus acidophilus* product in capsule or tablet form, and simply place one or two in the vagina before going to bed every other night for 2 weeks. Cotton underpants and a light sanitary pad can be worn to bed:
  ■ for cleansing, try a *Lactobacillus acidophilus* douche: empty 2 capsules of *L. acidophilus* into a travel-size douche bag, half fill the bag with lukewarm water, swirl around to mix the solution, finish filling the bag, and use immediately.

■ *Hydrastis canadensis* (goldenseal) tea: women who develop bladder infections after intercourse should wash their labia and urethra with a strong (2 tsp per cup) goldenseal tea, both before and after sexual relations. If this is inadequate, a dilute solution of povidone-iodine will usually prove effective.

Dermatitis herpetiformis

2

DESCRIPTION

A chronic skin inflammation characterized by clusters of small, itching blisters, dermatitis herpetiformis typically affects the skin of the elbows, knees, shoulders, arms, legs, and bottom of the spine (sacrum). Dermatitis herpetiformis is neither contagious nor cancerous but tends to occur in individuals with a family history of the disorder. Middle-aged Caucasian males are those most commonly afflicted; however, dermatitis herpetiformis may occur in individuals of any age.

FREQUENT SIGNS AND SYMPTOMS

- Small clusters of 5–20 blisters, called lesions. Blisters usually measure 2–6 mm in diameter.
- Lesions typically appear on both sides of the body in the same places.
- Lesions itch, but are usually not painful, although a burning or stinging sensation may be felt.

CAUSES

- **Gluten:** when evaluated, 75–90% of patients with dermatitis herpetiformis show signs of intestinal damage characteristic of "celiac" disease. Many studies have conclusively shown that when all sources of gluten are eliminated from the diet, both the rash and intestinal damage are healed or improve significantly in virtually all patients, but return when gluten is reintroduced.
- **Food allergy:** about 35% of patients are not completely healed simply by removing gluten from their diets:
  - this is probably due to the presence of additional food allergies that developed when the intestines, damaged by gluten, allowed other potential allergens to leak into the body.
  - in addition to wheat and rye (the primary sources of gluten), the most common offending foods are dairy products (cow's milk, cheese, yogurt), and egg whites.

RISK INCREASES WITH

- Gluten sensitivity: gluten is a protein found in wheat and other grains that cannot be digested by some persons because of their genetic makeup.
- Family history of wheat allergy and/or dermatitis herpetiformis.
- Exposure to heat and humidity.

PREVENTIVE MEASURES

- Identify and eliminate all food allergens.
- For more information see the chapter on Food allergy.

Expected outcomes

Since not only gluten but other food allergies may also be contributing to this condition, patience is necessary since complete resolution may take from several weeks to 6 months.

TREATMENT

A gluten-free diet is the primary treatment for dermatitis herpetiformis since it offers numerous advantages over dapsone, the most widely prescribed drug for this condition. While dapsone is often associated with severe side effects, on a gluten-free diet:

- well over 65% of patients experience complete and permanent cure, and the rest are substantially improved
- the damage to the intestinal wall is healed
- harsh medications can be reduced or eliminated
- most patients feel substantially healthier.

Diet

- **Eliminate gluten from the diet:** wheat and rye contain the highest amounts of gluten, but it is also found in other grains including oats, millet and rice.
- **Identify and remove other allergenic foods:** in addition to wheat and rye, the most common offending foods are dairy products (cow's milk, cheese, yogurt), and egg whites.

■ **After eliminating gluten and allergens**, consume a nutrient-dense diet rich in whole, unprocessed, preferably organic foods, especially plant foods (vegetables, fruits, beans, seeds and nuts), and cold-water fish (for more detailed information, see Appendix 1).

Nutritional supplements
■ **Para-aminobenzoic acid (PABA):** helpful in controlling symptoms but not in repairing damage to the intestinal wall, PABA is best used in unresponsive or particularly severe cases for symptom relief; dosage: 5 g q.d. until remission or for a maximum of 3 months.

Topical medicine
■ Soak in cool water or use cool-water compresses to relieve itching.

Diabetes mellitus

DESCRIPTION

Diabetes is a chronic disorder of carbohydrate, fat, and protein metabolism characterized by elevations in fasting blood sugar (glucose) levels. Diabetes occurs if the pancreas does not secrete enough insulin or if the cells of the body become resistant to insulin, the hormone responsible for transporting sugar from the bloodstream into cells. In either case, diabetes results in high levels of sugar in the bloodstream and inadequate levels of sugar entering cells. This situation leads to serious complications including a greatly increased risk of heart disease, stroke, kidney disease, loss of vision, senile cataracts, gangrene in the legs and feet, and impotence in men.

When the pancreas does not secrete enough insulin, the disease is categorized as type I or insulin-dependent diabetes mellitus (IDDM). IDDM is associated with complete destruction of the insulin manufacturing *beta-cells* of the pancreas. IDDM patients require lifelong insulin to control their blood sugar levels. About 10% of all diabetics are type I, which has also been called juvenile-onset diabetes since onset typically occurs in children and adolescents.

When the cells of the body become insulin resistant, the disease is categorized as type II or non-insulin-dependent diabetes mellitus (NIDDM). Although NIDDM used to be called adult-onset diabetes, onset of this form is now occurring in younger individuals. Of all diabetics, 90% are type II, and 90% of type II diabetics are obese, which underscores the fact that NIDDM is a disease caused by diet and lifestyle. NIDDM can usually be controlled by diet alone. In most cases, achieving ideal body weight results in restoration of normal blood sugar levels.

Besides IDDM and NIDDM, other conditions associated with abnormal blood sugar control include the following:

- **Secondary diabetes:** a form that is secondary to certain conditions and syndromes, such as pancreatic disease, hormone disturbances, drugs, and malnutrition.
- **Gestational diabetes:** glucose intolerance that occurs during pregnancy.
- **Impaired glucose tolerance:** a condition in which glucose tolerance testing reveals blood glucose levels that are not clearly abnormal, but are higher than normal.
- **Reactive hypoglycemia:** many practitioners consider reactive hypoglycemia to be a prediabetic condition. Overconsumption of refined carbohydrates sets the stage for reactive hypoglycemia. Refined carbohydrates are quickly absorbed into the bloodstream, causing a rapid rise in blood sugar. The body reacts by greatly increasing insulin secretion, which rapidly drives blood sugar down (hypo = low, glycemia = blood sugar). In response to the rapid fall in blood sugar, the adrenal glands secrete adrenaline, causing another rapid increase in blood sugar. Eventually, the adrenal glands become exhausted and can no longer respond. If blood sugar mechanisms continue to be stressed, the body will become insensitive to insulin and/or the pancreas will become exhausted. In either case, reactive hypoglycemia will evolve into diabetes.

Diabetes is now the seventh leading cause of death in the United States, and the number of Americans with diabetes is increasing. Rates of type II diabetes rose a striking 6% among adults in 1999. The Centers for Disease Control has linked climbing NIDDM rates with a similar increase in obesity, which rose 5.6% in 1999. More than 16 million Americans now have NIDDM, and about one-third don't even know they have it.

At the current rate increase of 6% per year, the number of persons with diabetes will double every 15 years. Population studies have linked type II diabetes to diet and lifestyle. It is uncommon in places where people consume their native, whole foods diets, but when indigenous peoples switch to the highly processed, Standard American Diet, their rate of diabetes increases, eventually reaching the same levels as seen in the United States.

FREQUENT SIGNS AND SYMPTOMS

The classic symptoms of diabetes are:
- frequent urination
- excessive thirst
- excessive appetite.

Because these symptoms are not very serious, many people do not seek medical care. Of the more than 16 million Americans with diabetes, about one-third of those afflicted are unaware that they have the disease.

CAUSES

Type I, juvenile-onset diabetes (IDDM)

- **Hereditary predisposition:** although the exact cause is unknown, current theory suggests a genetic predisposition to injury in the insulin-producing beta-cells coupled with some defect in the ability of the pancreas to regenerate new beta-cells:
  - in IDDM, the body's immune system apparently begins to attack the pancreas. Antibodies for beta-cells are present in 75% of all cases of IDDM, compared to 0.5–2% of non-diabetics.
  - probable causes of initial injury include free radicals, viral infection, chemicals, and food allergy. Injury triggers an autoimmune reaction in which antibodies to beta-cells are produced, leading to their destruction.
- **Smoked or cured meats:** smoked and cured meats contain N-nitroso-compounds similar in structure and function to a compound (streptozotocin) that is used to induce diabetes in studies with animals.
- **Viruses:** viral diseases such as mumps, hepatitis, infectious mononucleosis, congenital rubella, and Cocksackie virus infections are capable of infecting pancreatic beta-cells and inducing antibody attack.
- **Exposure to cow's milk protein in infancy:** exposure to a protein in cow's milk (bovine albumin peptide) in infancy may trigger the autoimmune process. Patients with type I diabetes are more likely to have been breast-fed for under 3 months and to have been exposed to cow's milk or solid foods before the age of 4 months. If the mother consumes cow's milk, cow's milk protein can be found in her breast milk, so in cases of family history of diabetes, it is recommended that the mother avoid cow's milk while breast-feeding.

Type II, adult-onset diabetes (NIDDM)

- **Genetic factors:** genetic factors increase susceptibility to NIDDM, but diet and lifestyle factors are required to trigger it.
- **Standard American Diet:** blood sugar problems are strongly associated with the so-called "Western diet" which is rich in refined sugar, fat, and animal products, and low in dietary fiber. It is widely accepted that refined carbohydrates are among the most important contributing factors to diabetes and reactive hypoglycemia (as well as obesity).
- **Obesity:** obesity is associated with insulin insensitivity. Weight loss, especially fat loss, improves all aspects of diabetes and may result in cure.
- **Dietary fat:** the percentage of calories from fat, especially saturated fat, in the diet is associated with NIDDM. A high-fat, low carbohydrate diet (ironically, the diet used in the past for dietary management of diabetes) increases the risk of developing NIDDM.
- **Chromium deficiency:** the trace mineral, chromium, is a critical component in "glucose-tolerance factor", a cofactor in all insulin-regulating activities. Chromium deficiency is widespread in the US. Supplementation with chromium has been shown to significantly improve insulin action, decrease fasting glucose, cholesterol and triglyceride levels; and increase the high density lipoprotein (good) cholesterol level by increasing insulin sensitivity in normal, elderly, and NIDDM patients.

RISK INCREASES WITH

Type I, IDDM

- Family history of diabetes mellitus
- Exposure to cow's milk protein in infancy

Type II, NIDDM

- Standard American Diet
- Obesity
- Chromium deficiency
- A diet high in fat and/or refined carbohydrates
- Reactive hypoglycemia
- Pregnancy
- Use of certain drugs including oral contraceptives, thiazide diuretics, cortisone or phenytoin.
- Prenatal factors: overconsumption of calories during pregnancy may increase the risk for diabetes in the unborn fetus later in life. Studies done in Berlin have shown that in adults born during the "hypocaloric war and postwar period (1941–48)", incidence of diabetes is 50% less than in those born before and after this period.

PREVENTIVE MEASURES

Type I, IDDM

- Avoid exposure to cow's milk protein in infants younger than 1 year.
- If IDDM is present in the family, avoid exposure to cow's milk for 1.5–2 years.
- Mothers should also avoid cow's milk while breast-feeding.

Type II, NIDDM

- Achieve ideal body composition by losing excess fat weight. This can be accomplished by following the dietary recommendations given below along with strength-training exercise that builds muscle mass.

■ A high-potency multiple vitamin and mineral supplement providing all of the known vitamins and minerals, including 200–400 μg of chromium. A good multiple should also include 400 μg of folic acid, 400 μg of vitamin B_{12}, and 50–100 mg of vitamin B_6. (Folic acid supplementation should always be accompanied by vitamin B_{12} supplementation to prevent folic acid from masking a vitamin B_{12} deficiency.)

■ A health-promoting diet rich in whole, unprocessed, preferably organic foods, especially plant foods (fruits, vegetables, whole grains, beans, nuts [especially walnuts] and seeds), and cold-water fish (for more detailed information, see Appendix 1).

Expected outcomes

Currently, patients with IDDM require insulin throughout life, although hope exists that the technology to restore pancreatic beta-cells will eventually be developed. NIDDM can frequently be controlled with diet and weight (fat) loss alone.

TREATMENT

It is important to recognize that as the suggestions described in this handout are employed, drug dosages will need to be lowered.

Diet

Dietary modification is essential for the successful treatment of both IDDM and NIDDM. Frequency of diabetes is highly correlated with the fiber-depleted, highly refined carbohydrate diet of "civilization". Epidemiological evidence indicting the Western diet and lifestyle as the ultimate cause of diabetes is overwhelming.

The dietary goal is to eat a balanced whole foods diet, while reducing all factors that increase insulin levels.

■ While basic guidelines follow below, until you are aware of which foods and food combinations excessively raise your insulin levels, the best approach is to monitor your blood sugar at home with a blood sugar monitoring device.

■ Check your insulin levels seven times each day: before you eat, an hour after you eat, and at bedtime. Write down what you eat, your blood sugar levels, activities and any observations. You will soon have a personal guide that will help you tailor the generic whole foods diet to best meet your individual needs.

A balanced whole foods diet that will optimize insulin control in both IDDM and NIDDM includes the following:

■ **Protein:** average minimum requirement for women is 60–70 g q.d.; men need 70–80 g q.d. Spread protein intake throughout the day, consuming some protein at every meal:

■ whenever possible buy hormone-free, antibiotic-free, range-fed meat and poultry, and eggs from chickens fed a diet rich in omega-3 essential fatty acids (DHA).

■ at least three times each week, choose deep-sea, cold-water fish such as salmon, mackerel, herring, and halibut. In addition to protein, these fish are excellent sources of omega-3 fats, which offer significant protection against hardening of the arteries, enhance insulin sensitivity in NIDDM, and insulin secretion in IDDM.

■ **Fats:** *real* fats are necessary for health and do not raise insulin levels. Do not be afraid to eat real fats in moderation, including butter, and cold or pure pressed oils (heat processes used to extract oils damage the fats, making them harmful), especially flaxseed oil (high in essential fatty acids) and extra virgin olive oil (a very stable monounsaturated fat that is the best choice for cooking):

■ do not eat damaged fats. Fats used in deep-frying, oils derived by heat processing, and hydrogenated or *trans* fats are damaging to your health. Hydrogenated fats are mutated into abnormal chemical structures the body cannot use for normal metabolic functions. Fats subjected to the high temperatures of deep-frying and oils derived via processing at high heat are both mutated and oxidized, which turns them into free radicals.

■ all fats should be refrigerated to prevent oxidation.

■ when purchasing oils, look for cold-pressed oils sold in opaque containers that lessen oxidation caused by exposure to light.

■ saturated (butter) and monounsaturated (olive oil) fats are more resistant to damage from heat, so are best used for cooking.

■ all proteins (meat, poultry, eggs, fish) should be cooked at low, even temperatures to avoid damaging the fats they contain.

■ **Non-starchy vegetables:** non-starchy vegetables contain no more than 5 g of carbohydrate per 1/2 cup serving:

■ eat as many non-starchy vegetables as desired. Try to consume at least 6–8 servings of non-starchy vegetables daily.

■ commonly eaten non-starchy vegetables include: asparagus, bell peppers, broccoli, Brussels sprouts, cabbage, carrots (raw), cauliflower, celery, cucumber, eggplant, green beans, greens (beet greens, chicory greens, dandelion greens, mustard greens, etc.), jicama (raw), jalapeno peppers, kale, lettuce, mushrooms, onions, parsley, radishes, snap beans, snow peas, spinach, spaghetti squash, summer squash (crookneck, scallop, zucchini), Swiss chard, tomatoes, watercress.

■ non-starchy vegetables (along with fruits, discussed next) provide vitamins, minerals and fiber. The vitamins and minerals are used as coenzymes in virtually all the chemical reactions involved in metabolism. Fiber slows down the digestive process, lowering the glycemic index of the entire meal, and is essential for a healthy digestive system.

■ the glycemic index of a food is a measure of how fast insulin rises after the food has been eaten. The faster a food is digested, the faster its sugars arrive, and the higher the food's glycemic index:

● in general, proteins, fats, and non-starchy vegetables have a low glycemic index; complex carbohydrates have a higher glycemic index; and refined carbohydrates have a high glycemic index.

■ a balanced meal composed of protein, fat, non-starchy vegetables and complex carbohydrates will not only provide each of the types of nutrients a body needs to function properly, but the glycemic index of the meal will also be balanced, so insulin levels will not rise excessively.

■ **Carbohydrates:** carbohydrates should never be eaten alone and should be thought of as fuel. If sedentary and/or overweight, eat fewer carbohydrates; if active, eat more carbohydrates:

■ if suffering from NIDDM, begin construction of a balanced whole foods diet by eating each day:

● three balanced meals containing protein, fat, non-starchy vegetables, and a carbohydrate selection containing 15 g of carbohydrate

● plus two balanced snacks containing protein, fat, non-starchy vegetables, and a carbohydrate selection containing 7.5 g of carbohydrate.

■ as insulin levels normalize, choose between 15 g (sedentary or needing to lose excess fat) and 80 g (very active) of carbohydrates per meal, depending upon immediate energy needs.

■ always eat carbohydrates with protein and fat. If you are eating only 15 g of carbohydrate per meal, you must eat three small meals and two snacks per day. If you are eating more than 15 g of carbohydrate per meal, snacks are optional.

■ if already depressed and becoming more depressed, add 7.5 g more carbohydrate to each meal and snack. This small additional carbohydrate will slightly raise insulin levels. Insulin assists in the transfer of tryptophan from the circulatory system

into the brain, where it is used to make *serotonin*, a neurotransmitter necessary for a healthy mood or emotional state.

■ as suggested above, monitor the effects of the meals you consume on your blood sugar levels to develop an understanding of how much and which carbohydrates you can tolerate.

■ do not eat refined carbohydrates, examples of which include:

● products made from refined grains such as wheat flour or white rice, e.g., bagels, cold cereal, noodles, pancakes, pasta, pizza dough, pie crust, spaghetti, waffles, white bread, English muffins, hamburger buns, white rice.

● sugar: check labels for sucrose, fructose, maltose, dextrose, polydextrose, corn syrup, maple syrup, molasses, sorbitol, maltodextrin.

● desserts: flavored yogurts, fruit leathers, granola and other snack bars, as well as cakes, candy, cookies, ice cream, etc.

● processed snack foods including corn chips, pork skins, potato chips, pretzels, tortilla chips, trail mix.

● condiments containing sugar and chemicals including barbecue sauces, fish sauces, Hoisin sauce, ketchup, relishes, sweet pickles, Worcestershire.

■ best carbohydrate choices include:

● starchy vegetables: e.g., acorn and butternut squash, artichokes, beets, cooked carrots, corn, green peas, lima beans, potatoes, rutabagas, yams, turnips.

● legumes: e.g., black beans, garbanzo beans, kidney beans, lentils, navy beans, pinto beans, soybeans (see below), split peas.

● fruits: choose fresh or frozen fruits without added sugar. Examples of fruit servings include: 1 small apple, 1/2 medium banana, 3/4 cup blueberries, 1 cup (with pits) cherries, 1/2 large grapefruit, 15 grapes, 1 large kiwi, 1/2 medium cantaloupe, 1 1/2 cups diced honeydew, 1 medium orange, 1 medium peach, 1/2 large pear, 3/4 cup pineapple, 2 tbsp raisins, 1 cup raspberries, 1 1/2 cups strawberries, 2 small tangerines, 1 medium tomato, 1 1/4 cups diced watermelon.

● whole grains and products made from whole grain flours: whole grains are preferable to products made from their flours as whole grains are more slowly digested. Examples of whole grains include: brown rice, wild rice, buckwheat kasha, bulgur (tabouli), corn grits, couscous farina, millet, oats, polenta, popcorn, quinoa, rye, wheat berries. A 1/3 cup serving of most grains contains approximately 15 g of carbohydrate. Examples of products made from whole grains include: whole wheat bread or crackers, sprouted wheat bread (Essene bread), whole rye bread, corn tortilla, whole grain crackers). A slice of bread, a corn tortilla, $1/2$ English muffin, 2 brown rice cakes, 2 rye wafers, or 4 small whole wheat crackers contains approximately 15 g of carbohydrate.

- ■ **Protein foods which contain carbohydrates:**
  - ▪ nuts, nut butters and seeds are good sources of healthful fats and protein. An average serving of most nuts (25 g [1 oz] of nuts or 2 tbsp of nut butter) and seeds contains approximately 6 g of carbohydrate.
  - ▪ soy products are excellent sources of high quality protein. A typical serving of soy products (1 cup soy milk, 1 cup tofu, 38 g [1.5 oz] soy protein) contains approximately 15 g of carbohydrate.
  - ▪ organic whole milk yogurt (whole milk is preferable because the fat content lowers the glycemic index of this healthful food) contains approximately 15 g of carbohydrate.

For more detailed information on controlling insulin levels through a whole foods diet, we recommend *The Schwarzbein Principle* by Diana Schwarzbein MD, and Nancy Deville (Health Communications, Inc.; Deerfield Beach, Florida, 1999).

Nutritional supplements

IDDM

- ■ **Insulin:** since insulin is not absorbed orally, it must be injected. Insulin preparations come in concentrations of 10 units/ml (U-100) and 500 units/ml (U-500), but can differ in their source (beef, pork, or human synthetic insulin), duration of action (rapid, intermediate, or long-acting) and solubility (crystalline versus soluble):
  - ▪ human synthetic insulin is gaining wider acceptance as the preferred source, and *intensified insulin therapy* as the preferred regimen for insulin administration, since it significantly reduces the diabetes-induced development of other chronic diseases (e.g., heart and kidney disease).
  - ▪ intensified insulin therapy requires either multiple daily injections (3–5 q.d.) or the use of an "insulin pump", which, by administering a continuous supply of insulin, most closely mimics natural insulin production.

IDDM and NIDDM

Individuals with either IDDM or NIDDM have a greatly increased need for many nutrients. Supplying additional key nutrients has been shown to improve blood sugar control and to help prevent or ameliorate many of the major complications of diabetes.

- ■ **Chromium:**
  - ▪ chromium is the mineral component in glucose tolerance factor, a molecule that helps the cells respond appropriately to insulin.
  - ▪ clinical studies of diabetics have shown that chromium supplementation can decrease fasting blood glucose levels, improve glucose tolerance, lower insulin levels, and decrease total cholesterol and triglyceride levels, while increasing high density lipoprotein (HDL) (good) cholesterol levels.
  - ▪ marginal chromium deficiency is common in the United States.
  - ▪ chromium levels are depleted by consuming refined sugars, white flour products, and lack of exercise.
  - ▪ no recommended dietary intake (RDI) has been established for chromium, but at least 200 μg each day appears necessary for optimal sugar regulation.
  - ▪ dosages used in studies range from 100 μg of chromium picolinate b.i.d. to 500 mg b.i.d.
- ■ **Vitamin C:**
  - ▪ vitamin C is essential for wound repair, healthy gums, the prevention of excessive bruising, immune function, the manufacture of certain nerve-transmitting substances and hormones, and the absorption and utilization of other nutritional factors.
  - ▪ transport of vitamin C into cells is facilitated by insulin, so many diabetics do not have enough vitamin C inside their cells despite adequate dietary consumption.
  - ▪ in diabetics, inadequate vitamin C leads to an increased tendency to bleed (increased capillary permeability), poor wound healing, vascular disease, elevations in cholesterol levels, and a depressed immune system.
  - ▪ at high doses (2,000 mg q.d.) vitamin C has been shown to reduce *sorbitol* accumulation in the red blood cells of diabetics and to inhibit the binding of sugar to protein (glycosylation), both of which are linked to many complications of diabetes, especially eye and nerve diseases:
    - ● sorbitol is a by-product of glucose metabolism formed within the cell by the enzyme aldose reductase. In non-diabetics, sorbitol is broken down into fructose and excreted, but, in diabetics, sorbitol accumulates and causes numerous problems.
  - ▪ vitamin C-rich foods are high in flavonoids and carotenes, which enhance the effects of vitamin C, plus further promote insulin secretion and inhibit

sorbitol accumulation. The best dietary sources of vitamin C include broccoli, peppers, potatoes, Brussels sprouts, and citrus fruits.

- dosage: vitamin C: 500–1,000 mg t.i.d. Mixed flavonoids: 1,000–2,000 mg q.d.

■ **Niacin and niacinamide:**

- like chromium, niacin is an essential component of glucose tolerance factor. In addition, niacinamide has been shown to play a role as an antioxidant, and to inhibit damage to the beta-cells by the immune system.
- clinical trials in experimental animals have shown that niacin in the form of niacinamide can help restore beta-cells or at least slow their destruction if given soon enough at the onset of diabetes, thus preventing type I diabetes from developing.
- some newly diagnosed type I diabetics have experienced complete reversal of their diabetes with niacinamide supplementation.
- niacin has also been effectively used to lower cholesterol levels.
- daily dose of niacinamide is based on body weight: 25 mg/kg. Studies in children used 100–200 mg q.d.
- niacin may cause acute skin flushing, but sustained or timed-release products developed to avoid this problem are more toxic to the liver.
- a better and safer form of niacin is *inositol hexaniacinate*. This form has long been used in Europe to lower cholesterol levels in dosages ranging from 600–1,800 mg t.i.d. with no patients reporting any adverse reactions.
- dosage: 600–1,000 mg t.i.d. of inositol hexaniacinate is usually sufficient to produce an 18% reduction in total cholesterol, a 26% reduction in triglycerides, and a 30% increase in HDL (good) cholesterol levels.

■ **Biotin:**

- biotin supplementation has been shown to enhance insulin sensitivity and increase the activity of *glucokinase*, the enzyme responsible for the first step in the utilization of glucose by the liver.
- glucokinase concentrations are typically very low in diabetics.
- biotin supplementation in IDDM at dosages greater than 1 mg q.d. may require adjustments in insulin dosages.
- dosage: 4 mg q.d. or discuss with your physician.

■ **Vitamin B$_6$:**

- offers significant protection against the development of diabetic nerve disease, and inhibits the binding of sugar to proteins (*glycosylation*), a major contributing factor in the development of diabetic complications.

- individuals with long-standing diabetes or who are developing signs of peripheral nerve abnormalities should be supplemented with B$_6$.
- B$_6$ supplementation should also be used as a safe treatment for gestational diabetes. In one study of women with gestational diabetes, taking 100 mg of B$_6$ for 2 weeks resulted in complete cure in 12 of the 14 women.
- dosage: 100 mg q.d.

■ **Vitamin B$_{12}$:**

- deficiency of B$_{12}$ is characterized by numbness of the feet, pins-and-needles sensations, or a burning feeling – symptoms typical of diabetic neuropathy.
- abnormal B$_{12}$ metabolism is frequently seen in diabetics.
- a deficit of B$_{12}$ in the nerve cells usually precedes anemia, often by several years, so blood levels of B$_{12}$ are a more reliable indicator of B$_{12}$ status.
- dosage: oral supplementation of methylcobalamin (the active form of B$_{12}$) with 1,000–3,000 µg q.d. is usually sufficient, but IM injections may be necessary in some cases.

■ **Vitamin E:**

- vitamin E protects cells membranes from oxidants. In diabetics, this translates into improving insulin's ability to cross cell membranes in glucose transport.
- in persons without diabetes, low levels of vitamin E are associated with a 3.9 times greater risk of developing diabetes.
- in patients with NIDDM, high doses of vitamin E (800–1,200 IU q.d.) have been shown significantly to improve glucose tolerance and insulin sensitivity.
- dosage: 800–1,200 IU q.d. of mixed tocopherols.

■ **Magnesium:**

- magnesium is involved in several areas of glucose metabolism and is commonly deficient in diabetics, with lowest levels in diabetics with severe retinopathy (a degenerative eye disease).
- recommended daily allowance for magnesium is 350 mg q.d. for men and 300 mg q.d. for women. Diabetics may need twice that amount.
- magnesium is abundant in whole foods but is largely processed out of refined foods. The best dietary sources of magnesium include tofu, legumes, seeds, nuts, whole grains, and green leafy vegetables.
- in addition to eating a magnesium-rich diet, supplementation with 300–500 mg of magnesium as magnesium aspartate or citrate is recommended.
- without adequate B$_6$, magnesium will not get inside the cell, so diabetics should also take at least 50 mg of B$_6$ q.d.

- dosage: magnesium citrate or aspartate, 250 mg b.i.d.–t.i.d. plus B_6, 50 mg q.d.
- **Manganese:**
  - manganese is a cofactor in many enzyme systems involved in blood sugar control, energy metabolism, and thyroid hormone function.
  - diabetics have been shown to have only one-half the manganese of normal individuals.
  - dosage: 30 mg q.d.
- **Zinc:**
  - zinc is involved in virtually all aspects of insulin metabolism: synthesis, secretion, and utilization, and also has a protective effect against beta-cell destruction.
  - zinc has been shown to improve insulin levels and wound healing in type I and type II diabetics.
  - dosage: 30 mg zinc picolinate (a well-absorbed form) q.d.
- **Essential fatty acids (EFAs):**
  - the omega-6 EFA gamma-linolenic acid (GLA) has been shown to offer significant protection against development of diabetic neuropathy:
    - diabetes is associated with a problem in EFA metabolism, specifically, the production of GLA from its precursor linoleic acid. Providing GLA in the form of borage, evening primrose, or black-currant oils is therefore recommended.
  - omega-3 EFAs (EPA and DHA), which are found in cold-water fish and flaxseed oil, are well known to protect against hardening of the arteries and enhance insulin secretion in NIDDM.
  - increase consumption of cold-water fish (e.g., salmon, herring, mackerel, halibut) rather than consuming fish oil supplements:
    - fish oil supplements may contain high levels of oxidized fats, which deplete antioxidants when ingested.
    - in one study (1,800 mg q.d. of fish oil supplements for 8 weeks), blood sugar control deteriorated and cholesterol levels increased significantly.
    - in diabetics fish consumption has been shown to produce improved glucose tolerance and blood viscosity with no adverse effects.
  - dosage: consume at least two 90 g (3.5 oz) servings of cold-water fish per week and supplement the diet with 480 mg of GLA and 1 tbsp of flaxseed oil q.d.
- **Carnitine:**
  - carnitine is involved in the breakdown of fats for energy.
  - carnitine supplementation has resulted in significantly decreased total serum lipid (blood fats) and

increased HDL (good) cholesterol levels in diabetic patients.
- dosage: 500 mg q.d.

Botanical medicines

- ***Gymnema sylvestre* extract:** *Gymnema* extract has been shown to reduce insulin requirements and fasting blood sugar levels, and to improve blood sugar control in both type I and type II diabetes. In type I diabetics, gymnema appears to enhance the action of insulin. In a study of type II diabetics given gymnema along with their oral hypoglycemic drugs, 21 of 22 patients were able to reduce their drug dosage considerably, while five were eventually able to discontinue their medication and maintain blood sugar control with gymnema alone. No side effects have been reported from *Gymnema* extract; dosage: 200 mg b.i.d.

If diabetic retinopathy is present:

- **Bilberry (or grape seed extract):** bilberry flavonoids provide numerous benefits in diabetics. Specifically, they increase intracellular vitamin C levels, decrease the leakiness and breakage of small blood vessels (especially in the eye), prevent easy bruising, and act as potent antioxidants; dosage: 80–160 mg t.i.d.

If diabetic neuropathy is present:

- ***Ginkgo biloba* extract:** ginkgo improves blood flow to the arms, legs, fingers and toes, and has been of significant benefit in peripheral vascular disease due to diabetes; dosage: *Ginkgo biloba* extract (24% ginkgo flavonglycosides) 40–80 mg t.i.d.

Drug–herb interaction cautions

- ***Ginkgo biloba*:**
  - plus *aspirin*: may induce spontaneous bleeding when combined with chronic use of aspirin. Increased bleeding potential reported after *Ginkgo biloba* usage in a chronic user (2 years) of aspirin.

Physical medicine

Exercise improves many parameters and is recommended in both IDDM and NIDDM. Benefits include: enhanced insulin sensitivity, diminished need for supplemental insulin, improved glucose tolerance, reduced total serum cholesterol and triglycerides with increased HDL (good) cholesterol levels, and improved weight loss in obese diabetics.

Many of the beneficial effects of exercise may be the result of improved chromium metabolism. Exercise increases tissue levels of chromium in rat studies, and increases the number of insulin receptors in IDDM patients.

Epididymitis

DESCRIPTION

Epididymitis is a painful inflammation of the *epididymis*, a C-shaped structure attached to the upper part of each testicle. In the average adult male, the epididymis is 5–7 cm long, 1 cm in diameter, and hugs the back border of the testicle. Sperm mature, developing their ability to fertilize, within the epididymis, which continues on as the vas deferens (the secretory duct of the testicle), joining the spermatic cord and eventually the ejaculatory duct.

FREQUENT SIGNS AND SYMPTOMS

- Rapid onset of pain, heat, and swelling at the back of one testicle (sometimes both)
- Gradual onset of swelling and pain (sometimes)
- Enlarged, hardened, painful testicle
- Fever or a slight elevation in temperature
- Severe scrotal pain and swelling (testicles can double in size)
- Tenderness of the second testicle (sometimes)
- Inflammation of the urethra, causing burning on urination
- Pus in the urine

CAUSES

- **Bacterial infection:** epididymitis is usually a complication of a bacterial infection elsewhere in the body, most often in the genitourinary tract, e.g., an infection in the urethra, prostate, bladder or kidneys.
- **Sexually transmitted diseases (STDs):** epididymitis may be caused by sexually transmitted organisms including *Chlamydia trachomatis*, and, during anal intercourse, *Escherichia coli.*
- **Mumps:** inflammation of the epididymis and testicle occurs in 20% of postpubertal men with mumps.
- **Trauma (rare):** the scrotum will typically "roll away" from injuries. If trauma is a cause, the scrotum will be discolored, while if infection is the cause, it will not.
- **Allergy:** generally seen in children, epididymitis resulting from allergy produces swelling in both testicles. Pain is due to an inflammation of the skin,

so there is no deep tenderness. Redness may extend beyond the scrotum to the perineum or inner thigh.
- **Strenuous exercise or straining with a full bladder:** the stress may cause urine to flow back through the ejaculatory ducts into the vas deferens, which is the continuation of the epididymis.

RISK INCREASES WITH

- Recent illness, especially of the genitourinary tract, e.g., chronic prostatitis, urethritis, or urinary tract infection
- Mumps
- Urethral scar tissue due to the insertion of medical instruments into the urethra
- Indwelling urethral catheter
- Numerous sexual partners
- Anal intercourse

PREVENTIVE MEASURES

- Use rubber condoms during intercourse.
- Don't engage in sexual activity with persons who have venereal disease.
- Don't engage in anal intercourse.
- Avoid urethral catheters if possible.

Expected outcomes

Symptoms should begin to decrease within 48 hours. Pain and swelling can be relieved within 2 weeks, but it typically takes 4 weeks, and as long as 3 months for the scrotum to return to normal size. All treatments (except for ice and bedrest) need to be continued for at least 1 week after the scrotum has returned to normal size.

TREATMENT

General considerations

- If an STD is the cause, men and their partners must be effectively treated as soon as possible. If a positive response to therapy does not occur immediately, antibiotics should be used, and repeat cultures taken to ensure that the offending organism has been eradicated.

■ Wait at least 1 month after all symptoms disappear before resuming normal sexual relations.

■ Always empty your bladder prior to strenuous activity. Interrupt strenuous activity to void if there is a sensation of a full bladder.

■ All treatments outlined below should be continued for at least 1 week after the scrotum has returned to normal size.

Diet

■ Drink large amounts of fluids (preferably diluted vegetable juices, soups, and herb teas).

■ Limit consumption of simple sugars (primarily found in refined carbohydrates but also including fruit sugars) to less than 50 g q.d.

■ Don't drink alcohol, tea, coffee or carbonated beverages. These irritate the urinary tract.

■ To prevent constipation, eat natural laxative foods such as wholegrain cereals, nuts and flaxseed meal.

Nutritional supplements

■ **Vitamin C:** directly antiviral and antibacterial, vitamin C's main claim to fame is its many different immune-enhancing effects including white blood cell response and function, increasing levels of interferon (a special chemical factor that fights viral infection and cancer), and increasing secretion of hormones from the thymus gland (the major gland of the immune system); dosage: 1,000 mg q.i.d.

■ **Vitamin A:** known as the "anti-infective vitamin", vitamin A plays a variety of essential roles in immune function including maintaining the surfaces of the skin, respiratory tract, and gastrointestinal tract and their secretions – all of which constitute a barrier that is the body's first line of defense against microorganisms – and stimulating and/or enhancing numerous immune processes including white blood cell function and antibody response; dosage: 5,000 IU q.d.

■ **Beta-carotene:** called "pro-vitamin A" since it can be converted into vitamin A, beta-carotene is a more powerful antioxidant than vitamin A and exerts additional immune-stimulating effects, including enhancing thymus function. Specifically, beta-carotene has been shown to increase the production of helper/inducer T cells by 30% after 7 days and all T cells after 14 days; dosage: 200,000 IU q.d.

■ **Bromelain:** a variety of inflammatory agents are inhibited by the action of bromelain, a group of sulfur-containing proteolytic (protein-digesting) enzymes

obtained from the pineapple plant. The rapid decrease in inflammation results in a faster recovery; dosage: (1,200–1,800 MCU) 250–500 mg q.i.d. between meals.

Botanical medicines

■ ***Echinacea* species:** the two most widely used species are *Echinacea angustifolia* and *Echinacea purpurea*, both of which exert numerous immune-enhancing effects:

■ one of *Echinacea*'s most important immune-stimulating components is *inulin*, a large polysaccharide that activates the *alternative complement pathway*, part of the immune system's first line of defense, and increases the production of immune chemicals that activate macrophages. The result is increased activity of many key immune parameters: production of T cells, macrophage phagocytosis, antibody binding, natural killer cell activity, and levels of circulating neutrophils.

■ in addition to immune support, echinacea is directly antiviral and helps prevent bacterial infection by inhibiting the bacterial enzyme hyaluronidase. Bacteria secrete hyaluronidase to break through the body's first line of defense – its protective membranes such as the skin or mucous membranes – so the bacteria can enter the body.

■ chose one of the following forms and take the recommended dosage t.i.d.:

● dried root or as tea: 0.5–1 g

● freeze-dried plant: 325–650 mg

● juice of aerial portion of *E. purpurea* stabilized in 22% ethanol: 2–3 ml

● tincture (1 : 5): 2–4 ml

● fluid extract (1 : 1): 2–4 ml

● solid (dry powdered) extract (6.5 : 1 or 3.5% echinacoside): 150–300 mg.

■ ***Hydrastis canadensis* (goldenseal):** goldenseal is a remarkably safe and effective natural antibiotic. Its most active alkaloid constituent, *berberine sulfate*, exhibits a broad range of antibiotic action against a wide variety of bacteria (including *Chlamydia* and *E. coli*), protozoa and fungi. Its action against some of these pathogens is actually stronger than that of commonly used antibiotics, but unlike antibiotic drugs, goldenseal does not destroy the protective bacteria (lactobacilli) in the intestine:

■ berberine is a more effective antimicrobial agent in an alkaline environment. Alkalinity can be increased by consuming fewer animal products and more plant foods, especially fruits. Although most fruits are acidic, digestion uses up their acid components leaving behind an alkaline residue.

Natural Medicine Instructions for Patients

■ choose one of the following forms and take the recommended dosage t.i.d.:
- dosage should be based on berberine content; standardized extracts are recommended
- dried root or as infusion (tea): 2–4 g
- tincture (1 : 5): 6–12 ml (1.5–3 tsp)
- fluid extract (1 : 1): 2–4 ml (0.5–1 tsp)
- solid (dry powdered) extract (4 : 1 or 8–12% alkaloid content): 250–500 mg.

Drug–herb interaction cautions
None.

Topical medicine
■ Rest in bed and apply an ice bag to the inflamed parts until fever, pain and swelling improve, usually within 48 hours.

■ Roll a soft bath towel and place it between the legs under the inflamed area to support the weight of the scrotum and testicles.

■ Wear an athletic supporter or two pairs of athletic briefs when you resume normal activity, and restrict activity until there is no pain.

Epilepsy

DESCRIPTION

A disorder caused by episodic abnormalities in the electrical activity of the brain, epilepsy is characterized by recurrent sudden seizures. Epilepsy can affect both sexes and all ages, although seizures usually begin between the ages of 2 and 14 years. Epilepsy is not contagious. About 10 : 1,000 persons experience chronic, recurrent epilepsy, and 2–5% of the population will have a seizure unrelated to fever at some point in their lives. An additional 2–5% of children will experience fever-related seizures during the first several years of life. About 10% of these children, especially those in whom the fever-induced seizure is prolonged, will develop epilepsy later in life.

FREQUENT SIGNS AND SYMPTOMS

Epileptic seizures, also called fits or convulsions, appear in several forms, each with its own characteristics.

- **Petit mal (or absence):** usually affects children. The child stops activity and stares around blankly unaware of his or her surroundings for a minute or two.
- **Grand mal:** affects all ages. The person loses consciousness, stiffens, then twitches and jerks uncontrollably, and may lose bladder control. Grand mal seizures last several minutes and are typically followed by confusion and deep sleep. Warning signals may occur prior to the seizure. The person may feel tense, experience visual disturbances, smell a bad odor, or hear strange noises.
- **Focal epilepsy:** uncontrollable twitching begins in a small part of the body and spreads until it may involve the whole body, but the person does not lose consciousness.
- **Temporal lobe epilepsy:** the person suddenly behaves out of character or inappropriately, e.g., becoming suddenly violent or angry, laughing for no reason, or making agitated or bizarre body movements, such as odd chewing movements.

CAUSES

Although 70–80% of epilepsy is characterized as idiopathic (i.e., of unknown cause), probable causes can be determined by age of onset of seizures.

Age of onset	Presumptive causes
Birth to 2 years	Birth injury, degenerative brain disease
2–19 years	Congenital birth injury, a fever-induced blood clot, head trauma, infection (meningitis or encephalitis)
20–34 years	Head trauma, brain tumor (benign or cancerous)
35–54 years	Brain tumor, head trauma, stroke
55 years and older	Stroke, brain tumor

Other causative factors in epilepsy
- **Brain damage** before birth.
- **Central nervous system infections:** these include brain abscess, rabies, neurosyphilis, tetanus, malaria, toxoplasmosis (infection with the parasite *Toxoplasma gondii*), and infection with *Taenia solium*, a type of tapeworm.
- **Metabolic disorders, including:**
  - hypocalcemia (abnormally low levels of circulating calcium)
  - hypoglycemia (abnormally low levels of sugar in the blood)
  - hypoparathyroidism (inadequate secretion of parathyroid hormones)
  - phenylketonuria (a hereditary error of metabolism that results in the accumulation of phenylalanine and its metabolites, which can produce brain damage, often with seizures).
- **Withdrawal** from alcohol and drugs.
- **Exposure** to neurotoxic chemicals in the environment.
- **Food allergy:** epileptic patients may have allergic reactions in the brain similar to the inflammatory chemical reactions seen at other sites of local allergic reactions:
  - in epileptics who suffer from multiple other symptoms of food allergy including recurrent headaches, hyperkinetic behavior, and abdominal pains, food allergy should be considered.
  - several studies, mostly of children, are highly suggestive of a causative link between food allergy,

especially celiac disease, and epilepsy. In each of four studies involving 2, 24, 43, and 63 children with epilepsy, allergy-free diets led to either significant reduction in symptoms or complete cessation of seizures, while reintroduction of allergenic foods caused recurrence.

- **Homocystinuria:** a genetically inherited inability to detoxify a by-product of metabolism called homocysteine, which accumulates and can be neurotoxic:
  - homocystinuria can be corrected with supplemental vitamin B_6, vitamin B_{12} and folic acid.

Epilepsy should not be diagnosed on the basis of a solitary seizure. The recurrence rate after a single seizure is approximately only 27% over 3 years.

RISK INCREASES WITH

- Family history of seizure disorders: the prevalence of seizures in close relatives is three times that of the overall population.
- Excess alcohol consumption.
- Certain prescription medications increase the risk of seizures.
- Hypoglycemia (low blood sugar): some researchers believe hypoglycemia is the most important metabolic cause of seizures. It is thought that low blood sugar may impair the production of ATP, the energy currency of the body. Without adequate ATP production, nerve cell membranes become electrically unbalanced, rendering the nerve cells trigger-happy. Researchers have found that:
  - blood sugar levels are unusually low prior to a seizure
  - 50–90% of epileptics have constant or periodic low blood sugar
  - 70% or more of epileptics have abnormal glucose tolerance tests.
- Use of mind-altering drugs.
- Exposure to environmental toxins: heavy metals such as lead, mercury, cadmium, and aluminum can induce seizures. Many neurotoxic chemicals have been and continue to be released into the environment, for example, cigarette smoke, car exhaust fumes, pesticides, solvents, food additives such as tartrazine, etc.
- Birth trauma.
- History of prior head injury.
- Celiac disease or other food allergy.

PREVENTIVE MEASURES

- Avoid alcoholic beverages and alcohol-containing over-the-counter drugs (e.g., cough syrup, mouthwash).

- Do not use mind-altering drugs.
- Minimize exposure to toxic fumes (e.g., car exhaust, cigarette smoke) and other neurotoxic chemicals. If your employment involves chemical exposure, wear a respirator or change your line of work.
- Take a high-potency multiple vitamin and mineral supplement: a daily multiple providing all of the known vitamins and minerals serves as a foundation upon which to build an individualized health-promotion program. Any good multiple should include $400\,\mu g$ of folic acid, $400\,\mu g$ of vitamin B_{12}, and $50–100\,mg$ of vitamin B_6.
- Eliminate food allergens from the diet: for more information, see the chapter on Food allergy.

Expected outcomes

In the poorly controlled epileptic, a significant reduction in seizures should be expected within 3 months of appropriate therapy.

TREATMENT

Diet
- **Ketogenic diet:** the ketogenic diet consists of large amounts of fat, and minimal amounts of protein and carbohydrate:
  - the ketogenic diet has a long history of use for the reduction of seizures. In one recent study of 27 children aged 1–16 years, 40% experienced a 50% reduction in seizures, with 25% becoming seizure free. This success rate greatly exceeds that of anticonvulsant drugs, the side effects are fewer, and the diet is cheaper.
  - the beneficial effects of the ketogenic diet are thought to result from it putting the body in an acid state, which corrects a tendency of epileptics to be more alkaline. The acid state is thought to normalize nerve cell membranes and nerve cell activity.
  - drawbacks: a high-fat diet is well known to increase the risk for cardiovascular disease, and is especially unhealthy for a growing child.
- **A health-promoting diet:** after identifying and removing allergenic foods from the diet, choose a health-promoting diet rich in whole, unprocessed, preferably organic foods, especially plant foods (non-starchy vegetables, beans, nuts [especially walnuts], and seeds), cold-water fish (high in omega-3 fats, which are necessary for healthy nerve cell membranes), and organically fed animal products and eggs. If possible, choose eggs from chickens fed flaxseed as their eggs will be high in omega-3 fats.

Nutritional supplements

- **A high-potency multiple vitamin and mineral supplement:** a daily multiple providing all of the known vitamins and minerals serves as a foundation upon which to build an individualized health-promotion program. Any good multiple should include 400 µg of folic acid, 400 µg of vitamin B_{12}, and 50–100 mg of vitamin B_6. These three nutrients are particularly important in persons with epilepsy as they are necessary for the conversion of homocysteine, a potentially neurotoxic by-product of cellular metabolism, into methionine, an amino acid necessary for numerous detoxification processes.

- **Vitamin B_6:** in susceptible newborns and infants less than 18 months of age, inadequate amounts of vitamin B_6 may lead to seizure. In some infants, seizures are promptly corrected by the administration of dietary amounts of B_6, while others need high or IV dosage:
  - vitamin B_6 is a necessary cofactor in the metabolism of a variety of neurotransmitters including the important inhibitory neurotransmitter GABA (gamma-aminobutyric acid).
  - the adult dosage for B_6 is 50 mg t.i.d., but this must be reduced proportionally for children.
  - dosage: the use of vitamin B_6 must be supervised by a physician. Daily doses in the range of 80–400 mg have been shown to interfere with commonly used anticonvulsant drugs.

- **Thiamin (vitamin B_1):** when nerve fibers are stimulated in test tubes, they lose significant amounts of thiamin, which suggests that thiamin plays an important role in nerve-to-nerve communication:
  - thiamin deficiency may also be accompanied by low concentrations of GABA, a neurotransmitter important in inhibiting seizures. Particularly in late-onset epilepsy, thiamin deficiency should be considered as a possible cause.
  - dosage: 25 mg q.d.

- **Taurine:** one of the most abundant amino acids in the brain, taurine has demonstrated significant anticonvulsive activity in numerous studies since the 1970s:
  - taurine stabilizes nerve cell membranes, acts like the inhibitory neurotransmitter GABA, and also increases levels of GABA itself.
  - epileptics commonly have significantly lower levels of taurine in platelets (blood components involved in inflammation and clotting) than control patients.
  - in one study of patients who were unresponsive to anticonvulsant drugs, taurine decreased seizures by more than 30% in 11 of 34 subjects.
  - dosage: 500 mg t.i.d.

- **Magnesium:** without adequate ATP production, nerve cell membranes become electrically unbalanced, rendering the nerve cells trigger-happy. Magnesium stabilizes nerve cell membranes and is necessary for ATP production:
  - epileptics have been shown to have significantly lower blood magnesium levels than controls.
  - magnesium deficiency has been shown to induce muscle tremors and convulsive seizures; 30 epileptic patients were able to control seizure activity when supplemented with 450 mg q.d. of magnesium.
  - dosage: 450 mg q.d., in divided doses, of magnesium citrate.

- **Manganese:** manganese is a critical cofactor in the neuron's use of glucose, the brain's primary fuel, and is also involved in neurotransmitter control:
  - low whole blood and hair levels of manganese have been found in epileptics, with those with the lowest levels of manganese typically having the highest seizure activity.
  - dosage: 10 mg t.i.d.

- **Zinc:** children with epilepsy commonly have significantly lower levels of zinc than controls:
  - although the exact role of zinc is not clearly understood, it appears to involve either the storage or building of the inhibitory neurotransmitter, GABA.
  - anticonvulsants may cause zinc deficiency.
  - dosage: 25 mg q.d.

- **Vitamin E:** vitamin E deficiency is known to produce seizures, antiepileptic drugs have been shown to decrease vitamin E levels, and studies have shown vitamin E to be low in epileptic patients:
  - in a double-blind, placebo-controlled study of 24 epileptic children who were not responding to antiepileptic drugs, supplementation with 400 IU q.d. of vitamin E significantly reduced seizures in 10 of the 12 children in the vitamin E group, and the 2 children who did not respond did not take the vitamin E. The 12 children who did not receive vitamin E did not improve.
  - dosage: 400 IU q.d. of mixed tocopherols.

- **Selenium:** selenium and vitamin E frequently work together synergistically. In addition, selenium is a component of glutathione peroxidase, an antioxidant made by the body that is perhaps its most important detoxifying agent:
  - in one study, four children with low levels of glutathione peroxidase who had intractable seizures starting within the first 6 months of life, and who were unresponsive to anticonvulsant drugs, all improved when anticonvulsants were discontinued and selenium was administered.
  - dosage: 100 µg q.d.

Botanical medicines

- **Saiko-Keishi-To (SK):** clinical research using SK, a Chinese herbal medicine combination formula, has shown benefit in epileptic patients. One study reported that 8 out of 28 epileptics experienced a 25% reduction in seizures after 8 weeks of treatment; dosage: 300 ml before bedtime.
- ***Coleus forskohlii*:** an important plant medicine in the Ayurvedic treatment of epilepsy, *Coleus forskohlii* increases cyclic AMP, a brain chemical that depresses electrical activity in the brain, thus inhibiting seizures; dosage: based upon forskolin content, 5–10 mg b.i.d.–t.i.d.

Drug–herb interaction cautions
None.

Erythema multiforme

DESCRIPTION

An acute inflammatory disorder of the skin and *mucous membranes* (thin moist tissues that line the body cavities), erythema multiforme typically first appears as a rash on the palm of the hand, then spreads to the soles of the feet, and other areas of the arms and legs, and may spread to the face and rest of the body. Erythema multiforme can be primarily a skin disorder, or it can be the skin's manifestation of an infection that has spread throughout the body, or of a chronic inflammatory disease. In the majority of cases, it is self-limiting and relatively benign, but it can be potentially severe. The severe form is known as *Stevens–Johnson syndrome* or erythema multiforme major; the less severe form is labeled *erythema multiforme minor*.

FREQUENT SIGNS AND SYMPTOMS

- Sudden onset of an itchy skin rash, characterized by lesions that are symmetrical, raised, fluid-filled red spots.
- Rash typically first appears on the palm of the hand, then spreads to the soles of the feet, arms and legs, with minimal or no appearance on the face and rest of the body.
- Rash is sometimes painful or has a burning sensation.
- Rash evolves into blister-like "target lesions" with clear centers and concentric red rings.
- Rash may develop into hives or become ulcerated.
- Lesions may gradually darken to purple, then fade to yellowish-brown before finally clearing in 2–3 weeks.
- In the major form, the mucous membranes of the mouth, eyes, and genitals become inflamed.
- Fever
- Headache
- Sore throat
- Diarrhea
- Tendency to recur in spring and fall.

CAUSES

- Viral infections, particularly herpes simplex virus
- Medications such as sulfonamides, penicillins, anticonvulsants, salicylates, barbiturates; reaction to the drug may not occur until 7–14 days after first using it

- Bacterial infections
- Protozoan infections
- Collagen vascular disease
- Malignancy
- Radiation therapy
- Pregnancy
- Premenstrual hormone changes

RISK INCREASES WITH

- Previous history of erythema multiforme
- Use of medications that can cause the disorder
- Underlying infection
- Premenstrual syndrome
- Herpes simplex outbreaks (both type I: blisters on the lips, and type II: genital blisters)
- Frequent infections
- Disease-promoting diet: immune function is directly related to the quality of the foods routinely ingested. A diet based on processed foods, with little consumption of fresh vegetables, legumes, fruits, nuts and seeds, whole grains, and cold-water fish is low in protective, anti-inflammatory factors – antioxidants, flavonoids, vitamin and mineral cofactors, essential fatty acids – and high in factors that promote inflammation and suppress immune function – refined carbohydrates, *trans* fats (also called partially hydrogenated oils), and chemical additives.

PREVENTIVE MEASURES

- **Initiating factor:** if possible, determine the initiating factor. If it is a drug, avoid it. If it is an underlying infection, treat it promptly and comprehensively. Chronic infections may signal a suppressed immune system and the need for a complete program of immune support and detoxification.
- **Prompt treatment** of any illness or infection.
- **Avoid** unnecessary use of medications that can cause erythema multiforme
- **Avoid** herpes outbreaks by avoiding sun exposure and reducing stress.
- **A health-promoting diet:** after identifying and removing allergenic foods from the diet, choose a

balanced diet composed of whole, unprocessed, preferably organic foods, especially plant foods (fruits, vegetables, whole grains, beans, nuts [especially walnuts], and seeds), and cold-water fish (for more detailed information, see Appendix 1).

- **A high-potency multiple vitamin and mineral supplement:** this should include 400 μg of folic acid, 400 μg of vitamin B_{12}, and 50–100 mg of vitamin B_6. (Folic acid supplementation should always be accompanied by vitamin B_{12} supplementation to prevent folic acid from masking a vitamin B_{12} deficiency.) A daily multiple providing all of the known vitamins and minerals serves as a foundation upon which to build an individualized health-promotion program.

Expected outcomes

Rash evolves over 1–2 weeks, usually clearing in 2–3 weeks, although complete healing may take as long as 5–6 weeks. Any eye involvement should be carefully monitored.

TREATMENT

- A careful search should be made to determine the initiating cause.
- Underlying infections should be treated.
- Unnecessary medications should be stopped.
- An anti-inflammatory program tailored to the causes should be initiated.
- Bed rest is indicated if fever is present.
- Any eye involvement should be carefully monitored. Eyewashes or other topical medications may be prescribed.

Diet

- Follow the recommendations given above for a health-promoting diet.
- If mouth sores are present, a soft or liquid diet may be better tolerated. Smoothies made from milk (soy, almond or rice milk if cow's milk allergy is suspected), protein powder, fresh or frozen fruit, and flaxseed meal can provide needed protein. Vegetable juices, soups, and herb teas are also good choices.
- Limit consumption of simple sugars (primarily found in refined carbohydrates but also including fruit sugars) to less than 50 g q.d.

Nutritional supplements

- **A high-potency multiple vitamin and mineral supplement** (as described in Preventive Measures above).
- **Potassium iodide:** potassium iodide has a long history of use for a variety of inflammatory skin disorders. Recent clinical studies have documented dramatic success, most likely resulting from potassium iodide's suppression of inflammatory reactive oxygen species, a type of free radical:
  - **caution:** iodine therapy has occasionally been associated with adverse skin reactions and gastrointestinal discomfort. Iodine therapy should never be used in pregnant women in the last trimester.
  - dosage: 100 mg t.i.d. for 4–6 weeks. Discontinue if any adverse reactions occur.
- **Vitamin C:** directly antiviral and antibacterial, vitamin C's main claim to fame is its many different immune-enhancing effects including white blood cell response and function, increasing levels of interferon (a special chemical factor that fights viral infection and cancer), and increasing secretion of hormones from the thymus gland (the major gland of the immune system); dosage: 500 mg q.i.d.
- **Vitamin A:** known as the "anti-infective vitamin", vitamin A plays a variety of essential roles in immune function including maintaining the surfaces of the skin, respiratory tract, and gastrointestinal tract and their secretions – all of which constitute a barrier that is the body's first line of defense against micro-organisms – and stimulating and/or enhancing numerous immune processes including white blood cell function and antibody response; dosage: 5,000 IU q.d.
- **Beta-carotene:** called "pro-vitamin A" since it can be converted into vitamin A, beta-carotene is a more powerful antioxidant than vitamin A and exerts additional immune-stimulating effects, including enhancing thymus function. Specifically, beta-carotene has been shown to increase the production of helper/inducer T cells by 30% after 7 days and all T cells after 14 days; dosage: 100,000 IU q.d.
- **Bromelain:** a variety of inflammatory agents are inhibited by the action of bromelain, a group of sulfur-containing proteolytic (protein-digesting) enzymes obtained from the pineapple plant. The rapid decrease in inflammation results in a faster recovery; dosage: (1,200–1,800 MCU): 250–500 mg between meals q.i.d.

Topical medicines

- Wet dressings and soaks or lotions to soothe the skin.
- Bathing in lukewarm to cool water three times a day for 30 min.
- Zinc sulfate: If herpes simplex virus is a possible cause, a 0.025–0.5% solution of zinc sulfate should be applied topically at the site of infection, both to help heal the infection and to prevent relapse.

Fibrocystic breast disease

DESCRIPTION

A common condition in the female breast that occurs in 20–40% of menstruating women, fibrocystic breast disease (FBD) is characterized by multiple non-malignant lumps, which vary in size throughout the month and are frequently accompanied by premenstrual breast pain and tenderness. A benign component of PMS (premenstrual syndrome), FBD is considered a risk factor for breast cancer, but is not as significant a risk factor as family history, early onset of menstruation, and late or no first pregnancy.

FREQUENT SIGNS AND SYMPTOMS

- Multiple lumps, typically in both breasts (solitary lumps may occur, but multiple lumps are more common).
- Lumps offer resistance when pressed and may be tender.
- Lumps often enlarge before menstrual periods, then shrink afterwards.
- Lumps vary in size. Larger lumps near the surface can be moved freely within the breast; lumps deep within the breast may be indistinguishable from lumps due to breast cancer.
- Generalized breast pain and tenderness.
- Nipple discharge.
- Consult a physician immediately if a breast lump of any kind is noticed. Although pain, cyclic variations in size, high mobility, and multiplicity of lumps indicate FBD, these clinical criteria do not definitively differentiate FBD from breast cancer. Non-invasive procedures, such as ultrasound, can help aid conclusive diagnosis, but at this time, definitive diagnosis depends upon biopsy.

CAUSES

- **Increased estrogen-to-progesterone ratio:** excessive estrogen is responsible for numerous feminine ills, including FBD.
- **B vitamin deficiency:** a well-supported theory, initially proposed in the 1940s by Dr Morton Biskind, suggests that excessive estrogen levels are the result of decreased detoxification and elimination of estrogen by the liver due to B vitamin deficiency. The liver uses various B vitamins to detoxify estrogen and excrete it in the bile.
- **Elevated levels of other hormones** (e.g., prolactin): estrogens, both internally produced and ingested as birth control pills or Premarin, are known to increase prolactin secretion by the pituitary gland. In women with FBD, levels of prolactin are typically found to be elevated, but not to levels high enough to cause *amenorrhea* (loss of menstruation).
- **A high-fat diet**, particularly saturated fat, significantly increases the level of circulating estrogens.
- **Environmental estrogens in food:** there has been widespread environmental contamination by a group of compounds known as *halogenated hydrocarbons*. Included in this group are the toxic pesticides DDT, DDE, PCB, PCP, dieldrin, and chlordane. These chemicals are stored in fat cells, mimic estrogen in the body, and are thought to be a major factor in the growing epidemics of estrogen-related health problems including FBD.
- **Caffeine and other methylxanthines:** population studies, experimental evidence, and clinical evaluations indicate a strong association between caffeine consumption and FBD:
  - caffeine, theophylline, and theobromine are all members of a family of compounds known as methylxanthines, which promote the production in breast tissue of the fibrous tissue and cyst fluid evidenced in FBD.
  - coffee, tea, cola, chocolate and caffeinated medications are sources of methylxanthines.
- **Sugar:** a high intake of sugar impairs estrogen metabolism and is associated with higher estrogen levels. Incidence of PMS as well as FBD is much higher in women who consume a sugar-laden diet.
- **Low-fiber diet:** women who have fewer than three bowel movements per week have a 4.5 times greater rate of FBD than women who have at least one bowel movement per day. This probably results from the action of unfriendly bacterial flora in the large intestine, which can transform excreted steroids into toxic derivatives or allow these excreted steroids to be reabsorbed.

■ **Hypothyroidism and/or iodine deficiency:**
- ■ an absence of iodine makes breast cells more sensitive to estrogen, which leads the breast ducts to produce small cysts and later fibrosis (hardening of the tissue because of deposition of fibrin similar to the formation of scar tissue).
- ■ thyroid hormone replacement therapy in patients with low or even normal thyroid function has been shown to decrease breast pain, serum prolactin levels, and breast nodules.
- ■ experimental iodine deficiency in rats results in changes very similar to FBD.

RISK INCREASES WITH

■ Disease-promoting diet: the liver's ability to detoxify and eliminate estrogen is directly related to the quality of foods routinely eaten. A diet based on animal products and processed foods, with little consumption of fresh vegetables, legumes, fruits, nuts and seeds, whole grains, and cold-water fish, is low in factors that promote estrogen's clearance from the body – B vitamins, fiber, vitamins A and E, and essential fatty acids – and high in factors that promote excessive estrogen – sugars, saturated fats, and environmental estrogens from pesticide residues in foods and animal growth stimulators.

■ Use of oral contraceptives

■ Consumption of caffeine and other methylxanthines

■ Constipation

■ Low thyroid function.

PREVENTIVE MEASURES

■ A high-potency multiple vitamin and mineral supplement including 400 µg of folic acid, 400 µg of vitamin B_{12}, and 50–100 mg of vitamin B_6. (Folic acid supplementation should always be accompanied by vitamin B_{12} supplementation to prevent folic acid from masking a vitamin B_{12} deficiency.) A daily multiple providing all of the known vitamins and minerals serves as a foundation upon which to build an individualized health-promotion program.

■ Consume a nutrient-dense, high-fiber diet rich in whole, unprocessed, preferably organic foods, especially plant foods (fruits, vegetables, beans, seeds and nuts), and cold-water fish, and low in animal products (for more detailed information, see Appendix 1).

■ If using oral contraceptives, switch to another form of birth control.

■ Limit consumption of coffee, tea, cola, chocolate and caffeinated medications.

Expected outcomes

Progressive reduction in signs and symptoms with maximum benefit achieved within 6 months.

TREATMENT

Diet

■ The diet should be primarily vegetarian with large amounts of dietary fiber. Emphasize whole, unprocessed, fiber-rich foods, such as whole grains, legumes, vegetables, fruits, nuts, and seeds.

■ Eliminate all methylxanthines (coffee, tea, cola, chocolate and caffeinated medications) until symptoms are alleviated; they may then be reintroduced in small amounts.

■ Avoid animal products with high estrogen content such as meats raised with the help of growth stimulators etc.

■ Substitute soy foods such as tofu, tempeh, soyburgers, soymilk, soynuts, etc. as an excellent source of protein and phytoestrogens. Phytoestrogens are often called antiestrogens because their estrogenic effect is only 2% as strong as human estrogen. Because they are capable of binding to estrogen receptors, phytoestrogens prevent estrogen from binding, thus decreasing its effects.

■ Drink at least 2 L (3 US pints) of water daily.

Nutritional supplements

■ **High-potency multiple vitamin and mineral supplement** (as described in Preventive Measures above).

■ **Lipotropic factors:** these are substances that hasten the removal or decrease the deposition of fat and bile in the liver through their interaction with fat metabolism, thus improving liver function. Estrogens are excreted from the body via the bile:
- ■ dosage: choline: 500–1,000 mg q.d.; methionine: 500–1,000 mg q.d.

■ **Vitamin B_6:** the liver requires B_6 (along with folic acid and other B vitamins in the multiple formula and in the healthful diet outlined above) to detoxify estrogen by binding (conjugating) it to glucuronic acid, so it can be excreted in the bile:
- ■ B_6 has been used in the management of women's cyclical conditions since the early 1970s. At least a dozen double-blind, placebo-controlled trials have demonstrated positive effects of B_6 supplementation in relieving PMS symptoms, including FBD.
- ■ dosage: 25–50 mg t.i.d.

■ **Vitamin E:** vitamin E has been shown to normalize circulating hormone levels in PMS and FBD patients,

relieving many symptoms of these conditions:
- while vitamin C protects the body's water-soluble areas, vitamin E is the primary antioxidant in the fat-soluble compartments such as cell membranes and fatty molecules like cholesterol.
- vitamin E also significantly enhances both types of immune defenses: non-specific or cell-mediated immunity and specific or humoral immunity. Cell-mediated immunity is the body's primary mode of protection against cancer.
- dosage: 400–800 IU q.d.

- **Vitamin C:** an essential antioxidant found in all body compartments composed of water, vitamin C strengthens and maintains normal epithelial integrity, improves wound healing, enhances immune function, and inhibits carcinogen formation:
  - vitamin C works synergistically with vitamin E, regenerating vitamin E after it has used up its antioxidant potential.
  - dosage: 500 mg t.i.d.

- **Beta-carotene:** also known as pro-vitamin A since it can be converted to vitamin A in the body, beta-carotene is a powerful antioxidant essential to epithelial health. A strong inverse correlation has been shown between serum levels of beta-carotene and cancer. Studies have also found that the higher the intake of beta-carotene, the lower the risk for cancer; dosage: 50,000 IU q.d.

- **Iodine (caseinate or liquid iodine):** breast cells lacking sufficient iodine are hypersensitive to estrogen stimulation. Iodine deficiency leads the breast ducts to produce small cysts and later fibrotic (lumpy) tissue:
  - in clinical trials, iodine has been an effective treatment in FBD in about 70% of subjects.
  - iodine was, however, associated with a high rate of side effects (altered thyroid function in 4%; iodine poisoning, characterized by a watery nose, weakness, excessive salivation, and bad breath, in 3%; and acne in 15%).
  - the most significant side effect was short-term increased breast pain, which was viewed as a positive sign since it corresponded with a softening of the breast and disappearance of the fibrous tissue.

- dosage: 70–90 µg of iodine (caseinate or liquid iodine) per kg of body weight q.d. (other forms of iodine 500 µg daily).

- **Zinc:** zinc is required for proper action of many body hormones, including sex hormones. Low zinc levels promote prolactin secretion, whereas high zinc levels inhibit its release. Zinc levels are frequently low in women with PMS:
  - dosage: 15–30 mg q.d. (Target dosage to address elevated prolactin levels is actually 30–45 mg q.d., which should be reached by the combined amounts of zinc in the multiple supplement recommended above plus this additional dose.)

- **Flaxseed:** flaxseed promotes a healthy menstrual cycle, alleviating numerous ills associated with hormonal imbalances, and providing protection against cancer:
  - flaxseeds contain a group of phytoestrogens called *lignans* with weak estrogenic and antiestrogenic effects; these promote normal ovulation and lengthen the second half of the menstrual cycle, in which progesterone is the dominant hormone, thus helping to restore hormonal balance.
  - lignan-rich fiber has also been shown to decrease insulin resistance, which also reduces bioavailable estrogen.
  - flaxseed oil: women with PMS are frequently deficient in vitamin B_6, magnesium and zinc, nutrients necessary for essential fatty acid metabolism. Providing these nutrients along with adequate levels of essential fatty acids should normalize essential fatty acid metabolism. Flaxseed oil is nature's richest source of essential fatty acids.
  - dosage: 2 tbsp of flaxseed meal and 1 tbsp flaxseed oil q.d. Both are highly perishable, should be kept in opaque containers in the refrigerator, and never heated.

- ***Lactobacillus acidophilus***: lactobacilli are friendly bacteria with numerous beneficial effects on intestinal health, one of which is that they supplant less friendly bacteria, such as those which transform excreted estrogen into a form which can be reabsorbed; dosage: 1–2 billion live organisms q.d.

Food allergy

DESCRIPTION

A food allergy is an adverse reaction to the consumption of a food. Food allergies may be a reaction to a protein, a starch, a contaminant found in the food (e.g., pesticide residues) or a food additive (e.g., colorings, preservatives, flavor enhancers, etc). A classic food allergy is, by definition, mediated (controlled and influenced) by the immune system, but in sensitive persons, adverse reactions may also occur in response to naturally occurring chemicals in foods. For example, phenolic compounds in red wine and aged cheese have been linked to migraine headaches in some individuals.

Other terms commonly used to refer to adverse reactions to food include: food hypersensitivity, food sensitivity, and food intolerance. Food allergies have been implicated in a wide range of medical conditions, affecting virtually every part of the body – from mildly uncomfortable symptoms such as indigestion and gastritis, to severe illnesses such as celiac disease, arthritis, and chronic infection. Allergies have also been linked to central nervous system disorders including depression, anxiety, and chronic fatigue.

The frequency of food allergies and the number of persons affected has increased dramatically. For example, eczema, an allergic condition of the skin often caused by food allergy, now affects between 10–15% of the population at some time in their lives. Adverse food reactions and food allergies are now reported in 25% of young children. Some physicians believe food allergies are the leading cause of undiagnosed symptoms and that at least 60% of Americans suffer from symptoms due to adverse food reactions.

From a clinical perspective, naturopathic and other nutrition-oriented physicians recognize two basic types of food allergy: cyclic and fixed. Cyclic allergies, which account for 80–90% of food allergies, develop slowly in response to the frequent consumption of a food. If the food is avoided for a period of time (typically about 4 months), it may be reintroduced and tolerated, but only if it is not eaten too frequently. Fixed allergies occur whenever a food is eaten, no matter how much time has elapsed since the last ingestion, and remain throughout a person's life.

FREQUENT SIGNS AND SYMPTOMS

- Dark circles under the eyes ("allergic shiners")
- Puffiness under the eyes
- Horizontal creases in the lower eyelid
- Chronic (non-cyclic) fluid retention
- Chronic swollen glands
- Frequent infections
- Frequent digestive upset

In addition to these typical signs, food allergy has been linked to many common symptoms and health conditions as shown in the table below.

Symptoms and diseases commonly associated with food allergy

System	Symptoms and diseases
Gastrointestinal	Canker sores, celiac disease, chronic diarrhea, duodenal ulcer, gastritis, irritable bowel syndrome, malabsorption, ulcerative colitis
Genitourinary	Bed-wetting, chronic bladder infections, nephrosis
Immune	Chronic infections, frequent ear infections
Mental/emotional	Anxiety, depression, hyperactivity, inability to concentrate, insomnia, irritability, mental confusion, personality change, seizures
Musculoskeletal	Bursitis, joint pain, low back pain
Respiratory	Asthma, chronic bronchitis, wheezing
Skin	Acne, eczema, hives, itching, skin rash
Miscellaneous	Arrhythmia, edema, fainting, fatigue, headache, hypoglycemia, itchy nose or throat, migraines, sinusitis

CAUSES

Immune response to food antigens

Most food allergies are a result of interactions between ingested food, the digestive tract, and the immune system. In classic (immune system-controlled) food allergy, the body sees an ingested food molecule as an *antigen* – a foreign substance. This triggers the immune system to send an *antibody* to bind to the antigen. Antibodies are protein molecules made by the immune system that latch on to foreign substances, in this case the food antigen. There are five major types of antibody: IgE (Ig = immunoglobulin, so IgE = immunoglobulin E), IgD, IgG, IgM and IgA, and four distinct types of immune-mediated reaction: Type I, immediate hypersensitivity reactions; Type II, cytotoxic reactions; Type III, immune complex-mediated reactions; and Type IV, T-cell-dependent reactions. IgE is involved in immediate hypersensitivity reactions, which occur within 2 hours after exposure. The other antibodies are involved in delayed reactions, which may occur up to 72 hours after exposure.

Type I: immediate hypersensitivity reactions

IgE antibodies are involved in these classic immediate reactions, which occur within 2 hours after the food is consumed. The IgE antibody binds to the antigen and then to specialized white blood cells called *mast cells* and *basophils,* which release histamine, causing swelling and inflammation. A variety of allergic symptoms result depending on the location of the mast cell: in the nasal passages, this causes sinus congestion; in the bronchioles, asthma; in the skin, hives and eczema; in the synovial cells that line the joints, arthritis; in the intestinal mucosa, inflammation with resulting poor absorption of nutrients, bloating, diarrhea, etc.; in the brain, headaches, loss of memory, and "spaciness". Immediate hypersensitivity reactions are, however, thought to account for only 10–15% of food allergy reactions.

Type II: cytotoxic reactions

These delayed reactions involve the binding of either IgG or IgM antibodies to antigens that have attached themselves to cells, a binding that signals the immune system to activate factors that destroy the cell. It has been estimated that at least 75% of all food allergy reactions are accompanied by cell destruction. Normally, the destroyed cells are intestinal since that is where the immune system and food antigen typically meet. Damage to the intestinal wall allows more antigens to leak into the circulation, leading to a vicious cycle of more antibody production, intestinal damage, and the production of additional food allergies.

Type III: immune complex-mediated reactions

Immune complexes are formed when antibodies attach to antigens. White blood cells (called macrophages) located in the liver and spleen usually clear the immune complexes from the circulation. However, if a lot of complexes are circulating and/or if histamines and other amines (which make blood vessels more permeable) are present, then the immune complexes can be deposited in and injure tissues. The response is also delayed in this type of allergy, which typically involves IgG and IgG$_4$ antibodies; 80% of food allergy reactions are thought to be of this type.

Type IV: T cell-dependent reactions

This delayed reaction does not involve antibodies but is controlled primarily by a type of white blood cell called a T lymphocyte. It occurs when an allergen contacts the skin, respiratory tract, gastrointestinal tract, or other body surface and stimulates sensitized T cells, causing inflammation 36–72 hours later. Examples of this type of allergy include poison ivy (contact dermatitis), allergic colitis, and regional ileitis.

Factors that increase the probability of an antibody response to foods

■ **Genetic predisposition:** individuals with a tendency to develop food allergies have nearly 50% more of a special type of white blood cell known as a T lymphocyte or T cell than non-allergic persons. T cells help other white blood cells make antibodies. Because these individuals have more circulating T cells, their allergic response is much more easily triggered.

■ **Overexposure to a limited number of foods:** these are often hidden as ingredients in commercially prepared foods.

■ **Food additives:** numerous preservatives, stabilizers, artificial colorings, and flavorings are now added to a wide variety of foods resulting in overexposure.

■ **Environmental toxins:** increased chemical pollution in our air, water, and food; for example, food contamination following the use of pesticides in farming.

■ **The use of formula, rather than breastfeeding infants:** breast milk is much less likely to contain antigens than formula. An infant's digestive tract is highly permeable, which allows antigens to leak into the general circulation and provoke allergic reactions.

■ **Weaning:** earlier weaning and earlier introduction of solid foods to infants.

■ **Genetic manipulation of plants:** this can result in food components with greater allergenic properties.

■ **Impaired digestion:** when improperly chewed and digested, dietary protein can cross the intestinal barrier and be absorbed into the bloodstream, activating an immune response (see below) that can occur either immediately at the intestinal barrier or at distant sites throughout the body. Impaired digestion may be due to:

- *lack of hydrochloric acid*: Hydrochloric acid is secreted by the stomach to digest food. Our ability to secrete hydrochloric acid lessens with age and can be disrupted by stress. *Hypochlorhydria* (inadequate secretion of hydrochloric acid) creates a hospitable environment for the bacterium that is responsible for duodenal ulcers, *Helicobacter pylori*.
- *Helicobacter pylori*, a pathogenic bacterium that further damages the lining of the stomach and disrupts digestive function, thus increasing the likelihood that dietary protein will leak into the bloodstream.
- *insufficient pancreatic enzymes*: Common symptoms of pancreatic insufficiency include abdominal discomfort and bloating, gas (flatulence), indigestion, and the passing of undigested food in the stool.
- **Stress:** during prolonged stress, levels of secretory IgA drop. Secretory IgA (sIgA), an antibody in the lining of the intestinal tract, prevents foreign substances from entering the body. When sIgA levels are low, the absorption of food allergens and microbial antigens increases dramatically:
  - stressors that can disrupt immune function include physical or emotional trauma, excessive use of drugs, immunization reactions, excessive frequency of consumption of a particular food, and/or environmental toxins.

RISK INCREASES WITH

- Inherited susceptibility: when both parents have allergies, a 67% chance exists that their children will also have allergies. When only one parent has allergies, the chance of a child being allergy-prone drops to 33%.
- Stress: physical or emotional stress, immunizations, drug use, environmental toxins.
- Frequent consumption of a limited number of foods, particularly allergenic foods such as wheat, dairy products, corn, soy, peanuts.
- Exposure to environmental toxins.
- *Helicobacter pylori* infection.
- Hypochlorhydria and/or pancreatic enzyme insufficiency: as we age, our ability to secrete these digestive aids diminishes.

PREVENTIVE MEASURES

- Try to consume a highly varied selection of foods rather than the same foods every day.
- If prone to allergies, try to rotate food families as well as individual foods. This is important because if a person is allergic to one food in a food family, the person will produce antibodies that can react with other foods in that family. The food family taxonomic table below provides a summary of common food families.

Edible plant and animal kingdom taxonomic table

Vegetables

Legumes	Mustard	Parsley	Potato	Grass	Lily
Beans	Broccoli	Anise	Chili	Barley	Asparagus
Cocoa bean	Brussels sprout	Caraway	Eggplant	Corn	Chives
Lentil	Cabbage	Carrot	Peppers	Oat	Garlic
Licorice	Cauliflower	Celery	Potatoes	Rice	Leek
Peanut	Mustard	Coriander	Tomato	Rye	Onions
Peas	Radish	Cumin	Tobacco	Wheat	
Soybean	Turnip	Parsley			
Tamarind	Watercress				
Laurel	Sunflower	Beet	Buckwheat		
Avocado	Artichoke	Beet	Buckwheat		
Camphor	Lettuce	Chard	Rhubarb		
Cinnamon	Sunflower	Spinach			

Fruits

Gourds	Plums	Citrus	Cashew	Nuts	Beech
Cantaloupe	Almond	Grapefruit	Cashew	Brazil nut	Beechnut
Cucumber	Apricot	Lemon	Mango	Pecan	Chestnut
Honeydew	Cherry	Lime	Pistachio	Walnut	Chinquapin nut

table continues

Edible plant and animal kingdom taxonomic table (continued)

Gourds	Plums	Citrus
Melons	Peach	Mandarin
Pumpkin	Plum	Orange
Squash	Persimmon	Tangerine
Zucchini		

Banana	Palm	Grape	Pineapple	Rose	Birch
Arrowroot	Coconut	Grape	Pineapple	Blackberry	Filberts
Banana	Date	Raisin		Loganberry	Hazelnuts
Plantain	Date sugar			Raspberry	
				Rosehips	
				Strawberry	

Apple	Blueberry	Pawpaws
Apple	Blueberry	Papaya
Pear	Cranberry	Pawpaw
Quince	Huckleberry	

Animals

Mammals (meat/milk)	Birds (meat/egg)	Fish	Crustaceans	Mollusks
Cow	Chicken	Catfish	Crab	Abalone
Goat	Duck	Cod	Crayfish	Clams
Pig	Goose	Flounder	Lobster	Mussels
Rabbit	Hen	Halibut	Prawn	Oysters
Sheep	Turkey	Mackerel	Shrimp	Scallops
		Salmon		
		Sardine		
		Snapper		
		Trout		
		Tuna		

Expected outcomes
Symptoms should be dramatically reduced within 10 days. Within 4 months, cyclic allergens may be reintroduced and, if tolerated, consumed every fourth day.

TREATMENT

After identification of allergenic foods using either (1) elimination diet and food challenge or (2) laboratory methods such as blood tests, follow the dietary suggestions below.

Diet
- Avoid allergenic foods to the fullest extent possible. Avoidance means not only avoiding the food in its most identifiable state (e.g., eggs in an omelet), but also in its hidden state (e.g., eggs in salad dressing, bread, baked goods, ice cream).
- For severe reactions, closely related foods with similar antigenic components may also need to be eliminated (e.g., other grains including rice and millet in persons with severe wheat allergy).

- Particularly for those who are experiencing allergic reactions to a large number of foods, completely eliminating allergenic foods may not be practical:
  - common allergens such as wheat, corn and soy are components of many processed foods
  - when eating away from home, it is difficult to determine what ingredients are used in purchased foods and prepared meals
  - it may be difficult (psychologically, socially, and nutritionally) to eliminate a large number of common foods from a person's diet.
- The best solution may be to follow a "rotary diversified diet" consisting of a highly varied selection of foods eaten in a definite rotation to prevent the formation of new allergies and control existing ones:
  - tolerated foods are eaten at regularly spaced intervals of 4–7 days. For example, if wheat is eaten on Monday, no foods containing wheat should be consumed until Friday.
  - for strongly allergenic foods, all members of the food family should be avoided.
  - not just tolerated foods, but the food families in which they occur, must be rotated (see the sample four-day rotation diet below).

■ After the first few months, dietary restrictions can be relaxed, though some individuals may require a rotation diet indefinitely.

Four-day rotation diet

Food family	Food
Day 1	
Citrus	Lemon, orange, grapefruit, lime, tangerine, kumquat, citron
Banana	Banana, plantain, arrowroot (musa)
Palm	Coconut, date, date sugar
Parsley	Carrots, parsnips, celery, celery seed, celeriac, anise, dill, fennel, cumin, parsley, coriander, caraway
Spices	Black and white pepper, peppercorn, nutmeg, mace
Subucaya	Brazil nut
Bird	All fowl and game birds, including chicken, turkey, duck, goose, guinea, pigeon, quail, pheasant, eggs
Juices	Juices (preferably fresh) may be made and used from any fruits and vegetables in the taxonomic table, in any combination desired, without adding sweeteners.
Day 2	
Grape	All varieties of grapes, raisins
Pineapple	Juice-pack, water-pack, or fresh
Rose	Strawberry, raspberry, blackberry, loganberry, rosehips
Gourd	Watermelon, cucumber, cantaloupe, pumpkin, squash, other melons, zucchini, pumpkin or squash seeds
Beet	Beet, spinach, chard
Legume	Pea, black-eyed pea, dry beans, green beans, carob, soybeans, lentils, licorice, peanut, alfalfa
Cashew	Cashew, pistachio, mango
Birch	Filberts, hazelnuts
Flaxseed	Flaxseed
Swine	All pork products
Mollusks	Abalone, snail, squid, clam, mussel, oyster, scallop
Crustaceans	Crab, crayfish, lobster, prawn, shrimp
Juices	Juices (preferably fresh) may be made and used without added sweeteners from any fruits, berries, or vegetables listed in the taxonomic table, in any combination desired, including fresh alfalfa and some legumes.
Day 3	
Apple	Apple, pear, quince
Gooseberry	Currant, gooseberry

Food family	Food
Buckwheat	Buckwheat, rhubarb
Aster	Lettuce, chicory, endive, escarole, globe artichoke, dandelion, sunflower seeds, tarragon
Potato	Potato, tomato, eggplant, peppers (red and green), chili pepper, paprika, cayenne, ground cherries
Lily (onion)	Onion, garlic, asparagus, chives, leeks
Spurge	Tapioca
Herb	Basil, savory, sage, oregano, horehound, catnip, spearmint, peppermint, thyme, marjoram, lemon balm
Walnut	English walnut, black walnut, pecan, hickory nut, butternut
Pedalium	Sesame
Beech	Chestnut
Saltwater fish	Herring, anchovy, cod, sea bass, sea trout, mackerel, tuna, swordfish, flounder, sole
Freshwater fish	Sturgeon, salmon, whitefish, bass, perch
Juices	Juices (preferably fresh) may be made and used without added sweeteners from any fruits and vegetables listed in the taxonomic table, in any combination desired.
Day 4	
Plum	Plum, cherry, peach, apricot, nectarine, almond, wild cherry
Blueberry	Blueberry, huckleberry, cranberry, wintergreen
Pawpaws	Pawpaw, papaya, papain
Mustard	Mustard, turnip, radish, horseradish, watercress, cabbage, Chinese cabbage, broccoli, cauliflower, Brussels sprouts, kale, kohlrabi, rutabaga
Laurel	Avocado, cinnamon, bay leaf, sassafras, cassia buds or bark
Sweet potato or yam	
Grass	Wheat, corn, rice, oats, barley, rye, wild rice, cane, millet, sorghum, bamboo sprouts
Orchid	Vanilla
Protea	Macadamia nut
Conifer	Pine nut
Fungus	Mushrooms and yeast (brewer's yeast etc.)
Bovid	Milk products – butter, cheese, yogurt, beef and milk products, oleomargarine, lamb
Juices	Juices (preferably fresh) may be made and used without added sweeteners from any fruits and vegetables listed in the taxonomic table, in any combination desired.

Nutritional supplements

Incompletely digested proteins can impair the immune system, leading to long-term allergies and frequent infections. Supplementation with hydrochloric acid and pancreatic enzymes, the body's digestive factors, is often helpful for individuals with food allergy.

Hydrochloric acid supplementation

- Begin by taking 1 tablet or capsule, containing 10 grains (600 mg) of hydrochloric acid, at the next large meal. If this does not aggravate allergy symptoms, at every subsequent meal of the same size, take one more tablet or capsule (1 at the next meal, 2 at the meal after that, then 3 at the next meal). When taking a number of tablets or capsules, do not take them all at once. Space them throughout the meal.
- Continue to increase the dose up to 7 tablets or until a feeling of warmth in the stomach is experienced, whichever occurs first. A warm feeling in the stomach means that too many tablets have been taken for that meal, and that one less tablet should be taken for a meal of that size. It is a good idea, however, to try the larger dose again at another meal to make sure that the HCl was what caused the warmth, and not something else.
- After identifying the largest dose that can be taken at large meals without feeling any stomach warmth, maintain that dose at all meals of a similar size. Take less at smaller meals.
- As the stomach begins to regain the ability to produce the amount of HCl needed to digest food properly, the warm feeling will be noticed again and the dose level should be cut down.

Pancreatic enzymes

- **Dosage:** use a $10 \times$ USP pancreatic enzyme product and take 350–1,000 mg t.i.d. immediately before meals.
- **Use a non-enteric-coated enzyme product:** enzyme products are often *enteric*-coated to prevent digestion in the stomach, so the enzymes will be liberated in the small intestine. However, numerous studies have shown that non-enteric-coated enzyme preparations actually outperform enteric-coated products if they are taken prior to a meal.
- **For vegetarians**, *bromelain* and *papain* (protein-digesting enzymes from pineapple and papaya, respectively) can substitute for pancreatic enzymes in the treatment of pancreatic insufficiency. However, best results are obtained if they are used in combination with pancreatin and ox bile.

Gallstones

DESCRIPTION

Gallstones form in the gallbladder (an organ under the liver that stores bile) when an imbalance, typically an elevation in cholesterol levels, occurs among the constituents of bile. Bile (composed of bile salts, bilirubin, cholesterol, phospholipids, fatty acids, water, electrolytes, and other substances) is produced in the liver, stored in the gallbladder, and secreted into the small intestine where it is essential for the absorption of fats, oils, and fat-soluble vitamins. When an imbalance develops among bile components, bile not only loses its solubility, but also attracts particulate matter, initiating stone formation. Once a stone begins to form, its radius increases at an average rate of 2.6 mm a year, eventually reaching a size of a few millimeters to a centimeter. Symptoms occur an average of 8 years after formation begins.

In the US, 80% of gallstones are "mixed", that is, they are composed primarily of cholesterol and its derivatives, but also contain bile salts, bile pigments, and inorganic salts of calcium. The remaining 20% of stones, called "pigmented" gallstones, are composed entirely of minerals, principally calcium salts, although some stones contain oxides of aluminum and silicon. Pure stones, composed only of either cholesterol or pure pigment (calcium bilirubinate), are extremely rare.

Gallstones may occur in adolescents, but are more common in adults. In the US, autopsy studies have shown that gallstones exist in approximately 20% of women and 8% of men over the age of 40. Although gallstones may be present without causing symptoms, more than 300,000 gallbladders are removed each year in the US because of gallstones.

FREQUENT SIGNS AND SYMPTOMS

- No symptoms in about 40% of cases; ultrasound provides definitive diagnosis
- Periods of colicky, intense pain in the upper right abdomen
- Pain typically radiates to the upper back between the shoulder blades
- Nausea and vomiting
- Bloating or belching, especially after eating fatty foods
- Jaundice

CAUSES

Mixed gallstones

- **Elevations of cholesterol within the gallbladder:** for bile to do its job, it must be soluble, and its solubility is based on its relative concentrations of cholesterol, bile acids, lecithin, and water. Since free cholesterol is not water soluble, it must be incorporated into a lecithin–bile salt mixture. If cholesterol secretion increases, or if bile acid or lecithin secretion decreases, the result is insoluble bile that is supersaturated with cholesterol. Once this supersaturated bile forms, it attracts particulate matter, and stone formation begins.
- **Fiber-depleted refined foods:** a diet high in refined carbohydrates and fat, and low in fiber leads to a reduction in the synthesis of bile acids by the liver and a lower bile acid concentration in the gallbladder:
  - fiber also reduces the absorption of *deoxycholic acid*, a compound made from bile acids by bacteria in the intestine that greatly lessens the solubility of cholesterol in bile. Fiber both decreases the formation of deoxycholic acid and binds to it, thus promoting its excretion in feces.
- **In susceptible individuals, diets rich in legumes:** Chileans, Pima Indians and other North American Indians have the highest prevalence rates for cholesterol gallstones. All consume a diet high in legumes. Legume intake can increase the saturation of bile with cholesterol as a result of legumes' high content of compounds called saponins.

Pigmented gallstones

In Asia:
- parasitic infection of the liver and gallbladder by a variety of organisms, including the liver fluke (*Clonorchis sinesis*).

In the United States:
- chronic destruction of red blood cells (hemolysis)
- alcoholic cirrhosis of the liver.

RISK INCREASES WITH

Risk factors for mixed gallstones and those composed of cholesterol

- **A low-fiber, high-fat diet:** this results in lower bile acid concentration in the gallbladder and increased production of deoxycholic acid, a compound made by bacteria in the intestines that renders cholesterol much less soluble in bile.
- **Sex:** the frequency of gallstones is 2–4 times higher in women than in men, either because of increased cholesterol synthesis or suppression of bile acids by estrogens. All causes of elevated estrogen levels including pregnancy, the use of oral contraceptives, and hormone replacement, greatly increase the incidence of gallstones.
- **Genetic factors:** some ethnic groups are more susceptible. Nearly 70% of Native American women over age 30 have gallstones. In contrast, only 10% of black women over 30 have gallstones. The difference reflects the extent of cholesterol saturation of the bile; however, controlling the dietary factors that contribute to gallstone formation can prevent genetic susceptibility from becoming actualized as disease.
- **Obesity:** obesity causes increased cholesterol synthesis with the result that more cholesterol ends up secreted in the bile.
- **Rapid weight loss:** during active weight reduction, the concentration of cholesterol in the bile initially increases. Secretion of all bile components is reduced during weight loss, but bile acids decrease more than cholesterol. Since bile acids keep cholesterol in solution, the risk of gallstone formation or accelerated growth greatly increases. Once weight is stabilized, bile acid output returns to normal while cholesterol output remains low, so the final outcome of weight loss is a significant improvement in bile solubility:
  - *low calorie dieting*: in two studies of obese patients on low calorie diets (605 calories q.d., 925 calories q.d.), a significant portion (11% and 12.8% respectively) developed gallstones. Those who developed gallstones had higher initial triglyceride and cholesterol levels and also a significantly greater rate of weight loss.
  - *weight loss program*: anyone on a weight loss program who is losing more than 0.5 kg (1 lb) per week, especially an individual with elevated triglycerides and/or cholesterol, should follow the recommendations for increasing bile solubility given below.
- **Elevated estrogen levels:** estrogens suppress the secretion of bile acids. Any cause of elevated estrogen levels greatly increases the incidence of gallstones.

Elevated estrogen levels may be caused by:
- estrogen replacement
- oral contraceptives
- pregnancy
- obesity.

- **Gastrointestinal diseases (especially Crohn's disease and cystic fibrosis):** normally, about 98% of the bile acids secreted during digestion are reabsorbed in the terminal portion of the small intestine (the ileum). Gastrointestinal diseases result in impaired reabsorption of bile acids, reducing the bile acid pool and greatly increasing the risk of gallstones.
- **Drugs:** some cholesterol-lowering drugs, especially the fibric acid derivatives such as clofibrate and gemfibrozil, increase the risk of gallstone formation. These drugs lower blood cholesterol levels but greatly increase the level of cholesterol in the bile.
- **Age:** although gallstones have been reported from fetus to extreme old age, the average patient is 40–50 years old. Frequency of gallstone occurrence increases with age.
- **Inflammation of the gallbladder:** gallstones are present in 95% of patients who have *cholecystitis* (inflammation of the gallbladder).
- **Sunbathing:** activation of the pigmentary system by sunlight may contribute to gallstone formation. In a study of 206 white-skinned individuals, those who liked to sunbathe had twice the risk for gallstones as those who did not. Those who always burned after long sunbathing had a 25.6 times greater risk of gallstones compared with those who did not sunbathe.
- **Nutrient deficiencies:** deficiencies of either vitamin E or vitamin C have been shown to cause gallstones in experimental animals.
- **High-calorie, high-sugar, or high-fat diet:** a high intake of refined sugar is a risk factor for gallstones as well as bile duct cancer due to the effects of sugars in increasing levels of blood lipids. People with gallstones typically consume more calories, primarily as a result of refined carbohydrates (sugars) in women and fats in men.
- **A diet high in animal proteins:** animal proteins, such as casein from dairy products, have been shown to increase gallstone formation in animals while vegetable proteins, such as soy, were protective against gallstone formation.
- **Food allergies:** food allergies have been linked to gallbladder pain. In one study, 100% of allergy patients on a basic elimination diet (one containing low or no allergenic foods) were free from symptoms, while reintroduction of allergenic foods caused gallbladder attacks. The mechanism proposed to explain this association is that ingestion of allergenic

substances causes swelling of the bile ducts, resulting in impairment of bile flow from the gallbladder.

Risk factors for pigmented gallstones

- Parasitic infection of the liver and gallbladder by a variety of organisms, including the liver fluke (*Clonorchis sinesis*); common in Asia
- Chronic destruction of red blood cells (hemolysis)
- Alcoholic cirrhosis of the liver

PREVENTIVE MEASURES

- If obese, lose excessive weight gradually (0.5 kg/1 lb per week). It is important to follow the recommendations given below for increasing bile solubility.
- Do not fast or severely restrict calories.
- Identify and eliminate food allergens.
- Reduce consumption of saturated fats, cholesterol, sugar, and animal proteins.
- Avoid all fried foods.
- If you have gallstones and are of American Indian descent, reduce consumption of saponin-rich legumes (beans).
- A health-promoting diet: after identifying and removing any allergenic foods from the diet, choose a high-fiber, low-fat diet composed of whole, unprocessed, preferably organic foods, especially plant foods (fruits, vegetables, whole grains, beans, nuts [especially walnuts], and seeds), and cold-water fish (for more detailed information, see Appendix 1).
- If on estrogen replacement, or have food allergies, Crohn's disease, cystic fibrosis or other gastrointestinal disease, follow the recommendations below for increasing bile secretion and solubility.
- If on oral contraceptives, consult with a physician and choose another form of birth control.
- If fair-skinned, wear sunscreen and minimize sunbathing.
- If using cholesterol-lowering drugs, especially the fibric acid derivatives such as clofibrate and gemfibrozil, discuss other means of lowering cholesterol with a physician.
- A high-potency multiple vitamin and mineral supplement: a daily multiple providing all of the known vitamins and minerals serves as a foundation upon which to build an individualized health-promotion program. Look for a multiple containing 200 IU of vitamin E (in the form of mixed tocopherols) and 1,000 mg of vitamin C. Any good multiple should also include 400 μg of folic acid, 400 μg of vitamin B_{12}, and 50–100 mg of vitamin B_6. (Folic acid supplementation should always be accompanied by vitamin B_{12} supplementation to prevent folic acid from masking a vitamin B_{12} deficiency.)

Expected outcomes

- Gallstones are easier to prevent than reverse. In most cases, a healthy diet rich in dietary fiber, especially if combined with reducing the controllable risk factors noted above, will prevent gallstone formation.
- Once gallstones have formed, avoiding aggravating foods and employing the recommendations below that increase the solubility of cholesterol in bile may result in symptom-free gallstones. While the chance of experiencing symptoms is cumulative – 10% at 5 years, 15% at 10 years, and 18% at 15 years – if controllable risk factors are eliminated or reduced, a person with a silent gallstone should never experience discomfort.
- Several non-surgical alternatives for the treatment of gallstones now exist and are described below; however, these therapies often take several years.
- If symptoms persist or worsen, surgical removal of the gallbladder should be considered.

TREATMENT

Diet

- Follow the high-fiber, low-fat diet described above in Preventive Measures.
- Increase intake of vegetables, fruits, and dietary fiber, especially the gel-forming or mucilaginous fibers (flaxseed, oat bran, guar gum, pectin, etc.)
- Reduce consumption of saturated fats, cholesterol, sugar, and animal proteins.
- Avoid all fried foods.
- Drink 6–8 glasses of water each day to maintain the water content of bile.
- Coffee, decaffeinated as well as regular, induces gallbladder contractions, so should be avoided until gallstones are resolved.
- **Caution:** if you have gallstones, do not try an olive oil "liver flush":
  - consuming a large quantity of oil will result in contraction of the gallbladder, which may increase the likelihood of a stone blocking the bile duct. This may result in an immediate need for surgery to prevent death.
  - oleic acid, the main component of olive oil, has been shown to increase the development of gallstones in rabbits and rats by increasing the content of cholesterol in the gallbladder.

Nutritional supplements

- **Vitamin C:** deficiencies of vitamin C have been shown to cause gallstones in animal studies. Supplementation with 2,000 mg q.d. has produced positive effects on bile composition and reduced cholesterol stone formation; dosage: 500–1,000 mg t.i.d.

- **Vitamin E:** deficiencies of vitamin E have also been shown to cause gallstones in animal studies; dosage: 200–400 IU mixed tocopherols q.d.
- **Phosphatidylcholine (lecithin):** increasing the lecithin content of bile increases the solubility of cholesterol in the bile:
  - **note:** the level of cholesterol in the bile does not correlate with total cholesterol levels in the blood. Higher levels of high density lipoprotein cholesterol do not signify more soluble bile, nor does a higher low density lipoprotein cholesterol level signify less soluble cholesterol in the bile. Increased serum triglyceride levels, however, are associated with less soluble bile.
  - dosage: 100 mg t.i.d.
- **Lipotropic factors:** lipotropic factors, such as choline and methionine, hasten the removal or decrease the deposition of fat in the liver:
  - dosage: choline: 1,000 mg q.d.; L-methionine: 1,000 mg q.d.
- **Fiber supplement (guar gum, pectin, psyllium, oat bran):** minimum of 5 g q.d.
- **Bile acids** (combination of *ursodeoxycholic* and *chenodeoxycholic* acid): bile acids promote increased cholesterol solubility and have been used to chemically dissolve gallstones. However, this often takes several years and is associated with mild diarrhea and possible liver damage:
  - ursodeoxycholic acid, alone or in combination with chenodeoxycholic acid, appears to be more effective and has fewer side effects than chenodeoxycholic acid.
  - combined therapy with plant terpenes (see Botanical medicines below) appears to give the best results, and allows for a lower dosage of bile acids.
  - dosage: 1,000-1,500 mg q.d.

Botanical medicines

- **Gallstone-dissolving formula:** the following combination of plant terpenes has been shown to effectively dissolve gallstones and to be safe even when used for up to 4 years:
  - menthol: 30 mg
  - menthone: 5 mg

  - pinene: 15 mg
  - borneol: 5 mg
  - camphene: 5 mg
  - cineole: 2 mg
  - citral: 5 mg
  - dosage: 1–2 capsules (0.2 ml/capsule) t.i.d. between meals
  - peppermint oil in an enteric-coated capsule can be used instead of the above formula.
- **Terpenes:** although terpenes have been found to be effective when used alone, the best results have been achieved when they were used in combination with oral bile acids (see Nutritional supplements above).
- **Herbal choleretics:** choleretics increase bile secretion by the liver. Choleretics appropriate to use in the treatment of gallstones include extracts of:
  - *Silybum marianum* (milk thistle): may offer the greatest benefit of all the choleretic herbs:
    - dosage depends upon the level of silymarin in the product and should be sufficient to yield 70–210 mg of silymarin q.d.
  - *Taraxacum officinale* (dandelion): choose one of the following forms and take the recommended dosage t.i.d.:
    - dried root: 4 g
    - fluid extract (1 : 1): 4–8 ml
    - solid extract (4 : 1): 250–500 mg.
  - *Cynara scolymus* (artichoke):
    - dosage: extract containing 15% cynarin, 500 mg t.i.d.
  - *Curcuma longa* (turmeric): use turmeric liberally as a spice:
    - dosage: curcumin extract, 300 mg t.i.d.
  - *Peumus boldo* (boldo): choose one of the following forms and take the recommended dosage t.i.d.:
    - dried leaves or by infusion: 250–500 mg
    - tincture (1 : 10): 2–4 ml
    - fluid extract (1 : 1): 0.5–1.0 ml.

Drug–herb interaction cautions
- ***Taraxacum officinale* (dandelion root):**
  - plus *lithium*: enhanced sodium excretion from the diuretic effect of the roots and leaves (in rats) may cause sodium depletion, which then might worsen lithium toxicity.

Glaucoma

DESCRIPTION

Glaucoma is a condition of increased pressure within the eye, which results when the flow of fluid that normally drains into and out of the eye (the aqueous humor) is obstructed. Normal *intraocular pressure* (pressure within the eye) is 10–21 mmHg. In chronic glaucoma, intraocular pressure is usually mildly to moderately elevated at 22–40 mmHg. In acute glaucoma, intraocular pressure is greater than 40 mmHg. If untreated, even mild elevation in intraocular pressure can damage the optic nerve, causing loss of vision.

Glaucoma is a major cause of blindness in adults. Approximately two million people in the United States have glaucoma, 25% of which is undetected. Ninety percent is of the chronic type. Nearly 2% of people over age 40 have glaucoma, and by age 70, over 10% have glaucoma. Although vision is typically not permanently impaired if glaucoma is treated, glaucoma is a serious condition that requires strict attention. Since chronic glaucoma causes no pain, and persons with glaucoma sometimes have no symptoms, it is important that regular eye examinations be included in an annual checkup after the age of 60. Acute glaucoma is a medical emergency. Unless adequately treated within 12–48 hours, an individual with acute glaucoma will become permanently blind within 2–5 days. Anyone showing signs of glaucoma should consult an ophthalmologist immediately.

FREQUENT SIGNS AND SYMPTOMS

Acute glaucoma
- Increased pressure within the eye (intraocular), usually on one side only
- Severe throbbing pain in the eye with markedly blurred vision
- Pupil moderately dilated and fixed
- Nausea and vomiting is common

Chronic glaucoma
Early stages:
- usually no symptoms apparent in the initial stages
- persistent elevation of the pressure within the eye
- loss of peripheral vision in small areas, gradually resulting in tunnel vision
- blurred vision on one side toward the nose.

Advanced stages:
- larger areas of vision loss, usually in both eyes
- hard eyeball
- halos frequently seen around electric lights
- vague visual disturbances accompanied by mild headaches
- blind spots
- trouble adapting vision from light to dark
- poor night vision.

CAUSES

- **Poor collagen integrity and function:** collagen is the most abundant protein in the body, including the eye. In the eye, it provides support and integrity to all eye structures. When collagen structures weaken, the eyeball is not properly supported, the flow of aqueous humor is blocked, and intraocular pressure becomes elevated.
- **Corticosteroid drugs, such as prednisone (prednisolone):** these drugs, used in severe allergic and inflammatory conditions, weaken collagen structures throughout the body.
- **Frequent medication use:** drugs such as cold and allergy pills, antihistamines, tranquilizers, and remedies for stomach and intestinal problems increase intraocular pressure.

RISK INCREASES WITH

- **Corticosteroid drugs:** these drugs weaken collagen structures throughout the body, including in the eye.
- **Medications:** frequent use of medications that increase intraocular pressure (see Causes above).
- **Diabetes mellitus:** high blood sugar levels damage the collagen structures of the eye.
- **Increasing age:** adults over 60 should have annual eye examinations.

PREVENTIVE MEASURES

- Unless medically necessary, do not use corticosteroid drugs or medications that raise intraocular pressure.
- Consume a diet rich in fresh fruits and vegetables, especially those high in vitamin C and flavonoids. Flavonoids also exert numerous beneficial effects on collagen. Berries are the best sources of flavonoids. Citrus fruits, strawberries, broccoli, tomatoes, red peppers, and spinach are all good sources of vitamin C.
- Regular consumption of cold-water fish (e.g., salmon, mackerel, herring, halibut) because of their high content of omega-3 fatty acids. Omega-3 fats have been shown to lower intraocular pressure, probably via the same mechanisms by which they lower blood pressure.

Expected outcomes

Treatment should halt progression of symptoms. Glaucoma may improve slowly within 6 months to 1 year.

TREATMENT

Diet

- **Identify and eliminate any food allergens:** exposure to a food or environmental allergen has been shown to result in an immediate rise in intraocular pressure of up to 20 mmHg, in addition to other symptoms of allergy. Chronic glaucoma has been successfully treated by eliminating allergies (follow the guidelines given in the chapter on Food allergies).
- **A diet rich in fresh fruits and vegetables, especially those high in vitamin C and flavonoids:** berries are the best sources of flavonoids. Citrus fruits, strawberries, broccoli, tomatoes, red peppers, and spinach are all good sources of vitamin C.
- **Regular consumption of cold-water fish:** (e.g. salmon, mackerel, herring, halibut) because of their high content of omega-3 fatty acids. Omega-3 oils lower intraocular pressure, most likely via the same mechanisms by which they lower blood pressure.

Nutritional supplements

- **Vitamin C:** optimal tissue concentrations of vitamin C are essential for improving collagen integrity. Vitamin C has demonstrated effectiveness in lowering intraocular pressure in many clinical studies, even in patients who were unresponsive to common glaucoma drugs:
  - in one study, 500 mg of vitamin C per kg (2.2 lb) of body weight reduced intraocular pressure in patients with glaucoma an average of 16 mmHg.
  - dosage: minimum of 2,000 mg q.d. in divided doses (effective dosage may be as high as 35 g q.d.).

- **Bioflavonoids (mixed):** bioflavonoid supplementation, particularly with *anthocyanosides* (the blue-red pigments found in berries), enhances the effects of vitamin C, improves capillary integrity, and stabilizes the collagen matrix by preventing free radical damage, inhibiting enzymes from cleaving the collagen matrix, and directly cross-linking with collagen fibers to form a more stable collagen matrix:
  - dosage: 1,000 mg q.d.
- **Magnesium:** Nature's calcium-channel blocker, magnesium relaxes the arteries and improves blood supply in a manner similar to the channel blocker drugs used in the treatment of glaucoma:
  - in one study, after 4 weeks of supplementation with magnesium, both the blood supply and visual field improved in glaucoma patients.
  - dosage: 200–600 mg q.d.
- **Chromium:** chromium increases the sensitivity of cells' insulin receptors to blood sugar. When insulin receptors do not function properly, as is the case in diabetes, sugar stays in the blood, causing blood sugar levels to rise. High blood sugar levels are very damaging to the collagen structures of the eye, which is why diabetics are at greater risk for glaucoma:
  - in a study of 400 patients, deficiencies of either vitamin C or chromium were associated with elevated intraocular pressure.
  - dosage: 200–400 µg q.d.
- **Flaxseed oil:** flaxseed is the richest vegetable source of omega-3 oils. Animal studies suggest that omega-3 oils may lower intraocular pressure via the same mechanisms by which they lower blood pressure:
  - dosage: 1 tbsp q.d. Flaxseed oil should be sold in an opaque container, kept refrigerated, and should not be heated.

Botanical medicines

- ***Vaccinium myrtillus* (bilberry) extract:** European bilberry is especially rich in the flavonoid and anthocyanidin compounds that improve collagen integrity:
  - dosage: bilberry extract (25% anthocyanidin content): 80 mg t.i.d.
- ***Ginkgo biloba* extract:** *Ginkgo* also contains flavonoid compounds that improve collagen integrity:
  - dosage: *Ginkgo* extract (24% ginkgo flavonglycosides): 40–80 mg t.i.d.

Drug–herb interaction cautions

- *Ginkgo biloba*:
  - plus *aspirin*: may induce spontaneous bleeding when combined with chronic use of aspirin. Increased bleeding potential reported after *Ginkgo biloba* usage in a chronic user (2 years) of aspirin.

Gout

DESCRIPTION

A common type of arthritis, with onset typically involving the first joint of the big toe, gout is due to an increased concentration of *uric acid* in biological fluids. Uric acid is the end product of the metabolism of *purine*, one of the nucleic acid units in DNA and RNA. In gout, uric acid crystals (*monosodium urate*) deposit in joints, tendons, kidneys, and other tissues, causing considerable inflammation and damage. Kidney involvement may lead to kidney failure.

The first attack of gout, although usually involving only one joint, is characterized by intense pain. The first joint of the big toe is afflicted in 50% of initial attacks and is involved at some time in over 90% of individuals with gout. First attacks usually occur at night and are typically preceded by a specific event, such as dietary excess, alcohol consumption, trauma, certain drugs (mainly chemotherapy drugs, certain diuretics, and high doses of niacin), or surgery. Fever and chills often appear as the attack progresses. Subsequent attacks are the norm, with most gout patients experiencing another attack within 1 year. However, nearly 7% never have a second attack, and chronic gout is extremely rare today, due to dietary therapy and drugs that lower uric acid levels. Nearly 90% of subjects with gout experience some degree of kidney dysfunction as a result of uric acid deposits, and the risk for kidney stones is also increased. Gout affects both sexes but is 20 times more prevalent in men than in women.

FREQUENT SIGNS AND SYMPTOMS

- Sudden onset of severe pain in the inflamed joint, usually the base of the big toe but may involve other large joints such as the elbow, knee, hand, foot, ankle, or shoulder
- Afflicted joints are red, hot, swollen, and extremely tender and sensitive
- Skin over the affected joint is red and shiny
- Fever and chills sometimes develop as the attack progresses
- Periods without symptoms between acute attacks
- Elevated serum uric acid level

- Identification of uric acid crystals in joint fluid
- Aggregated deposits of urate crystals in and around the joints of the arms and legs, and also in subcutaneous tissue, bone, cartilage and other tissues
- Uric acid kidney stones

CAUSES

- Increased production of purines caused by:
  - idiopathic (unknown): the majority of gout patients
  - increased purine intake
  - specific enzyme defects.
- Increased production of purines due to some other factor causing excessive breakdown of cells, such as:
  - chemotherapy/cytotoxic drugs, radiation treatment
  - catabolic (tissue-destroying) or inflammatory diseases such as cancer, leukemia, polycythemia, thyroid problems, anemia, hyperlipidemia, high blood pressure, diabetes, vascular disease, psoriasis
  - excessive exercise
  - trauma, surgery.
- Decreased uric acid excretion:
  - diuretic therapy for high blood pressure: thiazide drugs
  - low-dose aspirin therapy: salicylate drugs
  - kidney disease
  - increased lactic acid production due to alcoholism, toxemia of pregnancy
  - chronic lead intoxication: in the body, lead can cause a decrease in uric acid secretion. Historically, lead-related gout (*saturnine gout*) was the result of consumption of alcoholic beverages stored in crystal decanters. Lead concentration increases with storage time, but even a few minutes in a crystal glass results in a measurable increase in the level of lead in wine.

RISK INCREASES WITH

- Use of diuretic drugs, such as furosemide and hydrochlorothiazide
- Low-dose aspirin therapy
- Alcohol consumption

- Use of some antibiotics
- Trauma, surgery
- Catabolic (tissue-destroying), inflammatory diseases (see Causes above)
- Obesity
- Men over 60
- Family history of gout
- A diet high in purine, which raises uric acid levels, e.g., alcohol, fats, refined carbohydrates, anchovies, sardines, meats (especially organ meats: sweetbreads, kidney, liver), poultry, yeast, excessive calories:
  - the dietary contribution to the blood level of uric acid is usually only 10–20% of the total, but dietary purines can tip the scales, increasing the formation of uric acid crystals in tissues.
- High doses of niacin (greater than 50 mg q.d.) or vitamin C (greater than 3,000 mg q.d.): niacin competes with uric acid for excretion. Vitamin C may increase uric acid production in a small percentage of people.

PREVENTIVE MEASURES

- Avoid use of diuretics, antibiotics, and aspirin unless medically necessary.
- Avoid known dietary triggering factors, such as heavy alcohol consumption, organ meats, excessive calories, fats, refined carbohydrates.
- Maintain a healthful weight: if overweight, go on a gradual weight-loss program (see Diet below)
- Exercise regularly, but not excessively.
- Try to drink 2 l (3 US pints) of fluid (water, diluted juice, herb teas) every day: liberal fluid intake keeps joint tissue hydrated, dilutes urine and improves kidney function.
- Avoid high doses of niacin (greater than 50 mg q.d.) and vitamin C (greater than 3,000 mg q.d.). Niacin competes with uric acid for excretion and vitamin C may increase uric acid production in a small percentage of people.
- A high-potency multiple vitamin and mineral supplement including 400 µg of folic acid, 400 µg of vitamin B_{12}, and 50–100 mg of vitamin B_6. (Folic acid supplementation should always be accompanied by vitamin B_{12} supplementation to prevent folic acid from masking a vitamin B_{12} deficiency.) A daily multiple providing all of the known vitamins and minerals serves as a foundation upon which to build an individualized health-promotion program.

Expected outcomes
The first attack may last for a few days. By following the treatment protocol given below, the uric acid level in the blood should drop, preventing any further attacks.

TREATMENT

Individuals with gout are typically obese, prone to hypertension and diabetes, and at greater risk for cardiovascular disease. Attaining ideal body weight (through a healthful, low-purine diet and moderate exercise) is the therapeutic goal that has the most impact in preventing recurrent gout. Nutritional supplements and botanical medicines are also used to prevent further attacks.

Diet
- **Eliminate alcohol:** alcohol consumption hits the gout-prone individual with a double negative whammy, often precipitating an acute attack. Alcohol accelerates purine breakdown, thus increasing uric acid production. At the same time, alcohol increases lactate production, which impairs kidney function, thus reducing uric acid excretion. For many individuals, just eliminating alcohol will reduce uric acid levels and prevent gout.
- **Eliminate foods with high purine levels:** organ meats, meats, shellfish, yeast (brewer's and baker's), herring, sardines, mackerel, and anchovies.
- **Restrict consumption of foods with moderate purine levels:** dried legumes, fish, poultry, spinach, asparagus, and mushrooms.
- **Consume a high-fiber diet:** after eliminating high-purine foods from your diet, follow a high-fiber, low-fat diet rich in whole, unprocessed, preferably organic foods, especially plant foods (fruits, vegetables, whole grains, nuts [especially walnuts], and seeds).
- **Minimize** consumption of refined carbohydrates, simple sugars, and saturated fats:
  - simple sugars (refined sugar, honey, maple syrup, corn syrup, fructose, etc.) increase uric acid production.
  - saturated fats decrease uric acid excretion.
- **Protein:** protein intake should be adequate (0.8 g/kg of body weight) but not excessive:
  - adequate protein intake provides amino acids that decrease reabsorption of uric acid in the renal (kidney) tubes, thus increasing uric acid excretion and reducing blood levels of uric acid.
  - high protein intake, however, has been shown to accelerate uric acid synthesis in both normal and gouty patients.
- **Increase** consumption of omega-3 essential fatty acids by consuming flaxseed oil (1 tbsp q.d.): flaxseed is the richest vegetable source of omega-3 oils:
  - flaxseed oil is highly perishable, and should be sold in an opaque container, kept refrigerated, and not heated.

- **Drink** at least 2 L (3 US pints) of water each day: liberal fluid intake keeps urine diluted, promotes excretion of uric acid, and reduces the risk of kidney stones.

Nutritional supplements

- **A high-potency multiple vitamin and mineral supplement:** see Preventive Measures above.
- **EPA (eicosapentaenoic acid):** an omega-3 oil, EPA limits the production of inflammatory messengers called leukotrienes, responsible for much of the inflammatory and tissue damage observed in gout; dosage: 1.8 g q.d. (or 1 tbsp of flaxseed oil q.d.).
- **Vitamin E:** vitamin E is helpful in the treatment of gout because of its anti-inflammatory effects, both as an antioxidant and via its (mild) inhibition of leukotriene production; dosage: 400–800 IU (mixed tocopherols) q.d.
- **Folic acid:** a derivative produced in the body from folic acid has been shown to inhibit *xanthine oxidase*, the enzyme responsible for the production of uric acid, even more effectively than the drug allopurinol – the most widely used drug for gout:
  - dosage: 10–40 mg q.d.
  - **caution:** high-dose folic acid therapy should only be utilized under the care of a physician. High doses of folic acid may interfere with some drugs used to treat epilepsy and may also mask the symptoms of vitamin B$_{12}$ deficiency.
- **Bromelain:** a proteolytic enzyme complex from pineapple, bromelain has demonstrated significant anti-inflammatory effects in clinical human studies and is a side-effect-free alternative to the prescription anti-inflammatory agents used to treat gout:
  - to maximize bromelain's anti-inflammatory effects, bromelain should be taken between meals to ensure its enzymes are not used in digesting food.
  - dosage: 200–400 mg b.i.d.–t.i.d. between meals.
- **Quercetin:** this flavonoid inhibits uric acid production through a mechanism similar to that of the drug allopurinol; quercetin also inhibits the manufacture of inflammatory compounds:
  - for best results, take quercetin with bromelain (which may help enhance quercetin's absorption) between meals.
  - dosage: 200–400 mg b.i.d.–t.i.d. between meals.
- **Alanine, aspartic acid, glutamic acid, glycine:** these amino acids have been shown to increase excretion of uric acid, probably by decreasing uric acid reabsorption in the renal tubule (kidney):
  - best taken via supplemental minerals like magnesium and calcium bound to aspartate (aspartic acid).
  - dosage: 1,000 mg of a magnesium–calcium aspartate supplement daily.
  - **Caution:** avoid high intake of niacin (greater than 50 mg q.d.) and vitamin C (greater than 3,000 mg q.d.). Niacin competes with uric acid for excretion and vitamin C may increase uric acid production in a small percentage of people.

Botanical medicines

- **Anthocyanidins and proanthocyanidins:** these flavonoid compounds, found in highest amounts in cherries, hawthorn berries, blueberries, and extracts of bilberry (*Vaccinium myrtillus*), grape seed (*Vitis vinifera*) and pine bark (*Pinus maritima*), have been shown to be very effective in lowering uric acid levels and preventing attacks of gout via several beneficial actions, including:
  - prevention of collagen destruction, antioxidant activity, and inhibition of leukotriene formation.
  - dosage: 225 g (8 oz) of fresh, frozen or canned cherries per day or 150–300 mg q.d. of flavonoid-rich extracts from bilberry, grape seed, or pine bark.
- ***Harpagophytum procumbens* (devil's claw):** in clinical trials, devil's claw has been found to relieve joint pain, and to reduce serum cholesterol as well as uric acid levels:
  - some animal studies suggest that devil's claw possesses an anti-inflammatory and pain-relieving effect comparable to the potent drug phenylbutazone, while other studies have shown little anti-inflammatory activity. Although further clinical research is needed to clarify these inconsistent results, devil's claw may be useful in short-term management of gout. Simple dietary changes will prevent gout over the long term in most cases.
  - dosage: choose one of the following forms and take the recommended dosage t.i.d.:
    - tincture (1 : 5): 4–5 ml
    - dry solid extract (3 : 1): 400 mg
    - dried powdered root: 1–2 g

Drug–herb interaction cautions
None.

Physical medicine
- Use warm or cold compresses on painful joints.
- Keep the weight of bedclothes off any painful joint by making a frame that raises sheets off the feet.

Hemorrhoids

DESCRIPTION

Hemorrhoids are *varicose* (abnormally large, dilated) veins in the rectum (the final portion of the digestive tube) or *anus* (the lower opening of the digestive tract through which feces are eliminated). If located inside the anal canal, hemorrhoids are classified as internal. If located at the anal opening, they are called external hemorrhoids.

In the US and other industrialized countries, hemorrhoids are extremely common. Over one-third of the total US population has hemorrhoids to some degree, and 50% of persons over age 50 have symptomatic hemorrhoidal disease. Most individuals begin to develop hemorrhoids in their 20s, but symptoms are typically not apparent until the 30s.

FREQUENT SIGNS AND SYMPTOMS

- **Rectal bleeding:**
  - bright red blood may appear on the surface of the stool, adhering as streaks on toilet paper, or as a slow trickle following bowel movements. The toilet water is almost always tinged red.
- **Pain, burning, inflammation, swelling:**
  - pain does not usually occur unless external hemorrhoids are severely inflamed.
  - since no sensory nerves are found above the *anorectal line* – the point in the 3 cm long anal canal where the skin lining changes to mucous membrane – internal hemorrhoids rarely cause pain.
- **Itching followed by mucous discharge after bowel movements:**
  - itching is rarely caused by hemorrhoids, except when internal hemorrhoids prolapse (sink down) and extrude their mucous membrane covering (hence the mucous discharge) outside the body cavity.
  - common causes of anal itching are tissue trauma from excessive use of harsh toilet paper, yeast (*Candida albicans*) or parasite infections, and food allergies.
- **Bleeding and seepage:**
  - bleeding is almost always associated with internal hemorrhoids and may occur before, during, or after defecation.

- when bleeding occurs from an external hemorrhoid, it is due to rupture of blood clots within the hemorrhoid.
- **Anemia:** bleeding hemorrhoids can produce iron-deficiency anemia due to chronic blood loss.
- **A lump** that can be felt in the anus.
- **Large hemorrhoids** may cause a sensation that the rectum has not fully emptied after a bowel movement.

CAUSES

- **A low-fiber diet, high in refined foods:**
  - hemorrhoids are rarely seen in parts of the world where diets are rich in unrefined, high-fiber foods.
  - individuals eating a low-fiber diet strain more during bowel movements since their stools are smaller, harder and more difficult to pass.
  - straining increases pressure in the abdomen, which obstructs blood flow, and intensifies pressure in the veins.
  - veins in other parts of the body contain valves that help contain increased pressure. Veins in the anal and rectal area have no valves, so factors that increase congestion and pressure more easily weaken these veins, resulting in hemorrhoid formation.

RISK INCREASES WITH

Anything that results in increased pelvic congestion or pressure in the anal or rectal veins including:
- a low-fiber diet
- prolonged sitting or standing
- obesity
- pregnancy
- constipation
- loss of muscle tone in old age
- rectal surgery or episiotomy
- liver disease
- anal intercourse
- colon malignancy
- portal hypertension (high blood pressure in the primary vein of the liver).

PREVENTIVE MEASURES

- A high-fiber diet.
- Drink 8–10 glasses of water each day.
- Avoid straining.
- Don't hurry bowel movements but avoid prolonged sitting on the toilet.
- Clean the anal area gently with soft, moist paper after each bowel movement.
- When bathing or showering, do not scrub the anal area. Cleanse gently and apply a light oil, such as sesame oil, to the area after cleansing.
- Lose weight if overweight.
- Avoid sitting or standing for prolonged periods. Get up and move around for a few minutes every hour.
- Exercise regularly to maintain muscle tone. Exercises that strengthen the abdominal muscles and, for women, Kegel exercises, which strengthen the pelvic floor, are recommended.

Expected outcomes

Hemorrhoids should shrink and symptoms abate within 2 months.

TREATMENT

Diet
- **A high-fiber diet:**
  - a diet rich in vegetables, fruits, legumes, and whole grains promotes *peristalsis* (the contractions of the intestine that propel fecal matter to the anus for evacuation).
  - many components of fiber attract water to form a gelatinous mass that keeps feces soft, bulky, and easy to pass.

Nutritional supplements
- **Bulking agents:** natural bulking compounds such as flaxseed meal, psyllium seed and guar gum possess mild laxative action due to their ability to attract water and form a soft, gelatinous stool:
  - flaxseed meal is an especially good choice as it contains beneficial anti-inflammatory essential fatty acids in addition to fiber.
  - avoid wheat bran and other cellulose-fiber products as these can irritate already inflamed tissues.
  - dosage: 1–2 tbsp q.d. Follow package directions.
- **Vitamin C:** optimal tissue concentrations of vitamin C are essential for improving collagen integrity. Collagen is the most abundant protein in the body, providing the structural tissue for all body parts, including the veins. When collagen structures weaken, the veins are much more susceptible to hemorrhoid formation:
  - dosage: 500–1,000 mg t.i.d.
- **Flavonoids:** flavonoid preparations have been shown to relieve hemorrhoids by strengthening the veins. In studies of varicose veins and hemorrhoids, a potent type of flavonoid called hydroxyethylrutosides (HER) has been of great benefit in hemorrhoids both associated and not associated with pregnancy. Rutin and citrus bioflavonoid preparations provide similar, if not as potent, benefits:
  - dosage: HER: 1,000–3,000 mg q.d.; citrus bioflavonoids, rutin, and/or hesperidin: 3,000–6,000 mg q.d.
- **Aortic glycosaminoglycans (GAGs):** supplementation with a mixture of bovine-derived GAGs, which are structural components also naturally present in the human aorta, has been shown to protect and promote normal artery and vein function:
  - in two double-blind studies of GAGs' effects on hemorrhoids and varicose veins, the aortic extract produced such good results that researchers suggested they be used as the "drug of first choice" in the non-surgical treatment of acute hemorrhoidal pain and disease.
  - dosage: 100 mg q.d.

Botanical medicines
- ***Ruscus aculeatus* (Butcher's broom):** the active components in Butcher's broom, ruscogenins, have demonstrated a wide range of pharmacological actions, including anti-inflammatory and vasoconstrictor effects. Butcher's broom is used extensively in Europe, both internally and externally, to treat varicose veins and hemorrhoids:
  - most of the clinical research has been on Butcher's broom extract in combination with vitamin C and *hesperidin* (a bioflavonoid).
  - dosage: Butcher's broom extract (9–11% ruscogenin content): 100 mg t.i.d.
- For additional botanicals, see the chapter on Varicose veins. Any of the botanical medicines discussed there will also be helpful for hemorrhoids.

Drug–herb interaction cautions
None.

Topical medicines
- Topical over-the-counter products containing natural ingredients will provide temporary relief. Look for products containing natural ingredients such as witch hazel (Hamamelis water), shark liver oil, cod liver oil, cocoa butter, Peruvian balsam, zinc oxide, live yeast cell derivative, and allantoin.

- To reduce pain and swelling of a blood clot or protruding hemorrhoid, stay in bed for 1 day and apply ice packs to the anal area.

Physical medicine

- Hydrotherapy: a warm sitz bath – a partial immersion bath for the pelvic region – may provide soothing, if short-lived relief of painful symptoms. Sit in 20–25 cm (8–10 in) of warm water (water temperature should be between 100 and 105°F) for 10–20 min several times a day.
- Placing the feet on a low footstool when sitting on the toilet will aid bowel movement.
- Regular abdominal and pelvic floor exercise will improve muscle tone, thus also aiding bowel movement.

Hepatitis

DESCRIPTION

An inflammation of the liver, hepatitis can be caused by many drugs and toxic chemicals, but in most instances, is caused by a virus. The most common hepatitis viral types are A, B, and C. Other less common viral causes of hepatitis include hepatitis viruses D, E, and G, as well as herpes simplex virus, cytomegalovirus, and Epstein–Barr virus.

Hepatitis A is transmitted primarily through fecal contamination. Groups most at risk for hepatitis A infection are international travelers, persons living in American Indian reservations or Alaska Native villages, homosexually active men, and injecting drug users. The Centers for Disease Control (CDC) estimates 125,000–200,000 infections with hepatitis A occur annually in the United States, and that 33% of Americans have evidence of past infection (immunity). Approximately two-thirds (84,000–134,000) of hepatitis infections are symptomatic. Hepatitis A typically surfaces in large nationwide outbreaks every decade or so (the last outbreak occurred in 1989). Although hepatitis A does not evolve into chronic infection, it is responsible for 100 deaths each year in the US, and prolonged or relapsing hepatitis develops in 15% of cases.

Hepatitis B, which is shed in saliva, semen and vaginal secretions, is transmitted through sexual contact and also through infected blood or blood products. Hepatitis B can live on dry surfaces for at least 7 days; it is one of the most communicable diseases and the ninth cause of death worldwide. According to the CDC, approximately 1.25 million Americans are carriers of hepatitis B; 140,000–320,000 new cases are reported each year, about half of which (70,000–160,000) are symptomatic, and 70% of which occur in individuals between the ages of 15 and 39 years. In addition, 22,000 pregnant women are infected with hepatitis B and can transmit it to their newborns. About 93% of adults who contract hepatitis B recover within 6 months, but approximately 5–10% of adults and 75–90% of children under the age of 5 years who are infected with hepatitis B are unable to clear the virus within 6 months and are considered chronically infected.

Hepatitis C is primarily blood-borne but can also be transmitted sexually and by an infected mother to her newborn. Hepatitis C is responsible for roughly 90% of all cases of hepatitis contracted through blood transfusions. In the past, before the blood supply was checked for hepatitis, approximately 10% of persons receiving blood transfusions developed hepatitis C. Now, only 4% of hepatitis C cases are the result of transfusions; 60% of cases are due to illegal intravenous drug use. According to the CDC, 3.9 million Americans have been infected with hepatitis C, of whom 2.7 million are chronically infected. Of this group, 70% will develop serious liver damage, and 20–30% of these will develop liver cancer or liver failure requiring a liver transplant. Hepatitis C contributes to the deaths of 8,000–10,000 Americans each year, a much higher mortality toll than other forms of hepatitis, and one that is expected to triple by 2010 and exceed the number of annual deaths due to AIDS.

FREQUENT SIGNS AND SYMPTOMS

As noted above, a large percentage of hepatitis infections are asymptomatic.

Early stages
Symptoms occur 2 weeks to 1 month before liver involvement, depending upon the virus' incubation period.
- Flu-like symptoms
- Fatigue
- Intermittent nausea
- Abdominal pain
- Vomiting
- Loss of appetite

Several days later
- Jaundice (yellow eyes and skin) caused by a buildup of bile in the blood
- Dark urine due to elevated bilirubin levels
- Light, "clay-colored" whitish stools
- Tender, enlarged liver
- Fever

Laboratory findings
- Normal-to-low white blood cell count
- Markedly elevated liver enzymes (enzymes such as SGPT, GGPT, SGOT, and alkaline phosphatase leak into the blood when liver cells are damaged)

- The type of virus is determined by identifying viral antigens (compounds recognized as being foreign to the body), or antibodies (defensive molecules specifically developed by the immune system to bind to the antigens).

Chronic Hepatitis B or C
- Symptoms may be virtually non-existent
- Chronic fatigue
- Serious liver damage, including cirrhosis of the liver or liver cancer
- Chronic hepatitis B infection is monitored by continued blood evaluation of antibody levels
- Hepatitis C is monitored, in addition to liver enzymes, by the presence of the hepatitis C viral-RNA by polymerase chain reaction. The higher the level of HCV-RNA, the more aggressive the chronic infection.

CAUSES

- **Types A and E:** poor sanitation; consumption of water or food, especially raw shellfish, which has been contaminated by sewage.
- **Type B:** usually sexually transmitted through contact with the body fluids of an infected person, through contaminated blood transfusions, or from injections with non-sterile needles or syringes. An infected mother can pass it on to her newborn.
- **Type C:** usually transmitted through intravenous drug use, blood transfusions and other exposures to contaminated blood and blood products. In 40% of cases, mode of transmission is unknown.
- **Type D:** always associated with hepatitis B infection.
- **Type G:** usually blood-borne, similar to Type C.

RISK INCREASES WITH

Hepatitis A
- Travel to areas with poor sanitation or regions with endemic hepatitis A (American Indian reservations, Alaska Native villages)
- Children of immigrants from disease-endemic areas
- During outbreaks – day care centers or residential programs
- Poor nutrition
- Lowered resistance due to other illness

Hepatitis B and C
- Children of immigrants from disease-endemic areas
- Infants born to infected mothers
- Health care workers – hospital, dental

- Heterosexuals with multiple sex partners
- Homosexually active men
- Oral–anal sexual practices
- Injecting drug users
- Hemodialysis (kidney dialysis) patients
- Poor nutrition
- Lowered resistance due to other illness

Hepatitis C
- Blood transfusions before July 1992
- Recipient of clotting factors made before 1987

PREVENTIVE MEASURES

- When possible, avoid risks listed above.
- Vaccination: recommended for individuals in high-risk occupations, such as members of the medical and dental field who are regularly exposed to blood and other body fluids, and individuals traveling to disease-endemic areas or areas with poor sanitation.
- HBIG (hyperimmune globulin) injection: in the case of acute exposure to hepatitis B (HBV), HBIG – a concentrated solution of immune globulins specific to HBV – is administered by injection. HBIG confers immediate but short-lived (3 months) immunity. Two doses given within 2 weeks of exposure confer protective immunity in 75% of exposed individuals.
- Newborns whose mothers are positive for hepatitis surface antigen (HBsAG) should receive HBIG vaccine (0.5 ml) shortly after birth, at 3 months, and at 6 months.
- Anyone sexually exposed to someone with hepatitis should seek medical advice about receiving HBIG injections.
- If suffering from hepatitis or caring for someone with hepatitis, hands should be washed carefully and often, especially after bowel movements.
- An individual with hepatitis should have separate eating and drinking utensils or use disposable ones.

Expected outcomes

Acute hepatitis
- Acute viral hepatitis can be an extremely debilitating disease requiring bed rest.
- Jaundice and other symptoms peak and then gradually disappear over 3–16 weeks.
- Most people in good general health recover completely in 1–4 months (usually by 9 weeks for type A and 16 weeks for types B, C, D, and G). However, liver failure, cirrhosis of the liver, liver cancer, and even death are possible outcomes.

■ Death occurs in approximately $1:100$ infected individuals.

Chronic hepatitis

■ Currently, 10% of hepatitis B and 10–40% hepatitis C cases develop into chronic hepatitis.

■ Hepatitis C contracted from a transfusion is associated with a 70–80% chance of developing into chronic hepatitis.

■ Persons with chronic hepatitis may look well and not realize they are infected, but they are potentially infectious carriers to their household and sexual contacts.

TREATMENT

Diet

Acute phase

■ Do not drink alcohol. Alcohol stresses detoxification processes and can lead to liver damage and immune suppression.

■ Ensure adequate fluid intake by consuming a minimum of 8 glasses of fluid per day: water, vegetable broths, diluted vegetable juices (diluted by half with water), herbal teas.

■ Restrict solid foods to brown rice, steamed vegetables, and moderate intake of lean protein sources, e.g., legumes, fish.

Chronic Phase

■ **Avoid:**
  ▪ alcohol – the most common cause of impaired liver function.
  ▪ saturated fats (animal products) – these increase the risk of fatty infiltration of the liver or cholestasis, a condition in which the excretion of bile (a carrier substance for toxins) is inhibited.
  ▪ simple carbohydrates (sugar, white flour, [processed foods containing sugar and/or white flour], fruit juice, honey, maple syrup, etc.) – simple carbohydrates suppress immune function.
  ▪ oxidized fatty acids (fried foods, refined oils) – these damaged fats cause cellular damage and contribute to cholestasis
  ▪ foods containing iron – hepatitis C combines with iron molecules to form potent free radicals that seriously damage liver cells.

■ **Choose:**
  ▪ a high-fiber diet based on plant foods (for more information, see Appendix 1).
  ▪ foods rich in factors that help protect the liver from damage and improve liver function, including:
    ● high-sulfur content foods – garlic, legumes, onions, eggs
    ● foods containing water-soluble fibers – pears, oat bran, apples, legumes
    ● cabbage-family vegetables – broccoli, Brussels sprouts, cabbage
    ● artichokes, beets, carrots, dandelion
    ● herbs and spices – turmeric, cinnamon, licorice

Nutritional supplements

■ **A high-potency, iron-free, multiple vitamin and mineral supplement:**
  ▪ includes antioxidant vitamins such as vitamin C, beta-carotene, and vitamin E, which help protect the liver from damage.
  ▪ includes B vitamins, calcium and trace minerals, which are critical in the elimination of toxic compounds from the body.
  ▪ is iron-free: iron promotes hepatitis-induced liver injury.
  ▪ for more detailed information see Appendix 2.

■ **Vitamin C:** Robert Cathcart MD has demonstrated, and other studies have confirmed, that high doses of vitamin C (40–100 g q.d. IV) greatly diminish acute viral hepatitis in 2–4 days, with jaundice clearing within 6 days:
  ▪ when hospitalized patients (at higher risk for exposure to hepatitis) received 2 g of vitamin C q.d., they did not develop hepatitis, while 7% of the control patients (who received less than 1.5 g q.d.) did.
  ▪ dosage: 1,000 mg t.i.d. (in acute cases: IV vitamin C, 50–100 g q.d.).

■ **Selenium:** a cofactor in the production of glutathione (a critically important antioxidant and detoxifying agent in liver cells), selenium has been shown to reduce the incidence of hepatitis B and C:
  ▪ epidemiological studies: in areas of China with high rates of hepatitis B and primary liver cancer, high levels of dietary selenium significantly (35%) reduced hepatitis B infection and liver cancer incidence (in a group of 226 hepatitis B positive people, selenium supplementation reduced liver cancer incidence to zero).
  ▪ animal studies: selenium supplementation reduced hepatitis B infection by 77.2% and precancerous liver lesions by 75.8%.
  ▪ dosage: 200 µg b.i.d.–t.i.d.

■ **N-acetylcysteine (NAC):** an amino acid that, along with selenium, is a key component of glutathione; dosage: 600 mg t.i.d.

■ **Alpha-lipoic acid:** alpha-lipoic acid is an extremely powerful antioxidant that scavenges hydroxyl radicals (the most dangerous type of free radicals found in the body), chelates (binds and removes) heavy metals, recycles other antioxidants, and induces significantly increased intracellular levels of glutathione:

- in recent studies, when alpha-lipoic acid was added to various types of animal and human cells in tissue culture, including liver and kidney cells, it caused a 30–70% increase in cellular glutathione levels.
- dosage: 250 mg b.i.d.

■ **Liver extracts:** numerous scientific investigations into the therapeutic effectiveness of liver extracts have demonstrated that they promote liver regeneration and are very effective in treating chronic liver disease, including hepatitis; dosage: 500–1,000 mg crude polypeptides q.d.

■ **Thymus extracts:** thymus extract induces broad-spectrum immune enhancement via improving the activity of the thymus gland, the master gland of the immune system:

- in several double-blind studies of acute and chronic type B viral hepatitis, thymus extracts produced accelerated decreases of liver enzymes, elimination of the virus, and a higher rate of formation of anti-HBe (the antibody against hepatitis B), signifying clinical remission.
- dosage: equivalent to 120 mg pure polypeptides with molecular weights less than 10,000 or roughly 750 mg of the crude polypeptide fraction q.d.

Botanical medicines

■ *Glycyrrhiza glabra* **(licorice):** licorice exerts a variety of beneficial actions in chronic as well as acute hepatitis treatment, including: protecting the liver; enhancing the immune system; boosting interferon (the body's own antiviral and immune-enhancing agent); and promoting the flow of bile to and from the liver:

- dosage: choose one of the following forms and take the recommended dosage t.i.d.:
  - powdered root: 1–2 g
  - fluid extract (1 : 1): 2–4 ml
  - solid (dry powdered) extract (5% glycyrrhetinic acid content): 250–500 mg.
- caution: in susceptible individuals, licorice has blood pressure elevating effects:
  - adverse effects are rarely seen at levels below 100 mg q.d., but are common at levels above 400 mg q.d.
  - prevention of side effects may be possible by following a high-potassium, low-sodium diet. Patients who normally consume high-potassium foods and restrict sodium intake, even those

with high blood pressure and angina, are typically free from the blood pressure elevation side effects of licorice.

- to ensure safety, licorice should probably not be used by patients with a history of hypertension or renal failure, or who are currently using digitalis preparations.
- if licorice is used in treatment of chronic hepatitis, intake of potassium-rich foods must be increased.

■ *Silybum marianum* **(milk thistle):** milk thistle contains *silymarin*, a mixture of flavonoids that is one of the most potent liver-protecting substances known. Silymarin has been found to be dramatically effective in reversing liver damage and in treating both acute and chronic hepatitis. Silymarin inhibits liver damage by:

- acting as a direct antioxidant and free radical scavenger
- increasing intracellular levels of glutathione and superoxide dismutase, two critically important liver antioxidants and detoxifying agents
- inhibiting the formation of leukotrienes (agents that promote inflammation and free radical generation)
- increasing bile flow
- stimulating liver cell regeneration
- dosage: best results are achieved at higher doses – 140–210 mg of a standardized extract of silymarin t.i.d.

■ **Silymarin phytosome:** research indicates that this new form of silymarin, which is bound to phosphatidylcholine, is better absorbed and produces better and more rapid clinical results than unbound silymarin; dosage for silymarin phytosome is 120 mg b.i.d.–t.i.d. between meals.

Drug–herb interaction cautions

■ *Glycyrrhiza glabra* **(licorice):**

- plus *digoxin, digitalis*: due to a reduction of potassium in the blood, licorice enhances the toxicity of cardiac glycosides. Interaction with these cardioglycoside drugs could lead to arrhythmias and cardiac arrest.
- plus *stimulant laxatives or diuretics* (thiazides, spironolactone or amiloride): licorice should not be used with these drugs because of the additive increase of potassium loss to potentially dangerous levels.

Herpes simplex

DESCRIPTION

Herpes simplex, a virus responsible for recurrent eruptions of small, usually painful blisters – often called "cold sores" when they appear around the mouth or on the lips, and lesions when they appear on the genitals or adjacent areas – is quite common in the US, with 20% of Americans experiencing recurrent herpes simplex virus (HSV) infections. Two types of HSV have been distinguished: HSV-1 and HSV-2.

HSV-1 is the strain responsible for oral herpes, and, although HSV-2 is the more frequent culprit in genital herpes, HSV-1 is also the cause of 10–40% of genital herpes cases. Both HSV-1 and HSV-2 can be transmitted by sexual contact, with crossinfection of both types most likely occurring during oral–genital sex. In addition to sexual transmission, exposure to HSV-1 can occur during kissing, and by eating or drinking from contaminated utensils.

Initial HSV-1 infection usually occurs in childhood, is not considered a sexually transmitted disease, and is extremely common: approximately 85% of adults have been exposed to HSV-1. Twenty-five percent of the US population has been exposed to HSV-2, which is considered a sexually transmitted disease. The risk of herpes infection after sexual contact with an individual with active herpes lesions is estimated to be 75%. Worldwide, 86 million people are thought to have genital herpes.

After the initial infection, the virus lies dormant in nerve cells but can be reactivated and cause recurring outbreaks. Recurrent attacks may be rare or so frequent they seem continuous. Men seem more susceptible to recurrences, although repeat infections in men are usually milder and of shorter duration than those in women. Reactivation is usually triggered by minor infections, trauma, stress, fatigue, menstruation or sun exposure. Genital lesions caused by HSV-1 have a recurrence rate of 14%, while in those due to HSV-2 the recurrence rate is 60%.

In women, the herpes virus has been implicated as a cause of cancer of the cervix, especially when human papilloma virus (the virus responsible for genital warts), is also present. During childbirth, active herpes on the genitals or in the birth canal can result in transmission of life-threatening systemic (whole body) herpes to the newborn.

Herpes is also a serious threat to a person whose immune system is compromised due to illness (e.g., AIDS, cancer) or who must take drugs that suppress the immune system (e.g., chemotherapy, radiation therapy, or high dose cortisone preparations). In these individuals, herpes may produce life-threatening infections in various organs including the liver (herpetic hepatitis) and brain (encephalitis).

FREQUENT SIGNS AND SYMPTOMS

Oral and genital herpes
- Itching, burning, tingling, and/or irritation often precede blister eruption.
- Incubation period is 2–12 days, averaging 7, after exposure to HSV, although sometimes HSV infection is acquired with no symptoms, and the outbreak delayed.
- Single or multiple clusters of painful, small red bumps appear about the mouth and lips or in the genital and rectal areas.
- The mouth can be a site of infection in both sexes.
- Ulcerated sores typically heal in 7–10 days, but may last up to 3 weeks.
- Regional lymph nodes may be tender and swollen.

Genital herpes
- In men, blisters appear on the shaft and head of the penis, scrotum, inner thighs, and anus.
- In women, blisters appear on the labia, but may extend into the vagina to the cervix and urethra, or may appear on the anus and inner thighs.
- Bumps change into water-filled blisters that eventually rupture, forming shallow painful ulcers with yellow crusts.
- During the first outbreak of genital herpes, headache, fever, swollen lymph nodes, general achiness, and decreased appetite – as well as localized symptoms in the area of blister eruption – are common.
- Pain and tenderness in the groin area.
- In men, difficult, painful urination, especially if the lesion is near the opening of the urethra.
- Women may also develop painful urination and/or vaginal discharge in genital herpes.

- Urinary frequency or urgency.
- Incontinence.
- Painful sexual intercourse.

CAUSES

- Oral herpes is caused by infection with herpes simplex virus type 1 (HSV-1):
  - HSV-1 can be transmitted during kissing, and by eating or drinking from contaminated utensils.
- Genital herpes is more frequently caused by HSV-2, but may also be due to HSV-1:
  - genital herpes is transmitted via contact with a sexual partner who has active herpes lesions. Lesions may be on the genitals, lips, mouth, or hands.

RISK INCREASES WITH

- Serious illness that has lowered resistance
- Use of drugs that suppress the immune system (anticancer drugs, cortisone preparations)
- Stress – diminishes immune response, increasing susceptibility to primary infection or recurrence. Stressors can be:
  - *emotional*: stress places heavy demands on the adrenal glands, which respond by releasing glucocorticoid hormones (cortisol, corticosterone, cortisone), all of which suppress immune function
  - *dietary*: a diet high in sugars, refined foods, and/or arginine-rich foods (see Preventive Measures and Diet below)
  - *environmental*: sunbathing, excessive exercise, fatigue.
- Minor infection of some other type, e.g., cold, flu, toothache, dental disease
- Genital trauma
- Menstruation
- Smoking
- Disease-promoting diet: immune function is directly related to the quality of the foods routinely ingested. A diet based on processed foods, with little consumption of fresh vegetables, legumes, fruits, whole grains, and cold-water fish is low in the factors necessary for effective immune response – antioxidants, vitamin and mineral cofactors, essential fatty acids, magnesium and potassium – and high in factors that suppress immunity – sugars, refined carbohydrates, saturated and *trans* fats, and chemical additives.

PREVENTIVE MEASURES

- **Avoid** sexual contact when genital blisters or sores are present.
- **Avoid** kissing or oral sexual contact when cold sores are present.
- **Avoid** sexual contact when experiencing genital itching, burning, tingling, or irritation, as this often precedes blister eruption.
- **Intercourse:** use a rubber condom during intercourse if either partner has inactive genital herpes, especially if an infected partner has frequent recurrences.
- **Pregnancy:** if pregnant, tell your doctor if you have had herpes or any genital lesions in the past, so precautions can be taken to prevent infection in your baby.
- **Don't smoke**
- **Minimize consumption of sugars, and refined foods:** consuming 75 g (3 oz) of sugar in one sitting in any form (sucrose, honey, fruit juice) depresses white (immune) cell activity by 50% for 1–5 hours.
- **Minimize consumption of arginine-rich foods:** chocolate, peanuts, seeds, almonds and other nuts. HSV needs arginine to replicate.
- **Increase consumption of lysine-rich foods:** most vegetables, legumes, fish, turkey, and chicken. Lysine suppresses HSV replication.
- **Diet/lifestyle:** take this opportunity to choose diet (see Diet below) and lifestyle practices (regular exercise, adequate sleep, meditation, prayer, counseling, etc.) that enhance your immune system's ability to respond effectively to stress.
- **Take a daily multiple vitamin and mineral supplement:** a deficiency of virtually any nutrient can render the body more susceptible to infection. A high-potency daily multiple providing all of the known vitamins and minerals serves as a foundation upon which to build an individualized health-promotion program. Any good multiple should include 400 µg of folic acid, 400 µg of vitamin B_{12}, and 50–100 mg of vitamin B_6. (Folic acid supplementation should always be accompanied by vitamin B_{12} supplementation to prevent folic acid from masking a vitamin B_{12} deficiency.)
- **Consume a nutrient-dense diet** rich in whole, unprocessed, preferably organic foods, especially plant foods (fruits, vegetables, beans, whole grains), and cold-water fish (for more detailed information, see Appendix 1).

Expected outcomes

While HSV infection is currently incurable, recurrence of symptoms can be significantly reduced (once a year or even less).

TREATMENT

Diet
- **High-lysine/low-arginine diet:** *in vitro* (test tube) studies have shown that HSV replication requires the manufacture of proteins rich in the amino acid *arginine*, and that arginine stimulates HSV replication, particularly when levels of the amino acid *lysine* are low. In addition, lysine has been shown to suppress HSV replication:
  - *foods high in arginine*: chocolate, peanuts, seeds, almonds and other nuts.
  - *foods high in lysine*: most vegetables, legumes, fish, turkey, and chicken.

Nutritional supplements
- **Vitamin C:** vitamin C stimulates white cells to fight infection and directly kills many bacteria and viruses. Vitamin C's main claim to fame is its many different immune-enhancing effects, including white blood cell response and function, increasing levels of interferon (a special chemical factor that fights viral infection and cancer), and increasing secretion of hormones from the thymus gland (the major gland of the immune system):
  - both oral consumption and topical application (see below) of vitamin C have been shown to significantly increase the rate of healing of herpes lesions.
  - dosage: 500 mg every 2 hours during initial stages of active infection; 2,000 mg q.d. during later stages and to prevent recurrence.
- **Bioflavonoids:** a group of plant pigments largely responsible for the colors of fruits and flowers, bioflavonoids are powerful antioxidants in their own right and, when taken with vitamin C, significantly enhance its absorption and effectiveness; dosage: 1,000 mg q.d.
- **Vitamin A:** known as the "anti-infective vitamin", vitamin A plays an essential role in immune function by: (1) maintaining the surfaces of the skin, respiratory tract, and gastrointestinal tract and their secretions – all of which constitute a defensive barrier against micro-organisms; (2) stimulating and/or enhancing numerous immune processes, including white blood cell function and antibody response; (3) direct antiviral activity; (4) preventing immune suppression due to stress-induced adrenal hormones, severe burns and surgery. Some of these latter effects are likely due to vitamin A's ability to prevent stress-induced shrinkage of the thymus gland and to promote thymus growth:
  - preliminary laboratory data suggest vitamin A directly inhibits HSV replication. Low serum concentrations of vitamin A have been correlated with a much higher incidence of HSV shedding (38%) versus normal (less than 2%).
  - dosage: 10,000 IU q.d.; *should not be taken by pregnant women.*
- **Zinc:** involved in vitamin A function, wound healing, immune system activity, inflammation control, and tissue regeneration, zinc boosts immunity by increasing circulating lymphocytes and antibody production:
  - dosage: 50 mg q.d. when infection is active, 30 mg q.d. when infection is dormant.
  - **caution:** long-term use of high amounts of zinc can suppress immune function. Do not take 50 mg q.d. for longer than 2 weeks at a time, then use 30 mg q.d. for 2 months before resuming a daily 50 mg q.d. dose if needed.
- **Lysine:** several double-blind studies have shown that low levels of lysine encourage HSV replication while adequate/higher levels of lysine suppress HSV, especially when sources of arginine – nuts, chocolate and gelatin – are restricted; dosage: 1,000 mg t.i.d.
- **Thymus extract:** substantial clinical data demonstrate that thymus extracts restore and enhance immune system function:
  - thymus extracts have been shown to be effective in preventing both the number and severity of recurrent infections in immune-suppressed individuals.
  - thymus extract has been shown to normalize the ratio of T helper cells to suppressor cells, whether the ratio is low (as in AIDS or cancer) or high (as in allergies or rheumatoid arthritis) and to boost cell-mediated immunity.
  - some evidence suggests that a defect of specific cell-mediated immunity is present even in apparently normal subjects with HSV. Thymus extract boosts cell-mediated immune response.
  - dosage: the equivalent of 120 mg of pure polypeptides with molecular weights less than 10,000, or roughly 500 mg of the crude polypeptide fraction q.d.

Topical medicines
- **Ascoxal:** a pharmaceutical formulation containing vitamin C (ascorbic acid), Ascoxal, applied to herpes ulcers with a soaked cotton pad t.i.d. for 2 min each time, has been shown to significantly lessen the number of days until scabs heal and result in fewer cases of worsening of symptoms.
- **Zinc sulfate solution:** topical application of zinc sulfate solution (0.025% solution, applied t.i.d.) has been shown effective in both relieving symptoms and inhibiting recurrence of HSV outbreak.
- ***Melissa officinalis* (lemon balm) cream:** *Melissa* contains several active components that work

together to prevent HSV from infecting human cells:

- results from comprehensive trials at three German hospitals and a dermatology clinic demonstrated that not a single recurrence took place when *Melissa* was used immediately during initial cold sore infection.
- melissa produced rapid interruption of the infection and promoted healing of herpes blisters much more rapidly than normal – 5 days versus 10 days for the control group, which received other topical creams.
- dosage: concentrated (70 : 1) extract of *Melissa*, apply thickly, b.i.d.–q.i.d. during active recurrences, b.i.d. to prevent recurrence.

- **Glycyrrhetinic acid:** a component of licorice root (*Glycyrrhiza glabra*), glycyrrhetinic acid inhibits HSV as well as several other viruses and has been shown in clinical studies to reduce healing time and pain associated with both oral and genital herpes lesions. Apply b.i.d.

- **Ice pack:** 10 min on, 5 min off for up to three cycles every 4 hours during initial symptoms.
- **Clothing:** Women should wear cotton underpants or pantyhose with a cotton crotch.
- **Urination:** to reduce pain during urination, urinate while showering or pour a cup of warm water over genitals while urinating.
- **Warm baths** with 1 tsp of salt added may ease some of the discomfort.

HIV/AIDS

DESCRIPTION

Infection with human immunodeficiency virus (HIV) causes a major failure in immune function, specifically cell-mediated immunity, which severely decreases the body's ability to fight infection and destroy abnormal cells (cancer). HIV targets special immune system blood cells (lymphocytes) and the immune cells of the organs (bone marrow, spleen, liver, and lymph glands). HIV itself does not kill; it cripples the immune system to such an extent that the person dies from severe infection or cancer. Acquired immune deficiency (AIDS) is a secondary syndrome, now recognized as a late stage of HIV infection.

Diagnosis of HIV is made by a blood test positive for HIV antigen and antibodies. Diagnosis of AIDS is made on the basis of the following criteria:

■ presence of one of the 23 *opportunistic infections* (an infection caused by an organism that the immune system would normally destroy) and cancers linked to AIDS, or
■ a positive HIV test plus a total helper lymphocyte (an important white blood cell) count (CD4 count) of less than 200 cells/μl, or
■ a percentage of helper cells to total lymphocytes (CD8 count) of less than 14%.

Classified as a retrovirus, HIV has the ability to transform its RNA into DNA through the activity of the enzyme *RNA reverse transcriptase*. The virus then incorporates this piece of DNA into the infected cell's DNA, taking over the cell's machinery to promote viral replication. The immune cells most affected by this process are the T4 inducer/helper subset of lymphocytes.

Helper T cells function in helping another type of lymphocyte to multiply in response to infection as well as helping these white blood cells to destroy bacteria, viruses, other organisms, and cancer cells. HIV is highly selective for helper T cells but is also found in other white blood cells, where it actively replicates, particularly when the T cells are themselves activated to fight an infection. This infection–replication process renders the T cells non-functional and eventually destroys them, ultimately producing the profound immune suppression of AIDS.

Current estimates are that over 1 million Americans are infected with HIV, and a little under 200,000 meet the requirements of having AIDS. Current average time between HIV infection and development of AIDS is 10 years.

At this time, we recommend that conventional drug therapies (protease inhibitors that slow HIV replication and antibiotics to help prevent infection) be used for all individuals with CD4 counts below 500. Along with drug therapies, however, natural measures that promote good health should be aggressively employed. In addition to supporting immune function, the natural medicine treatments below assist patients in improving nutritional status and gastrointestinal function, which significantly lightens the load on the immune system, slows disease progression, and optimizes health and quality of life.

FREQUENT SIGNS AND SYMPTOMS

■ **Initial infection with HIV may produce no symptoms:** laboratory studies of blood cells and HIV antibodies test may not become positive for 6 months after infection.
■ **Sudden onset (with duration up to 2 weeks):** fevers, night sweats, joint and muscle pain, tiring easily, headaches, sore throat, generalized swelling of lymph glands, and/or rash on the trunk.
■ **Slow onset:** unexplained fatigue, weight loss, fever, diarrhea, and/or generalized swelling of lymph glands.
■ **Recurrent respiratory and skin infections**
■ **Mouth sores**
■ **Opportunistic infections**, such as thrush (oral yeast infection) or pneumonia.
■ **Genital swelling:** the result of swollen lymph glands in the groin area.
■ **Enlarged spleen**
■ **Advanced stages:** neurological changes including dementia, partial paralysis, dizziness, visual disturbances.

CAUSES

Infection by HIV, a retrovirus that invades and destroys cells of the immune system, causes lowered resistance to infections and some cancers. HIV is considered a sexually transmitted disease, although the virus may also be contracted via needles contaminated by blood and blood products of persons infected with HIV/AIDS.

RISK INCREASES WITH

- Sexual contact with an HIV-infected person. (*Note*: usual non-sexual contact does not transmit HIV, so a person with HIV/AIDS is not a risk to the general population.)
- Male homosexual activity.
- Multiple heterosexual partners.
- Intravenous drug use involving needle sharing – needles may be contaminated.
- Being born to a mother infected with HIV.
- Transfusions of blood or blood products from a person with AIDS (rare).
- Exposure of hospital workers and laboratory technicians to blood, feces and urine of HIV-positive patients. Accidental needle injury poses the greatest risk.

PREVENTIVE MEASURES

To prevent HIV infection
- Restrict sexual activity to partners whose sexual histories are known.
- Use condoms for vaginal and anal intercourse. Effectiveness is not proven but consistent use may reduce transmission.
- Risk of oral sex is not known. Ejaculation into the mouth should be avoided.
- Avoid intravenous self-administered drugs. Do not share unsterilized needles.
- Avoid unscreened blood products (some foreign countries may not test blood as effectively as others).
- Infected persons and those in high-risk groups should not donate blood, sperm, organs or tissue.

To slow progression of HIV/AIDS
- Avoid exposure to individuals with easily transmitted infectious diseases, e.g., colds, flu.
- Avoid raw eggs, unpasteurized milk or other potentially contaminated foods.
- Do not smoke or consume alcohol.
- Follow the treatment protocol outlined below.

Expected outcomes
In HIV-positive individuals, an improvement in nutritional status and immune function will significantly delay and possibly prevent progression to AIDS.

TREATMENT

Diet
- **Elimination diet:** assume food sensitivities and try a trial elimination diet. Eliminate the most common food allergens – wheat, dairy products, corn, soy, and peanuts – for 2 weeks (for more information see the chapter on Food allergy).
- **A health-promoting diet:** after identifying and removing any allergenic foods from the diet, choose a nutrient-dense diet rich in whole, unprocessed, preferably organic foods, especially plant foods (fruits, vegetables, whole grains, beans, nuts [especially walnuts], and seeds), and cold-water fish (for more information, see Appendix 1).
- **Eliminate caffeine and alcohol**
- **Minimize consumption of sugars, and refined foods:** consuming 75 g (3 oz) of sugar in one sitting in any form (sucrose, honey, fruit juice) depresses white (immune) cell activity by 50% for 1–5 hours.
- **Optimal health smoothie:** try this nutrient-dense shake for breakfast or a light lunch or snack:
  - combine in blender: 2 scoops of protein powder, 1–2 tbsp nuts or nut butter (not peanuts), 1 cup yogurt, 1 cup fresh fruit/berries, 1 tbsp flaxseed oil, 1 tbsp spirulina, 1 tbsp flaxseed meal; thin with rice, almond, or soy milk. Blend.
- **Oat bran:** oat bran is rich in soluble fiber and glutamine. Glutamine, an amino acid that is the preferred fuel for intestinal cells, has been shown to significantly improve and/or safeguard intestinal health. Add 1–2 tbsp to other foods.

Nutritional supplements
- **HIV/AIDS patients require higher levels of virtually all known nutrients:**
  - the immune system requires a constant supply of nutrients to function properly. Malnutrition and/or nutrient deficiency is common in AIDS patients and frequently exacerbated by gastrointestinal tract infection.
  - since the immune system is suppressed in HIV-infected people, they are susceptible to inflammatory responses induced by oxidative stress resulting from exposure to viral and opportunistic pathogens and drugs. Inflammatory responses involve the formation of a variety of damaging free radicals (reactive oxygen species – ROS).
  - more than 29% of HIV-positive (HIV+) individuals are deficient in one or more of the antioxidant nutrients (beta-carotene, vitamin E, selenium, zinc, vitamin C).

- free radical damage contributes to HIV progression by destroying cells, lowering immune function, enhancing viral replication, increasing the toxic side effects of drugs, and contributing to weight loss.
- **Multiple vitamin and mineral supplement (without iron if viral load is high):**
  - a high-potency multiple vitamin and mineral supplement including 400 µg of folic acid, 400 µg of vitamin B_{12}, and 50–100 mg of vitamin B_6. (Folic acid supplementation should always be accompanied by vitamin B_{12} supplementation to prevent folic acid from masking a vitamin B_{12} deficiency.)
  - dosage: 2 capsules, b.i.d. with breakfast and lunch.
- **Beta-carotene:**
  - HIV+ patients are significantly depleted in all the carotenoids, including beta-carotene. Even asymptomatic HIV+ patients typically have severe beta-carotene deficiency.
  - low beta-carotene levels are associated with significant impairment of immune function. Carotene deficit allows free radicals to increase, which stimulates HIV replication and decreases immune response.
  - in a randomized controlled trial in HIV+ patients, beta-carotene supplementation increased CD4 counts by 17% in 4 weeks.
  - beta-carotene supplementation has been shown to decrease fever, nocturnal sweating, diarrhea, weight loss and improve CD4 counts.
  - **caution:** recent data indicate that synthetic beta-carotenoids may increase the risk of lung cancer in smokers. Use only natural carotenoids in non-smokers. Those who smoke can take two glasses of freshly prepared carrot juice instead of beta-carotene supplements.
  - dosage: 75,000 IU of natural beta-carotene b.i.d. (if possible use beta-carotene derived from palm oil, which is better absorbed and has much greater antioxidant activity).
- **Vitamin C:**
  - laboratory studies suggest that vitamin C can suppress HIV replication in both chronically and acutely infected immune cells (T lymphocytes).
  - studies show that HIV+ patients with the highest levels of vitamin C intake had the slowest progression to AIDS.
  - vitamin C significantly enhances the activity of natural killer cells and neutrophils, two types of immune cells that engulf and destroy enemies.
  - vitamin C diminishes HIV viral protein production in infected cells.
  - vitamin C works synergistically with N-acetylcysteine (see NAC below) in controlling HIV infection.

- **caution:** Information is conflicting, but high doses of vitamin C may impair lymphocyte function. The dosage recommended should safely promote vitamin C's beneficial effects.
- dosage: 500–1,000 mg t.i.d. between meals.
- **Vitamin E:**
  - vitamin E has demonstrated immune-enhancing and antioxidant properties.
  - vitamin E restores HIV-suppressed multiplication of spleen cells (the spleen produces immune cells called macrophages and acts as a blood filter) and the ability of natural killer cells to destroy infected cells.
  - vitamin E partially reverses the negative side effects of AZT (zidovudine) on the myelin sheath that protects nerve cells.
  - vitamin E inhibits activation of NF-kappa B, a chemical messenger that plays a critical role in initiating HIV replication.
  - reduced blood levels of vitamin E have been correlated with progression from HIV to AIDS. In one study, men with the highest levels of vitamin E in their blood showed a 34% decrease in their progression to AIDS compared to those with the lowest levels.
  - dosage: 400 IU mixed tocopherols q.d.
- **Selenium:**
  - selenium deficiency is common in HIV infection and AIDS.
  - selenium and beta-carotene improve the function of the body's enzymatic antioxidant system in the blood and levels of glutathione, the most important antioxidant in the liver and mitochondria (the energy-production factories in each cell) in HIV-infected patients.
  - when selenium is supplemented, glutathione activity increases and helps prevent HIV from replicating after exposure to reactive oxygen species (free radicals).
  - selenium inhibits NF-kappa B, an inflammatory agent that triggers HIV replication.
  - several studies have shown selenium status is a major determinant of how fast HIV will progress to AIDS. It has been proposed that the period between exposure to HIV and AIDS may be attributed to the period of time it takes to deplete the body of selenium storage.
  - dosage: 200–600 µg q.d.
- **N-acetylcysteine (NAC):**
  - intracellular levels of the important antioxidant, glutathione, and cysteine (an amino acid that is one of the components of glutathione) drop in HIV+ individuals, causing a lowering in CD4 count.

Supplementation with NAC has been shown to reverse this reduction in CD4 count.

- cysteine deficiency causes T-cell dysfunction. A series of clinical studies and laboratory investigations suggests that progression to AIDS may, in part, be the result of the HIV causing cysteine deficiency.
- treatment with NAC has been shown to improve cysteine and glutathione deficiency in AIDS patients.
- NAC has been shown to effectively suppress HIV replication in infected cells.
- when glutathione itself is taken orally, most of it is broken down in the stomach rather than absorbed into the bloodstream. Supplementing with NAC increases blood levels of glutathione.
- dosage: 1,000 mg b.i.d.

Lipoic acid:
- while other antioxidants act in either fat- or water-soluble areas, alpha-lipoic acid is unique in its ability to act in both fat- and water-soluble tissues.
- lipoic acid increases glutathione in human T-lymphocyte cells, thus preventing HIV activation, inhibits HIV replication by reducing the activity of reverse transcriptase – the enzyme responsible for manufacturing the virus from the DNA of lymphocytes – and increases T cell counts.
- lipoic acid also helps protect other antioxidants, such as vitamin C, increasing their levels in the blood of HIV+ patients.
- dosage: 150 mg t.i.d.

Vitamin B_1 (thiamin):
- thiamin is a coenzyme in many important reactions central to energy production and is vital for proper nervous system and neuronal (brain cell) function.
- a high intake of vitamins C, thiamin, and niacin has been associated in studies with a significantly decreased progression rate to AIDS.
- thiamin disulfide is a potent inhibitor of HIV virus production.
- dosage: up to 50 mg b.i.d.

Vitamin B_{12} (methylcobalamin – active B_{12}):
- decreased levels of B_{12} are frequently found in patients with HIV; low blood vitamin B_{12} concentrations are associated with faster progression to AIDS and worsening neurological symptoms.
- B_{12} has been shown to inhibit HIV infection of normal blood monocytes and lymphocytes and to inhibit HIV replication *in vitro* (test tubes).
- dosage: 2 mg b.i.d. of methylcobalamin (the active form of B_{12}).

Coenzyme Q_{10}:
- CoQ_{10} increases blood levels of CD4 lymphocytes and significantly increases levels of IgG, an important immune protein, in AIDS patients.

- dosage: 30–100 mg t.i.d.

Lactobacillus acidophilus:
- *Lactobacillus acidophilus* are friendly bacteria that supplant unfriendly bacteria and whose metabolic by-products provide nutrients needed by intestinal cells.
- any disturbance in intestinal microflora leaves the intestines vulnerable to colonization by unfriendly bacteria. When gut flora are not in healthful balance, intestinal health declines, so nutrients in food are not well absorbed.
- dosage: 1–2 billion live bacteria q.d.; typically 2 capsules, b.i.d. between meals.

Pancreatic enzymes:
- the pancreas is often infected or dysfunctional during HIV infection, and pancreatitis (inflammation of the pancreas) is a common cause of death in patients with AIDS.
- without adequate pancreatic enzymes, normal digestion cannot occur.
- digestive enzymes taken with meals help digest foods for absorption.
- dosage: 1–2 capsules t.i.d. with meals.

Glutamine:
- glutamine is an amino acid that is the preferred fuel for intestinal cells.
- glutamine supplementation decreases the spread of infection from the intestine to other tissues.
- glutamine deficiency is associated with atrophy of the small intestine, where nutrients are absorbed, and is thought to be a contributing cause of HIV-associated wasting.
- glutamine supplementation has been shown to significantly improve intestinal function and nutrient absorption. In addition, by preventing the influx of toxins that occurs when the intestinal wall is damaged, glutamine significantly lightens the load on the immune system, enabling better immune function.
- dosage: 300–500 mg/kg body weight.

Flaxseed oil: flaxseed oil is nature's richest source of omega-3 essential fatty acids, i.e., GLA and EPA:
- diets high in omega-3s decrease inflammation, a contributing factor to HIV replication, and encourage the production of antigens necessary for immune defenses.
- a deficiency in dietary GLA or EPA is thought to increase susceptibility to AIDS.
- GLA supplementation has effected a regression in early Kaposi's sarcoma.
- GLA has been shown to selectively kill HIV-infected cells, and prevent and treat intestinal inflammation.
- flaxseed oil is highly perishable, should be purchased in an opaque container, kept refrigerated,

and not heated. Add to smoothies, mix into spreads, use on bread, as a dressing for salads, etc.
- dosage: 1 tbsp q.d.–b.i.d.
- **Quercetin:**
  - quercetin works synergistically with vitamin C, increasing its anti-inflammatory and antioxidant effects.
  - a strong inhibitor of HIV-reverse transcriptase and HIV-integrase, quercetin inhibits HIV replication.
  - dosage: 2,000 mg q.d.

Botanical medicines

- *Glycyrrhiza glabra* (licorice root):
  - licorice exerts a variety of beneficial actions including: protecting the liver; enhancing the immune system; boosting interferon (the body's own antiviral and immune-enhancing agent); and promoting the flow of bile to and from the liver.
  - glycyrrhizin, the primary active component in licorice root, has been shown to inhibit several viruses including HIV, and replication of HIV-infected cells.
  - in several studies, HIV+ patients who took glycyrrhizin daily did not progress to AIDS, while several members in the control groups developed AIDS.
  - dosage: choose one of the following forms and take the recommended dosage t.i.d.:
    - powdered root: 1–2 g
    - fluid extract (1 : 1): 2–4 ml
    - solid (dry powdered) extract (5% glycyrrhetinic acid content): 250–500 mg.
  - **caution:** in susceptible individuals, licorice has blood pressure elevating effects, which can frequently be avoided by increasing intake of potassium-rich foods. Blood pressure should be monitored.
- *Curcuma longa* (turmeric):
  - curcumin inhibits HIV replication by blocking a gene in HIV's DNA called the long terminal repeat (LTR) gene. HIV remains inactive until signaled by LTR to replicate.
  - curcumin also inhibits the activity of HIV-integrase, the enzyme that integrates a double-stranded DNA copy of the RNA genome, synthesized by reverse transcriptase, into a host chromosome.
  - curcumin has also been shown to inhibit a chemical mediator of inflammation called tumor necrosis factor (TNF). TNF is used by the immune system to kill disease-causing organisms, but it also triggers the production of NF-kappa B, a chemical messenger that plays a critical role in initiating HIV replication.

- curcumin is a powerful antioxidant, showing activity as much as 300 times greater than that of vitamin E.
- curcumin should be taken with bromelain, which enhances curcumin's absorption.
- dosage: 400 mg five times a day with an equal amount of bromelain (1,200–1,800 MCU), preferably on an empty stomach.
- **Bromelain:**
  - bromelain is a natural protease inhibitor.
  - proteases are protein-digesting enzymes that, in HIV, are required to condense the viral protein core for subsequent replications. Protease-inhibitor drugs that inhibit this are showing tremendous benefit in the treatment of HIV and AIDS, but they are expensive and associated with many side effects.
  - when compared to protease-inhibiting drugs, bromelain demonstrated significantly better activity.
  - dosage: bromelain 1,200–1,800 MCU, five times a day, preferably on an empty stomach. Take bromelain with turmeric (curcumin).
- *Hypericum perforatum* (St John's wort):
  - St John's wort has been shown to inhibit binding and entry of HIV into host cells. In one study, incubation of HIV with St John's wort rendered the virus non-infectious.
  - St John's wort has the ability to cross the blood–brain barrier, especially important as HIV often attacks the brain.
  - *note*: while it is difficult to achieve sufficiently high blood levels of hypericin via oral administration to produce antiviral activity, it is highly recommended as an antidepressant for HIV+ patients. Hypericum can produce photosensitivity. Patients will tan and burn more rapidly and should wear sun block.
  - dosage: 3 capsules (300 mg each) q.i.d. standardized to contain 0.3% hypericin.

Drug–herb interaction cautions

- *Glycyrrhiza glabra* (licorice):
  - plus *digoxin, digitalis*: because of a reduction of potassium in the blood, licorice enhances the toxicity of cardiac glycosides. Interaction with these cardioglycoside drugs could lead to arrhythmias and cardiac arrest.
  - plus *stimulant laxatives or diuretics* (thiazides, spironolactone or amiloride): licorice should not be used with these drugs because of the additive increase of potassium loss to potentially dangerous levels.
- *Hypericum perforatum* (St John's wort):
  - plus *monoamine oxidase (MAO) inhibitors*: possible additive effects of St John's wort with these drugs, so physician monitoring is advised.

■ plus *selective serotonin reuptake inhibitors (SSRIs)*: possible additive effects of St John's wort with these drugs, so physician monitoring is advised. When replacement of an SSRI is desirable, either of two physician-supervized approaches may be used: (1) a trial for several weeks combining a reduced dose of St John's wort or the SSRI prior to withdrawal of the pharmaceutical medication, or (2) a 3-week wash-out period for the SSRI before switching to St John's wort.

Physical medicine

Long-term survivors with AIDS generally engage in physical fitness/exercise programs.

■ **Relaxation exercise:** perform some relaxation exercise, such as deep breathing, meditation, prayer, visualization, etc., for 10–15 min each day.
■ **Aerobic exercise:** an aerobic exercise program – a minimum of 20 min, three times a week – may enhance critical components of cellular immunity as well as acting as a buffer for the detrimental mood changes that typically accompany stress.
■ **Resistance exercise:** during the non-acute stage of HIV/AIDS, progressive resistance exercise (e.g., weight training) increases muscle mass and function.

Hypertension

DESCRIPTION

Elevated blood pressure is a major risk factor for a heart attack and is generally regarded as the greatest risk factor for a stroke. "Blood pressure" signifies the resistance produced each time the heart beats and sends blood coursing through the arteries. The peak pressure exerted by this contraction is the systolic pressure. Between beats, the heart relaxes, and blood pressure drops. The lowest pressure is referred to as the diastolic pressure. A normal blood pressure reading for an adult is: 120 (systolic)/80 (diastolic). High blood pressure is divided into different levels:

- borderline: 120–160/90–94 mmHg
- mild: 140–160/90–104 mmHg
- moderate: 140–180/105–114 mmHg
- severe: 160+/115+ mmHg

Physicians are primarily concerned with diastolic pressure (the second number in the blood pressure reading), but systolic pressure is also important. Individuals with a normal diastolic pressure (<82 mmHg) but elevated systolic pressure (>158 mmHg) have double the risk of death from heart attack or stroke compared to individuals with normal systolic pressures (<130 mmHg). Blood pressure typically goes up as a result of stress or physical activity, but in a person with high blood pressure, is elevated even at rest.

Over sixty million Americans have high blood pressure, including more than half (54.3%) of all Americans aged 65–74 years, and almost three-fourths (71.8%) of all African-Americans in the same age group.

Most patients (over 80%) with high blood pressure are in the borderline-to-moderate range, a group in which almost all cases of high blood pressure can be brought under control through changes in diet and lifestyle. In fact, in cases of borderline-to-mild hypertension, healthful changes in diet and lifestyle (discussed below) have proven superior to drugs in head-to-head comparisons.

In addition, in some people, the drugs typically prescribed to lower blood pressure produce the very thing they are trying to prevent: a heart attack. Several well-designed long-term clinical studies have found that people who take blood pressure lowering drugs (typically diuretics and/or beta-blockers) actually suffer from unnecessary side effects (e.g., fatigue, headaches, and impotence), including an increased risk of heart disease.

FREQUENT SIGNS AND SYMPTOMS

Usually none:

- typically discovered as part of a routine checkup
- blood vessels do not contain nerves, so no symptoms are felt unless disease is severe.

A hypertensive crisis may be indicated by:

- headache, drowsiness, confusion
- numbness and tingling in hands and feet
- coughing blood; nosebleeds
- severe shortness of breath.

CAUSES

Disease associations

- **Atherosclerosis (hardening of the arteries):** the health of the artery is critical to maintaining normal blood pressure. When the arteries harden due to the buildup of cholesterol-containing plaques, blood pressure rises.
- **Alcoholism:** excessive consumption of alcohol causes frequent steep rises in blood sugar and increases the production of free radicals, both of which damage the arteries. In addition, alcoholics eat poorly, so are depleted of the vitamins and minerals necessary for cardiovascular health.
- **Kidney disease:** the kidneys are responsible for removing excess fluid from the body. When they are not functioning properly fluid builds up, increasing blood pressure.

Lifestyle factors

- **Obesity:** leads to insulin insensitivity, and excessive sugar in the blood, which damages the arteries. High cholesterol levels and atherosclerosis are also common in obese individuals.
- **Sedentary lifestyle:** studies have shown that an unfit individual has an eight times greater risk of a heart attack or stroke than a physically fit individual.

Researchers estimate that for every hour of exercise, there is a 2-hour increase in longevity.

■ **Stress:** inability to cope effectively with stress has been shown to promote atherosclerosis and to lower magnesium levels. Magnesium, Nature's relaxant, causes blood vessels to dilate, and works with potassium to pump sodium out of cells. Inside cells, excessive sodium causes fluid retention, increasing blood pressure.

■ **Smoking:** according to the US Surgeon General, "Cigarette smoking should be considered the most important risk factor for coronary heart disease". It is well documented that smoking causes atherosclerosis and high blood pressure.

Dietary factors

■ **Coffee consumption:** caffeine (and nicotine – another reason not to smoke) is a stimulant that promotes the fight-or-flight response, releasing stress hormones that elevate blood pressure.

■ **Alcohol intake:** in susceptible individuals, even moderate alcohol consumption causes a steep rise in blood sugar and increases the production of free radicals, both of which damage arteries.

■ **High sodium-to-potassium ratio:** excessive consumption of dietary sodium chloride (table salt), coupled with diminished dietary potassium, is a common cause of high blood pressure, especially in "salt-sensitive" individuals:

■ numerous studies have shown that sodium restriction alone does not improve blood pressure control in most people; it must be accompanied by a high potassium intake.

■ in our society, only 5% of sodium intake comes from the natural ingredients in food. Prepared foods contribute 45% of our sodium intake, 45% is added in cooking, and another 5% is added as a condiment. All the body requires in most instances is the salt that is naturally present in food.

■ most Americans have a potassium-to-sodium (K : Na) ratio of less than 1 : 2. This means that most people ingest twice as much sodium as potassium.

■ researchers recommend a dietary potassium-to-sodium ratio of greater than 5 : 1 to maintain health. This is 10 times higher than the average intake. Even this may not be optimal. A natural diet rich in fruits and vegetables can produce a K : Na ratio greater than 100 : 1, as most fruits and vegetables have a K : Na ratio of at least 50 : 1.

■ **Low-fiber, high-sugar diet:** excessive sugar in the blood causes damage to arterial walls. Low fiber is associated with atherosclerosis.

■ **A diet low in calcium, magnesium, and vitamin C:** epidemiological and clinical studies have found numerous links between inadequate amounts of these three nutrients (discussed below) and high blood pressure.

■ **High saturated-fat intake:** a high intake of saturated fats has been conclusively linked to high cholesterol levels and atherosclerosis.

■ **Low intake of essential fatty acids:** population and autopsy studies have demonstrated that people who consume a diet rich in omega-3 oils from either fish or vegetable sources have the least, and conversely, those who consume the least omega-3 oils have the highest degree of cardiovascular disease.

RISK INCREASES WITH

■ **Any of the above causative factors.**
■ **Genetic factors:** hypertension is most common among blacks.
■ **Family history of hypertension, stroke, heart attack or kidney failure.**
■ **Use of contraceptive pills, steroids, and some appetite suppressants or decongestants.** These drugs alter metabolism, promoting high blood pressure.
■ **Soft water:** chronic exposure to lead from environmental sources, including drinking water, is associated with high blood pressure and increased cardiovascular mortality. Areas with a soft water supply have higher lead concentrations in drinking water due to the acidity of the water. Soft water is also low in calcium and magnesium – two minerals that protect against high blood pressure.

PREVENTIVE MEASURES

■ Don't smoke.
■ Reduce excess weight.
■ Minimize consumption of alcohol and caffeine.
■ Consume a nutrient-dense diet rich in whole, unprocessed, preferably organic foods, especially plant foods (fruits, vegetables, beans, seeds and nuts), and cold-water fish, and low in animal products (for more detailed information, see Appendix 1).
■ Exercise regularly – a minimum of 30 min, at least three times a week. A carefully graded, progressive aerobic exercise program is essential. Walking is a good exercise with which to start.
■ Learn how to control anger or express it appropriately. The following subjective suggestions will help:
■ be kind to yourself; make time to give and receive love in your life.

- be an active listener. Allow others to really share their feelings and thoughts uninterrupted. Empathize. Put yourself in their shoes.
- if you find yourself being interrupted, relax. If you are courteous and let others speak, they will eventually respond in kind (unless they are extremely rude). If they don't, point out to them that they are interrupting the communication process (you can only do this if you have been a good listener).
- avoid aggressive or passive behavior. Be assertive, but express your thoughts and feelings in a kind way, as you would wish to be treated, to help improve relationships at work and at home.
- avoid excessive stress as best you can by avoiding excessive work hours, poor nutrition, and inadequate rest.
- avoid stimulants like caffeine and nicotine that promote the fight-or-flight response and tend to make people more irritable.
- take time to build your long-term health by performing stress-reduction techniques and deep-breathing exercises.
- be patient and tolerant of others, and yourself. Remember you, and they, are human and will make mistakes, which are always opportunities to learn and grow.

Expected outcomes

Treatment and outcome vary according to the severity of hypertension.

Mild hypertension (140–160/90–104)

If, after following the dietary and lifestyle recommendations, plus the supplement recommendations given for mild hypertension, for 3–6 months, blood pressure has not returned to normal, seek professional advice about further non-drug recommendations.

Moderate hypertension (140–180/105–114)

If, after following all the recommendations given for moderate hypertension for 1–3 months, blood pressure has not dropped below 140/105, seek professional advice about selecting the most appropriate medication. If a prescription drug is necessary, calcium channel blockers or ACE inhibitors appear to be the safest.

Severe hypertension (160+/115+)

- Consult a physician immediately.
- Employ all the measures listed for mild and moderate hypertension. A drug may be necessary to achieve initial control. When satisfactory control over the high blood pressure has been achieved, work with your physician to taper off the medication.

TREATMENT

Diet

- **Increase consumption of plant foods:** vegetarians generally have lower blood pressure, and a lower incidence of high blood pressure and other cardiovascular diseases, than non-vegetarians:
  - vegetarians and non-vegetarians consume similar amounts of sodium, but vegetarians consume more potassium, complex carbohydrates, essential fatty acids, fiber, calcium, magnesium, and vitamin C, and less saturated fat and refined carbohydrates, all of which have been shown to have a favorable influence on blood pressure.
- **Increase consumption of green leafy vegetables:** green leafy vegetables are fat-free, rich sources of calcium and magnesium, both of which have beneficial effects on blood pressure.
- **Increase consumption of whole grains and legumes:** a high fiber diet helps lower cholesterol levels.
- **Increase consumption of broccoli and citrus fruits:** these foods are rich in vitamin C. Population-based and clinical studies show that the higher the intake of vitamin C, the lower the blood pressure.
- **Consume four stalks of celery daily:** a compound found in celery, 3-n-butyl phthalide, has been shown to lower blood pressure:
  - in animals, a very small amount of 3-n-butyl phthalide lowered blood pressure by 12–14%, and also lowered cholesterol levels by about 7%. Four stalks of celery supply the equivalent dose in humans.
- **Consume both garlic and onions liberally:** the sulfur-containing compounds in garlic and onions have been shown to lower blood pressure in cases of hypertension. Garlic supplements may also be of benefit (see Botanical medicines below).
- **Avoid saturated fats** (found mainly in animal products), margarine and foods containing *trans* fatty acids (found in processed foods). Extensive research links these fats to heart disease, strokes, and cancer.
- **Avoid processed foods:** their primary ingredients – sugars, refined carbohydrates, and *trans* fats – elevate cholesterol levels, blood pressure, and risk for obesity and diabetes.
- **Increase consumption of omega-3 essential fatty acids** by consuming flaxseed oil (1 tbsp q.d.) and/or eating cold-water fish – salmon, mackerel, tuna, herring, halibut (110 g [4 oz] at least three times a week). These fats "thin" the blood and have numerous beneficial effects on cardiovascular health.

Dietary supplement recommendation summary

- **Mild hypertension (140–160/90–104):** supplement the diet with:
  - high-potency multiple vitamin and mineral formula
  - omega-3 essential fatty acids (flaxseed oil): 1 tbsp q.d.
  - magnesium citrate or aspartate: 800–1,200 mg in divided doses q.d.
  - vitamin C: 500–1,000 mg t.i.d.
  - vitamin E: 400–800 IU q.d.
  - garlic: the equivalent of 4,000 mg of fresh garlic q.d.
- **Moderate hypertension (140–180/105–114):** employ all the measures listed for mild hypertension and add:
  - coenzyme Q_{10}: 50 mg b.i.d.–t.i.d.
  - hawthorn extract (10% procyanidins or 1.8% vitexin-4'-rhamnoside): 100–250 mg t.i.d.

Nutritional supplements

- **A high-potency multiple vitamin and mineral supplement:** this should include 400 µg of folic acid, 400 µg of vitamin B_{12}, and 50–100 mg of vitamin B_6. (Folic acid supplementation should always be accompanied by vitamin B_{12} supplementation to prevent folic acid from masking a vitamin B_{12} deficiency.) A daily multiple providing all of the known vitamins and minerals serves as a foundation upon which to build an individualized health-promotion program.
- **Omega-3 essential fatty acids:** over 60 double-blind studies have demonstrated that either fish oil supplements or flaxseed oil, the two best sources of omega-3s, are very effective in lowering blood pressure:
  - fish oils have typically produced a more pronounced effect than flaxseed oil because the dosage of fish oils used was quite high (equal to 10 fish oil capsules q.d.). Flaxseed oil may be the better choice for lowering blood pressure, especially when cost-effectiveness is considered.
  - along with reducing the intake of saturated fat, 1 tbsp q.d. of flaxseed oil should lower both the systolic and diastolic readings by up to 9 mmHg.
  - one study found that for every absolute 1% increase in body content of the omega-3 oil, alpha-linolenic acid (ALA), systolic, diastolic and mean blood pressure decreased by 5 mmHg.
  - dosage: flaxseed oil: 1 tbsp q.d.
- **Potassium:** several studies show that potassium supplementation alone can produce significant reductions in blood pressure in hypertensive subjects. Typically, these studies have utilized dosages ranging from 2.5–5.0 g of potassium q.d. Significant drops in both systolic and diastolic values have been achieved:
  - in one study, potassium supplementation lowered systolic blood pressure by an average of 12 mmHg and diastolic blood pressure by an average of 16 mmHg.
  - potassium supplementation may be especially useful in the treatment of high blood pressure in persons over the age of 65, who often do not fully respond to blood pressure lowering drugs. In one double-blind study of 18 patients whose average age was 75, with a systolic blood pressure of greater than 160 mmHg and/or a diastolic blood pressure of greater than 95 mmHg, those who received potassium chloride (supplying 2.5 g of potassium) q.d. for 4 weeks experienced a drop of 12 mmHg in systolic and 7 mmHg in diastolic pressure – results comparable to drug therapy without its negative side effects.
  - **caution:** check with a physician before taking potassium:
    - individuals with kidney disease do not handle potassium in the normal way and are likely to experience heart disturbances and other consequences of potassium toxicity.
    - potassium supplementation is contraindicated when using a number of prescription medications, including digitalis, potassium-sparing diuretics, and the angiotensin-converting enzyme-inhibitor class of blood pressure lowering drugs.
    - people with kidney disease or severe heart disease should not take magnesium or potassium unless under the direct advice of a physician.
    - using foods or food-based potassium supplements to meet the human body's high potassium requirements rather than pills is suggested since potassium salts can cause nausea, vomiting, diarrhea, and ulcers when given in pill form at high dosages. These effects are not seen when potassium levels are increased through diet alone.
- **Magnesium:** magnesium is second only to potassium in its concentration within cells and it interacts with potassium in many body systems. Studies suggest that low intracellular potassium levels may be the result of low magnesium intake:
  - population studies provide considerable evidence that a high intake of magnesium is associated with lower blood pressure.
  - numerous studies have demonstrated an inverse correlation between water "hardness" (water high in magnesium) and high blood pressure. Where magnesium content of the water was high, there were fewer cases of high blood pressure and heart disease.
  - dietary studies found the same results: when magnesium levels were high, blood pressure was lower.

- additional studies have shown that magnesium supplementation is particularly helpful in lowering blood pressure if:
  - the individual is taking a diuretic, since diuretics cause magnesium depletion
  - high blood pressure is associated with a high level of *renin* – an enzyme released by the kidneys that leads to the formation of *angiotensin* and the release of *aldosterone* – compounds that cause blood vessels to constrict and blood pressure to increase
  - the patient has elevated intracellular sodium or decreased intracellular potassium levels (as measured by red blood cell studies).
- absorption studies indicate that magnesium is easily absorbed orally, especially when bound to citrate. In addition, while inorganic magnesium salts often cause diarrhea at higher dosages, organic forms of magnesium (magnesium citrate or aspartate) generally do not.
- dosage: 800–1,200 mg magnesium citrate or aspartate in divided doses q.d.
- **Vitamin C:** studies have shown that the higher the intake of vitamin C the lower the blood pressure:
  - one of the ways vitamin C helps to keep blood pressure in the normal range is by promoting the excretion of lead. Chronic exposure to lead from environmental sources, including drinking water, is associated with high blood pressure and increased cardiovascular mortality.
  - areas with a soft water supply have higher lead concentrations in drinking water as a result of the acidity of the water. Soft water is also low in calcium and magnesium – two minerals that protect against high blood pressure.
  - dosage: 1,000–2,000 mg q.d. in divided doses.
- **Vitamin E:** of all the antioxidants, the fat-soluble antioxidant, vitamin E, may offer the most protection against hardening of the arteries because it is easily incorporated into the low density lipoprotein (LDL) cholesterol molecule where it prevents free radical damage:
  - vitamin E not only reduces LDL peroxidation, but also improves plasma LDL breakdown, inhibits excessive platelet aggregation, increases high density lipoprotein (HDL) cholesterol levels, and increases the breakdown of fibrin, a clot-forming protein.
  - dosage: 400–800 IU mixed tocopherols q.d.
- **Coenzyme Q$_{10}$:** CoQ$_{10}$ is an essential component of the mitochondria – the factories where energy is produced in our cells:
  - although CoQ$_{10}$ can be synthesized within the body, deficiency has been found in 39% of patients with high blood pressure.

- in several studies, CoQ$_{10}$ has been shown to lower blood pressure approximately 10% in patients with hypertension, although not until after 4–12 weeks of therapy.
- CoQ$_{10}$ seems to lower blood pressure by: (1) lowering cholesterol levels, and (2) stabilizing the vascular system via its antioxidant properties. These actions reduce resistance to blood flow through the arteries.
- dosage: 50 mg b.i.d.–t.i.d.

Additional supplements that may be recommended
- **Vitamin B$_6$:** B$_6$ influences the nervous system in a manner that leads to reduction in blood pressure:
  - vitamin B$_6$ supplementation has resulted in significant reductions in systolic and diastolic blood pressure as well as serum levels of the stress-induced hormone, norepinephrine (noradrenaline).
  - the effects of B$_6$ may have tremendous clinical significance, as the systolic pressure dropped from 167 to 153 mmHg and the diastolic pressure dropped from 108 to 98 mmHg in a 4-week study.
  - dosage: dosage used in the above study was 5 mg/kg body weight for 4 weeks.
- **Calcium:** while epidemiological data have demonstrated that calcium supplementation can lower blood pressure in cases of hypertension, clinical studies have been inconsistent:
  - currently it appears that calcium supplementation produces effective reductions in blood pressure in Blacks, in patients who are salt sensitive (but not in patients who have salt-resistant hypertension), and in elderly hypertensives. In one study, over a period of 24 hours, the mean systolic and diastolic blood pressures declined by 13.6 mmHg and 5.0 mmHg, respectively, in elderly patients whose diet was supplemented with 1 g of elemental calcium.
  - dosage: 1 g elemental calcium (calcium citrate is recommended as it is more effectively absorbed).

Botanical medicines
- **Garlic:** commercial preparations that provide a daily dose of at least 10 mg alliin, or a total allicin potential of 4,000 µg, have been shown to result in a drop of roughly 8–11 mmHg for the systolic and 5–8 mmHg for the diastolic blood pressure within 1–3 months; dosage: the equivalent of 4,000 mg of fresh garlic q.d.
- ***Crataegus monogyna* (hawthorn):** studies in Europe, where extracts of hawthorn are widely used by physicians, have demonstrated that hawthorn extracts are effective in lowering blood pressure and in

improving heart function:

- it usually requires 2–4 weeks before hawthorn begins to exert an effect, and in general, its blood pressure lowering effect is mild.
- dosage: hawthorn extract (10% procyanidins or 1.8% vitexin-4'-rhamnoside): 100–250 mg t.i.d.

Drug–herb interaction cautions

- **Garlic:**
  - plus *insulin*: animal studies suggest insulin dose may require adjusting due to hypoglycemic effects of whole garlic (in rats) and its constituent allicin (in rabbits).
  - plus *warfarin*: the anticoagulant activity of warfarin is enhanced as a result of increased fibrinolytic activity and diminished platelet aggregation caused by garlic components allicin, ajoene, trisulfides, and adenosine.
- ***Crataegus monogyna* (hawthorn):**
  - plus *digitalis*: hawthorn enhances the activity of cardiotonics such as digitalis, and the cardiac glycosides such as digitoxin (*in vitro*), as a result of its polymeric procyanidins, while reducing their toxicity by its coronary vasodilating and antiarrhythmic effects.

Physical medicine

In addition to the suggestions given above (Preventive Measures) to reduce stress, relaxation techniques, such as deep-breathing exercises, biofeedback, transcendental meditation, yoga, progressive muscle relaxation, and hypnosis, have all been shown to have some value in lowering blood pressure.

Diaphragmatic breathing

- One of the most powerful methods of reducing stress and increasing energy in the body is diaphragmatic breathing. When volunteers with normal blood pressure were taught how to breathe very shallowly, measurement of the amount of sodium and potassium excreted in their urine indicated that shallow breathing led to the retention of sodium in the body, which is a cause of high blood pressure.
- Producing deep relaxation with any technique requires learning how to breathe. One of the most powerful ways to decrease stress and increase energy in the body is by breathing with the diaphragm. By using the diaphragm to breathe, a person's physiology can be dramatically changed, literally activating the relaxation centers in the brain.
- To learn to breathe with your diaphragm:
  - find a quiet, comfortable place to sit or lie down.
  - place your feet slightly apart. Place one hand on your abdomen near your navel. Place the other hand on your chest.
  - inhale through your nose and exhale through your mouth.
  - concentrate on your breathing. Notice which hand is rising and falling with each breath.
  - gently exhale most of the air in your lungs.
  - inhale while slowly counting to four. As you inhale, slightly extend your abdomen, causing it to rise about 2.5 cm (1 in). Make sure that you are not moving your chest or shoulders.
  - as you breathe in, imagine the warmed air flowing in. Imagine this warmth flowing to all parts of your body.
  - pause for 1 sec, then slowly exhale to a count of four. As you exhale, your abdomen should move inward.
  - as the air flows out, imagine all your tension and stress leaving your body.
  - repeat the process until you achieve a sense of deep relaxation.

Hyperthyroidism

DESCRIPTION

Hyperthyroidism refers to overactivity of the thyroid, an endocrine gland situated in the front of the neck, just below the larynx (voice box), that regulates the metabolism of every cell of the body, and therefore, all body functions. Excessive production of thyroid hormone (T_4), most commonly (85% of cases) results in an autoimmune disorder (a disorder in which the individual's immune system produces antibodies that attack the body's own tissues) called Graves' disease. Graves' disease occurs much more frequently in women than men (a ratio of 8 : 1), and typically begins between the ages of 20 and 40 years.

FREQUENT SIGNS AND SYMPTOMS

- Nervousness, anxiety, restlessness, irritability
- Sweating
- Feeling warm or hot all the time, heat intolerance
- Pounding, rapid, irregular heartbeat
- Sleeplessness
- Tremors
- Weight loss, despite a good appetite (older persons may gain weight)
- Frequent stools
- Loose stools, diarrhea (sometimes)
- Hair thinning or loss (sometimes)
- Protruding eyes (*exophthalmos*) and double vision (sometimes)
- Non-painful goiter (chronic swelling of the thyroid) (sometimes)
- *Vitiligo* (the appearance of white patches on otherwise normal skin) (sometimes)
- Nails may be thickened and spoon-shaped or may separate prematurely from the nail bed (sometimes)

CAUSES

- **Autoimmune disorder:** the immune system develops antibodies that stimulate excessive production of thyroid hormones.

RISK INCREASES WITH

- **Female gender:** the female to male ratio is 8 : 1.
- **Stress:** onset of Graves' disease often follows some kind of emotional shock, in particular some sort of loss such as divorce, death, or difficult separation. Risk for Graves' disease is increased 6.3 times after such a negative life event.
- **Heredity/genetic susceptibility:** identical twins have a 50% chance, and fraternal twins a 9% chance of manifesting Graves' if one twin is affected. Risk for developing Graves' disease is increased 3.6 times if a family member has the disease.
- **Left-handedness:** 70% of Graves' disease patients have some degree of left-handedness compared to 24% of controls.
- **Smoking:** risk for Graves' disease increases 1.5 times for smokers, especially if other eye problems (protruding eyes, double vision) are present.
- **Mercury and cadmium exposure:** exposure to toxic levels of cadmium or mercury will induce immediate hyperthyroidism.
- **Drugs:** especially in older patients whose intake of iodine is low, a toxic reaction to prescription drugs – particularly the use of the antihypertensive (high blood pressure) drug, amiodarone – may induce hyperthyroidism. In older adults, the most common symptoms are apathy; rapid, irregular heartbeat; and weight loss.
- **Iodine:** although iodine deficiency is still a problem worldwide, iodine excess is more common in developed countries:
  - *excessive iodine supplementation*: dietary iodine supplementation – through mandatory consumption of iodized salt – in areas where iodine intake is sufficient has been shown to increase incidence of Graves' disease in susceptible individuals.
  - *sources of iodine include*: additives to food products (e.g., salt and iodine are used to sterilize pipes in dairies), and in medical washes (e.g., Betadine washes, and iodine-containing drugs such as amiodarone).

PREVENTIVE MEASURES

- **Learn to cope with stress effectively:**
  - prioritize – then live according to your values.

- avoid excessive work hours, poor nutrition, and inadequate rest.
- avoid stimulants like caffeine and nicotine that promote the fight-or-flight response and tend to make people more irritable.
- take time to build your long-term health. Meditate, pray, learn deep-breathing exercises, exercise regularly.
- join a church, synagogue, or other group that provides spiritual and social support.
- focus on what you can be thankful for and give thanks daily. Keep a gratitude journal.
- be patient and tolerant of others, and yourself. Everyone makes mistakes, which are always opportunities to learn and grow.

- **Don't smoke**
- **Minimize intake of caffeine**
- **Ensure iodine intake is not excessive:** minimize intake of iodized salt.
- **Minimize mercury exposure:**
  - if mercury dental fillings are present, consider their removal. Silver amalgam fillings contain between 48 and 55% mercury, which does leach into the system. One recent study found that frequent gum chewers with amalgam fillings had twice the amount of mercury in their blood and three times the amount of mercury in their urine and breath exhalation as non-frequent gum chewers.
  - tuna, sea bass, oysters (Gulf of Mexico), marlin, halibut, pike, walleye, white croaker, and largemouth bass are all fish that may contain potentially harmful levels of mercury.
- **A health-promoting diet:** consume a nutrient-dense diet rich in whole, unprocessed, preferably organic foods, especially plant foods (fruits, vegetables, beans, seeds and nuts), and cold-water fish, and low in animal products (for more detailed information, see Appendix 1).
- **Take a high-potency multiple vitamin and mineral supplement:** a daily multiple providing all of the known vitamins and minerals serves as a foundation upon which to build an individualized health-promotion program. Any good multiple should include 400 μg of folic acid, 400 μg of vitamin B_{12}, and 50–100 mg of vitamin B_6. (Folic acid supplementation should always be accompanied by vitamin B_{12} supplementation to prevent folic acid from masking a vitamin B_{12} deficiency.)

Expected outcomes

The chief objective of the natural treatment of Graves' disease and hyperthyroidism is to provide supportive care to conventional medicines in reducing symptoms while trying to reestablish normal thyroid status. About 20% of patients with Graves' disease experience spontaneous remission. Most patients with Graves' disease ultimately develop hypothyroidism either as a result of medical treatment or simply the progressive autoimmune destruction of the thyroid gland.

TREATMENT

Diet

- Consume a balanced whole foods diet composed of unprocessed, preferably organic foods, especially plant foods (fruits, vegetables, whole grains, beans, nuts [especially walnuts], and seeds), and cold-water fish (for more detailed information, see Appendix 1).
- The diet should be high in calories to compensate for the increased metabolic rate of hyperthyroidism.
- Eat small, frequent meals to provide a source of fuel throughout the day. Each mini-meal should contain protein as well as complex carbohydrates, fat, and fiber.
- If weight loss has been significant, supplement with additional protein. Try this nutrient-dense shake as a mini-meal or snack:
  - combine in blender: 2 scoops of protein powder, 1–2 tbsp nuts or nut butter, 1 cup yogurt, 1 cup fresh or frozen fruit/berries (bananas and blueberries are especially good), 1 tbsp flaxseed oil, 1 tbsp spirulina, 1 tbsp flaxseed meal; if desired, thin with rice, almond, soy or cow's milk. Blend.
- Avoid caffeine-containing foods and other stimulants.

Nutritional supplements

- **Vitamin A:** in large amounts, vitamin A inhibits thyroid function and has been shown to lessen the symptoms of Graves' disease:
  - in animal studies, large amounts of vitamin A inhibit the cells' uptake of thyroid hormone by lowering the capacity of the cells' receptors for T_3 (the active form of thyroid hormone).
  - dosage: 50,000 IU q.d.
- **Vitamin C:** abnormalities in thyroid hormone levels are associated with a reduction in the ascorbic acid (vitamin C) content of the serum, blood, liver, adrenal, thymus, and kidney. Supplementation is recommended to help normalize vitamin C levels and ameliorate the symptoms and metabolic effects of excessive thyroid activity; dosage 2,000 mg b.i.d.
- **Vitamin E:** higher amounts of free radical production are associated with hyperthyroidism. Supplemental vitamin E is recommended to protect against oxidative damage; dosage: 800 IU mixed tocopherols q.d.

- **Calcium:** calcium metabolism is altered in hyperthyroidism, and Graves' patients are more susceptible to osteoporosis; dosage: 1,000–1,500 mg q.d.
- **Zinc:** blood levels of zinc are decreased in patients with hyperthyroidism, most probably because the increased breakdown of tissue that occurs because of the elevated metabolic rate of hyperthyroidism results in greater urinary excretion of zinc. Hyperthyroidism also causes less zinc to be assimilated by tissues after zinc-containing foods are eaten; dosage: 30–45 mg q.d.

Botanical medicines

- ***Lycopus* species (*Lithospermum officinale* and/or *Melissa officinalis*):** these plants have been traditionally used in the treatment of hyperthyroidism. The results of both *in vitro* (test tube) and *in vivo* (in rats) studies support their use. *Lycopus* spp. have been shown to block thyroid stimulating hormone receptors, and to block conversion of thyroid hormone (T_4) to its more active form (T_3). Dosage: choose one of the following forms and take the recommended dosage t.i.d.:
  - dried herb: 1–3 g or by infusion
  - tincture (1 : 5): 2–6 ml
  - fluid extract (1 : 1): 1–3 ml.

Drug–herb interaction cautions

Lycopus species plants may interfere with thyroid hormone medications.

Physical medicine
- **Hydrotherapy:**
  - place cold packs on the throat (over the thyroid) for 15 min t.i.d.
  - tepid baths, particularly before bed, are calming. A few drops of lavender essential oil may be added for a soothing aromatherapy treatment.
  - an ice bag placed over the heart will reduce heart rate but should not be overused.

Mind/body medicine

Stress control is the single most important action you can take to help thyroid function return to normal.
- Avoid anything that excites and agitates.
- Utilize the stress reduction suggestions given above (see Preventive Measures).
- Get counseling to help prevent a return to stress-generating life strategies.
- Increase rest: take a daily nap after lunch as well as getting a full night's sleep.

Hypoglycemia

DESCRIPTION

Hypoglycemia is low (hypo) blood sugar (glycemia). Normally, the body maintains blood sugar levels within a narrow range through the coordinated teamwork of several glands and their hormones. However, when these finely balanced control mechanisms are disrupted, hypoglycemia (low blood sugar) or diabetes (high blood sugar) may result.

Normally, as food is digested, levels of blood sugar (glucose) gradually rise, signaling the beta-cells of the pancreas, which respond by secreting the hormone *insulin*. Insulin lowers blood glucose levels by increasing the rate at which cells recognize and admit sugar. When blood glucose levels drop because food is not consumed (e.g., overnight), or because energy needs are increased (e.g., exercise), another hormone called *glucagon* is secreted by the alpha cells of the pancreas. Glucagon stimulates the release of glucose that has been stored in body tissues, especially the liver, as *glycogen*. Glycogen is also released when a rapid drop in blood sugar levels, such as that caused by anger, fright, or stress, stimulates the secretion of the adrenal gland's flight-or-fight hormones, *epinephrine* and *corticosteroids*, which rapidly break down glycogen for immediate energy needs.

Because the Standard American Diet is loaded with refined carbohydrates, which are stripped of both fiber (which slows down their absorption) and nutrients (which help the body metabolize sugars), large amounts of glucose are dumped into the bloodstream after virtually every meal and snack, overloading normal sugar delivery control mechanisms, until malfunction – in the form of hypoglycemia, and eventually, diabetes – results.

Although numerous organizations, including the US government, recommend that not more than 10% of a person's total calories come from refined sugars added to foods, these added sugars account for about 30% of the diets of most Americans. The average American consumes over 45 kg (100 lb) of sucrose and 18 kg (40 lb) of corn syrup each year. It is therefore not surprising that faulty blood sugar control is becoming an increasingly common factor in a cluster of related disease processes. The term "syndrome X" has been coined to describe a progression of abnormalities initiated by a high intake of refined carbohydrates, leading to the development of hypoglycemia, excessive insulin secretion, and glucose intolerance, and followed by diminished insulin sensitivity, which leads to high blood pressure, elevated cholesterol levels, obesity, and ultimately, type II diabetes. Hypoglycemia is divided into two main types: *reactive* and *fasting*. Reactive hypoglycemia, by far the more common, is characterized by the development of symptoms 3–5 hours after a meal (but may also be caused by the drugs commonly used to treat diabetes). Fasting hypoglycemia is rare, only appearing in severe disease states such as pancreatic tumors, extensive liver damage, prolonged starvation, various cancers, or as a result of excessive insulin injections in diabetics.

In hypoglycemia, the brain is the first organ affected. Almost all of the energy used by the brain is supplied by glucose derived from the blood, and most of this is derived second by second, with a total of only about a 2-min supply of glucose, stored as glycogen, in the brain cells. And, although it accounts for only 2% of the body's total mass, the brain is a very hungry organ, using up 15% of all the glucose in the body. Mental symptoms, which can range from mild to severe, include headache, depression, anxiety, irritability, psychological disturbances, confusion, incoherent speech, bizarre behavior, and convulsions.

FREQUENT SIGNS AND SYMPTOMS

Symptoms vary greatly in frequency and severity.
- Weakness or faintness
- Sweating
- Excessive hunger
- Craving for sweets
- Feeling tired or weak if a meal is missed
- Feeling tired an hour or so after eating
- Dizziness when standing suddenly
- Occasional shakiness
- Afternoon fatigue
- Occasional blurry vision
- Overweight
- Frequent headaches: hypoglycemia has been known to be a common trigger for migraines since 1993

- Poor memory (forgetfulness) or concentration
- Confusion
- Frequent anxiety, nervousness and trembling hands
- Depression or mood swings
- Premenstrual syndrome (PMS): symptoms including increased appetite, craving for sweets, headache, fatigue, fainting spells, and heart palpitations have been linked to hypoglycemia.
- Personality changes: several controlled studies of psychiatric patients and habitually violent and impulsive criminals have shown that reactive hypoglycemia is common in both populations. Several large studies involving over 6,000 inmates in 10 penal institutions have demonstrated that the elimination of refined sugars significantly reduced antisocial, aggressive, and self-damaging behavior in males.
- Atherosclerosis, intermittent claudication (a painful cramp in the calf muscle due to lack of oxygen), angina (chest pain): a high sugar intake leads to elevations in triglyceride and cholesterol levels. Abnormal glucose tolerance tests and high insulin levels are common findings in patients with heart disease.
- Heart palpitations or irregularities (rare)
- Fainting, loss of consciousness (rare)
- Seizures (sometimes)

CAUSES

- **Excessive intake of refined carbohydrates:** this is the most common cause of hypoglycemia and triggers the pancreas to secrete too much insulin, the hormone responsible for removing glucose from the bloodstream.
- **Heavy exercise:** can rapidly deplete available energy stores.
- **Pregnancy:** providing for the metabolic needs of the rapidly developing fetus places additional demands on sugar control mechanisms.
- **Drugs that decrease blood sugar levels:**
  - tobacco
  - caffeine
  - alcohol
  - aspirin
  - prescription drugs: sulfonylurea medications; metformin; haloperidol; chlorpromazine; propranolol; pentamidine; disopyramide and the prescription painkiller Darvocet, in which propoxyphene is combined with acetaminophen
- **Diseases:**
  - tumor in the pancreas (rare)
  - chronic kidney failure

RISK INCREASES WITH

- A diet too high in refined carbohydrates/sugars
- Stress
- Smoking
- Use of drugs, especially those listed above
- Fatigue or overwork
- Skipping meals

PREVENTIVE MEASURES

- **Stop consuming the Standard American Diet (SAD):** the human body was not designed to handle the amount of refined sugar, salt, saturated and *trans* fats, and harmful chemical additives found in the processed foods typically consumed in the United States.
- A health-promoting diet: consume a nutrient-dense diet rich in whole, unprocessed, preferably organic foods, especially plant foods (fruits, vegetables, beans, seeds and nuts, and whole grains) and cold-water fish, and low in animal products and processed foods (for more detailed information, see Appendix 1).
- **A high-potency multiple vitamin and mineral supplement:** this should include 400 µg of folic acid, 400 µg of vitamin B_{12}, and 50–100 mg of vitamin B_6. (Folic acid supplementation should always be accompanied by vitamin B_{12} supplementation to prevent folic acid from masking a vitamin B_{12} deficiency.) A good daily multiple providing all of the known vitamins and minerals serves as a foundation upon which to build an individualized health-promotion program.

Expected outcomes

Blood sugar control should improve immediately, and all symptoms due to reactive hypoglycemia should resolve within 2–4 weeks.

TREATMENT

Diet

- **Follow the dietary recommendations** given in Preventive measures.
- **Consume a diet high in fiber and complex carbohydrates:**
  - blood sugar disorders have been conclusively shown to be related to inadequate dietary fiber intake.
  - water-soluble fibers slow digestion and absorption of carbohydrates (thus preventing rapid rises in blood sugar), increase cell sensitivity to insulin (thus preventing excessive insulin secretion), and

Natural Medicine Instructions for Patients

improve the uptake of glucose by the liver and other tissues (thus preventing a sustained elevation in blood sugar).

- best sources of water-soluble fiber: legumes, oat bran, nuts, seeds (especially flaxseed meal), psyllium seed husks, pears, apples, and most vegetables.
- a daily intake of 50 g of fiber is recommended.

■ **Legumes**, which are high in fiber, complex carbohydrates and protein, should be eaten regularly.

■ **Don't skip meals**

■ **Eat frequently:** frequent (five) small meals q.d. will stabilize blood sugar levels more effectively than three large meals.

■ **Avoid alcohol:** alcohol causes hypoglycemia by interfering with normal glucose utilization and increasing insulin secretion. The resulting drop in blood sugar produces a craving for foods that quickly elevate blood sugar, as well as a craving for more alcohol:

- hypoglycemia is a significant complication of alcohol abuse that aggravates the mental and emotional problems of the active or withdrawing alcoholic with symptoms such as sweating, tremor, dizziness, rapid heartbeat, headache, visual disturbance, decreased mental function, and depression.
- alcohol initially induces hypoglycemia, but eventually the body becomes desensitized to the excessive release of insulin caused by alcohol. In the long term, alcohol leads to hyperglycemia (high blood sugar) and diabetes.

■ **Minimize consumption of refined carbohydrates and sugars:** refined carbohydrates and sugars are quickly absorbed by the body, rapidly elevating blood sugar levels and stimulating a correspondingly excessive rise in blood insulin levels:

- virtually all the vitamin and trace mineral content has been removed from white sugar, white breads and pastries, and many breakfast cereals. Eating foods high in simple sugars in any form – lactose, maltose, glucose, sucrose, fructose, white grape juice concentrate, corn syrup, honey, maple syrup – is harmful to blood sugar control.
- currently, more than half the carbohydrates consumed in the US are in the form of these sugars added to processed foods. Read food labels and avoid these foods.

■ **Fructose** – the sugar found in whole fruits – may be well tolerated:

- fructose must be converted in the liver to glucose before it can be utilized, so does not raise blood sugar levels as quickly as sucrose (white table sugar) or white bread and other refined carbohydrates.
- fructose has been shown to enhance sensitivity to insulin.
- the sugars in whole foods (fruits and vegetables) are balanced by a wide range of nutrients that aid in their utilization, and are absorbed more slowly because they are contained within cells and are associated with fiber and other food elements.
- eating whole fruit may also help control sugar cravings and promote weight loss in overweight individuals. Studies have shown that eating aspartame (Nutrasweet), glucose, and sucrose actually increases sugar cravings. Fructose, however, decreases the amount of calories and fat consumed.

■ **Caution:** large amounts of fruit juice and even vegetable juice can cause problems for hypoglycemics because the cell wall disruption characteristic of juicing increases the absorption rate of the sugars in the juices.

Nutritional supplements
■ **Multiple vitamin and mineral supplement** (see Preventive measures).

■ **Chromium:** as a key constituent of *glucose tolerance factor*, chromium functions as a cofactor in all insulin-regulating activities, and plays a major role in the sensitivity of cells to insulin:

- marginal chromium deficiency is widespread in the US. In supplementation studies (b.i.d. for 3 months), chromium was shown to improve glucose tolerance test results and alleviate hypoglycemic symptoms.
- chromium supplementation should be combined with a regular exercise program for maximum effect (see below).
- dosage: 200–400 μg q.d.

Physical medicine
■ **Exercise:** regular exercise has been well documented to prevent type II diabetes by improving many aspects of glucose metabolism, including enhancing insulin sensitivity and improving glucose tolerance, even in persons with diabetes:

- some of the positive effects of exercise may stem from the fact that it increases tissue concentrations of chromium.
- follow an exercise program that elevates the heart rate to at least 60% of maximum for 30 min, three times a week.

Hypothyroidism

DESCRIPTION

Hypothyroidism refers to low function of the thyroid, an endocrine gland located in the front of the neck, just below the larynx (voice box). Through its production of thyroid hormones (T_4 and T_3), the thyroid gland activates over 100 cellular enzymes responsible for a multitude of functions in every cell of the body. Excessive secretion of thyroid hormones can increase metabolic rate up to 100% above normal, while if no thyroid hormone is produced, a 40% drop in metabolic activity can quickly occur. In most cases of hypothyroidism, thyroid function is simply less than optimal, but this results in a slowing down of cellular functions and a buildup of metabolic wastes in all body systems. Hypothyroidism ranges from a barely detectable (subclinical) lessening in thyroid hormone production and/or activity to a severe life-threatening deficiency state called myxedema.

The thyroid gland is not an isolated entity, but is part of a web of bodily systems whose other primary actors include: the hypothalamus, the pituitary, the liver, the kidneys, the adrenal glands, and a network of hormone-like substances called cytokines. Impairment in the activity of any of these components of the thyroid system may be an underlying cause of an individual's low thyroid activity.

The thyroid produces two main hormones: T_4, which is much less active, and T_3, the hormone that primarily regulates the metabolic machinery inside cells. The production of T_4 and T_3 is closely controlled by the thyroid's two supervisors, the pituitary and hypothalamus, two endocrine glands that are located in the brain. When T_3 levels in the blood drop, the hypothalamus secretes *thyrotropin-releasing hormone* (TRH), which in turn signals the pituitary to secrete *thyroid-stimulating hormone* (TSH). As its name implies, TSH stimulates the thyroid gland to combine iodine with the amino acid tyrosine, thus producing about 90% of the body's T_4 together with about 10% of its T_3. (T_4 is tyrosine plus four iodine molecules, while T_3 is tyrosine plus three iodine molecules.) If, for some reason, the hypothalamus does not secrete TRH, the pituitary has a fail-safe system. The pituitary double-checks the hypothalamus by sampling the level of T_3 in its own circulation when it converts inactive

T_4 into T_3 in its own cells. If its T_3 levels drop, the pituitary gland will secrete TSH, thus triggering the production and release of T_4 by the thyroid to quickly rectify this situation.

Once T_4 is in the blood, another physiologic network takes over, and, with the aid of cortisone, a hormone secreted by the adrenal gland, T_4 is converted to T_3 in the peripheral tissues, primarily the liver and kidneys, and sent into the bloodstream.

Although in the circulation, T_3 is still not home free. Its final target, where it actually affects metabolic functioning, is the interior of cells. To get inside the cells, T_3 has to pass through the cellular membranes and, by connecting with the correct receptor sites, gain entry into the mitochondria (the tiny organs in each cell where energy is produced) and/or the cell nucleus.

Lastly, proper thyroid function faces one other potential roadblock: cytokines. Cytokines are hormone-like substances secreted by various types of cell that direct immune responses and act as messengers in cell-to-cell communication. Some cytokines directly affect the hypothalamic–pituitary–thyroid axis and are also capable of blocking the conversion of T_4 to T_3.

What else can go wrong? If levels of iodine in the diet are inadequate, the thyroid cannot produce T_4. In this situation, the thyroid typically enlarges, swelling into a goiter, a characteristic sign of hypothyroidism in the developing world where iodine deficiency is common. Long-term stress, which uses up the adrenal glands' reserve of cortisone, may cause a problem. Even if the thyroid gland produces sufficient amounts of T_4, so that blood tests of T_4 levels (the test commonly used to evaluate thyroid activity) appear normal, if no cortisol is available for use in the liver and kidneys to convert T_4 to T_3, metabolism will slow down. Excessive levels of cytokines may also be the culprit here, as certain cytokines prevent the conversion of T_4 to T_3.

If a blood test finds low levels of T_4 along with low levels of TSH, this suggests that the pituitary is not doing its job. If, however, blood levels of TSH are elevated and T_4 levels are still low, this indicates that the pituitary has responded properly, but that the thyroid gland is not following the directions provided by TSH.

If T_3 levels are adequate, this suggests one of three possibilities: cellular membranes could be malfunctioning so T_3 cannot gain entry into the cells; T_3 could be just slightly malformed, so it cannot gain entry into the cell or, if it can gain entry to the cell, it cannot attach to the appropriate receptor sites once inside; or the receptor sites inside the cells are not functioning properly.

To sum up, hypothyroidism may be due to: (1) inadequate T_4 synthesis, either because the pituitary is not secreting TSH or because the thyroid gland is not responding to TSH and making T_4; (2) inadequate conversion of T_4 to T_3 in peripheral tissues; (3) an inability of T_3 to gain entry to the interior of cells because of a problem with cell membranes; or (4) an inability of T_3 to attach to receptors inside the cells and activate enzymes. Factors that may contribute to these four potential causes of hypothyroidism are discussed below.

It is estimated that as many as 13 million Americans have some disorder in their thyroid function, but more than half are undiagnosed, since many people mistake the signs of hypothyroidism for aging-associated declines. Mild thyroid failure occurs in 4–17% of women and 2–7% of men, with the risk increasing with age. The elderly are most susceptible, but hypothyroidism can affect people of all ages, even infants. One in 4,000 infants is born with congenital hypothyroidism.

If blood levels of T_4 are used as the only criterion, between 1 and 4% of the adult population has moderate to severe hypothyroidism, and another 10–12% has mild hypothyroidism. If, in addition to blood thyroid (T_4) levels, medical history, physical examination, and basal body temperature are used, the true incidence of hypothyroidism ranges somewhere near 25% of the population – about 20% of those affected being women and 5% men.

FREQUENT SIGNS AND SYMPTOMS

- Low basal body temperature (the temperature of the body at rest):
  - body temperature reflects metabolic rate which is largely determined by thyroid hormones.
  - should be between 97.6 and 98.2°F.
  - to check basal body temperature, shake down a thermometer to below 95°F and place it by the bed before going to sleep. Upon waking, place the thermometer under the armpit for a full 10 min. Remain as still as possible, resting with the eyes closed. Record the temperature for at least three consecutive mornings, preferably at the same time of day.
  - menstruating women must perform the test on the second, third, and fourth days of menstruation. Men and postmenopausal women can perform the test on any three consecutive days.
- Chronic lethargy, fatigue, weakness

- Overly sensitive to cold (cold hands or feet)
- Elevation in cholesterol and triglyceride levels: this greatly increases the risk of cardiovascular disease
- Muscle and joint aches
- Headaches
- Moderate weight gain, despite diminished appetite, and difficulty losing weight: hypothyroid patients generally show a moderate weight increase of 2–5 kg (5–10 lb), mainly from edema (fluid accumulation)
- Constipation
- Recurrent infections
- Loss of libido
- Heavy menstrual bleeding and shorter menstrual cycle (the time between periods) in premenopausal women
- Infertility
- Miscarriages, premature deliveries, stillbirths
- Rough, dry skin covered with fine, superficial scales
- Coarse, dry, brittle hair
- Thin brittle nails with transverse grooves
- Slight impairment of concentration and memory
- Depression
- Shortness of breath
- Impaired kidney function

Symptoms indicating significant thyroid dysfunction

- Edema resulting from increases in capillary permeability and slow lymphatic drainage
- Hardening of the arteries as a result of the increase in cholesterol and triglyceride levels
- Hypertension, reduced heart function, reduced heart rate
- Husky voice
- Numbness of arms and legs
- Muscle pain and weakness, causing carpal tunnel syndrome in some cases
- Joint stiffness, pain and tenderness
- Hearing loss
- Depression
- Mental confusion, difficulty concentrating, extreme forgetfulness/memory problems, especially in the elderly
- Unsteadiness
- Daytime sleepiness
- Obstructive sleep apnea: tissues in the upper throat collapse at intervals during sleep, blocking the passage of air
- Myxedema – a round puffy face, sleepy appearance, dry rough skin, loss of hair

Symptoms associated with pituitary tumor

- Any of the above symptoms
- Lowered sexual drive, impaired fertility

- Decreased adrenal gland function resulting in exhaustion, low blood pressure, salt craving
- Headaches and visual disturbances directly related to the pituitary tumor

CAUSES

- **Overtreatment of hyperthyroidism (excessive thyroid activity):** surgery, drugs and/or radiation can damage the thyroid resulting in hypothyroidism.
- **Disorders of the pituitary or hypothalamus glands (rare)**
- **Inadequate intake of iodine:** T_4 is made when the thyroid gland adds iodine to the amino acid tyrosine; if the diet is deficient in iodine, the body cannot manufacture T_4:
  - in developing nations worldwide, 200 million people have goiters. In all but 4% of these cases, the goiter is due to iodine deficiency.
- **Excessive iodine:** too much iodine inhibits the conversion of T_4 to T_3:
  - in developed nations such as the US where iodine has been added to salt, iodine deficiency is quite rare, yet some people still develop goiters. In these people, the goiter may be due to excessive consumption of foods, called *goitrogens*, that block iodine utilization (rare) or to nutrient deficiency (see below).
  - goitrogens include Brassica family foods (turnips, cabbages, rutabagas, mustard greens, radishes, horseradishes), cassava root, soybeans, peanuts, pine nuts, and millet.
  - cooking, however, usually inactivates goitrogens.
- **Deficiency in nutrient cofactors necessary for T_4 production:** zinc, copper, vitamins A, B_2, B_3, B_6, and/or C.
- **Deficiency in nutrient cofactors necessary for conversion of T_4 to T_3:** selenium, zinc.
- **Impaired cellular response to T_3:** due to iron or zinc deficiency, physical inactivity.
- **Metals and heavy metals, including lead, mercury, dental amalgams:** these metals can cause alterations in cellular membranes and receptor sites, thus preventing T_3 from gaining entry to the cell's interior or mobilizing enzymes once inside:
  - the destructive effects of heavy metals on the endocrine organs, including the thyroid gland, are well documented. Both lead and mercury (dental amalgams are 50% mercury, and the teeth are only a short distance from the thyroid gland) commonly invade the thyroid gland and interfere with the

production of thyroid hormones, or induce minute alterations in their molecular structure, so that the hormones are no longer recognized by, and admitted into, cells.
  - heavy metals can also impair liver and kidney function, thus decreasing conversion of T_4 to T_3.
- **Stress:** chronic stress may result in a state of adrenal exhaustion in which supplies of cortisone are depleted. Cortisone is necessary for the conversion of T_4 to T_3 in the liver and kidneys. Sources of stress may be emotional as well as physical, including head or body injury, chronic allergies or infections, anxiety, poor diet, lack of sleep.
- **Pesticide-contaminated water exposure:** tap water can be contaminated with low levels of insecticides, weed killers, and artificial fertilizer. Pesticides have been shown to interfere with thyroid function and to increase cancer risk:
  - people not only drink and cook with water, but also bathe and shower in it, thus absorbing chemicals through the digestive tract, skin and by breathing in the vapors, through the lungs.
  - the likelihood of pesticide contamination of water is highest in agricultural areas.
- **Fluoride:** it is well documented that fluoride is a direct antagonist to, and therefore inhibits utilization of, iodine. Although fluoridation of water supplies is controversial, many experts believe fluoride, like mercury, is a chemical toxin that should be avoided.
- **Xenobiotics:** the term *xenobiotic* is used to describe toxins that come into our bodies from the environment. These include pesticides, hormone and antibiotic residues in meat and dairy products, food-borne bacteria; chemicals in cleaning products, food additives, cosmetics; the metabolic by-products of unfriendly gut bacteria, etc.
  - xenobiotics can impair the activity of the liver and kidneys, thus decreasing conversion of T_4 to T_3.
  - xenobiotics have been shown to increase the production of reverse T_3 – a form of T_3 in which the iodide group normally removed from T_4 is left on and another iodide is removed instead. Since reverse T_3 is shaped differently from normal T_3, it does not produce the same effects.
- **Autoimmune disease:** in autoimmune disease, the body's immune system develops antibodies that attack its own cells – in this case, the cells in the thyroid gland. Experts are not certain why the immune system starts to attack the thyroid:
  - two current theories are:
    - *a virus or bacterium* with a protein resembling a thyroid protein triggers the immune attack. This theory is backed up to some extent by the

association between hepatitis C, for instance, and the onset of autoimmune hypothyroidism.

- *a genetic defect or susceptibility* leads to the development of abnormal thyroid cells that provoke an attack by T cells, important agents in the immune system.

■ *Hashimoto's thyroiditis*, a common form of hypothyroidism, is an autoimmune disease linked to genetic susceptibility. Named after the Japanese physician who first described the condition, it presents with a goiter, and results in damage to the thyroid gland, therefore requiring life-long treatment.

■ *atrophic thyroiditis* is a variation on Hashimoto's thyroiditis in which no goiter is present.

■ *postpartum thyroiditis*: In 1 : 2,000 women, hypothyroidism may develop during or after pregnancy. These women develop antibodies to their own thyroid during pregnancy, causing a thyroid inflammation that typically develops 4–12 months after delivery. Fortunately, this type of hypothyroidism usually resolves on its own, although bouts of hyperthyroidism may also occur before thyroid function normalizes. Women who experience recurrent episodes of postpartum thyroiditis after multiple pregnancies, or who have other autoimmune disorders, may develop permanent hypothyroidism.

■ *Riedel's thyroiditis* is a rare disorder in which patients develop a hard stony mass that suggests cancer, but which responds well to thyroid replacement.

■ **Drugs:** many drugs contain iodine or have properties that disrupt thyroid function, although the effects are almost always reversible when the drugs are stopped:

■ *lithium*: widely used to treat psychiatric disorders, lithium has multiple effects on thyroid hormone synthesis and secretion. Up to 50% of patients who take lithium develop goiter, and another 20–30% develop subclinical hypothyroidism.

■ *amiodarone (Cordarone)*: a drug used to treat abnormal heart rhythms that contains iodine and can induce hypothyroidism.

■ *certain antidepressants* may cause hypothyroidism.

■ *epilepsy drugs*, including phenytoin and carbamazepine, reduce thyroid hormone levels.

■ **X-rays:** ionizing radiation from medical and dental X-rays, particularly those received in childhood, can adversely affect thyroid function.

■ **Radioactive iodine:** high-dose radiation for cancers of the head or neck, or for Hodgkin's disease causes hypothyroidism in up to 65% of patients within 10 years after treatment.

■ **Frequent "yo-yo" dieting:** the body reacts to any significant reduction in calories consumed by turning

down the conversion of T_4 to T_3 – its metabolic thermostat.

■ **Pituitary tumor (rare):** a pituitary tumor will disrupt normal production of TSH, the hormone that stimulates the thyroid to produce T_4.

RISK INCREASES WITH

■ **Sex and age:** women are three to eight times more likely than men to develop hypothyroidism. Some experts estimate that as many as 10% of women over 50 have low thyroid function.

■ **Depression:** a recent study indicates that the active form of thyroid hormone (T_3) and L-tryptophan (a precursor of the neurotransmitter serotonin, a chemical important for feelings of well-being) are taken up by red blood cells using the same carrier. Alterations in one substance may affect the other.

■ **Radiation treatment** for cancers of the head or neck, or Hodgkin's disease.

■ **Frequent dieting**

■ **Surgery for hyperthyroidism**

■ **High intake of goitrogens** (foods that impair the use of iodine).

■ **Use of prescription drugs** including lithium, amiodarone, phenytoin, carbamazepine: so many drugs affect the thyroid that anyone taking drugs for the treatment of chronic disease should discuss the impact these on thyroid function with their physician.

■ **Disease-promoting diet:** thyroid function is dependent upon adequate amounts of a number of vitamins and minerals. A diet based on processed foods, with little consumption of fresh vegetables, legumes, fruits, nuts and seeds, whole grains, and cold-water fish is low in the factors necessary for T_4 production and conversion to T_3 – vitamins A, B_2, B_3, B_6, and C, and trace minerals zinc and selenium.

■ **Genetic susceptibility:** about half of those whose close relatives have chronic autoimmune disease have antibodies to the thyroid. Thyroid disease will often skip generations; someone with low thyroid function may have parents with normal thyroid activity, but grandparents who had thyroid problems:

■ *Turner's syndrome*: approximately half of those with Turner's syndrome, one of the most common genetic diseases in women, have hypothyroidism, usually the autoimmune form called Hashimoto's thyroiditis.

■ **Smoking, especially during pregnancy:** pregnant women with subclinical hypothyroidism who smoke between one and two packs of cigarettes daily are at risk for even lower thyroid function as well as decreased action of TSH in areas outside the thyroid, such as the liver. These women may also develop significantly higher levels of total cholesterol and low density lipoprotein (LDL) (bad) cholesterol than non-smoking women with subclinical hypothyroidism.

- **Autoimmune disease, especially during pregnancy:** women with insulin-dependent diabetes (type I) or other autoimmune conditions have a 25% risk for hypothyroidism during pregnancy. A miscarriage during early pregnancy may indicate the presence of antithyroid antibodies, and the risk for autoimmune-induced hypothyroidism is significantly elevated during the subsequent year.
- **Anorexia or bulimia:** people with anorexia or bulimia are at risk for hypothyroidism; in these cases, however, reduced thyroid function may be an adaptation to malnutrition. Treatment of the eating disorder will likely result in normalization of thyroid function.
- **Childhood X-ray treatments:** Everyone who has had head and neck radiation should have their thyroid glands examined regularly. Between 1920 and 1960, 2 million Americans, mostly children, received X-ray treatments to the head or neck for acne, enlarged thymus gland, recurrent tonsillitis, or chronic ear infections. Their risk of developing thyroid nodules and thyroid cancers is increased, particularly in those who have developed hypothyroidism, and cancer can develop as long as 40 years after the original treatment.
- **Atherosclerosis:** hypothyroidism is associated with atherosclerosis (commonly known as hardening of the arteries) and heart disease. Individuals with hypothyroidism are at higher risk due to their typically high levels of LDL (bad) cholesterol, even in subclinical hypothyroidism, and elevated levels of the cholesterol-carrying molecule lipoprotein(a), or Lp(a). Treatment of hypothyroidism can significantly reduce total cholesterol, LDL, and Lp(a), helping to prevent hardening of the arteries.
- **High blood pressure:** hypothyroidism may also slow the heart rate to less than 60 bpm and reduce the heart's pumping capacity. Although a recent study found no association between hypothyroidism and high blood pressure in older women, hypothyroidism does increase the risk for high blood pressure in pregnant women.
- **Disease associations:** hypothyroidism is associated with Addison's disease, iron deficiency anemia, respiratory problems, myasthenia gravis, ovarian failure, sleep apnea, premature gray hair, left-handedness, insulin-dependent diabetes, rheumatoid arthritis, and glaucoma.

PREVENTIVE MEASURES

- Avoid excessive consumption of goitrogens: Brassica family foods (turnips, cabbages, rutabagas, mustard greens, radishes, horseradishes), cassava root, soybeans, peanuts, pine nuts, and millet. When eating these foods, be certain they are well cooked as cooking usually inactivates goitrogens.
- Minimize drug use and use natural alternatives whenever possible.
- Avoid X-ray treatments unless medically necessary.
- Replace mercury-containing dental amalgams: amalgam fillings should be removed by a biologically trained dentist and replaced with non-metal (composite) fillings.
- Minimize exposure to xenobiotics. Eat whole organically grown foods, check your water supply and, if necessary, install water filters to ensure clean water.
- Exercise regularly and get adequate (an average of 8 hours per night) sleep.
- If chronic allergies or infections are present, work with a physician to develop a health-promotion program that heals these conditions.
- If weight loss is needed, don't diet. Work with a physician to develop an individualized version of the health-promoting diet described below that will enable weight loss without endangering health.
- Ensure adequate intake of key nutrients needed for production of T_4 and its conversion to T_3 by:
  - consuming a nutrient-dense diet rich in whole, unprocessed, preferably organic foods, especially plant foods (fruits, vegetables, beans, seeds and nuts, and whole grains) and cold water fish, and low in animal products and processed foods (for more detailed information, see Appendix 1).
  - taking a high-potency multiple vitamin and mineral supplement including 400 µg of folic acid, 400 µg of vitamin B_{12}, and 50–100 mg of vitamin B_6. (Folic acid supplementation should always be accompanied by vitamin B_{12} supplementation to prevent folic acid from masking a vitamin B_{12} deficiency.) A daily multiple providing all of the known vitamins and minerals serves as a foundation upon which to build an individualized health-promotion program.

Expected outcomes

In mild cases, hypothyroidism may be curable in 2–3 months, once underlying causal factors have been identified and an appropriate dietary, supplement, and exercise protocol instituted. Even in more severe cases, improvement in symptoms should be seen within 2–4 weeks.

TREATMENT

Diet

- Avoid goitrogens: Brassica family foods (turnips, cabbages, rutabagas, mustard greens, radishes, horseradishes), cassava root, soybeans, peanuts, pine nuts, and millet.
- After removing goitrogens from your diet, choose a balanced diet composed of whole, unprocessed, preferably organic foods, especially plant foods (fruits, vegetables, whole grains, beans, nuts [especially walnuts], and seeds), and cold-water fish (for more detailed information, see Appendix 1).

Nutritional supplements

- **Armour desiccated thyroid:** complete with all the thyroid hormones, not just T_4, supplements made from desiccated natural thyroid gland are preferred over synthetic hormones, which typically contain only isolated T_4:
  - using thyroid hormone replacement should be a last resort after attempting to restore normal function to the various components of the thyroid system. T_4 and T_3 replacement may suppress the patient's own hypothalamic–pituitary–thyroid axis and/or desensitize T_3 receptors to the body's own T_3, leading to dependency on thyroid hormone replacement.
  - because of the serious potential consequences of taking too much thyroid hormone, these preparations are available only by prescription from a physician.
- **Thyroid extracts sold in health food stores:** while much weaker, since licensing authorities require that they be virtually free of T_4, thyroid support formulas sold in health food stores still do contain minimal amounts of thyroid hormone and may provide adequate support for mild hypothyroidism. In addition, most health food store products contain the other key nutrients the body requires to manufacture T_4 and convert it to T_3, including iodine, zinc, and tyrosine.

- **Iodine and tyrosine:** T_4 is made from iodine and the amino acid tyrosine. Iodine's only function in the body is the synthesis of T_4, but too much iodine can actually inhibit this synthesis. Average intake of iodine in the US is estimated to be over 600 µg q.d.:
  - dosage: neither dietary levels nor supplementation of iodine should exceed 600 µg q.d.
- **Trace minerals:** the trace minerals zinc and copper, and the vitamins A, B_2 (riboflavin), B_3 (niacin), B_6 (pyridoxine), and C are all needed for the production of T_4. Of the three enzymes that convert T_4 to T_3, one is dependent on the trace mineral, selenium, while the activity of another is increased by vitamin A. Dosages per day (which should be found in any high-quality multiple):
  - zinc: 15–45 mg
  - copper: 1–2 mg
  - selenium: 100–200 µg
  - vitamin A (retinol): 5,000 IU (women of childbearing age should not exceed 2,500 IU q.d. if becoming pregnant is a possibility due to the risk of birth defects)
  - B_2 (riboflavin): 10–50 mg
  - B_3 (niacin): 10–100 mg
  - B_6 (pyridoxine): 25–100 mg
  - vitamin C: 1,000–2,000 mg.

Physical medicine

- Ensure a full 8 hours sleep each night.
- Exercise daily for 30–60 min:
  - exercise stimulates thyroid gland secretion and increases tissue sensitivity to thyroid hormone.
  - exercise is essential for overweight hypothyroid individuals who are dieting. Dieting has consistently been shown to cause a decrease in metabolic rate as the body strives to conserve fuel. Exercise prevents this decline in metabolic rate in response to dieting.
  - both weight training (which builds muscle mass) and aerobic exercise (which improves the body's use of oxygen) should be part of a regular exercise program.

Inflammatory bowel disease

DESCRIPTION

Inflammatory bowel disease (IBD) is a general term for a group of chronic inflammatory disorders of the intestines characterized by recurrent inflammation in specific parts of the intestines. The two main types of IBD are Crohn's disease and ulcerative colitis.

In Crohn's disease, the ileum (the final part of the small intestine) is the primary area affected, although the inflammatory reaction may also involve the mucosa of the mouth, esophagus, stomach, duodenum (the first part of the small intestine), jejunum (the middle portion of the small intestine), colon (the large intestine), the mesentery (outside covering of the intestines), or the lymph nodes in the abdominal region. In ulcerative colitis, the lining of the colon is the area affected.

IBD may occur at any age, but initial appearance is typically between the ages of 15 and 35 years, and women are affected slightly more often than men. Caucasians develop IBD two to five times more often than people of African or Asian descent, and individuals of Jewish descent have a three to six times higher incidence compared with other Caucasians. Ulcerative colitis is more common than Crohn's disease, averaging between 70 and 150 cases per 100,000 people. The average incidence of Crohn's disease is 20–40 cases per 100,000; however, the rate of Crohn's disease is increasing in the West, possibly due to excessive antibiotic use and the Western diet (discussed below).

FREQUENT SIGNS AND SYMPTOMS

Crohn's disease
- Cramping abdominal pain, especially after eating
- Pain may be in the right lower abdomen, mimicking appendicitis
- Nausea and diarrhea
- Fever, generally ill feeling
- Loss of appetite and weight
- Tender abdomen, often with a palpable abdominal mass
- Bloody stools (sometimes)
- Growth retardation in children

Ulcerative colitis
- Pain in the left side of the abdomen (the location of the colon) that improves after bowel movements
- Attacks of bloody diarrhea with mucus, alternating with symptom-free intervals
- Up to 10–20 bowel movements a day
- Dehydration
- Sweating, nausea
- Severe cramps and pain around the rectum
- Bloated abdomen
- Fever as high as 104°F (40°C)
- Loss of appetite and weight

Complications of IBD
- **Malnutrition:** unhealthy weight loss and malnutrition are prevalent in 65–75% of IBD patients. Contributing factors include:
  - decreased food intake (most common cause)
  - diarrhea-induced nutrient loss (especially electrolytes, minerals and trace mineral loss)
  - malabsorption in patients with extensive small intestine involvement or who have had surgical resection of the small intestine resulting in decreased absorptive surface and/or bile salt deficiency
  - overgrowth of unfriendly bacteria in the small intestine
  - fat malabsorption, which results in significant loss of calories and fat-soluble vitamins (vitamins E, A, D, K), and all minerals, including calcium, magnesium, potassium, and trace minerals is common
  - protein loss due to increased turnover and shedding of intestinal cells:
    - a significant loss of blood proteins across the damaged and inflamed intestinal mucosa occurs that may exceed the ability of the liver to replace, even with a high protein intake. Chronic loss of blood often leads to iron depletion and anemia.
  - common drugs – the corticosteroids – used in treatment of IBD significantly contribute to malnutrition:
    - corticosteroids (e.g., prednisone [prednisolone]) stimulate protein breakdown (catabolism); depress protein synthesis; decrease absorption of calcium and phosphorus; increase urinary

excretion of vitamin C, calcium, potassium and zinc; increase levels of blood glucose, serum triglycerides, and serum cholesterol; increase requirements for vitamin B_6, vitamin C, folate, and vitamin D; decrease bone formation; and impair wound healing.

- **Rheumatoid arthritis:** occurs in about 25% of IBD patients, typically affecting the knees, ankles, and wrists. Severity of symptoms is usually proportional to disease activity.
- **Rheumatoid arthritis of the spine:** this is similar to ankylosing spondylitis but is infrequent:
  - symptoms are low back pain and stiffness with eventual limitation of motion.
  - may precede bowel symptoms by several years.
- **Skin lesions:** occur in about 15% of patients, can be severe (gangrene or painful red lumps), but more typically are annoying, like canker sores. Canker sores occur in 10% of patients with IBD.
- **Serious liver disease:** affects 3–7% of people with IBD, can be severe (e.g., sclerosing cholangitis, chronic active hepatitis, cirrhosis):
  - if liver abnormalities are present, patients should take *Silybum marianum* (see Botanical medicines below).
- **Disease associations:** inflammation of blood vessels, impaired blood flow to fingers or toes, inflammatory eye conditions (episcleritis, iritis, uveitis), kidney stones, gallstones, and in children, failure to grow, thrive and mature normally.

CAUSES

No definitive agreement exists as to the causes of IBD. Theories include the following.
- **Genetic predisposition:** no specific genetic marker has been found, but genetic predisposition is likely since IBD is two to four times more common in Caucasians than non-Caucasians, and four times more common in individuals of Jewish descent than non-Jews. Also, in 15–40% of cases, multiple family members have IBD.
- **Infectious agent or agents:** numerous micro-organisms could potentially cause IBD. Favored candidates include mycobacteria and viruses such as rotavirus, Epstein–Barr virus, and cytomegalovirus. Other candidates include pseudomonas-like organisms, *Chlamydia*, and *Yersinia enterocolitica*.
- **Antibiotic exposure:** prior to the 1950s, when penicillin and tetracycline became available in oral form, Crohn's disease was found only in isolated groups and had a strong genetic component. Since

then, the number of Crohn's disease cases has risen rapidly in developed countries, especially the US, and in countries that had virtually no reported cases:
- the annual increase in prescriptions for antibiotics parallels the annual increase in incidence of Crohn's disease.
- comparative statistics show that wherever antibiotics are used early and in large quantities, the incidence of Crohn's disease escalates.
- one possible explanation is that Crohn's disease is caused by an infectious agent that is a normally innocuous resident in the intestines, but when subjected to sublethal doses of antibiotics, increases its production of toxins and becomes invasive:
  - such behavior is typical of microbes. When not given a lethal dose of antibiotics, their usual response is to adapt, become more aggressive and multiply.
- **Immune system abnormality:** although immune disturbances are evident in IBD, they are most likely a result rather than a cause of the disease process.
- **Dietary factors:** several lines of evidence strongly support dietary factors as the most important causative factor:
  - incidence of Crohn's disease is increasing in countries where people consume the Western diet (high in saturated fats, refined carbohydrates and sugars), while it is virtually nonexistent where a more "primitive" diet (high fiber, whole foods) is consumed.
  - food is the major factor in determining the intestinal environment.
  - when the pre-illness diets of people who develop Crohn's disease are analyzed, they habitually eat more refined sugar and less raw fruit, vegetables, and dietary fiber than healthy people.
    - patients with ulcerative colitis, however, do not show an increased consumption of refined carbohydrates compared with controls. In these patients, food allergy may be the most important causative factor.
- **Emotional factors:** while not an initiating cause, psychological factors can significantly affect the course of the disease.

RISK INCREASES WITH

- **History:** family history of IBD.
- **Antibiotics:** early and/or frequent use of antibiotics.
- **Disease-promoting Western diet:** a diet based on animal products and processed foods, with little consumption of fresh vegetables, legumes, fruits, nuts and

seeds, and whole grains is low in fiber and protective factors such as antioxidants and essential fatty acids, and high in factors associated with IBD, specifically Crohn's disease – sugar and refined carbohydrates, and saturated and *trans* fats (also called partially hydrogenated oils).

- **Food allergies:** numerous studies have demonstrated that common allergens, especially wheat and dairy products, are significant contributing factors in IBD.

PREVENTIVE MEASURES

- **Minimize** consumption of sugars and refined foods.
- **A health-promoting diet:** after identifying and removing any allergenic foods from the diet, choose a balanced diet composed of whole, unprocessed, preferably organic foods, especially plant foods (fruits, vegetables, whole grains, beans, nuts [especially walnuts], and seeds), and cold-water fish (for more detailed information, see Appendix 1).
- **A high-potency multiple vitamin and mineral supplement:** this should include 400 μg of folic acid, 400 μg of vitamin B_{12}, and 50–100 mg of vitamin B_6. (Folic acid supplementation should always be accompanied by vitamin B_{12} supplementation to prevent folic acid from masking a vitamin B_{12} deficiency.) A daily multiple providing all of the known vitamins and minerals serves as a foundation upon which to build an individualized health-promotion program.
- **Antibiotics:** use antibiotics only when truly necessary.
- **Regular exercise:** among its many mental and physical benefits, regular exercise tones muscles, improving bowel function.

Expected outcomes

Crohn's disease
Significant improvement in nutritional status and reduced frequency of acute attacks. Complete remission is quite possible. In several controlled studies of Crohn's disease, a significant percentage of patients (approximately 20% at 1 year and 12% at 2 years) who were given a placebo experienced spontaneous remission. The rate of spontaneous remission was dramatically higher in patients who had no previous history of steroid therapy: 41% achieved remission after 17 weeks, and 23% of this group continued in remission after 2 years, compared to only 4% of the group with a prior history of steroid use. Once remission is achieved, the majority of patients can maintain their health using natural, non-drug therapy.

Ulcerative colitis
In most cases, significant clinical improvement and/or complete resolution are seen within the first 3 months following the protocol. Complete resolution of signs and symptoms are much more likely in this form of IBD compared to Crohn's disease.

TREATMENT

Optimize diet and correct nutritional deficiencies.

Diet
- Identify and eliminate food allergens.
- Eliminate alcohol, caffeine, and sugar: all exacerbate inflammation.
- Drink at least 2 L (3 US pints) of clean water (filtered if your tap water has not been tested and found to be pure) daily to prevent dehydration.
- Reduce or eliminate consumption of meat and dairy products, while increasing consumption of cold-water fish (salmon, mackerel, herring, halibut):
  - meat and dairy products are the highest sources of arachidonic acid, a type of omega-6 essential fatty acid that the body uses to create inflammatory compounds called leukotrienes. Leukotrienes amplify the inflammatory process and cause intestinal cramping and pain.
  - cold-water fish are the best sources of the anti-inflammatory omega-3 essential fatty acids, EPA (eicosapentaenoic acid) and DHA (docosahexanoic acid).
- Avoid all foods containing *carrageenan*:
  - carrageenan, a compound extracted from red seaweeds, is used by researchers to experimentally induce ulcerative colitis in animals, including primates.
  - carrageenan compounds are widely used by the food industry as stabilizing and suspending agents in milk and chocolate milk products (ice cream, cottage cheese, milk chocolate, etc.) because of their ability to stabilize milk proteins.
  - in healthy human subjects and animals whose intestines are germ-free, carrageenan does not cause ulcerative colitis.
  - the bacterium *Bacteroides vulgatus*, an organism typically found in high concentrations (six times higher than normal) in the fecal cultures of patients with ulcerative colitis, appears to be responsible for facilitating carrageenan-induced damage in the intestines.
- Patients with IBD typically require as much as, or even more than, 25% more protein than the usual

recommended dietary allowance (see Complications of IBD, Malnutrition above).

- an elemental diet is often an effective alternative to corticosteroids in IBD:
  - an elemental diet contains all essential nutrients, with protein provided in the form of predigested or isolated amino acids.
  - improvement may be due to allergy elimination.
- Elimination (*oligoantigenic*) diets: these eliminate potentially offending foods:
  - most common offending foods in IBD are wheat and dairy products.
  - see the chapter on Food allergy for more information on elimination diets and various methods of determining food allergy or sensitivity.
- High-complex carbohydrate, high-fiber diet:
  - a high-fiber diet has been shown to have beneficial effects in both Crohn's disease and ulcerative colitis.
  - dietary fiber exerts numerous beneficial effects on the digestive tract:
    - provides food for health-promoting intestinal flora
    - soluble fiber slows transit time in individuals with diarrhea
    - binds to and removes toxins via feces.
  - foods rich in fiber (legumes, fruits, vegetables) and unrefined carbohydrates (starchy vegetables such as potatoes, corn, and whole grains such as rice, barley, millet, quinoa, spelt) should be emphasized.
  - best additional fiber choices are oat bran and flaxseed meal, both of which provide soluble fiber:
    - flaxseed meal also contains anti-inflammatory omega-3 essential fatty acids
    - wheat bran should not be consumed as it is too rough and irritating.
  - food allergens should be identified and avoided.

Nutritional supplements

- **Flaxseed oil:** take 1 tbsp of flaxseed oil q.d.:
  - flaxseed oil contains the omega-3 essential fatty acid ALA (alpha-linolenic acid), which the body converts to the anti-inflammatory fatty acid, EPA.
  - **caution:** flaxseed oil should always be refrigerated and should not be used in cooking as its essential fatty acids are very susceptible to oxidation/rancidity.
- **Probiotics:** friendly intestinal flora are needed to repopulate the intestines, both for their numerous beneficial effects on intestinal health and also because they compete with, and therefore lessen the effects of, less friendly bacteria whose cell components promote destruction of intestinal cells; dosage: 1–10 billion viable *Lactobacillus acidophilus* and *Bifidobacterium bifidum* cells q.d.

- **A high-potency multiple vitamin and mineral supplement** (see Preventive Measures above) is essential.
- **Additional antioxidants:** vitamins C and E are the two primary antioxidants in the body. Vitamin C is found in all body compartments composed of water, while vitamin E is found in the fat-soluble compartments (all cell membranes, and fat-containing molecules such as cholesterol). Recommended dosages for patients with IBD (including the amount found in the multiple vitamin and mineral formula) are:
  - vitamin E (mixed tocopherols): 400–800 IU q.d.
  - vitamin C: 1,000–3,000 mg q.d.
- **Zinc:** zinc deficiency is a well-known complication in both Crohn's disease and ulcerative colitis, occurring in approximately 45% of patients, as a result of low dietary intake, poor absorption, and excessive fecal loss:
  - many complications of IBD may be due to zinc deficiency, including poor healing of fissures and fistulas, skin lesions, decreased sexual development, growth retardation, retinal (eye) dysfunction, lowered immune function, and loss of appetite.
  - many patients appear to have a defect in tissue transport that prevents them from responding to oral or even intravenous zinc supplementation.
  - zinc picolinate, a form of zinc bound to a molecule secreted by the pancreas, appears to be best absorbed and utilized.
  - dosage: zinc picolinate 30–45 mg q.d.
- **Folic acid:** deficiency is quite common in IBD, ranging from 25–64% of patients:
  - the drug sulfasalazine is a frequent cause of folic acid deficiency.
  - folic acid deficiency results in abnormalities in the structure of the intestinal mucosal cells, thus promoting further malabsorption and diarrhea. The turnover of intestinal mucosal cells for which a constant supply of folic acid is needed, is very rapid (1–4 days).
  - dosage: 400–800 µg q.d.
- **Vitamin B_{12}:** B_{12} is absorbed in the portion of the intestine most commonly affected in Crohn's disease (the terminal ileum):
  - abnormal B_{12} absorption is found in 48% of patients with Crohn's disease.
  - often the terminal ileum is surgically removed (resected) in Crohn's disease patients. If the length removed is less than 60 cm, or the extent of the inflammatory lesion is less than 60 cm, adequate absorption of B_{12} may occur. Otherwise, monthly B_{12} injections (1,000 mg IM) are necessary.

- vegetarians should also supplement with a sublingual form of B_{12}.
- dosage: 400 µg q.d.
- **Pancreatic extracts:** pancreatic enzymes can reduce the inflammation of IBD and help with digestion; dosage: use a 10×USP pancreatic enzyme product and take 350–750 mg t.i.d. between meals.

Botanical medicines

IBD

- **Robert's Formula:** a naturopathic remedy with a long history of effectiveness in treating IBD, Robert's Formula may be purchased in health food stores. It is composed of:
  - *Althea officinalis* (marshmallow root): a soothing demulcent
  - *Baptista tinctora* (wild indigo): used for gastrointestinal infections
  - *Echinacea angustifolia* (purple coneflower): antibacterial, used to support immune function
  - *Geranium maculatum* (geranium): astringent action helps heal ulcerations
  - *Hydrastis canadensis* (goldenseal): inhibits the growth of many disease-causing bacteria
  - *Ulmus fulva* (slippery elm): soothing demulcent.

Ulcerative colitis

- **Demulcent herbs** such as deglycyrrhizinated licorice (DGL), marshmallow root, and slippery elm:
  - demulcent herbs contain glycoproteins (proteins with sugar molecules attached) called *mucins* that are largely responsible for the viscous and elastic character of secreted mucus.
  - mucin abnormalities are typical in ulcerative colitis patients (but not in Crohn's disease) and are a major factor in their increased risk of colon cancer.

- in ulcerative colitis, the mucus content of the intestinal goblet (mucus-producing) cells dramatically decreases, as does the production of sulfur-containing mucin.
- demulcent herbs soothe irritated mucous membranes and promote mucus secretion.

IBD with liver disease

- ***Silybum marianum* (milk thistle):** milk thistle contains silymarin, a mixture of flavonoids that is one of the most potent liver-protecting substances known. Silymarin is dramatically effective in reversing liver damage and in treating both acute and chronic hepatitis. Silymarin inhibits liver damage by:
  - acting as a direct antioxidant and free radical scavenger
  - increasing intracellular levels of glutathione and superoxide dismutase, two critically important liver antioxidants and detoxifying agents
  - inhibiting the formation of leukotrienes (agents that promote inflammation and free radical generation)
  - increasing bile flow
  - stimulating liver cell regeneration
  - dosage: best results are achieved at higher doses – 140–210 mg of a standardized extract of silymarin t.i.d.
- **Silymarin phytosome:** research indicates that this new form of silymarin, which is bound to phosphatidylcholine, is better absorbed and produces better and more rapid clinical results than unbound silymarin; dosage for silymarin phytosome is 120 mg b.i.d.–t.i.d. between meals.

Drug–herb interaction cautions

None.

Insomnia

DESCRIPTION

Sleep disturbance including any or any combination of the following: difficulty in falling asleep, difficulty remaining asleep, intermittent wakefulness, early morning awakening. Insomnia is typically transitory if due to a life crisis or lifestyle change, but may be chronic, especially if the result of medical or psychological problems or drug intake. In the course of a year, insomnia affects one out of every three people in the US, particularly the elderly. Each year, roughly 10 million people in the US receive prescriptions for sedative hypnotics (sleeping pills). Insomnia is closely associated with depression, and psychological factors (depression or anxiety) account for 50% of all insomnias evaluated in sleep laboratories.

FREQUENT SIGNS AND SYMPTOMS

- Sleep-onset insomnia: restlessness and difficulty falling asleep
- Sleep-maintenance insomnia:
  - brief sleep followed by wakefulness
  - frequent awakening throughout the night
  - fall asleep normally but wake early (3–4AM), unable to return to sleep
- Periods of sleeplessness alternating with periods of excessive sleep or sleepiness at inconvenient times

CAUSES

Sleep-onset insomnia
- Anxiety or tension caused by stress
- Depression
- New environment or location
- Emotional arousal
- Fear of insomnia
- Fear of sleeping
- Disruptive environment: noise, including a snoring partner. Light either entering the room from outside or caused by illuminated clocks, radios, etc.
- Pain or discomfort, e.g., from fibromyositis or arthritis
- Jet lag

- Daytime napping
- Prescription and over-the-counter drugs: well over 300 drugs can interfere with normal sleep. Some specific examples are given under Sleep-maintenance insomnia immediately below.
- Caffeine, a natural stimulant, is found not only in coffee, but in soft drinks, chocolate, coffee-flavored ice cream, hot cocoa, and tea:
  - while some people's liver detoxification system can quickly eliminate caffeine from the body, others, because of a much slower elimination, are extremely sensitive to caffeine's stimulant effects. In these individuals, even the small amount of caffeine found in decaffeinated coffee or chocolate may cause insomnia.
- Alcohol disrupts sleep by:
  - causing the release of adrenaline, the fight-or-flight hormone
  - impairing the transport of the amino acid tryptophan into the brain. Tryptophan is the precursor to serotonin, a neurotransmitter that initiates sleep, so by blocking tryptophan, alcohol disrupts serotonin levels.
- Lack of physical exercise: physical exercise reduces cortisol levels and increases levels of mood-elevating beta-endorphins, thus increasing the amount of available tryptophan while decreasing tension and anxiety.

Sleep-maintenance insomnia
- Depression (usually characterized by early morning wakefulness)
- New environment or location
- Disruptive environment (snoring partner, any source of light in the room):
  - exposure to light short-circuits the body's production of the sleep inducing hormone, melatonin.
- Allergies and early morning wheezing
- Urinary or gastrointestinal problems that require urination or bowel movements during the night
- Heart or lung conditions that cause shortness of breath when lying down, e.g., congestive heart failure, emphysema
- Overactivity of the thyroid gland
- Sleep apnea (ceasing to breathe while sleeping)

- Nocturnal muscle cramps: may be due to inadequate levels of magnesium
- Low nighttime blood sugar level (nocturnal hypoglycemia): when blood sugar drops, this triggers the release of hormones (adrenaline, glucagons, cortisol, and growth hormone) that regulate blood sugar levels. These hormones signal the brain that it is time to eat:
  - both hypoglycemia and diabetes are common in the United States as a result of overconsumption of refined carbohydrates.
  - to keep blood sugar levels steady throughout the night, good bedtime snacks are oatmeal and other wholegrain cereals, wholegrain breads or other complex carbohydrates such as starchy vegetables or beans.
  - complex carbohydrates not only maintain blood sugar levels but also help promote sleep by increasing the level of serotonin in the brain.
- Sleep dysfunctions such as sleep apnea (ceasing to breathe while sleeping), restless legs syndrome (RLS):
  - *nocturnal myoclonus*: almost all patients with RLS have nocturnal myoclonus, a neuromuscular disorder characterized by repeated contractions of one or more muscle groups, typically in the legs, during sleep.
  - family history of RLS is common, and, when present, a high dose of folic acid (35–60 mg q.d.) can be helpful. Dosage this high requires a prescription as licensing authorities limit the amount of folic acid per capsule to 800 µg.
  - if there is no family history of RLS, iron deficiency may be the cause:
    - the best way to check for iron deficiency is to measure the amount of the iron-storage protein *ferritin* in the blood. Iron deficiency (low ferritin levels) can be present even without anemia.
- Pain or discomfort
- Drugs: a wide variety of drugs can disrupt normal sleep patterns, including natural stimulants (caffeine), over-the-counter antihistamines, decongestants, diet pills (dextroamphetamines), and sleep-inducing drugs.
- Sleeping pills: the use of sleep-inducing drugs for more than a week or two can disrupt sleep patterns:
  - two primary types of drugs are used – antihistamines and benzodiazepines. Antihistamines – Benadryl, Nytol – are available over-the-counter. Benzodiazepines – Valium, Halcion – are given by prescription. Both are effective short term but cause problems long term.
  - benzodiazepines are addictive and cause abnormal sleep patterns. Antihistamines also disrupt sleep patterns.
  - **caution:** if a benzodiazepine has been taken for more than 4 weeks, the drug should not be stopped suddenly. Work with a physician to gradually taper off the drug to avoid potentially dangerous withdrawal symptoms, including anxiety, irritability, headache, panic, insomnia, nausea, impaired concentration, memory loss, depression, extreme sensitivity to the environment, seizures, hallucinations, and paranoia.
- Withdrawal from addictive substances
- Alcohol

RISK INCREASES WITH

- **Smoking:** nicotine stimulates adrenal hormone secretion, including cortisol. Cortisol activates tryptophan oxygenase, resulting in less tryptophan being delivered to the brain. Tryptophan is necessary for the production of serotonin, a neurotransmitter that is an important initiator of sleep. Serotonin and melatonin are the two hormones involved in normal circadian (waking–sleeping) cycles.
- **Stress:** increases levels of stress hormones, e.g., cortisol.
- **Depression:** low levels of serotonin are common in depression, and one of the earliest signs of depression is a disruption in sleep patterns.
- **Lack of physical exercise:** physical exercise lowers cortisol levels.
- **Obesity:** obesity is associated with higher levels of cortisol and lower levels of melatonin.
- **Alcohol consumption:** alcohol increases adrenal hormone output (cortisol) and interferes with normal brain chemistry, thus interfering with normal sleep cycles.
- **Drug use**, including sleeping pills.

PREVENTIVE MEASURES

- Avoid caffeine for at least 6 hours before bedtime. If sensitive to caffeine, eliminate it entirely.
- Don't smoke. Smokers should initiate a program to quit and avoid smoking for at least 2 hours before bedtime.
- Learn to deal with stress constructively. Meditate, pray, learn stress reduction techniques, exercise. Taking the time to discover which practices help and to integrate them into a lifestyle will significantly benefit not just sleeping patterns, but will improve overall health, joy in living, and longevity.
- Get regular exercise, but do not exercise for at least 3 hours before bedtime.
- Establish regular bedtime and waking hours and stick to them, even on weekends.
- Don't work in your bedroom. This room should be a place of calm and rest.

- Stop working and tune down for at least 1 hour before going to bed.
- Ensure your bedroom is dark and quiet. Wear an eye mask and/or earplugs if necessary.

Expected outcomes

In cases of chronic insomnia with identification and effective elimination of a causative factor, most people experience significant improvement in sleep quality and maintenance within 7–10 days. In cases where no factor could be easily identified, improvements can be experienced with the use of natural sedatives, but it may require significant trial and error to determine which natural therapy offers the greatest benefit. A trial of at least 4 nights is required before abandoning a natural sedative.

TREATMENT

Diet

While healthful for all, these guidelines are especially important for persons suffering from stress or anxiety.

- Eliminate or restrict intake of caffeine. Do not consume caffeine for at least 3–4 hours before bedtime.
- Eliminate or restrict intake of alcohol. No alcohol should be consumed for at least 3–4 hours before bedtime.
- Eliminate refined carbohydrates (most processed foods) from the diet.
- Eat regular planned meals in a relaxed environment.
- Identify and remove food allergens from the diet.

Nutritional supplements

Once causative factors have been identified and addressed, and a normal sleep pattern has been re-established, dosages of these recommended supplements should be slowly decreased.

Take the following 45 min before bedtime:

- **Niacin:** tryptophan is the precursor to niacin, so niacin supplementation results in more available tryptophan for conversion into serotonin; dosage: 100 mg (decrease dose if uncomfortable flushing interferes with sleep induction).
- **Vitamin B$_6$:** B$_6$ plays an important role in the reactions that occur in the conversion of tryptophan to serotonin; dosage: 50 mg.
- **Magnesium:** nature's most soothing mineral, magnesium helps dilate blood vessels and is necessary for muscle relaxation; dosage: magnesium citrate 250 mg.

Choose one of the following, and take 45 min before bedtime:

- **5-Hydroxytryptophan (5-HTP):** 5-HTP is the immediate precursor of serotonin, a neurotransmitter that is an important initiator of sleep. Numerous double-blind clinical studies have demonstrated that 5-HTP supplementation decreases the time required to get to sleep and the number of night-time awakenings, while increasing rapid eye movement (REM) and deep-sleep stages 3 and 4, the most important stages of sleep:
  - enhance the sedative effects of 5-HTP by taking it with a source of carbohydrate such as a small piece of fruit or small glass of fruit juice.
  - dosage: 100–300 mg.
- **Melatonin:** melatonin is only effective as a sedative when body melatonin levels are low:
  - melatonin is a hormone produced by the pineal gland. Normally, melatonin levels rise just before sleep onset, but as we age, melatonin production drops and in some individuals, especially the elderly, melatonin production is quite low.
  - dosage: 3 mg.

Botanical medicines

Once causative factors have been identified and addressed, and a normal sleep pattern has been re-established, dosages of these recommended supplements should be slowly decreased.

Take the following 45 min before bedtime:

- ***Valeriana officinalis*** **(valerian):** double-blind studies have confirmed valerian's long history of use as a sedative that improves sleep quality and relieves insomnia. In one study of insomniacs, a valerian/ *Melissa officinalis* preparation was shown to be as effective as benzodiazepines with none of the drug's negative side effects (daytime sleepiness, diminished concentration, impairment of physical performance):
  - dosage: choose one of the following forms:
    - dried root (or as tea): 2–3 g
    - tincture (1 : 5): 4–6 ml (1–1.5 tsp)
    - fluid extract (1 : 1): 1–2 ml (0.5–1 tsp)
    - dry powdered extract (0.8% valerenic acid): 150–300 mg.
- ***Passiflora incarnata*** **(passionflower):** a constituent of passionflower, harmine, can inhibit the breakdown of serotonin, thus promoting sleep. Because of its effects on serotonin, passionflower would add to the effectiveness of 5-HTP:
  - best used with 5-HTP.
  - dosage: choose one of the following forms:
    - dried herb (or as tea): 4–8 g
    - tincture (1 : 5): 6–8 ml (1.5–2 tsp)

- fluid extract (1 : 1): 2–4 ml (0.5–1 tsp)
- dry powdered extract (2.6% flavonoids): 300–450 mg.

Drug–herb interaction cautions

■ *Valeriana officinalis* (valerian):

 ■ plus *phenobarbital, thiopental*: in mice, a component of valerian, valerenic acid, increased sleeping time induced by phenobarbital and thiopental.

■ *Passiflora incarnata* (passionflower):

 ■ plus *pentobarbital*, hexobarbital: in rats and mice, the active sedative component maltol increases sleeping time induced by pentobarbital and hexobarbital.

Physical medicine

■ **Progressive relaxation:** a popular and easy-to-use technique to promote relaxation, progressive relaxation is based on a simple procedure of comparing tension to relaxation, which clearly shows what it feels like to relax, and can be used to help fall asleep:

 ■ forcefully contract one muscle group for 1–2 sec, then let the muscles completely relax.

 ■ begin by contracting the muscles of the face and neck for 1–2 sec, then relax. Next, contract and relax the upper arms and chest, followed by the lower arms and hands. Progress down the body, i.e., the abdomen, buttocks, thighs, calves, and feet.

 ■ repeat the whole process two to three times, or until asleep.

■ **Exercise:** improves sleep quality and general health and reduces negative effects of stress:

 ■ exercise in the morning, afternoon or early evening, but not before bedtime.

 ■ daily aerobic exercise of moderate intensity (a heart rate between 60 and 75% of maximum – approximately 220 minus age in years) for 20 min is sufficient.

Intestinal dysbiosis

DESCRIPTION

Intestinal dysbiosis, the growth of unfriendly organisms or overgrowth of normally harmless organisms in the gastrointestinal tract, is a widespread but frequently unrecognized cause of chronic disorders throughout the body. Normally, more than 500 different species of friendly or neutral microflora live in the digestive tract; in fact, there are nine times as many bacteria in the digestive tract as there are cells in the human body! We couldn't live without the help of our friendly microflora, which are called probiotics (pro-life). Probiotics perform numerous functions essential for our health including metabolizing nutrients, vitamins, drugs, hormones, and carcinogens; synthesizing food for intestinal cells; preventing unfriendly organisms from attaching to and colonizing the mucosal lining of the digestive tract; and stimulating normal immune responses. When unfriendly organisms, such as viruses, parasites and unfriendly bacteria, do manage to gain entry, or when normally neutral organisms, such as the yeast *Candida albicans*, overgrow, normal gut ecology is upset, and a wide variety of problems can occur. These problems include digestive disorders such as indigestion, diarrhea, constipation, inflammatory bowel disease, irritable bowel syndrome, food intolerances and food allergies, but are not limited to the digestive tract. Intestinal dysbiosis is a causative factor in numerous chronic degenerative diseases such as arthritis, autoimmune diseases, colon and breast cancer, psoriasis, eczema, cystic acne, and chronic fatigue.

FREQUENT SIGNS AND SYMPTOMS

- Frequent indigestion
- Bloating
- Belching
- Flatulence
- Diarrhea
- Constipation
- Nausea after taking supplements
- Food allergies or intolerances
- Irritable bowel syndrome
- Crohn's disease
- Celiac disease
- Gastritis
- Inflammatory skin diseases such as psoriasis, eczema, acne, hives
- Autoimmune diseases
- Arthritis
- Asthma
- Rectal itching
- Undigested food in the stools
- Foul smelling stools
- Weight loss: poor absorption of nutrients resulting in malnutrition

CAUSES

- **Western diet:** the Western diet is high in fat, meat, sugars and refined carbohydrates, and low in fruits, vegetables and fiber:
  - a diet high in fat and meat and low in fiber results in putrefaction in the intestinal tract and promotes the growth of unfriendly bacteria such as *Bacteroides* spp. The metabolic by-products produced by these bacteria activate enzymes whose activity promotes colon and breast cancer.
  - soluble fiber is the food eaten by the cells that compose the lining of the intestines. When the diet is lacking in fiber, these cells starve, and the gut wall literally develops tiny holes. This "leaky gut" then allows undigested food molecules as well as pathogens to leak into the bloodstream. Food allergies, autoimmune diseases, and infection can result.
  - excessive consumption of refined carbohydrates promotes the overgrowth of normally benign bacteria in the small intestine. When these bacteria ferment carbohydrates, the result is bloating, flatulence, diarrhea, constipation, and general feelings of malaise.
- **Antibiotic use:** antibiotics kill not only unfriendly but also friendly microflora, leaving the intestinal tract wide open to colonization by pathogens.
- **Food allergies:** when an allergenic food is consumed, an inflammatory immune response occurs that can result in damage to the lining of the intestines.

■ **Lack of digestive secretions:** when food is not properly broken down, it becomes available for unfriendly bacteria or can contribute to the overgrowth of normally benign bacteria. In addition, when proteins are not digested, they activate an immune response, which can lead to the development of food allergies.

■ **Intestinal infections:** unfriendly bacteria such as *Helicobacter pylori* (now known to cause ulcers), as well as parasites, fungi and viruses can upset gut ecology and damage the digestive tract.

■ **Laxative abuse:** laxatives work by irritating the gut, thus triggering forceful contractions (*peristalsis*) of the intestines in an effort to purge the irritant. Laxative abuse can damage the intestinal lining and also results in nutrient malabsorption.

RISK INCREASES WITH

■ **Stress:** disrupts digestive secretions.

■ **Food allergies:** consumption of allergenic foods triggers an inflammatory immune response that can damage the intestinal lining.

■ **Disease-promoting diet:** a diet based on animal products and processed foods, with little consumption of fresh vegetables, legumes, fruits, nuts and seeds, and whole grains is low in factors that promote gut health – fiber, vitamins and minerals, antioxidants, and essential fatty acids – and high in damaging factors – meat, saturated fat, *trans* fats (also called partially hydrogenated oils), sugars and refined carbohydrates.

■ **Antibiotic/drug therapy:** in addition to antibiotics, which wipe out friendly microflora, numerous drugs damage the intestinal lining, e.g., non-steroidal anti-inflammatory drugs such as aspirin, ibuprofen.

■ **Decreased immune function:** a compromised immune system cannot mount as effective a defense against pathogens.

PREVENTIVE MEASURES

■ **A health-promoting diet:** after identifying and removing any allergenic foods from the diet, choose a nutrient-dense, fiber-rich diet of whole, unprocessed, preferably organic foods, especially plant foods (fruits, vegetables, whole grains, beans, nuts [especially walnuts], and seeds), and cold-water fish. Minimize consumption of meats and processed foods (for more detailed information, see Appendix 1).

Expected outcomes

Intestinal dysbiosis represents a syndrome with a very broad spectrum. In minor disturbances, clinical signs of improvement can often be seen within the first week. If disturbances in the intestinal flora are moderate to severe, up to 3–6 months may be needed to see significant changes in bacterial counts and/or clinical symptoms.

TREATMENT

A stool analysis is usually performed to check for pathogens including bacteria, yeasts, fungi, and parasites. Depending upon the organism(s) founds, appropriate natural antimicrobial agents may be prescribed.

Diet

■ **A health-promoting diet:** consume a diet primarily composed of non-starchy vegetables, fruits, cold-water fish, nuts and seeds.

■ **Decrease sugar consumption:** sugar depresses immune function. Many unfriendly organisms thrive on sugar.

■ **Avoid starchy foods:** these can be fermented by unfriendly organisms in the digestive tract:
  ▪ grains, e.g., wheat, rice, oats, barley, rye
  ▪ legumes high in starch, e.g., chickpeas, garbanzo beans, soybeans, fava beans
  ▪ starchy vegetables, e.g., potatoes, yams, corn.

■ **Increase dietary fiber:**
  ▪ in addition to non-starchy vegetables and fruits, especially good sources of fiber include whole prunes, flaxseed meal.

■ **Drink** 6–8 glasses of fluid (clean water, diluted fruit juices, herbal teas) daily.

Nutritional supplements

■ **Digestive factors:** supplementation with hydrochloric acid and pancreatic enzymes can improve digestion.

■ **Hydrochloric acid supplementation:**
  ▪ begin by taking 1 tablet or capsule, containing 10 grains (600 mg) of hydrochloric acid, at your next large meal. If this does not aggravate your symptoms, at every subsequent meal of the same size, take 1 more tablet or capsule (one at the next meal, two at the meal after that, then three at the next meal). When taking a number of tablets or capsules, don't take them all at once. Space them throughout the meal.
  ▪ continue to increase the dose until you reach seven tablets or until you experience a feeling of warmth in your stomach, whichever occurs first. A warm feeling in the stomach means that you have taken too many tablets for that meal, and you need to take one less tablet for a meal that size. It is a good idea, however, to try the larger dose again at another

meal to make sure that the HCl was what caused the warmth, and not something else.

■ after you have found the largest dose you can take at your large meals without feeling any stomach warmth, maintain that dose at all meals of a similar size. You will need to take less at smaller meals.

■ as your stomach begins to regain the ability to produce the amount of HCl needed to properly digest your food, you will notice the warm feeling again and will have to cut down the dose level.

■ **Pancreatic enzymes:**
  ■ dosage: use a $10 \times$ USP pancreatic enzyme product and take 350–1,000 mg t.i.d. immediately before meals.
  ■ use a non-enteric-coated enzyme product. Enzyme products are often *enteric*-coated to prevent digestion in the stomach, so the enzymes will be liberated in the small intestine. However, numerous studies have shown that non-enteric-coated enzyme preparations actually outperform enteric-coated products if they are taken prior to a meal.

  ■ for vegetarians, *bromelain* and *papain* (protein-digesting enzymes from pineapple and papaya, respectively) can substitute for pancreatic enzymes in the treatment of pancreatic insufficiency. However, best results are obtained if they are used in combination with pancreatin and ox bile.

■ **Probiotics:** friendly intestinal flora are needed to repopulate the intestines, both for their numerous beneficial effects on gut health (see Description above) and also to compete with, thereby preventing colonization by, unfriendly organisms or the overgrowth of normally benign organisms such as *Candida albicans*; dosage: 1–10 billion viable *Lactobacillus acidophilus* and *Bifidobacterium bifidum* cells q.d.)

Botanical medicines

Depending upon the results of the stool analysis, botanical agents effective against the organisms found may be recommended.

Irritable bowel syndrome

DESCRIPTION

Irritable bowel syndrome (IBS) is characterized by recurrent irritation and inflammation of the large intestine, resulting in abdominal bloating and pain that is relieved by bowel movements. A functional disorder with no evidence of accompanying structural defect in the intestines, IBS is the most common gastrointestinal disorder in the US; 30–50% of referrals to gastroenterologists are for IBS. Approximately 15% of Americans have IBS complaints, with women reporting IBS symptoms twice as often as men. Symptoms usually begin in early adult life and may last for days, weeks or months.

FREQUENT SIGNS AND SYMPTOMS

- Cramp-like pain in the middle or to one side of the lower abdomen
- Pain usually relieved with bowel movements
- Loose or more frequent painful bowel movements
- Diarrhea or constipation, usually alternating
- Symptoms of upset stomach: flatulence, nausea, loss of appetite
- Headache, backache
- Rectal pain
- Fatigue
- Varying degrees of anxiety or depression
- Excessive secretion of colonic mucus

CAUSES

It is extremely important to consult a physician for a proper diagnosis of IBS. The following conditions may mimic IBS and must be ruled out:

- cancer
- diverticular disease
- infectious diarrhea, such as amebiasis or giardiasis
- inflammatory bowel disease
- intestinal candidiasis (yeast overgrowth)
- lactose intolerance
- malabsorption diseases, such as pancreatic insufficiency and celiac disease
- mechanical causes, such as fecal impaction
- metabolic disorders, such as adrenal insufficiency, diabetes, or hyperthyroidism.

Physiological, psychological and dietary factors

- **Disturbed bacterial microflora as a result of antibiotic or antacid usage:**
  - antibiotics wipe out the friendly as well as unfriendly bacteria, disrupting normal gut ecology.
  - antacids decrease hydrochloric acid, which is necessary for proper digestion and also destroys unfriendly bacteria in the stomach.
- **Laxative abuse:** laxatives are irritants that work by triggering forceful contractions (*peristalsis*) of the intestines in the body's effort to purge these offending substances. Laxative abuse can damage the intestinal lining and also results in nutrient malabsorption.
- **Stress and emotional conflict that results in anxiety or depression:**
  - stress disrupts the secretion of the body's digestive factors: hydrochloric acid and pancreatic enzymes.
  - attacks are often preceded by significant stress: obsessive worry about everyday problems, marital tension, fear of loss of a beloved person or object, death of a loved one.
- **Food allergy:** approximately two-thirds of patients with IBS have at least one food allergy. Most common allergens are wheat and dairy products.
- **Response to dietary factors** that interfere with digestion, such as excessive consumption of tea, coffee, carbonated beverages, and simple sugars.
- **Refined sugars:** excessive consumption of refined sugar may be the most important contributing factor to IBS in the US:
  - a diet high in refined sugar quickly raises blood sugar levels, causing a sharp decrease in intestinal peristalsis – the rhythmic contractions of the intestine that propel food through the digestive tract.
  - since sugar is primarily absorbed in the first sections of the small intestine (*duodenum* and *jejunum*), this portion of the digestive tract is constantly ordered to stop contracting and eventually becomes *atonic* (paralyzed).
  - when partially digested food sits in the small intestine, bacteria have an abnormally long time to feed. The result is bacterial overgrowth.

RISK INCREASES WITH

- **Stress:** disrupts digestive secretions.
- **Disease-promoting diet:** a diet based on animal products and processed foods, with little consumption of fresh vegetables, legumes, fruits, nuts and seeds, and whole grains is low in factors that promote gut health – fiber, vitamins and minerals, antioxidants, and essential fatty acids – and high in damaging factors – meat, saturated fat, *trans* fats (also called partially hydrogenated oils), sugars and refined carbohydrates.
- **Drug therapy:** in addition to antibiotics, which wipe out friendly microflora as well as their intended targets, thus leaving the gut wide open to colonization by pathogenic organisms, numerous commonly used drugs irritate the intestinal lining, e.g., laxatives, non-steroidal anti-inflammatory drugs such as aspirin, ibuprofen.
- **Excess alcohol consumption:** alcohol is an irritant that increases gut permeability to toxins and potentially allergenic foods. In addition, alcohol increases the adrenal gland's secretion of stress hormones, including cortisol, which disrupt digestive secretions.
- **Smoking:** nicotine stimulates the adrenal glands to secrete stress hormones.
- **Fatigue, overwork:** both signify increased stress.
- **Poor physical fitness:** physical exercise reduces cortisol (stress hormone) levels and increases levels of mood-elevating beta-endorphins, thus decreasing tension and anxiety.
- **Other family members with IBS:** family members typically share eating patterns and may also share behavioral patterns, i.e., reacting to stressful situations by shutting off the production of digestive factors.

PREVENTIVE MEASURES

- Avoid caffeine, alcohol, carbonated beverages, and simple sugars (refined foods).
- Get adequate sleep (8 hours nightly). Poor sleep quality correlates with an increase in both the severity and frequency of IBS symptoms (for information on improving sleep, see the chapter on Insomnia).
- Don't smoke.
- Learn to deal with stress constructively. Meditate, pray, learn stress reduction techniques, exercise. Taking the time to discover which practices help and to integrate them into a lifestyle will significantly benefit overall health, joy in living, and longevity.
- Choose a health-promoting diet rich in whole, unprocessed, preferably organic foods, especially plant foods (fruits, vegetables, whole grains, beans, nuts [especially walnuts], and seeds), and cold-water fish (for more detailed information, see Appendix 1).

Expected outcomes

Irritable bowel syndrome has a broad spectrum of clinical severity. In minor cases, improvements can be seen within the first few days of treatment. The key is identifying and eliminating the underlying factors. In moderate to severe cases of IBS, most patients will experience significant improvements within 4–6 weeks.

TREATMENT

Diet

In addition to the health-promoting diet recommended above:

- **Eliminate alcohol, caffeine, carbonated beverages and simple sugars (refined, processed foods):** all exacerbate inflammation and interfere with normal digestion, promoting bacterial overgrowth.
- **Increase dietary fiber from fruit and vegetable sources:** wheat and other grains are among the most commonly implicated foods in malabsorptive and allergic conditions:
  - in IBS, a condition in which the intestines are irritated and highly susceptible to potentially allergenic proteins leaking into the general circulation, food allergy is frequently a significant factor.
- **Identify and eliminate allergenic foods:** approximately two-thirds of patients with IBS have at least one food allergy:
  - most common allergens are dairy products (40–44%), and grains (40–60%).
  - many IBS patients have related symptoms consistent with food allergy/intolerance reactions including vascular instability, heart palpitation, hyperventilation, fatigue, excessive sweating, and headaches.
  - most reactions are IgG mediated (i.e., related to prostaglandin synthesis), so skin tests and the IgE-RAST test, which tests for IgE reactions, are inappropriate in these patients. The ELISA ACT or ELISA IgE/IgG$_4$ are preferred tests.

Nutritional supplements

- **Probiotics:** friendly intestinal flora (probiotics) are needed to repopulate the intestines:
  - probiotics perform numerous functions essential for intestinal health including: metabolizing nutrients, vitamins, drugs, hormones, and carcinogens;

synthesizing food for intestinal cells; preventing unfriendly organisms from attaching to and colonizing the mucosal lining of the digestive tract; and stimulating normal immune responses.

- probiotics compete with, thereby preventing colonization by, unfriendly organisms or the overgrowth of normally benign organisms such as *Candida albicans*.
- dosage: 1–10 billion viable *Lactobacillus acidophilus* and *Bifidobacterium bifidum* cells q.d.

- **Fiber:** use fiber derived from fruit and vegetable sources, not potentially allergenic grains; dosage: 3–5 g q.d. at bedtime.

Botanical medicines

- **Enteric-coated volatile oil preparations** (e.g., peppermint oil): peppermint oil inhibits gastrointestinal smooth muscle action so effectively it is used to reduce colonic spasm during endoscopy (a procedure in which a tube with a lens is inserted up the rectum to view the surface of the colon):
  - enteric-coated peppermint oil capsules not only relax and soothe the intestines, but are also antimicrobial and effective against the yeast, *Candida albicans*. *C. albicans* overgrowth is common in those who consume large amounts of sugar.
  - in double-blind, placebo-controlled studies, enteric-coated peppermint oil has demonstrated significant symptom relief (pain reduction) in IBS patients after 4 weeks of use.
  - enteric-coated peppermint oil capsules are necessary because, without enteric-coating, menthol (the major constituent of peppermint oil) is so rapidly absorbed that esophageal reflux and heartburn can result.
  - in some patients using enteric-coated peppermint oil, a transient burning sensation may be felt in the rectum during defecation due to unabsorbed menthol.
  - dosage: 0.2–0.4 ml b.i.d. between meals.

Drug–herb interaction cautions
None.

Physical medicine

- **Daily, leisurely 20-min walks:** many people with IBS find daily walks markedly reduce symptoms, probably due to the stress-reducing effects of exercise.
- **An effective stress-reduction program:** psychotherapy in the form of relaxation therapy, biofeedback, hypnosis, counseling, or stress-management training has been shown to reduce symptom frequency and enhance the results of standard medical treatment of IBS. Biofeedback, in which the patient learns how to initiate the "relaxation response", may be particularly helpful.

Kidney stones

DESCRIPTION

Crystallized particles that form in one or both kidneys and may travel into the *ureters* (the slender muscular tubes that carry urine from the kidneys to the bladder), kidney stones may be as tiny as a grain of sand or as large as a golf ball, and one or several may be present. Large stones usually remain in the kidney without causing symptoms, although they may damage the kidney. Tiny stones pass easily through the ureter to the bladder and are voided in the urine. Stones small enough to enter the ureter but too big to pass easily cause excruciating pain, until they are voided, typically in a few days. If a stone lodges and blocks the flow of urine, it must be removed to prevent kidney damage. Fortunately, a variety of non-surgical options now exist including chemical dissolution, and various forms of *lithotripsy* (the crushing of a stone with focused sound energy).

The frequency of stone formation has increased dramatically during the last few decades, paralleling the rise in other diseases associated with the Western diet, e.g., heart disease, high blood pressure and diabetes. It is now estimated that 10% of all American males will develop a kidney stone in their lifetime, with an annual frequency of 0.1–6.0% of the general population. In the US, one out of every thousand hospital admissions is for kidney stones. Kidney stones usually occur in adults over age 30 and affect both sexes, but are more common in men than in women.

In the US, stones are most often composed of calcium salts (75–85%), followed by struvite (non-calcium containing crystals, 10–15%), and uric acid (5–8%). Diagnosing the type of stone is critical as therapy differs for each type. Normally, components of human urine remain in solution as a result of pH control and the secretion of inhibitors of crystal growth. However, when the concentration of stone components increases or when protective factors decrease, kidney stones can develop.

FREQUENT SIGNS AND SYMPTOMS

- Usually no symptoms until the stone becomes dislodged
- Episodes of excruciating, intermittent, radiating pain, originating in the flank or kidney

- Pain usually first appears in the back, just below the ribs (the location of the kidneys), and, over several days, migrates, following the stone's course through the ureter to the groin. Pain stops when the stone passes.
- Nausea, vomiting, abdominal distension
- Chills, fever, urinary frequency accompanied by infection
- Traces of blood in the urine, which may appear cloudy or dark
- Diagnosed by ultrasound

CAUSES

- **Western diet:** Western dietary patterns are directly causative of calcium-containing stones:
  - low in fiber:
    - vegetarians, who typically consume high amounts of fresh fruits and vegetables, have a decreased risk of developing stones. Even meat eaters who eat large amounts of fruits and vegetables have a lower incidence of stone formation.
    - bran supplementation, as well as the change from white to whole wheat bread, has resulted in a lowering of urinary calcium levels.
  - high in refined carbohydrates, alcohol consumption, animal protein, fat.
  - high intake of high-calcium, low-magnesium, vitamin D-enriched milk products.
- **Excess weight and insulin insensitivity:** both lead to increased urinary excretion of calcium and are high risk factors for stone formation.
- **Sugar:** an exaggerated increase in urinary calcium oxalate content following high sugar meals occurs in approximately 70% of people with recurrent kidney stones.
- **Magnesium deficiency:** magnesium increases the solubility of calcium oxalate and inhibits both calcium phosphate and calcium oxalate stone formation:
  - a magnesium-deficient diet is used in studies to quickly induce kidney stones in rats.
  - supplemental magnesium alone has been shown to prevent recurrences of kidney stones.

- **Vitamin B$_6$ deficiency:** vitamin B$_6$ reduces the production and excretion of oxalates. Many patients with recurrent oxalate stones show laboratory signs of B$_6$ deficiency:
  - an important way in which vitamin B$_6$ reduces the production of calcium oxalate stones is by transporting the nonessential amino acid, glutamine, from the intestines into the general circulation, and thence to the kidneys.
  - the kidneys use glutamine to produce ammonia, an important part of a buffering system in the kidneys that prevents urine from becoming too acidic. An acidic urine promotes the precipitation (falling out of solution) of calcium oxalate, which then forms stones.
  - glutamine supplementation in rats greatly reduces the incidence of kidney stones, but when levels of vitamin B$_6$ are adequate, glutamine supplementation will likely be unnecessary.
- **Purines:** frequent consumption of foods high in *purines* (a component of the nucleic acids, DNA and RNA), including organ meats, meats, shellfish, yeast (brewer's and baker's), herring, sardines, mackerel, and anchovies:
  - high purine consumption increases the rate of urinary uric acid excretion
  - elevation of the purine content of uric acid is a causative factor in the formation of recurrent calcium oxalate stones.
- **Heavy metal toxicity:** many heavy metals (mercury, gold, uranium, and especially cadmium) are toxic to the kidneys:
  - a prospective study of coppersmiths showed a 40% incidence of kidney stones, which correlated with elevated serum cadmium levels.
- **Excessive sodium consumption:** urinary calcium excretion increases approximately 1 mmol (40 mg) for each 100 mmol (2,300 mg) increase in dietary sodium in normal adults. People who tend to form kidney stones excrete even more urinary calcium with an increase in salt intake.

RISK INCREASES WITH

- **Excess weight and insulin insensitivity:** excess weight frequently indicates problems with carbohydrate metabolism. Both excess weight and insulin insensitivity lead to increased urinary excretion of calcium.
- **High sugar intake:** urinary calcium levels rise following a meal high in sugar.

- **Low magnesium status:** a low urinary magnesium-to-calcium ratio is an independent risk factor in stone formation.
- **Calcium restriction:** most doctors tell their patients to avoid calcium, but in actuality, calcium restriction enhances oxalate absorption, increasing the risk of calcium oxalate stone formation. A recent study that measured urinary oxalate excretion after calcium supplementation and the administration of oxalic acid has shown that calcium supplementation significantly reduces oxalate absorption and excretion.
- **Excessive consumption of alcohol:** causes a rapid increase in blood sugar levels, which causes urinary calcium levels to rise and leads to increased urinary excretion of calcium.
- **Western dietary patterns:** frequent consumption of highly refined carbohydrates, animal protein, fat, and vitamin D-enriched dairy products, along with low intake of fiber and green leafy vegetables.
- **Frequent consumption of foods high in purines:** organ meats, meats, shellfish, yeast (brewer's and baker's), herring, sardines, mackerel, and anchovies.
- **Excessive salt consumption:** people who form kidney stones excrete much higher amounts of urinary calcium when their intake of sodium is high.
- **Dehydration**: dehydration results in a much higher concentration of stone components in the urine.

PREVENTIVE MEASURES

For all types of kidney stones:
- Maintain ideal weight.
- Drink at least 3 L (6 US pints) of fluid, mostly purified water, each day to increase urine flow and dilute the urine.
- Avoid excessive sweating.
- Exercise regularly: exercise improves insulin sensitivity.
- Minimize intake of sugar, refined carbohydrates, and alcohol.
- Increase consumption of fiber by choosing wholegrain breads and cereals, fresh fruits and vegetables.
- Increase consumption of green leafy vegetables, a rich source of vitamin K, which is a powerful inhibitor of stone formation. Vitamin K may be one reason that vegetarians have a lower incidence of kidney stones.
- Consume a nutrient-dense diet rich in whole, unprocessed, preferably organic foods, especially plant foods (fruits, vegetables, beans, seeds and nuts, and whole grains) and cold-water fish, and low in animal products, fat, and processed foods (for more detailed information, see Appendix 1).

Expected outcomes

Prevention of future recurrence should be expected in virtually all cases.

TREATMENT

In addition to the preventive measures outlined above, specific treatments to prevent recurrence are determined by the type of stone.

Diet
Calcium stones

- Increase intake of fiber, complex carbohydrates, and green leafy vegetables.
- Decrease intake of simple carbohydrates and purines (meat, fish, poultry, yeast).
- Increase intake of high magnesium-to-calcium ratio foods (barley, bran, corn, buckwheat, rye, soy, oats, brown rice, avocado, banana, cashew, coconut, peanuts, sesame seeds, lima beans, potato).
- If stones are oxalate, reduce oxalate-containing foods (black tea, cocoa, spinach, beet leaves, rhubarb, parsley, cranberries, nuts).
- Limit intake of products made with milk, including ice cream, chocolate.

Uric acid stones

- Decrease consumption of purine-rich foods: organ meats, meats, shellfish, yeast (brewer's and baker's), herring, sardines, mackerel, and anchovies.
- Decrease consumption of foods with moderate levels of purines: dried legumes, spinach, asparagus, fish, poultry, mushrooms.

Cystine stones

- Avoid methionine-rich foods (soy, wheat, dairy products [except whole milk], fish, meat, lima beans, garbanzo beans, mushrooms, and all nuts except coconut, hazelnut, and sunflower seeds).

Nutritional supplements
Calcium stones

- **Vitamin B$_6$:** reduces the production and excretion of oxalates; dosage: 25 mg q.d.
- **Vitamin K:** is necessary for the body's synthesis of a molecule that is a powerful inhibitor of kidney stone formation; dosage: 2 mg q.d.
- **Magnesium:** increases the solubility of calcium oxalate and inhibits both calcium phosphate and calcium oxalate stone formation; dosage: 600 mg q.d.
- **Calcium citrate or malate**: calcium restriction enhances oxalate absorption while calcium supplementation reduces oxalate excretion; dosage: 300–1,000 mg q.d.
- **Citrate bound to magnesium or potassium:** citrate, which has the ability to reduce urinary saturation of calcium oxalate and calcium phosphate and retard the crystal growth of calcium salts, has been shown to be quite effective, ceasing stone formation in nearly 90% of subjects; dosage: based upon the level of elemental mineral, 500–1,000 mg q.d.
- **Avoid aluminum-containing antacids:** aluminum and alkali both cause excessive excretion of calcium.
- **Note:** numerous studies have demonstrated that vitamin C is rarely, if ever, a potential factor in the development of calcium oxalate stones. Administration up to 10 g q.d. has shown no effect on urinary oxalate levels.

Uric acid stones

- **Folic acid:** folic acid inhibits xanthine oxidase, the enzyme responsible for the production of uric acid; dosage: 5 mg q.d. (**Note**: to avoid masking a vitamin B$_{12}$ deficiency, also supplement with 1,000 µg of B$_{12}$ q.d.)
- **Bicarbonate or citrate:** uric acid stones form in an overly acidic urine. Bicarbonate or citrate can be used to alkalinize the urine; dosage: modify dosage to alkaline urine. Optimal pH is 7.5–8.0.

Magnesium ammonium phosphate stones

- **Ammonium chloride:** ammonium chloride is used to acidify urine:
  - the urine of individuals with magnesium ammonium phosphate stones is typically at a pH of less than 6.2, which signifies a bladder infection (for more information about eradicating bladder infections, see the chapter on Cystitis).
  - dosage: 100–200 mg t.i.d.

Botanical medicines
Acute obstruction

- ***Ammi visnaga* (khella) extract:** khella has been shown to be effective in relaxing the ureter, allowing the stone to pass; dosage: 12% khellin content, 250 mg t.i.d.
- ***Ruta graveolens* (gravel root):** contains similar compounds to khella and has also been used to ease the passage of kidney stones.

Calcium stones

- ***Aloe vera* or senna:** both *Aloe vera* and senna contain compounds called *anthraquinones* that bind calcium and significantly reduce the growth rate of urinary crystals when used in oral doses lower than the laxative dose:

- use at a dosage just below a level that will produce a laxative effect (this will vary from person to person).

- **_Vaccinium macrocarpon_ (cranberry):** cranberry juice or extracts have been shown to reduce the amount of ionized calcium in the urine by over 50% in patients with recurrent kidney stones:
  - most cranberry juice products are loaded with sugar, so cranberry juice extracts (in pill form) or unsweetened cranberry juice concentrates are preferable.
  - dosage: take the equivalent of 0.5 L (1 US pint) of cranberry juice daily.

Drug–herb interaction cautions

- **Senna:**
  - plus _analgesics_: may aggravate nephropathy from analgesics associated with dehydration (speculative).
  - plus _oral drugs_: may decrease absorption of oral drugs due to decrease in bowel transit time (speculative).
  - plus _diuretics_: aggravates loss of potassium associated with diuretic use.
  - plus _cardiac glycosides (digitalis)_: overuse or misuse of senna may cause potassium loss leading to increased toxicity of cardiac glycosides.

Leukoplakia

DESCRIPTION

A white plaque-like lesion appearing on the lips or in the delicate lining of the mouth or tongue, leukoplakia is not contagious. Generally, leukoplakia is a reaction to irritation caused by tobacco products or dentures, but may also be an early indication of impaired immune function in persons infected with HIV (human immunodeficiency virus). Leukoplakia affects all ages but is most common in men aged 50–70 years.

Leukoplakia is a precancerous lesion. Oral cancer is among the most common malignant cancers, with nearly 50,000 new cases and 12,000 deaths reported in the US annually. Since oral cancer has a 5-year survival of 50% (more than half the people who develop oral cancer die within 5 years of diagnosis), the primary preventive measures – giving up tobacco and increasing the intake of antioxidants – are strongly recommended.

FREQUENT SIGNS AND SYMPTOMS

- A small white patch anywhere on the inside of the cheek, floor or roof of the mouth, tongue, or palate.
- The patch feels firm, rough, and stiff.
- May be without symptoms until there is ulceration, fissuring, or malignant transformation.
- Diagnosis confirmed by biopsy.

CAUSES

- Excessive, chronic irritation combined with marginal or low levels of vitamin A, carotenoids, and/or antioxidants. Sources of irritation include:
  - tobacco: cigarettes, chewing tobacco, snuff, pipe or cigars
  - betel nut chewing
  - sunlight exposure
  - jagged teeth
  - poorly fitting dentures
  - habitually biting the inside of the cheek or lip
  - alcohol consumption
  - hot, spicy food.

RISK INCREASES WITH

- Use of tobacco products
- Betel nut chewing
- Alcohol consumption
- Excessive sun exposure
- Dentures, jagged teeth
- Frequent consumption of hot or highly spiced food
- Nervous habit of biting the inside of the cheek or lip
- Disease-promoting diet: a diet based on animal products and processed foods, with little consumption of fresh vegetables, legumes, fruits, nuts and seeds, and whole grains is low in protective factors – vitamin A, carotenoids, and antioxidants – and high in factors that suppress immune function – sugars, refined carbohydrates, saturated fat, *trans* fats (also called partially hydrogenated oils), and numerous chemical additives.

PREVENTIVE MEASURES

- Don't smoke or use tobacco products.
- Wear lip balm with sunscreen.
- Have regular dental checkups.
- If wearing dentures, ensure proper fit.
- Decrease consumption of hot or highly seasoned food if suspicious lesions develop.

Expected outcomes

Because the lining of the mouth (the oral mucosa) has excellent repair mechanisms, oral leukoplakias can be reversed quite quickly – 1–2 weeks with minor leukoplakias, and 1–2 months in deeper, more extensive lesions. The key is to eliminate the irritant in combination with providing the cells with the nutrition they need to heal.

TREATMENT

Diet

- Consume a nutrient-dense diet rich in whole, unprocessed, preferably organic foods, especially plant foods (fruits, vegetables, beans, seeds and nuts, and whole grains) and cold-water fish, and low in animal products and processed foods (for more detailed information, see Appendix 1).

- Eliminate potentially irritating hot or spicy foods.
- Increase consumption of foods rich in vitamin A and carotenes:
  - *rich food sources of vitamin A*: liver, carrots, cod liver oil, egg yolks, dried apricots, kale, sweet potatoes, parsley, spinach, beet greens, butternut squash, mangos, sweet red peppers, Hubbard squash, cantaloupe.
  - *rich food sources of carotenes*: dark green leafy vegetables and yellow and orange vegetables such as squash, yams, sweet potatoes, carrots.

Nutritional supplements

- **Vitamin A:** because of its importance in immune function and in epithelial and mucosal tissues, the fat-soluble nutrient, vitamin A, is critical in the treatment of leukoplakia and in the prevention of oral cancers:
  - the epithelium is a layer of cells forming the epidermis of the skin and the surface layer of mucous and serous membranes. All epithelial surfaces including those of the lips, tongue, and mouth rely upon vitamin A.
  - when vitamin A status is inadequate, keratin is secreted in epithelial tissues, transforming them from their normally pliable, moist condition into stiff dry tissue that is unable to carry out its normal functions, and leading to breaches in epithelial integrity that promote the development of lesions and oral cancers.
  - known as the "anti-infective vitamin", vitamin A promotes the functioning of the thymus gland (the master gland of the immune system), and stimulates or enhances numerous immune

processes, including white blood cell function and antibody response.
  - dosage: 5,000 IU q.d.
- **Beta-carotene:** also known as "pro-vitamin A" since it can be converted to vitamin A in the body, beta-carotene is a more powerful antioxidant than vitamin A and is essential to epithelial health:
  - a strong inverse correlation has been shown between serum levels of beta-carotene and cancer. Studies have also found that the higher the intake of beta-carotene, the lower the risk for cancer.
  - dosage: 30–90 mg q.d.
- **Vitamin C:** an essential antioxidant found in all body compartments composed of water, vitamin C strengthens and maintains normal epithelial integrity, improves wound healing, enhances immune function, and inhibits carcinogen formation:
  - vitamin C regenerates vitamin E after it has used up its antioxidant potential.
  - inadequate intake of vitamin C has been identified as an independent risk factor for the development of carcinoma *in situ*.
  - dosage: 1,000–3,000 mg q.d.
- **Vitamin E:** a powerful antioxidant, vitamin E plays an important role in protecting vitamin A and increasing its storage:
  - while vitamin C protects the body's water-soluble areas, vitamin E is the primary antioxidant in the fat-soluble compartments such as cell membranes.
  - vitamin E also significantly enhances both types of immune defense: non-specific or cell-mediated immunity and specific or humoral immunity. Cell-mediated immunity is the body's primary mode of protection against cancer.
  - dosage: 400 IU mixed tocopherols q.d.

Macular degeneration

DESCRIPTION

Macular degeneration is a progressive, age-related loss of vision due to the deterioration of the macula, the area of the retina where images are focused. Degeneration is a result of free radical damage, similar to the damage that causes cataracts.

The two most common types of age-related macular degeneration (ARMD) are the "dry" (*atrophic*) form and the "wet" (*neovascular*) form. Between 80 and 95% of people with ARMD have the dry form of the disease. In this form, cellular debris (*lipofuscin*) accumulates in the innermost layer of the retina, the *retinal pigmented epithelium* (RPE), eventually causing other tissue components beneath the RPE to extrude. The hallmark feature of ARMD is the appearance of this extrusion (referred to as *drusen*) when the eye is examined with the aid of an ophthalmoscope. Dry ARMD progresses slowly, and while central vision is lost, peripheral vision remains intact, with the result that people with dry ARMD can see peripherally but cannot see what is directly in front of them. Currently, no allopathic (conventional) medical treatment exists for dry ARMD.

Wet ARMD, which affects 5–20% of those with ARMD, is characterized by the growth of abnormal blood vessels and can be treated quite effectively with laser photocoagulation therapy. In wet ARMD, surgery should be performed as soon as possible because the disease can rapidly progress to a point where surgery can no longer be utilized.

ARMD is the leading cause of severe visual loss in persons aged 55 and older in both the United States and Europe. More than 150,000 Americans are legally blind as a result of ARMD, with 20,000 new cases occurring annually. Incidence increases with each decade over age 50, reaching more than 30% by age 75.

FREQUENT SIGNS AND SYMPTOMS

In both the dry and wet form of ARMD, patients may experience the following:
- blurred vision
- straight objects may appear distorted or bent

- a dark spot may appear near or around the center of the visual field
- while reading, parts of words may be missing
- eye examination may reveal spots of pigment near the macula and blurring of the macular borders
- drusen, extrusions beneath the retina:
  - *in dry ARMD*, drusen appear as discrete hard yellow deposits that can be seen in the macular region with the use of an ophthalmoscope (a piece of equipment physicians use to examine the eye).
  - *in wet ARMD*, drusen are soft, larger, paler and less distinct.

CAUSES

Free radical damage and poor oxygenation of the macula.

RISK INCREASES WITH

- **Smoking:** this significantly increases free radical exposure:
  - a 12-year study of 31,843 female nurses found those who currently smoked were 2.4 times more likely to get ARMD than those who had never smoked. Past smokers of 25 cigarettes or more per day still had twice the risk of those who never smoked, and risk did not return to the control level until 15 years after stopping smoking.
- **Aging:** beginning in early life and accumulating throughout life, cells of the innermost layer of the retina gradually accumulate sacs of cellular debris called lipofuscin. As lipofuscin accumulates, it causes the extrusions (drusen) that are the hallmark of ARMD.
- **Cardiovascular disease, e.g., atherosclerosis, high blood pressure:**
  - these are degenerative diseases in which free radical damage plays an important causative role and which result in suboptimal oxygenation throughout the body, including the macula.
  - in subjects younger than 85 years with atherosclerosis (hardening of the arteries), plaques in the

carotid arteries are associated with a 4.7 times greater frequency of ARMD. Lower extremity atherosclerosis is associated with a 2.5 times greater risk.

- for more detailed information about prevention and reversal of cardiovascular disease, see the chapters on Atherosclerosis and Hypertension.

- **Standard American Diet:** the Standard American Diet, which is based on animal products and processed foods with little consumption of fresh vegetables, legumes, fruits, nuts and seeds, and whole grains is low in protective factors – antioxidants, flavonoids, and carotenes such as *lutein, zeaxanthin,* and *lycopene* – and high in damaging factors that elevate cholesterol levels and blood pressure, and increase the risk for obesity and diabetes – saturated fat, *trans* fats (also called partially hydrogenated oils), sugars and refined carbohydrates.

- **A high-potency multiple vitamin and mineral supplement:** a daily multiple providing all of the known vitamins and minerals serves as a foundation upon which to build an individualized health-promotion program. Any good multiple should include 400 µg of folic acid, 400 µg of vitamin B_{12}, and 50–100 mg of vitamin B_6. (Folic acid supplementation should always be accompanied by vitamin B_{12} supplementation to prevent folic acid from masking a vitamin B_{12} deficiency.)

PREVENTIVE MEASURES

- Don't smoke.
- Moderate wine consumption may be protective.
- A diet rich in fruits and vegetables is associated with a lowered risk for ARMD.

Expected outcomes

Progression of macular degeneration should be stopped or, at the very least, significantly slowed within 4 weeks.

TREATMENT

Diet

- **Avoid fried and grilled foods** and other sources of free radicals.
- **Consume a nutrient-dense diet** rich in whole, unprocessed, preferably organic foods, especially plant foods (fruits, vegetables, beans, seeds and nuts), and cold-water fish, and low in animal products (for more detailed information, see Appendix 1).
- **Increase consumption of legumes** which are high in sulfur-containing amino acids used by the body in the generation of internally produced antioxidants.

- **Increase consumption of carotenes:**
  - *lycopene:* best sources include tomatoes (especial cooked tomato products), carrots, green pepper apricots, pink grapefruit
  - *zeaxanthin:* best sources include spinach, paprik corn, fruits
  - *lutein:* best sources include green plants, cor potatoes, spinach, carrots, tomatoes, fruits.
- **Increase consumption of flavonoids:** best sourc are berries including blueberries, blackberries, cherrie
- **Increase consumption of vitamin E:** best sourc are seeds, nuts, wheat germ, and green leafy vegetable
- **Increase consumption of vitamin C:** best sourc include sweet peppers, kale, parsley, broccoli, Brusse sprouts, cauliflower, persimmons, red cabbage, straw berries, papayas, spinach, oranges, lemons, ar grapefruit.

Nutritional supplements

- **Mixed carotenoids derived from palm o** carotenes, especially lutein, lycopene, and zeaxanthi which are found in high concentrations in the ma ula, have been found to be even more significant i protecting against ARMD than the well-know antioxidants vitamin C, vitamin E, and selenium:
  - when compared with healthy controls, individua with low levels of lycopene were twice as likely have macular degeneration.
  - the macula owes its yellow color to its high concer tration of lutein and zeaxanthin.
  - palm oil carotenes closely mirror the pattern carotenoids found in high-carotene foods and hav been shown to be 4–10 times better absorbed tha synthetic beta-carotene.
  - dosage: 50,000 IU mixed carotenoids (derived fron palm oil) q.d.
- **Lutein:** a yellow carotene found in especially hig concentration in the macula, particularly its centr portion (the *fovea*), which plays an important protec tive role in the area of the retina responsible for fin vision (the area that deteriorates in ARMD); dosag 5 mg q.d.
- **Vitamin C:** a water-soluble antioxidant, vitamin protects the aqueous environments in the body, bot inside and outside cells, and works with vitamin E an carotenes (its fat-soluble partners), as well as wit the body's internally produced antioxidant enzyme glutathione peroxidase, catalase, and superoxid dismutase:
  - vitamin C works synergistically with vitamin E regenerating vitamin E after it has used up it antioxidant potential.

- vitamin C is a critical nutrient in the prevention of cardiovascular disease, preventing the oxidation of low density lipoprotein (LDL) (bad) cholesterol (thought to be a primary initiating factor in atherosclerosis), strengthening the collagen structures of the arteries, lowering total cholesterol level and blood pressure, raising high density lipoprotein (HDL) (good) cholesterol levels, and inhibiting platelet aggregation.
  - dosage: 1 g t.i.d.
- **Vitamin E:** while vitamin C protects the body's water-soluble areas, vitamin E is the primary antioxidant in the fat-soluble compartments such as cell membranes and fatty molecules like cholesterol:
  - of all the antioxidants, vitamin E may offer the most protection against arteriosclerosis because it is easily incorporated into the LDL cholesterol molecule where it prevents free radical damage.
  - dosage: 600–800 IU mixed tocopherols q.d.
- **Bioflavonoids:** a group of plant pigments largely responsible for the colors of fruits and flowers, flavonoids are powerful antioxidants in their own right, and, when taken with vitamin C, significantly enhance its absorption and effectiveness; dosage: 1,000 mg q.d.
- **Selenium:** selenium and vitamin E work together synergistically. Selenium is also a component of glutathione peroxidase, an antioxidant made by the body that is perhaps its most important detoxifying agent; dosage: 400 μg q.d.
- **Zinc:** zinc is important to the functioning of numerous enzymes, is essential for retinal function, and is frequently deficient in the elderly; dosage: 15–30 mg q.d.

Botanical medicines

Flavonoid-rich extracts of *Ginkgo biloba*, bilberry, and grape seed all possess excellent antioxidant activity and have been shown to increase blood flow to the retina and improve visual processes. Clinical studies in humans have demonstrated all three can halt the progressive vision loss of dry ARMD and may even improve visual function.

Choose one of the following:

- ***Vaccinium myrtillus* (bilberry) extract (25% anthocyanosides):** the most effective of all three extracts, bilberry contains flavonoids with a strong affinity for the retinal pigmented epithelium (RPE), the functional portion of the retina that is affected in ARMD; dosage: 40–80 mg t.i.d.
- ***Ginkgo biloba* extract (24% ginkgo flavonglycosides):** especially helpful if poor blood flow to the brain (cerebrovascular insufficiency) is present. By increasing blood flow to the brain, *Ginkgo biloba* significantly improves oxygenation and glucose utilization; dosage: 40–80 mg t.i.d.
- ***Vitis vinifera* (grape seed) extract (95% procyanidin content):** may be particularly useful when poor night vision or significant sensitivity to light is present. Procyanidins are extremely potent antioxidants with effects 20–50 times stronger than vitamins C or E and have been used successfully in the treatment of both diabetic retinopathy and macular degeneration; dosage: 150–300 mg q.d.

Drug–herb interaction cautions

- ***Ginkgo biloba*:**
  - plus *aspirin*: may induce spontaneous bleeding when combined with chronic use of aspirin. Increased bleeding potential reported after *Ginkgo biloba* usage in a chronic user (2 years) of aspirin.

 Pizzorno L U, Pizzorno, Jr J E, Murray M T   Natural Medicine Instructions for Patients

Male infertility

DESCRIPTION

In the US, approximately 15% of all couples have difficulty conceiving a child. In about one-third of these cases, the man is infertile; in another one-third, both the man and woman are infertile; and in the remaining one-third, the woman is infertile. Current estimates suggest that 6% of men between the ages of 15 and 50 are infertile.

Male infertility is considered likely if, in the absence of female causes, a child is not conceived after 6 months of unprotected sex. In 90% of cases, male infertility is due to low sperm count. In an average ejaculate, a man will eject nearly two hundred million sperm, but because of the natural barriers in the female reproductive tract, only about 40 sperm ever reach the vicinity of the egg. A strong correlation exists, therefore, between fertility and the number of sperm in an ejaculate.

In about 90% of cases of low sperm count, the reason is deficient sperm production. Unfortunately, in about 90% of these cases, the reason sperm formation is low cannot be identified, so the condition is labeled *idiopathic oligospermia* (low sperm count for unknown reasons) or *azoospermia* (complete absence of living sperm in the semen).

Semen analysis for sperm concentration and quality is the most widely used test to estimate a man's fertility potential. Total sperm count and quality have been deteriorating over the last few decades; men now supply only about 40% of the number of sperm per ejaculate compared to 1940 levels. Substantial evidence supports the theory that this downward trend is the result of environmental, dietary, and lifestyle changes in recent decades.

As sperm counts have dropped in the general population, a parallel reduction has occurred in the accepted diagnostic line differentiating infertile from fertile men on the basis of sperm concentration, which has dropped from 40 million/ml to 5 million/ml. One positive reason for this drop is that researchers have learned that quality is more important than quantity. Numerous pregnancies have occurred involving men with very low sperm counts; in studies at fertility clinics, 40% of those with sperm counts as low as 5 million/ml are able to achieve pregnancy. On the other hand, if the majority of sperm are abnormally shaped or non-motile (inactive), a man can be infertile despite having a normal sperm concentration. Therefore, in addition to conventional sperm concentration analysis, functional tests should be used to evaluate the sperm's ability to achieve fertilization. One important test detects antisperm antibodies, which, when produced by the man, usually attack the sperm's tail, lessening its ability to move and penetrate the cervical mucus. The presence of these antisperm antibodies in semen analysis is usually a sign of past or current infection in the male reproductive tract.

When the cause of oligospermia (low sperm count) can be identified, standard medical treatment is often quite effective. If the cause of azoospermia (no sperm in the semen) is ductal obstruction, new surgical techniques are showing good results. When the cause is unknown, the rational approach is to focus on those factors that promote the production of healthy sperm: scrotal temperature and nutritional status. These factors, along with herbs that have been shown to increase sperm counts are discussed below.

FREQUENT SIGNS AND SYMPTOMS

- Inability to conceive a child after 6 months of unprotected sex in the absence of female causes
- A total sperm count of lower than 5 million/ml
- The presence of greater than 50% abnormal sperm
- Inability of sperm to impregnate an egg, as determined by the postcoital or hamster-egg penetration *in vitro* (test tube) tests:
  - *the postcoital test* measures the ability of sperm to penetrate the cervical mucus after intercourse.
  - *the hamster-egg penetration test* is based on the discovery that, under appropriate conditions, human sperm can penetrate hamster eggs. The sperm of fertile males exhibits a range of penetration of 10–100%. Less than 10% indicates infertility.
- Detection of antisperm antibodies in semen analysis:
  - when produced by the man, these antibodies attack the sperm's tail, impeding its ability to move and penetrate the cervical mucus.

- antisperm antibodies usually indicate past or current infection in the male reproductive tract.

CAUSES

Possible causes of low sperm counts

- **Increased scrotal temperature:** normally, the scrotal sac keeps the testes at a temperature between 94 and 96°F. Temperatures above 96°F greatly inhibit or stop sperm production completely:
  - infertile men typically have a higher scrotal temperature than fertile men.
  - scrotal temperature can be raised by tight-fitting underwear, tight jeans, hot tubs, and exercising (jogging, rowing or cross-country skiing machines, treadmills), especially if a man is wearing tight shorts or bikini underwear.
  - varicoceles (varicose veins that surround the testes): a large varicocele can cause scrotal temperatures high enough to inhibit sperm production and motility. Surgical repair may be necessary, but scrotal cooling (see Physical medicine below) should be tried first.
- **Increased environmental pollution and cigarette smoking:** many of the chemicals with which we have contaminated our environment over the last 50 years promote free radical production and/or are weakly estrogenic. Cigarette smoke is a significant source of oxidants (free radicals) and is associated with decreased sperm counts and motility as well as increased levels of abnormal sperm:
  - high levels of free radicals are found in the semen of 40% of infertile men.
  - sperm are extremely susceptible to damage from free radicals:
    - sperm cell membrane is primarily composed of polyunsaturated fatty acids, particularly omega-3 essential fatty acids, which are especially vulnerable to free radical damage.
    - sperm themselves generate high quantities of free radicals to help break down barriers to fertilization.
    - sperm lack their own defensive enzymes, so are completely dependent upon antioxidants for protection.
  - exposure to estrogenic chemicals during fetal development and puberty inhibits the multiplication of the Sertoli cells, the sperm-producing cells of the testes.
  - heavy metals (lead, mercury, arsenic, etc.): sperm are particularly susceptible to the damaging effects of heavy metals. A hair mineral analysis for heavy metals should be performed on all men with reduced sperm counts.
  - organic solvents: increased free radical production can cause abnormal fetal development.
  - pesticides (DDT, PCBs, DBCP, etc.): these weak estrogens are resistant to biodegradation and are recycled in the environment until they deposit in our bodies. For example, although DDT has been banned for 20 years, it is still frequently found in root vegetables, such as carrots and potatoes.
- **Diet:**
  - *increased exposure to synthetic estrogens:*
    - diethystilbestrol (DES) was given to several million pregnant women between 1945 and 1971 they had gestational diabetes or were likely to miscarry. DES given to pregnant mothers carrying a male fetus is now known to have caused developmental problems of the reproductive tract as well as decreased semen volume and sperm counts. DES and other synthetic estrogens were also used for 20–30 years to fatten livestock and increase their growth rates.
    - although DES is now outlawed, many livestock and poultry are still hormonally manipulated especially dairy cows, whose milk now contains substantial amounts of estrogen. The rise in consumption of dairy products since the 1940 parallels the drop in sperm counts.
    - estrogens have been detected in drinking water presumably having been recycled from excreted synthetic estrogens (birth control pills) at water treatment plants.
  - *increased intake of saturated fats from animal products:*
    - estrogens concentrate in the fat cells of animals.
    - healthy sperm membranes are primarily composed of very fluid fats (omega-3 essential fatty acids). In the typical Western diet, intake of saturated fats is high while that of essential fatty acids is very low. This results in the production of sperm that are much less motile due to their abnormally stiff membranes.
  - *reduced intake of dietary fiber:* without adequate fiber, excreted estrogens are reabsorbed from the intestines.
  - *reduced intake of fruits, vegetables, and whole grains* sources of dietary fiber.

Causes of temporary low sperm counts

- **Increased scrotal temperature**
- **Infections:**
  - infections in the male genitourinary tract (the epididymis, seminal vesicles, prostate, bladder,

urethra) are thought to play a major role in many cases of infertility. Functional testing that reveals the presence of antisperm antibodies is a good indicator of chronic infection.

■ a large number of bacteria, viruses and other organisms can infect the male genitourinary system, but the most common and most serious infection is caused by *Chlamydia trachomatis*, a sexually transmitted disease:
  ● between 28 and 71% of infertile men show evidence of chlamydial infection.
  ● chlamydial infection of the prostate or urethra typically presents as pain or burning sensations upon urination or ejaculation.
  ● chlamydial infection of the epididymis and vas deferens can result in serious scarring and blockage.
  ● during an acute chlamydial infection, antibiotics must be used. *Chlamydia* is sensitive to tetracyclines and erythromycin, but because it lives in human cells, it may be difficult to eradicate totally with antibiotics alone.
  ● chronic chlamydial infections of the urethra, seminal vesicles, or prostate may be present with few or no symptoms.
  ● the presence of antisperm antibodies may indicate a chronic chlamydial infection. Rectal ultrasonography and detection of antibodies against *Chlamydia* can confirm the diagnosis.
  ● if chlamydial infection is indicated, both partners should take the antibiotic.

■ **Overuse of alcohol, tobacco, or marijuana:** all of these drugs significantly increase production of free radicals. Sperm, which contain large amounts of essential fatty acids, are extremely susceptible to damage by free radicals.
■ **Many prescription drugs**
■ **Exposure to radiation:** generates tremendous amounts of free radicals.
■ **Exposure to solvents, pesticides, and other toxins:** these substances are estrogenic and/or increase free radical production.

RISK INCREASES WITH

■ **Standard American Diet:** a diet based on animal products and processed foods, with little consumption of fresh vegetables, legumes, fruits, nuts and seeds, and whole grains is low in factors necessary for the production of healthy sperm – fiber; antioxidants; essential fatty acids; vitamins C, E, B_{12} and folic acid; beta-carotene, and zinc – and high in damaging

factors that elevate estrogen levels and suppress immune function – saturated fat, sugars, pesticide residues, and chemical additives.
■ Wearing tight-fitting underwear, shorts or jeans.
■ Mother who was given DES during her pregnancy.
■ Mother who consumed a high fat, low fiber diet during pregnancy.
■ Multiple sexual partners: increased risk of sexually transmitted disease.
■ Smoking, alcohol consumption, use of marijuana.
■ Prescription drug use.
■ Exposure to solvents, pesticides and other toxins.

PREVENTIVE MEASURES

■ Take a cold shower after exercising and allow the testicles to hang free to allow recovery from heat build-up.
■ Wear loose underwear made of cotton.
■ Avoid activities that elevate testicular temperature, e.g., hot tubs.
■ Maintain scrotal temperatures between 94 and 96°F.
■ Avoid exposure to free radicals.
■ Identify and eliminate environmental pollutants.
■ Drink filtered water.
■ Stop or reduce consumption of all drugs, especially antihypertensives, antineoplastics such as cyclophosphamide, and anti-inflammatory drugs such as sulfasalazine.
■ Consume a nutrient-dense diet rich in whole, unprocessed, preferably organic foods, especially plant foods (fruits, vegetables, beans, seeds and nuts, and whole grains) and cold-water fish, and low in animal products and processed foods (for more detailed information, see Appendix 1).

Expected outcomes
Sperm production and motility should improve significantly within 1 month.

TREATMENT

Diet
■ Consume the nutrient-dense diet of organically grown foods recommended above in Preventive Measures. Emphasize dark-colored vegetables and fruits (good sources of protective antioxidant vitamins, carotenes and flavonoids), and nuts and seeds (good sources of essential fatty acids and zinc).
■ Consume daily: 8–10 servings of vegetables; 2–4 servings of fresh fruits; 75 g (3 oz) of raw nuts or seeds. (Once removed from their shells, nuts and seeds

should be refrigerated to prevent oxidation of their delicate essential fats.)

- Avoid hormone-fed animal products, especially cow's milk and other dairy products.
- Avoid foods containing fats that have been cooked at high temperature, e.g., fried foods, grilled meats. When fats are exposed to high temperatures, large amounts of free radicals are produced.
- Avoid saturated fats, hydrogenated oils, *trans* fats, and cottonseed oil. Sperm membranes are composed of essential fatty acids, the most fluid of all fats. Excessive consumption of saturated fats, combined with inadequate intake of essential fatty acids, results in the production of abnormally stiff sperm membranes, which significantly decreases sperm's mobility:
  - saturated fats are found in meat and animal products, coconut and palm oils, and *trans* fats.
  - cottonseed oil may contain toxic residues due to heavy spraying of cotton and its high levels of *gossypol*, a substance so effective in inhibiting sperm production that it is being investigated as a "male birth control pill". Antifertility research on cottonseed oil began when it was discovered that men who had used crude cottonseed oil as their cooking oil had low sperm counts followed by total testicular failure.
- Increase consumption of essential fatty acids: best sources are cold-water fish such as salmon, and nuts and seeds. These oils, the primary constituents of sperm membranes, are vitally important for sperm formation and activity.
- Drink purified or bottled water.
- Increase consumption of legumes, especially soy foods:
  - soy is a particularly good source of *isoflavonoids*. Isoflavonoids are also called *phytoestrogens* because of their ability to bind to estrogen receptors. Their weak estrogenic action (0.2% of the estrogenic activity of *estradiol*, the principal human estrogen) exerts an antiestrogenic effect by preventing the body's own estrogen from binding. In addition, phytoestrogens stimulate the production of sex hormone binding globulin, which binds to estrogen, reducing its potency.
  - soy and other legumes also contain *phytosterols* (plant compounds similar in structure to human hormones), which may aid in the manufacture of steroid hormones, including testosterone.

Nutritional supplements

- **A high-potency multiple vitamin and mineral supplement:** this should include 400 µg of folic acid, 400 µg of vitamin B_{12}, and 50–100 mg of vitamin B_6.

(Folic acid supplementation should always be accompanied by vitamin B_{12} supplementation to prevent folic acid from masking a vitamin B_{12} deficiency.) daily multiple providing all of the known vitamins and minerals serves as a foundation upon which to build an individualized health-promotion program.

- **Vitamin C:** the primary antioxidant in all water-soluble compartments in the body, vitamin C (ascorbic acid) plays an especially important role in protecting sperm's genetic material (DNA) from damage:
  - ascorbic acid levels are much higher in seminal fluid than in other body fluids, including blood. When dietary vitamin C was reduced from 250 mg q.d. to 5 mg q.d. in healthy human subjects, the seminal fluid ascorbic acid level dropped 50% and the number of sperm with damaged DNA rose 91%.
  - cigarette smoking greatly reduces vitamin C levels throughout the body. Smokers require twice as much vitamin C as non-smokers, and when smokers were given supplemental vitamin C in doses of either 200 or 1,000 mg q.d., their sperm quality improved proportional to the level of vitamin given.
  - non-smokers have also been shown to benefit significantly from vitamin C supplementation. When 30 healthy but infertile men were given 200 or 1,000 mg of vitamin C daily, after 1 week the 1,000 mg group demonstrated a 140% increase in sperm count, the 200 mg group a 112% increase, and the placebo group, no change. At the end of 60 days, all of the men receiving vitamin C had impregnated their wives, compared to none of the placebo group.
  - vitamin C may improve fertility by reducing the number of agglutinated (clumped together) sperm. Sperm agglutinate when antibodies produced by the immune system bind to the sperm. Such antibodies are often associated with genitourinary tract infection. In the study cited above, initially all three groups had over 25% agglutinated sperm. After 3 weeks, the number of agglutinated sperm in those receiving vitamin C had dropped to 11%.
  - vitamin C works synergistically with vitamin E and carotenes (its fat-soluble partners), as well as with antioxidant enzymes such as glutathione peroxidase, catalase, and superoxide dismutase. Vitamin C also regenerates oxidized vitamin E, enabling it to resume its antioxidant defense activities.
  - dosage: 500–3,000 mg t.i.d.
- **Vitamin E:** the primary antioxidant in all fat-soluble areas of the body including cell and sperm membranes, vitamin E has been shown to inhibit free radical damage of sperm membranes and to enhance

the ability of sperm to fertilize an egg in test tubes. During the course of one study, 11 of 52 infertile men given vitamin E impregnated their wives; dosage: 600–800 IU (mixed tocopherols) q.d.

■ **Beta-carotene:** a powerful fat-soluble antioxidant that works synergistically with vitamins C and E; dosage: 100,000–200,000 IU q.d.

■ **Folic acid:** folic acid is involved in the reactions that lead to the synthesis of nucleic acids (the components of DNA and RNA) and is therefore essential for the production of all germinal cells, including sperm; dosage: 400 μg q.d.

■ **Vitamin B$_{12}$:** B$_{12}$ is used by all DNA-synthesizing cells to facilitate the metabolic activities of folic acid. A deficiency of B$_{12}$ leads to reduced sperm counts and motility:
  ▦ even in infertile men without B$_{12}$ deficiency, B$_{12}$ supplementation has significantly improved sperm counts (in one study, from under 20 million/ml to over 100 million/ml).
  ▦ dosage: 1,000 μg q.d.

■ **Zinc:** a cofactor in numerous enzymatic reactions, zinc is involved in virtually every aspect of male reproduction including hormone metabolism, sperm formation, sperm motility, and prostate health:
  ▦ zinc deficiency results in many problems including decreased testosterone levels and sperm counts.
  ▦ zinc levels are typically much lower in infertile men with low sperm counts.
  ▦ studies show that infertile men with low sperm counts and low testosterone levels receive significant benefit from zinc supplementation. In one study that included 22 men who had been infertile for more than 5 years and whose sperm counts were less than 25 million/ml, zinc supplementation for 45–50 days resulted in an increase in mean sperm count from 8 million/ml to 20 million/ml. Nine out of the 22 wives became pregnant during the study. An additional 15 infertile men with normal testosterone levels participated in this study. Although their sperm counts increased slightly, no changes occurred in their testosterone levels, and no pregnancies occurred.
  ▦ dosage: 30–60 mg q.d.

■ **Arginine:** the amino acid arginine is required for cell replication. If sperm counts are higher than 20 million/ml, arginine may be of benefit, but arginine therapy should be reserved for use after other nutritional therapies have been tried; dosage: 4 g q.d. for 3 months.

■ **Carnitine:** a non-essential amino acid, carnitine is essential for the transport of fatty acids into the mitochondria, the energy production factories in the cells:
  ▦ carnitine concentrations are very high in the epididymis and sperm, both of which derive the majority of their energy from fatty acids.
  ▦ after ejaculation, the motility of sperm correlates directly with their carnitine content. The higher the carnitine content, the more motile the sperm. Conversely, when carnitine levels are low, sperm development, function, and motility are drastically reduced.
  ▦ carnitine supplementation was shown to increase sperm count and motility in 37 of 47 men with abnormal sperm motility.
  ▦ dosage: 1,000 mg t.i.d.

Botanical medicines

■ **Panax ginseng:** Chinese or Korean ginseng has a long history of use as a male tonic and, although no human clinical studies are available, it has been shown to promote growth of the testes, increase sperm formation and testosterone levels, and increase sexual activity and mating behavior in animal studies. Panax ginseng is regarded as the more potent ginseng in its effects, particularly its stimulant effects:
  ▦ dosage: choose one of the following forms and take the recommended dosage t.i.d.:
    ● high-quality crude ginseng root: 1.5–2 g
    ● standardized extract (5% ginsenosides): 100–200 mg.

■ ***Eleutherococcus senticosus* (Siberian ginseng):** Siberian ginseng has been shown to increase reproductive capacity and sperm counts in bulls:
  ▦ dosage: choose one of the following forms and take the recommended dosage t.i.d.:
    ● dried root: 2–4 g
    ● tincture (1:5): 10–20 ml
    ● fluid extract (1:1): 2.0–4.0 ml
    ● solid (dry powdered) extract (20:1): 100–200 mg.

■ ***Pygeum africanum*:** in men with diminished prostatic secretion, pygeum has led to increased levels of total seminal fluid as well as increases in alkaline phosphatase (an enzyme that maintains the proper pH of seminal fluid) and protein:
  ▦ *Pygeum* extract is most effective in cases in which the level of alkaline phosphatase is reduced (to less than 400 IU/cm^3), and there is no evidence of inflammation or infection (i.e., the absence of white blood cells or IgA).
  ▦ *Pygeum* extract can sometimes improve the capacity to achieve erections in patients with benign prostatic hyperplasia.

dosage: fat-soluble extract, standardized to contain 14% triterpenes including beta-sitosterol and 0.5% *n*-docosanol: 100–200 mg q.d. in divided doses.

Drug–herb interaction cautions
- **Panax ginseng:**
  - plus *monoamine oxidase inhibitor, phenelzine*: may produce manic-like symptoms
  - plus *caffeine*: long-term use (13 weeks) of large amounts (3 g q.d. on average) of ginseng may lead to hypertension in one person out of six
  - plus *insulin*: dosage may need adjusting because of ginseng's hypoglycemic effects in diabetic patients
  - plus *warfarin*: anticoagulant activity may be reduced.
- ***Eleutherococcus senticosus* (Siberian ginseng):**
  - plus *hexobarbital*: when injected into the peritoneal cavity in mice, Siberian ginseng increases the effect of hexobarbital due to inhibition of its metabolic breakdown.
  - plus *insulin*: when injected into the peritoneal cavity in mice, Siberian ginseng extract has hypoglycemic effects, so insulin dosage may need adjustment.

Topical medicine
- **Testicular hypothermia device:** also called a testicle cooler, this device looks like a jock strap from which long, thin tubes have been extended. The tubes are attached to a small fluid reservoir filled with cold water that attaches to a belt around the waist. The fluid reservoir contains a pump that circulates the water, which evaporates and keeps the scrotum cool. The reservoir must be refilled approximately every 6 hours. Most users claim that the testicle cooler is fairly comfortable and easy to conceal. It should be worn daily during waking hours.

Physical medicine
- After exercising, take a cold shower and allow the testicles to hang free to allow recovery from heat buildup.
- Wear boxer-type underwear and periodically take a cold shower or apply ice to the scrotum.

Menopause

DESCRIPTION

The permanent cessation of menstruation (menopause) may occur as early as age 40 or as late as 55, but the average age when menopause occurs is 51 years. The commonly accepted criterion for diagnosing menopause is 6–12 months without a menstrual period. Menopause is only one event in the "climacteric" a series of biological changes in body systems and tissue that occurs in both sexes between the mid-40s and mid-60s.

The time period, typically 2–3 years, prior to menopause is referred to as *perimenopause* ("peri" meaning "around"), while the time period after menopause is referred to as *postmenopause*. During perimenopause, many women ovulate irregularly due to fluctuations in estrogen secretion and/or resistance of the remaining egg follicles to ovulatory stimulus.

Menopause occurs when virtually no eggs remain in the ovaries. At birth, about one million eggs (or *ova*) are contained within the ovaries. At puberty, this number drops to 300,000–400,000, but only about 400 ova actually mature during the reproductive years. By the time a woman reaches 50, few viable ova remain. The absence of active follicles (the cellular housing of the eggs) results in reduced production of estrogen and progesterone. In response to this drop in estrogen, the pituitary gland increases its secretion of follicle-stimulating hormone (FSH) and luteinizing hormone (LH), which continue to be secreted in large quantities after menopause. Although no egg follicles remain to stimulate, FSH and LH stimulate the ovaries and adrenal glands to secrete increased amounts of androgens, which can be converted to estrogens by fat cells in the hips and thighs. In postmenopausal women, converted androgens provide some circulating estrogen, but total estrogen levels are far below those of menstruating women.

Although in the United States, menopause is associated with a variety of unpleasant symptoms and treated as a disease, in many cultures of the world, achieving menopause is synonymous with acceptance as a respected elder and relief from childbearing. In such traditional cultures, discomfort due to menopausal symptoms is reported far less frequently than in the US.

Menopausal symptoms are not, however, merely the result of negative social conditioning in the West. Of equal impact on a woman's transition through menopause are the physiological stresses imposed by the Standard American Diet and exposure to the wide variety of environmental toxins commonplace in the West. Not only are women in the West told that menopause is an "estrogen-deficiency disease", which will leave them sexless "caricatures of their former selves ... the equivalent of a eunuch", they must also traverse this period of significant physiological change while bombarded with literally thousands of potentially toxic chemicals (e.g., pesticides, cleaning products, cosmetics, food additives, and drugs), and while consuming a diet based on animal products and processed foods that is low in protective factors – antioxidants, essential fatty acids, vitamins and minerals – and high in damaging factors that elevate cholesterol levels, blood pressure, and risk for obesity, cancer and diabetes – saturated fat, *trans* fats (also called partially hydrogenated oils), sugars, refined carbohydrates, pesticide residues and chemical additives.

These negative factors need not dominate a woman's evolution through menopause. Natural medicine offers a variety of well-documented health-promoting therapies to support a graceful transition through the climacteric to the next phase of a vital, healthy life.

FREQUENT SIGNS AND SYMPTOMS

As the body attempts to maintain its former state of hormonal balance, hormone levels (particularly estrogen levels), may fluctuate widely causing the following symptoms.

- **Menstrual irregularity:**
  - periods may occur more frequently than normal (e.g., every 21–24 instead of 28 days) or may not occur for one to several months
  - spotting between periods
  - periods may be heavier or lighter than usual.
- **Hot flashes or flushes:** sensations of heat spreading from the waist or chest toward the neck, face and upper arms:
  - hot flashes are caused by a dilation of the peripheral blood vessels, which leads to a rise in skin temperature and flushing skin, especially of the head and neck.

Skin becomes red and warm for a few seconds to 2 min, with cold chills following.

- in the US, 65–85% of women experience hot flashes to some degree.
- hot flashes are often the first sign of approaching menopause, but are usually most frequent in the first and second years after menopause as the body adapts to decreased estrogen levels.
- **Headaches:** these are due to increased instability of blood vessels and often accompany hot flashes.
- **Dizziness, rapid irregular heartbeat:** also related to vascular instability and may accompany hot flashes.
- **Hypoglycemic symptoms:** suddenly feeling weak or shaky, breaking out in a cold sweat.
- **Atrophic vaginitis:** thinning and drying of the lining of the vaginal canal due to lack of estrogen. May cause painful intercourse, increased susceptibility to infection, and vaginal itching or burning.
- **Bloating** in the upper abdomen.
- **Frequent urinary tract infections:** about 15% of menopausal women experience frequent bladder infections due to a breakdown in the natural defense mechanisms that protect against bacterial growth in the urinary tract.
- **Bladder irritability**
- **Breast tenderness**
- **Cold hands and feet**
- **Mood changes**
- **Pronounced tension and anxiety**
- **Sleeping difficulty**
- **Forgetfulness, an inability to concentrate**
- **Depression or melancholy and fatigue**

CAUSES

Menopause
- A normal decline in ovarian function resulting in decreased levels of the female hormones, estrogen and progesterone
- Surgical removal of both ovaries

Menopausal symptoms
- **Diet:** consumption of the Standard American Diet and exposure to numerous environmental toxins significantly exacerbates the stress placed on a woman's system, which is attempting to maintain balance while undergoing physiological change to a new state of equilibrium.
- **Psychological:** cultural devaluation of older women in the West.

RISK INCREASES WITH

- **Smoking:** women who smoke have double the risk of early menopause (menopause beginning as early as age 44).

PREVENTIVE MEASURES

Menopause is a normal part of life that cannot be avoided, but the majority of negative effects frequently associated with menopause can be largely prevented or alleviated.

Atrophic vaginitis
- **Keep well hydrated:** drink at least 1.5 L (3 US pints) of clean (filtered) water daily.
- **Avoid substances that dry the mucous membranes:** these include antihistamines, alcohol, caffeine, diuretics.
- **Wear clothes made from natural fibers**, e.g., cotton, which allow the skin to breathe, thus preventing development of the hot, moist environment that favors vaginal infections.
- **Regular intercourse:** frequent sex increases blood flow to vaginal tissues, thus helping to improve tone and lubrication. If needed, maintain good lubrication with oil or K-Y jelly.

Bladder infections
- **Drink large quantities of fluids** (at least 2 L [4 US pints] q.d.), including at least 0.5 L (1 US pint) of *unsweetened* cranberry juice or 0.25 L (8 US fl oz) of blueberry juice each day to:
  - enhance the flow of urine by maintaining good hydration
  - prevent bacterial adherence to the lining of the bladder. In order for bacteria to infect, they must first adhere to the mucosal lining of the urethra and bladder. Components found in cranberry and blueberry juice reduce the ability of *Escherichia coli* to adhere.
- **Minimize consumption of sugars and refined foods:** consuming 75 g (3 oz) of sugar in one sitting in any form (sucrose, honey, fruit juice) depresses white (immune) cell activity by 50% for 1–5 hours, thus significantly increasing susceptibility to infection.
- For more detailed information, including several botanical medicines that can be employed against bladder infections, see the chapter on Cystitis.

Cold hands and feet
- **The three major causes** of cold hands and feet are hypothyroidism, low iron levels in the body, and poor circulation.

- The following tests may be suggested:
  - *basal body temperature test* (described in the chapter on Hypothyroidism) to evaluate thyroid activity
  - *serum ferritin levels*, a laboratory test that checks the amount of ferritin in the blood, the best indicator of body iron stores
  - *CBC (complete blood count) and chemistry panel* that includes low density lipoprotein (LDL)/high density lipoprotein (HDL) cholesterol levels
  - *a physical examination* for any other causes of decreased blood flow.

Forgetfulness and inability to concentrate

- These symptoms are often due to decreased oxygen and nutrient supply to the brain caused, not by menopause, but atherosclerosis (hardening of the arteries).
- Regular exercise, a health-promoting diet low in factors that damage the cardiovascular system (saturated and *trans* fats, alcohol, sugars, refined foods), and the botanical medicine, *Ginkgo biloba* – all discussed below – will significantly enhance the supply of oxygen and nutrients to the brain.

Expected outcomes

Most women will become virtually asymptomatic within 4–6 weeks after instituting the natural approach that targets the underlying causes of their symptoms.

TREATMENT

While hormone replacement therapy (HRT) is currently the standard allopathic treatment for menopausal symptoms, HRT is not without potentially serious adverse side effects. Rather than immediately using HRT to artificially counteract menopausal symptoms, the natural approach first focuses on improving physiology through diet, exercise, nutritional supplementation and botanical medicines.

Side effects of hormone replacement therapy

- The cancer-causing potential of HRT is a serious concern. Breast cancer, the most common cancer in women, is the form most likely to be exacerbated since estrogens play a critical role in the development of most breast cancers. Current estimates are that one in nine women in the US will develop breast cancer in her lifetime.
- Despite more than 50 studies, the cancer risk of HRT is still not clear, but experts have calculated that estrogen replacement therapy is associated with a 1–30% increase in breast cancer risk.

- Most of the studies showing that HRT increases cancer risk were conducted in Europe, while most of those in the US have found no increased risk. Several hypotheses have been advanced to explain this surprising difference including:
  - American researcher bias
  - the years-long US medical establishment's enthusiastic recommendation of estrogen replacement therapy
  - American women are already at such high risk for breast cancer that the effect of estrogen replacement is difficult to measure.
- In addition to possible increased risk for cancer, synthetic estrogen and progesterone products increase risk for gallstones and blood clots, and cause nausea, breast tenderness, symptoms similar to PMS, depression, liver disorders, enlargement of uterine fibroids, fluid retention, blood sugar disturbances, and headaches.
- In the Nurses Health Study of more than 23,000 women, postmenopausal women on synthetic hormone replacement were also found to be twice as likely to suffer from adult-onset asthma, this side effect being dose related. This finding is not surprising since the incidence of asthma in women soars at the onset of puberty when estrogen levels begin to increase.

Type of hormone replacement therapy

If, after weighing all the evidence with a physician, HRT is chosen – either for short-term relief or for long-term use because of a high risk for osteoporosis – natural hormone replacement using hormones identical to human estrogen and progesterone is recommended.

- Conjugated estrogens (e.g., Premarin, Genisis), which are derived from pregnant mares' urine, progestins (synthetic progesterone formulations) and medroxyprogesterone products (e.g., Provera, Cycrin, Amen) are not biochemically identical and do not produce effects identical to human hormones.
- Human estrogen is actually composed of three estrogens: estriol, estrone, and estradiol. Tri-Est, a formulation containing these three natural forms of human estrogen in a ratio equivalent to that found in the human body along with natural progesterone, derived from wild yam but biochemically identical to human progesterone, is preferred.
- A salivary hormone profile test to determine current hormone levels may be suggested, together with working with a compounding pharmacist to develop a natural hormone replacement prescription that meets specific needs.

Diet

- **Increase the amount of plant foods**, especially those high in phytoestrogens, e.g., soy, flaxseed and flaxseed oil, nuts, whole grains, apples, fennel, parsley, and alfalfa:
  - a diet rich in fruits and vegetables not only eases the transition through menopause, but also provides protection against chronic degenerative diseases including heart disease, breast cancer, arthritis, cataracts, etc.:
    - as estrogen levels drop, a woman's risk of heart disease increases significantly. Heart disease is the leading cause of death in women over 50.
  - phytoestrogens are plant compounds capable of binding to estrogen receptors that can help balance estrogen's effects whether estrogen levels are too high or too low:
    - particularly during perimenopause, estrogen levels may fluctuate widely as the body attempts to compensate for declining ovarian estrogen production. These abrupt shifts in estrogen levels are responsible for many of the symptoms associated with menopause in the West.
    - although phytoestrogens' activity is only 2% as strong as that of human estrogen, if estrogen levels are low, the net effect is an increase in estrogenic activity. If estrogen levels are too high, phytoestrogens lower estrogen's effects by binding to estrogen-receptor sites, thereby preventing estrogen from doing so.
  - increasing dietary intake of phytoestrogens helps decrease hot flashes, increase maturation of vaginal cells, and inhibit osteoporosis.
  - a diet rich in phytoestrogens results in decreased frequency of breast and colon cancer.
  - synthetic and even natural unopposed estrogen replacement pose significant health risks including increased risk of cancer, gallbladder disease, strokes and heart attacks:
    - phytoestrogen-containing foods and herbs have not been associated with any of these side effects, and in addition, have been found extremely effective in inhibiting breast cancer by occupying estrogen receptors and via other anticancer mechanisms.
- **Consumption of soy foods** reduces cancer risk, vaginal atrophy, and heart disease risk:
  - *genistein* and *daidzein*, the *isoflavones* (phytoestrogens) in soybeans produce a mild estrogenic effect. One cup of soybeans provides approximately 300 mg of isoflavone, the equivalent to 0.45 mg of conjugated estrogens, or one tablet of Premarin:
    - while Premarin therapy is associated with an increased risk of cancer, consumption of soy foods is associated with a significant reduction in cancer risk.
  - in one study of postmenopausal women, those who consumed enough soy foods to provide 200 mg of isoflavone q.d. had an increase in the number of superficial cells that line the vagina, thus preventing the vaginal drying and irritation common in postmenopausal women.
  - soy also protects LDL cholesterol from oxidation, an extremely important protective effect for the prevention of cardiovascular disease.
- **Soybeans' safety** is demonstrated by the fact that they have been cultivated as food for more than 13,000 years in China.
- **Consume products made from whole soybeans** (soy flour, whole soy) rather than those produced from soybean protein concentrates:
  - products made from whole soybeans are higher in isoflavonoid content.
  - soy protein isolates contain no isoflavones.

Nutritional supplements

Clinical studies have found the following nutrients effective in relieving hot flashes and atrophic vaginitis:

- **Vitamin E:** found primarily in the lipid (fatty) membrane of cells, which it protects from free radical damage, vitamin E is the main antioxidant in all fat-soluble areas of the body. A healthy cell membrane is essential for the passage of nutrients into and wastes out of cells, so an adequate supply of vitamin E is essential for healthy cellular metabolism. Vitamin E is particularly important during menopause as it not only relieves menopausal symptoms but also protects against cancer and heart disease:
  - in several clinical studies, vitamin E has been found to improve blood supply to the vaginal wall and to relieve atrophic vaginitis and hot flashes.
  - in premenstrual syndrome and fibrocystic breast disease, two other female complaints related to hormonal imbalances, vitamin E has been shown to normalize circulating hormone levels, relieving many symptoms.
  - of all the antioxidants, vitamin E may offer the most protection against cardiovascular disease. Vitamin E reduces LDL (bad) cholesterol peroxidation, improves plasma LDL breakdown, inhibits excessive platelet aggregation, increases HDL (good) cholesterol levels, and increases the breakdown of fibrin, a clot-forming protein.
  - vitamin E significantly enhances both types of immune defense: non-specific or cell-mediated immunity and specific or humoral immunity.

Cell-mediated immunity is the body's primary mode of protection against cancer.

- dosage: oral use – 800 IU (mixed tocopherols) q.d. until symptoms have improved, then 400 IU q.d.; topical use – vitamin E oil, creams, ointments or suppositories can be used topically for symptomatic relief of vaginal dryness and irritation.

- **Hesperidin:** like many other flavonoids, hesperidin improves vascular integrity, lessening excessive capillary permeability – a primary factor in hot flashes:
  - after 1 month's supplementation of hesperidin in combination with vitamin C, symptoms of hot flashes were relieved in 53% of patients and reduced in 34%. Nocturnal leg cramps, nosebleeds and easy bruising were also lessened. The only side effects were a slight body odor and a tendency for perspiration to discolor clothing.
  - dosage: 900 mg q.d. in combination with at least 1,200 mg vitamin C.

- **Vitamin C:** vitamin C, the body's primary antioxidant in all water-soluble areas inside and outside cells, works synergistically with vitamin E and carotenes (its fat-soluble partners):
  - as noted under hesperidin, vitamin C helps to alleviate hot flashes by strengthening the collagen structures of the vascular system, thus preventing excessive capillary permeability.
  - vitamin C regenerates oxidized vitamin E, enabling it to resume its many beneficial activities.
  - vitamin C is extremely effective in its own right in protecting against cardiovascular disease by preventing oxidation of LDL cholesterol, raising HDL cholesterol levels, lowering the total cholesterol level and blood pressure, and inhibiting platelet aggregation.
  - dosage: 1,200 mg q.d.

- **Gamma-oryzanol (ferulic acid):** a growth-promoting substance found in grains and isolated from rice bran oil, gamma-oryzanol has been shown to be effective in alleviating menopausal symptoms including hot flashes and also to lower blood cholesterol and triglyceride levels:
  - in treating hot flashes, gamma-oryzanol's primary action is to enhance pituitary function and promote release of endorphins by the hypothalamus.
  - an extremely safe, natural substance, gamma-oryzanol has produced no significant side effects in experimental or clinical studies.
  - dosage: 300 mg q.d.

Botanical medicines

The following botanicals are often referred to as uterine tonics. Their positive effects are thought to result from the phytoestrogens they contain and their ability to improve blood flow to the female organs. While effective individually, these herbs are often combined to produce even greater benefit.

- ***Angelica sinensis* (dong quai):** the predominant "female" remedy in Asia, dong quai is used to treat menopausal symptoms (especially hot flashes), as well as menstrual difficulties (painful menstruation, too frequent menstruation, lack of menstruation), and to ensure a healthy pregnancy and delivery:
  - dong quai's active components have both mild estrogenic effects and a stabilizing action on blood vessels, both of which contribute to its effectiveness in relieving hot flashes.
  - dosage: choose one of the following forms and take the recommended dosage t.i.d.:
    - powdered root or as tea: 1–2 g
    - tincture (1 : 5): 4 ml (1 tsp)
    - fluid extract: 1 ml (0.25 tsp).

- ***Glycyrrhiza glabra* (licorice):** during peri-menopause, estrogen levels fluctuate widely while progesterone levels consistently drop. Licorice increases the estrogen-to-progesterone ratio by lowering estrogen levels while simultaneously raising progesterone levels, thus restoring hormonal balance:
  - dosage: choose one of the following forms and take the recommended dosage t.i.d.:
    - powdered root or as tea: 1–2 g
    - fluid extract (1 : 1): 4 ml (1 tsp)
    - solid (dry powdered) extract (4 : 1): 250–500 mg.

- ***Vitex agnus-castus* (chasteberry):** chasteberry's profound effects on pituitary function, specifically altering LH and FSH secretion, are likely the cause of its beneficial effects on menopausal symptoms:
  - although traditionally used in countries around the Mediterranean to suppress libido of women of childbearing age, chasteberry does not reduce libido during menopause.
  - dosage: choose one of the following forms and take the recommended dosage t.i.d.:
    - powdered berries or as tea: 1–2 g
    - fluid extract (1 : 1): 4 ml (1 tsp)
    - solid (dry powdered) extract (4 : 1): 250–500 mg.

- ***Cimicifuga racemosa* (black cohosh):** a special extract of *Cimicifuga* standardized to contain 1 mg of triterpenes calculated as 27-deoxyactein per tablet (trade name Remifemin) is the most widely used and thoroughly studied natural alternative to HRT:
  - in 1997, 10 million monthly units of this extract were sold in Germany, the US, and Australia. A large open study involving 131 doctors and 629 patients found *Cimicifuga* extract produced clear improvement in menopausal symptoms (hot

flashes, depression, vaginal atrophy) in over 80% of patients within 6–8 weeks.

- additional studies that have compared *Cimicifuga* to conjugated estrogens (0.625 mg q.d.) or diazepam (a Valium-like drug) (2 mg q.d.) indicate *Cimicifuga* extract is far more effective than either drug in relieving hot flashes, vaginal atrophy, and the depressive mood and anxiety associated with menopause.
- *Cimicifuga* not only does not stimulate breast tumor cells, but even inhibits their growth:
  - when combined with tamoxifen (an antiestrogen drug often used to prevent a recurrence of breast cancer), *Cimicifuga* improved tamoxifen's effectiveness.
  - detailed toxicology studies have shown no mutagenic or carcinogenic effects, indicating that even long-term use is safe.
- dosage: in clinical studies, the dosage of *Cimicifuga* extract used is 2 mg of 27-deoxyactein (an important biochemical marker of therapeutic activity) b.i.d. If a non-standardized form of *Cimicifuga* is used, choose one of the following forms and take the recommended dosage b.i.d.:
  - powdered rhizome: 1–2 g
  - tincture (1 : 5): 4–6 ml
  - fluid extract (1 : 1): 3–4 ml (1 tsp)
  - solid (dry powdered) extract (4 : 1): 250–500 mg.
- ***Ginkgo biloba* extract:** ginkgo's effects of improving blood flow throughout the vascular system make it especially useful for the cold hands and feet and the forgetfulness that often accompany menopause:
  - in human clinical trials, *Ginkgo* extract has been shown to be effective in the treatment of Raynaud's disease, a peripheral vascular disease of the extremities characterized by very cold fingers and toes.
  - ginkgo is also very effective in improving mental health in patients with cerebral vascular insufficiency, working not only by increasing blood flow to the brain, but also by enhancing energy production within the brain, increasing the uptake of glucose by brain cells and even improving the transmission of nerve signals (memory is directly related to the speed at which the nerve impulse can be transmitted).
  - although most people report benefits within 2–3 weeks, *Ginkgo* should be taken for at least 12 weeks in order to determine effectiveness. The longer *Ginkgo* is taken, the more obvious and lasting its benefits.
  - dosage: 24% ginkgo flavonglycosides content, 40 mg q.d.

Drug–herb interaction cautions
- ***Ginkgo biloba*:**
  - plus *aspirin*: may induce spontaneous bleeding when combined with chronic use of aspirin. Increased bleeding potential reported after *Ginkgo biloba* usage in a chronic user (2 years) of aspirin.

Physical medicine
- ***Regular exercise*:** a minimum of 30 min, four times a week; 3–4 hours per week is recommended:
  - impaired endorphin activity within the hypothalamus is a major factor in provoking hot flashes. Regular exercise increases the production and secretion of endorphins thus reducing the frequency and severity of hot flashes:
    - endorphins, the body's internally produced mood-elevating and pain-relieving compounds, reduce hot flashes via their effects on the functioning of the hypothalamus.
    - located in the center of the brain, the hypothalamus serves as the bridge between the nervous system and the endocrine (hormonal) system, and controls many body functions including body temperature, metabolic rate, sleep patterns, libido, reactions to stress, mood, and the release of pituitary hormones including FSH, the hormone whose excessive secretion results in hot flashes.
    - in a study in Sweden of 79 postmenopausal women who took part in a regular exercise program, those who exercised an average of 3.5 hours per week experienced no hot flashes. Similar results have been reported in other studies of women both on and off HRT.
  - regular exercise provides numerous other benefits including: decreased blood cholesterol levels; decreased bone loss; improved ability to deal with stress; improved circulation; improved heart function; improved oxygen and nutrient utilization in all tissues; increased endurance and energy levels; increased self-esteem, mood and frame of mind; and reduced blood pressure.

Menorrhagia

DESCRIPTION

The average amount of blood loss during a menstrual period of normal length is 60 ml (2 US fl oz). Blood loss greater than 80 ml (2.5 US fl oz) that occurs during menstrual cycles of normal length or a prolonged period of menstrual flow (more than 7 days) is considered excessive menstrual bleeding or menorrhagia. A fairly common female complaint, menorrhagia may be a symptom of an underlying disorder, such as the presence of uterine fibroids, endometriosis, or hypothyroidism. If no underlying disorder is present, menorrhagia may occur because of functional abnormalities in the biochemical processes of the endometrium (the lining of the uterus) that can be prevented in most cases simply by ensuring appropriate nutrition.

FREQUENT SIGNS AND SYMPTOMS

- Excessive menstrual flow (varies greatly from woman to woman)
- Imbalance of female hormones: estrogen and progesterone
- Menstrual period lasting for more than 7 days
- Passage of large clots of blood
- Paleness and fatigue (anemia)

CAUSES

Underlying disorders
- **Chronic iron deficiency:** menstrual blood loss above 60 ml (2 US fl oz) is a common cause of chronic iron deficiency in women. Iron-containing enzymes are depleted before changes in the blood (anemia) are observed. Lack of these iron-dependent enzymes leads to a state of low energy metabolism in the uterine lining and excessive blood loss.
- **Anovulation (failure to release an egg each month):** in a normal menstrual cycle, after ovulation (the release of an egg), the follicle that held the egg becomes the *corpus luteum*, which remains in the ovary and produces progesterone. Progesterone, the hormone secreted during the second half of the menstrual cycle, stops the buildup of the *endometrium*, the lining of the uterus that is shed each month via the menstrual flow. When ovulation does not occur (*anovulation*), corpus luteum growth is impaired, and inadequate progesterone is secreted. Excessive endometrial tissue may accumulate leading to excessive menstrual flow.
- **Fibroids:** benign uterine tumors, fibroids may be symptomatic of an increased estrogen-to-progesterone ratio. Estrogen, the hormone produced during the first half of the menstrual cycle, promotes the growth of uterine tissue.
- **Endometriosis:** normally, during the first half of a woman's menstrual cycle, estrogen promotes a thickening of the lining of the uterus to prepare for implantation of a fertilized egg. If fertilization does not occur, the additional lining peels away from the uterus and is expelled in the menstrual flow. When estrogen levels are particularly high, this tissue may build up and pass backwards out of the fallopian tubes into the pelvic cavity where it can attach to other tissues. Each month, this transplanted tissue continues to react as if it were still in the uterus, thickening, peeling away, and creating new implants, eventually causing pain, cramps and excessive menstrual bleeding.
- **Pelvic infection:** a pelvic infection damages uterine tissue thus causing an increased amount of menstrual bleeding.
- **Intrauterine device (IUD):** an IUD may be a source of constant local trauma to the uterine lining.
- **Hypothyroidism:** the thyroid gland produces hormones that regulate the metabolism of every cell in the body. A common symptom of mild hypothyroidism in women is prolonged and heavy menstrual bleeding, with a shorter menstrual cycle (the time from one period to the next).

Functional disorder
- **Endometrium:** abnormalities in the biochemical processes of the *endometrium* (the lining of the uterus):
  - endometrial biochemical processes control the supply of the essential fatty acid *arachidonic acid*, which is used to manufacture *series 2 prostaglandins*, inflammatory hormone-like molecules.
  - the endometrium of women with menorrhagia concentrates arachidonic acid much more than is

normal, thus leading to the production of high levels of series 2 prostaglandins. This excessive concentration of arachidonic acid is thought to be the major factor in both the excessive bleeding and accompanying menstrual cramps of menorrhagia.

RISK INCREASES WITH

- **Obesity:** fat cells produce estrogen, further exacerbating an excessive estrogen-to-progesterone ratio.
- **Estrogen administration** (without progesterone)
- **An IUD**
- **Irregular ovulation:** young women who have not yet established a regular ovulation cycle may have higher than ideal amounts of estrogen.
- **Women approaching menopause:** during perimenopause, anovulation becomes more frequent, estrogen levels fluctuate, sometimes spiking quite high, and progesterone production decreases.
- **A diet high in animal products:** animal fats are the primary source of arachidonic acid, the essential fatty acid used to make the pro-inflammatory series 2 prostaglandins that are a major factor in excessive menstrual bleeding and cramps.
- **A diet low in green leafy vegetables:** green leafy vegetables contain vitamin K, which is necessary for blood clotting.

PREVENTIVE MEASURES

- Consume a nutrient-dense diet rich in whole, unprocessed, preferably organic foods, especially green leafy vegetables and cold-water fish, and low in animal products (for more detailed information, see Appendix 1).

Expected outcomes

Outcome will depend upon the underlying cause. For example, in case of large fibroids or endometriosis the goal may be simply to reduce the severity of the menorrhagia. If the menorrhagia is due to hypothyroidism, chronic iron deficiency, or other easily treatable cause, improvement and possibly complete resolution of menorrhagia may occur within 1 month.

TREATMENT

Diet

- **Essential fatty acids:** increase consumption of foods containing the essential fatty acids that the body uses

to produce anti-inflammatory prostaglandins. Decrease consumption of foods containing the essential fatty acids the body uses to produce pro-inflammatory prostaglandins:
- minimize consumption of land animals: beef, poultry, lamb, etc. Arachidonic acid, which is used to produce the pro-inflammatory series 2 prostaglandins, is derived from the fats of land animals.
- increase consumption of cold-water, fatty fish: salmon, mackerel, herring, halibut. EPA (eicosapentaenoic acid) and DHA (docosahexanoic acid), which are used to create anti-inflammatory series 3 prostaglandins, are derived from cold-water, fatty fish.
- take 1–2 tbsp of flaxseed oil q.d.:
  - EPA can also be synthesized from ALA (alpha-linolenic acid), which is found in flaxseed.
  - flaxseed oil should be refrigerated and never heated. Use in salad dressings, add to smoothies, add to already cooked soup, cereal or vegetables.
- **Increase consumption of green leafy vegetables:** these vegetables, particularly turnip greens, broccoli, lettuce, cabbage, and spinach, are good sources of vitamin K, the vitamin necessary for blood clotting.

Nutritional supplements

- **Iron:** menstrual blood loss above 60 ml (2 US fl oz) is a common cause of chronic iron deficiency in women. A number of studies suggest that chronic iron deficiency can cause menorrhagia:
  - iron-containing enzymes are depleted before changes in the blood (anemia) are observed. A result of low levels of these iron-dependent enzymes is a state of low energy metabolism in the uterine lining which results in excessive blood loss.
  - dosage: 100 mg of elemental iron q.d.
- **Vitamin C:** vitamin C helps to form a more stable collagen structure. Stronger collagen forms less fragile, permeable capillaries. Fragile capillaries are thought to play an important role in many causes of menorrhagia:
  - vitamin C also significantly increases iron absorption.
  - dosage: 500–1,000 mg t.i.d.
- **Bioflavonoids:** a group of plant pigments largely responsible for the colors of fruits and flowers, flavonoids, when taken with vitamin C, significantly enhance its absorption and effectiveness; dosage: 500–1,000 mg q.d.
- **Vitamin A:** the health of all epithelial tissue, including that which lines the uterus, cannot be properly maintained without adequate vitamin A:
  - **caution:** vitamin A should not be used if there is any chance of pregnancy or a risk of getting

pregnant. If at risk, use beta-carotene, which the body converts to vitamin A, instead. Dosage: 50,000 IU q.d.

- dosage: 25,000 IU b.i.d. for 2 weeks, then lower dosage to 25,000 IU q.d. thereafter until the situation normalizes.

■ **Vitamin E:** in a study of patients with an IUD, supplementation with vitamin E resulted in improvement in all patients by the end of 10 weeks:

- some studies suggest that free radicals play a causative role in endometrial bleeding, particularly if an IUD is present. Vitamin E is the body's primary fat-soluble antioxidant.
- vitamin E may also reduce bleeding by quenching the inflammatory processes that series 2 prostaglandins initiate.
- dosage: 200–400 IU (mixed tocopherols) q.d.

■ **Chlorophyll (fat soluble):** an excellent source of vitamin K, a fat-soluble vitamin necessary for the formation of the factors necessary for blood clotting; dosage: 25 mg q.d.

Botanical medicines

■ ***Capsella bursa pastoris* (shepherd's purse):** in addition to its long history of use to cause cessation of obstetric and gynecological bleeding, clinical studies have shown shepherd's purse to be effective in treating menorrhagia resulting from functional abnormalities and fibroids:

- dosage: choose one of the following forms and take the recommended dosage t.i.d.:
  - dried leaves by infusion (tea): 1.54 g
  - tincture (1 : 5): 4–6 ml
  - fluid extract (1 : 1): 0.5–2.0 ml
  - solid (dry powdered) extract (4 : 1): 250–500 mg.

Drug–herb interaction cautions
None.

Migraine headache

DESCRIPTION

Migraine is a neurological and often hereditary disease in which the most prominent symptom is an intense, pounding headache. The headache, itself called a migraine, is usually felt on one side of the head and is accompanied by other symptoms including nausea, vomiting, and visual disturbances.

During a migraine attack, blood vessels in the head become hyperreactive and enter into a repetitive cycle of extreme constriction followed by rapid dilation. While a full understanding of the process that produces a migraine headache has not yet been reached, most scientists believe in the following basic scenario: a variety of triggers, which differ from individual to individual, imbalance brain chemistry causing nerve pathway changes, specifically in a major nerve pathway in the brain called the *trigeminal system*. The trigeminal nerve releases neuropeptides, which inflame blood vessels causing them to constrict and then dilate. These blood vessel changes then restimulate trigeminal nerve endings to release more neuropeptides, initiating a vicious cycle. The result is a severe throbbing headache that may last anywhere from 2–72 hours.

Migraine headaches are generally classified as either "common" or "classic". Common migraines come on without warning, while classic migraines, which are more typical, are preceded by auras before the onset of pain. Auras usually last a few minutes and include blurring or bright spots in the vision, anxiety, fatigue, disturbed thinking, and numbness or tingling on one side of the body.

A surprisingly common disorder, migraines affect between 18 and 26 million Americans, 15–20% of men and 25–30% of women. Initial onset is often during the teen years, but migraines also commonly occur for the first time between the ages of 20 and 40. Frequency varies dramatically. In some people, migraines occur weekly, in others, less than once a year. Among female migraineurs (migraine sufferers), about 65% experience migraines immediately before, during, or immediately after their monthly period.

FREQUENT SIGNS AND SYMPTOMS

Classic migraine

Although the signs and symptoms of a migraine attack vary among individuals and even in the same individual over time, the symptoms of a "classic" migraine typically occur in the following sequence.

- An aura that may affect vision, hearing or smell precedes the headache.
- The most common aura symptom is an inability to see clearly, followed by seeing bright spots and zigzag patterns. Visual disturbances may last several minutes to several hours, but disappear once the headache begins.
- Other common preceding symptoms include a feeling of anxiety, fatigue, disturbed thinking, and/or numbness or tingling on one side of the body.
- Dull, boring pain begins in one temple and spreads to that entire side of the head, becoming intense, pounding or throbbing.
- Nausea, vomiting.

Common migraine

In a "common" migraine, the headache may occur without preceding aura symptoms.

In either classic or common migraine, the following symptoms may be present:
- pale skin
- bloodshot eyes
- runny nose or eyes (in some individuals)
- gastrointestinal upset, nausea and anorexia accompanying the headache
- drowsiness following the headache.

CAUSES

The proximate cause of migraine is a hyperreactivity of nerves in the head (the trigeminal system), which triggers constriction and then rebound dilation of blood vessels that go to the scalp and brain. Headache begins when these blood vessels dilate (widen) again. Several hypotheses have been advanced as to the why these nerves become hyperreactive including the following:

- **Inherited vascular instability:** migraine patients may have an inherited abnormality in their control of blood vessel constriction and dilation and/or may be abnormally sensitive to the effects of physical and chemical factors that cause these changes in blood vessels.
- **Platelet disorder:** platelets are small blood cells involved in the formation of blood clots. Migraine sufferers' platelets act differently from normal platelets:
  - migraineurs' platelets spontaneously clump together (aggregate) much more often than normal platelets.
  - migraineurs' platelets release serotonin differently from normal platelets:
    - serotonin is a compound used in the chemical transfer of information from one cell to another and also plays a role in vascular tone – the state of relaxation or constriction of blood vessels.
    - normal platelets release only a set amount of serotonin when they are stimulated.
    - platelets of migraineurs, in response to stimulation (such as from exposure to a chemical or food allergen), release higher and higher amounts of serotonin until a migraine is produced.
  - mitral valve prolapse: patients with classic migraine are twice as likely as normal individuals to have *mitral valve prolapse*, i.e., a leaky heart valve. With each beat of the heart, this leaky valve can damage platelets as they surge through, thus leading to the platelet disorder described above.
- **Excessive levels of estrogen:** estrogen contributes to migraines by increasing the uptake of magnesium into bone and soft tissues, thus decreasing the amount of magnesium available to stabilize brain cell membranes:
  - one of magnesium's most important jobs is stabilizing cellular membranes, thus regulating molecular traffic into and out of cells. When magnesium levels are low, brain cell membranes become much more permeable, rendering them hyperreactive and prone to a special kind of neuronal depression termed "spreading depression" that is the first phase of a migraine attack.
  - when estrogen levels are too high, too much magnesium is shunted into bone and soft tissue, leaving both brain and blood vessel cell membranes unstable, and prone to hyperreactivity.
  - estrogen may rise to abnormally high levels during a woman's menstrual cycle, particularly immediately before, during or immediately after menstruation:
    - high estrogen levels are a primary cause of premenstrual syndrome (PMS).
    - estrogen levels fluctuate widely during perimenopause, frequently spiking to higher than optimal levels.
    - supplemental estrogen from oral contraceptive use or hormone replacement therapy can also raise estrogen to problematic levels.
- when estrogen is prescribed to help prevent osteoporosis, high doses of calcium are also typically given, which exacerbates any magnesium inadequacy:
  - calcium and magnesium are usually maintained in a delicate balance necessary for the many enzymatic reactions that occur during normal cellular metabolism. Not only are these reactions disrupted, but excessive amounts of calcium, which competes with magnesium for entry into the cells, blocks magnesium's absorption.
  - in addition, the influx of calcium into blood vessel cells causes blood vessels to constrict.
- **Nerve disorder:** nerve cells in the blood vessels of migraineurs are more prone to release a compound termed "substance P", which triggers pain, dilates blood vessels, and signals the immune system's white blood cells, called *mast cells*, to release histamine and other allergic compounds. Chronic stress is thought to play an important role in hypersensitizing nerve cells.
- **Serotonin deficiency:** migraineurs have been found to have low levels of the neurotransmitter serotonin in their tissues. Low serotonin levels lead to a decrease in the pain threshold in patients with chronic headaches:
  - low serotonin is most likely due to higher than normal activity of MAO (monoamine oxidase). MAO, an enzyme found in the gut as well as in the brain, breaks down chemicals in foods that affect the tone of blood vessels, thus preventing the absorption of these chemicals into the bloodstream. Because serotonin, which acts as a neurotransmitter in the brain, is also a potent vasoconstrictor and stimulator of smooth muscle contraction in the gut, it is broken down by MAO.
  - many prescription drugs for migraine (e.g., sumatriptan) work by inhibiting MAO, thus increasing serotonin levels.
  - the serotonin system is, however, very complicated. Some serotonin receptors actually trigger migraines while others prevent them:
    - drugs that bind to serotonin 5-HT_{1c} receptors trigger migraines, while drugs that inhibit 5-HT_{1c} receptors or bind to 5-HT_{1d} receptors may prevent migraines.
    - the serotonin precursor 5-HTP (5-hydroxytryptophan) prevents migraines by gradually decreasing the sensitivity of 5-HT_{1c} receptors while increasing the sensitivity of 5-HT_{1d} receptors, the reason why 5-HTP becomes more

effective over time (better results are seen after 60 days than after 30 days).

- **Low levels of phenol-sulfotransferase (PST):** the enzyme PST normally breaks down serotonin and other chemicals in platelets that affect blood vessel tone. In addition to being in platelets, these chemicals, called amines, are found in certain foods such as red wine, chocolate, and cheese:
  - many migraineurs have been found to have significantly lower levels of PST, so they are more susceptible to the accumulation of amines, such as histamine. *Histamine*, an inflammatory amine known for its production of cold-like allergy symptoms, also causes blood vessels to expand, thus acting as a migraine trigger.
- **Low levels of diamine oxidase:** this enzyme breaks down histamine found in the lining of the small intestine before it can be absorbed into the circulation, travel to the head and cause blood vessel dilation:
  - diamine oxidase is a vitamin B_6-dependent enzyme. If a person is deficient in B_6 or ingests compounds that inhibit B_6, diamine oxidase activity is inhibited. Factors that inhibit B_6 include food coloring agents (specifically the hydrazine dyes such tartrazine, also called FD&C yellow #5), some drugs (isoniazid, hydralazine, dopamine, and penicillamine), birth control pills, alcohol, and excessive protein intake.
  - women have lower levels of diamine oxidase than men, which may explain their higher incidence of migraine.
  - during pregnancy, a woman's diamine oxidase levels increase by over 500% – one reason why remission of headaches is common during pregnancy.
- **A combination of causes:** migraines are most likely initiated when a combination of triggers builds to a threshold, after which the next stressor sets off the series of physiological reactions that produce a headache. Reaching this critical threshold is probably the result of a combination of decreased tissue serotonin levels, low levels of magnesium, changes in platelets, increased sensitivity to compounds such as substance P, and the buildup of histamine and other chemicals that cause inflammation.

Triggering factors

As explained above, in most cases, a single trigger will not cause a migraine, but when combined with other potential stressors will produce sufficient stimulus to provoke an attack.

An individual's triggers are often complex. To identify them, a daily diary should be kept recording foods eaten, weather conditions, medications taken, and any other potential triggers. Particular combinations of triggers may also increase the severity of a migraine.

Common triggers include the following.

- **Tension:** prolonged tension or stress causes an increase in the secretion of stress hormones and a shift of magnesium from inside of cells to the bloodstream:
  - stress hormones constrict blood vessels and stimulate platelets to aggregate more easily.
  - a lowering of the level of magnesium within cells renders them more permeable, thus more likely to become hyperreactive.
- **Drug reaction:** several clinical studies have estimated that 70% of patients with chronic headaches suffer from drug-induced headaches, of which there are two basic types: analgesic rebound and ergotamine rebound:
  - *analgesic-rebound headaches*: analgesic medications such as aspirin or acetaminophen constrict blood vessels. Rebound dilation may occur as their effects wear off:
    - in one study, migraineurs who took more than 30 analgesic tablets per month were found to have twice as many headaches as those who took fewer analgesics.
    - in another study, when 70 patients consuming 14 or more analgesic tablets per week discontinued their use, 66% were improved within 1 month, and 81% were improved within 2 months.
    - dosage that typically leads to rebound headache is 1,000 mg of either acetaminophen or aspirin.
    - withdrawal symptoms – nausea, abdominal cramps, diarrhea, restlessness, sleeplessness, anxiety – typically start within 24–48 hours and subside in 5–7 days.
  - *ergotamine-rebound headaches*: ergotamine is the most widely used drug for treatment of severe migraine and cluster headaches. Administered by IM injection, inhalation or suppository since it is poorly absorbed orally, ergotamine works by constricting blood vessels in the head:
    - although effective, ergotamine, even at prescribed doses, is associated with serious side effects including acute poisoning in about 10% of patients.
    - regular use is associated with dependency syndrome characterized by severe chronic headache.
    - migraines rarely occur more than once or twice a week, so an almost daily migraine headache in individuals taking ergotamine is a strong indicator of an ergotamine-rebound headache.
    - withdrawal symptoms – protracted, debilitating headache accompanied by nausea/vomiting – usually appear within 72 hours and may last another 72 hours.

- **Food allergy/intolerance:** the immune response that is activated by consumption of foods to which an individual is intolerant results in platelets releasing serotonin and histamine, thus triggering a migraine:
  - foods most commonly found to induce migraine include cow's milk, wheat, chocolate, egg, orange.
- **Foods high in amines:**
  - foods such as chocolate, cheese, beer, and wine (especially red wine) contain histamine and/or other compounds that cause blood vessels to expand:
    - red wine contains 20–200 times more histamine than white wine.
    - histamine stimulates platelets to release *vaso-active* compounds (compounds that affect blood vessel tone).
    - red wine also contains high amounts of flavonoids that inhibit PST, an enzyme that breaks down vasoactive amines and serotonin in platelets, before these substances can be released into the bloodstream where they cause blood vessel dilation.
    - red wine, citrus fruits, aged cheese, and chocolate all inhibit PST.
- **Factors that inhibit vitamin B$_6$:**
  - FD&C yellow dye #5 (tartrazine), drugs (isoniazid, hydralazine, dopamine, penicillamine), birth control pills, alcohol, and excessive protein intake inhibit vitamin B$_6$.
  - vitamin B$_6$ is necessary for the activity of diamine oxidase, an enzyme that breaks down histamine.
- **Foods containing certain additives:**
  - meats such as hot dogs and hams that contain nitrates; beer and red wines which contain nitrites; the chemicals used in pickled or marinated foods; foods prepared with monosodium glutamate; foods containing the artificial sweetener, aspartame.
  - in susceptible individuals, these chemicals trigger brain cell hyperreactivity.
- **Foods containing caffeine** such as chocolate, coffee and other caffeinated beverages:
  - caffeine causes blood vessels to constrict.
  - in susceptible individuals, a rebound blood vessel dilation occurs when caffeine is withdrawn from the system.
- **Missing meals:** the brain, the body's hungriest organ, relies on glucose for fuel. Missing meals may result in a less than optimal supply of glucose, a significant stressor for brain cells prone to hyperreactivity.
- **Light:** the stress caused by bright sunlight, fluorescent lights that cause glare, or eyestrain may act as the final straw for hyperreactive brain cells.
- **Chemical fumes:** chemicals in perfumes, cleaning products, gasoline, etc. may be a source of significant stress in susceptible individuals:
  - individuals' liver detoxification capabilities, which are composed of numerous enzyme systems, vary widely. Individuals with lesser amounts of various enzymes will not be able to clear these chemicals rapidly, which may then act as migraine triggers.
- **Fatigue:** a stressor that, in susceptible individuals, may increase the tendency of platelets to aggregate and release serotonin.
- **Menstrual cycles:** high levels of estrogen result in too much magnesium being shunted into bone and soft tissue, leaving both brain and blood vessel cell membranes unstable, and prone to hyperreactivity.

RISK INCREASES WITH

- **Stress:** increases secretion of stress hormones and depletes the amount of magnesium within cells:
  - stressors include intense emotions, such as grief or anger, exhaustion, muscle tension, poor posture.
  - weather changes (barometric pressure changes, sun exposure) may be physiological stressors in sensitive individuals.
- **Family history of migraines:**
  - possible inherited low production of enzymes that break down histamine.
  - food allergy and/or increased sensitivity to various triggers.
  - learned styles of coping with stress that are ineffective.
- **Food allergies or intolerances:** consumption of foods to which an individual reacts causes an immune response that involves the release of serotonin and histamine from platelets.
- **Smoking:** smoking causes blood vessel constriction and promotes platelet aggregation.
- **Use of oral contraceptives:**
  - oral contraceptives prevent conception by increasing estrogen levels.
  - birth control pills are known to increase the adverse effects of smoking and to decrease cellular levels of numerous nutrients including vitamin B$_6$, riboflavin, and magnesium. A deficiency in any of these nutrients can trigger a migraine in susceptible individuals.
- **Estrogen replacement therapy:** increases estrogen levels.
- **PMS:** often due to high levels of estrogen.
- **Perimenopause:** during menopause, estrogen levels fluctuate widely and may spike irregularly before subsiding.
- **Menstruation:** estrogen may rise to excessively high levels at various times during a woman's monthly cycle, e.g., immediately before, during or after menstruation.

- **Use of many prescription and non-prescription drugs:**
  - many commonly used drugs, antihistamines for example, constrict blood vessels; a rebound dilation may occur when these drugs are discontinued.
  - diuretics, often prescribed to lower blood pressure, do so by increasing urination, thus increasing the loss of minerals, including magnesium.
  - numerous commonly used drugs inhibit histamine breakdown. Histamine can trigger migraines in sensitive individuals by causing blood vessels to expand.
- **Alcohol consumption:** alcohol, especially red wine, inhibits histamine breakdown.

PREVENTIVE MEASURES

- Reduce stress where possible: exercise regularly, develop your spirituality, take regular vacations.
- Keep a "trigger diary" to identify factors that precede attacks, so that these can be avoided.
- Minimize drug use, especially oral contraceptives, antihistamines, diuretics, and analgesics (aspirin, acetaminophen).
- Don't smoke.
- Avoid alcohol consumption, especially red wine.
- Get adequate rest – 8 hours sleep per night.
- Ensure adequate intake of riboflavin, vitamin B_6 and magnesium. Good food sources include:
  - *riboflavin*: liver, brewer's yeast, almonds, wheat germ
  - *vitamin B_6*: brewer's yeast, sunflower seeds, wheat germ, soybeans, salmon, liver, walnuts
  - *magnesium*: kelp, wheat bran, wheat germ, almonds, cashews, blackstrap molasses, brewer's yeast, buckwheat, brazil nuts, dulse, filberts, peanuts.
- If high estrogen levels are suspect, refer to the chapters on the appropriate issue: Menopause, Menorrhagia, Premenstrual syndrome.

Expected outcomes
Headache frequency should begin to decrease within 2 weeks. Although this process may take several months, complete resolution of migraines can be expected after triggers have been identified and controlled.

TREATMENT

Diet
- Eliminate all food allergens and utilize a 4-day rotation diet.

- Initially, all foods containing vasoactive amines should be totally eliminated from the diet:
  - primary foods to eliminate are alcoholic beverages, cheese, chocolate, citrus fruits, and shellfish.
  - after symptoms have been controlled, these foods can be carefully reintroduced, one at a time. If, after 3 days, no reactions to the reintroduced food have occurred, this food may be eaten every fourth day, and another food may be reintroduced.
- The diet should be low in meat and dairy products since these contain animal fats:
  - domestically grown animal fats are our primary source of arachidonic acid, a fatty acid that is metabolized in the body to produce series 2 prostaglandins, which promote inflammation.
- Increase intake of flaxseed oil, and cold-water fish such as salmon, garlic and onion:
  - flaxseed oil and cold-water fish are excellent sources of omega-3 essential fatty acids. These fats are metabolized in the body to produce series 1 and 3 prostaglandins, both of which are anti-inflammatory. (Flaxseed oil, which is highly susceptible to oxidation, should be stored in an opaque container, refrigerated, and never heated.)
  - onions and garlic inhibit platelet aggregation, as they contain compounds that inhibit the enzymes responsible for metabolizing arachidonic acid into the pro-inflammatory prostaglandins and thromboxanes that promote platelet aggregation.
- Use fresh ginger liberally. Ginger can be added to juices, used as a spice in cooking, or steeped in hot water for tea:
  - ginger is a potent anti-inflammatory agent, which has also been shown to inhibit platelet aggregation.

Nutritional supplements
- **Magnesium:** one of magnesium's key functions is to stabilize cell membranes, thus preventing overexcitability of nerve cells and changes in blood vessel tone:
  - low tissue levels of magnesium are common in persons with migraine.
  - the tests which best indicate low tissue levels of magnesium are those for the level of magnesium in red blood cells (erythrocyte magnesium level), and the level of ionized magnesium (the most biologically active form) in serum:
    - serum (the blood minus all blood cells) magnesium is a very poor indicator of tissue levels of magnesium since most of the body's store of magnesium is within cells. Low serum magnesium reflects only end-stage deficiency.

- magnesium also improves mitral valve prolapse, which is linked to migraines since it leads to damage to blood platelets, which then release histamine, platelet-activating factor, and serotonin:
  - research shows that 85% of patients with mitral valve prolapse have chronic magnesium deficiency and that oral magnesium supplementation improves mitral valve prolapse.
- dosage: magnesium bound to citrate, malate or aspartate. 250–400 mg t.i.d.:
  - these forms are better absorbed and better tolerated than inorganic forms such as magnesium sulfate, hydroxide, or oxide, which tend to have a laxative effect.
  - if a loose stool results, cut back to a level that is tolerable.
- IV magnesium for acute migraine: in several studies, a dosage of 1–3 g of IV magnesium, given over a 10-min period, resulted in a nearly 90% resolution of headache in patients with low ionized magnesium levels.
- **Vitamin B$_6$**: B$_6$ increases the cellular accumulation of magnesium and is necessary for the activity of the enzyme diamine oxidase, which breaks down histamine in the lining of the small intestine, thus helping to prevent a migraine induced by foods containing histamine; dosage: 25 mg t.i.d.
- **Riboflavin:** in the mitochondria, the energy factories in every cell, riboflavin (vitamin B$_2$) acts as a coenzyme in the production of energy from fatty acids. When the amount of available riboflavin is inadequate, mitochondrial energy production drops. Decreased energy production in brain cells activates the trigeminal nerve, which then releases neuropeptides that cause blood vessel inflammation and dilation, triggering a migraine attack; dosage: 50 mg q.d.
- **5-Hydroxytryptophan (5-HTP):** 5-HTP increases levels of both serotonin (discussed under Causes above) and endorphins:
  - levels of endorphins, the body's own pain-relieving and mood-elevating substances, are typically low in migraineurs.
  - 5-HTP has been found to be as effective as drugs used to prevent migraines (methysergide, pizotifen, propranolol), but unlike these drugs, 5-HTP has no unpleasant side effects, plus it improves mood and helps alleviate, sleep disorders and feelings of depression.
  - 5-HTP is so safe, it has been used with excellent results to treat chronic headaches in children.
  - dosage: 100–200 mg t.i.d.

Botanical medicines

- ***Tanacetum parthenium* (feverfew):** feverfew has been shown in a number of clinical trials to reduce both frequency and intensity of migraine attacks:
  - feverfew works by inhibiting the release of blood vessel dilating substances from platelets, inhibiting the production of inflammatory substances, and re-establishing proper blood vessel tone.
  - effectiveness is dependent upon the presence of adequate levels of parthenolide, the active component in feverfew.
  - dosage: 0.25–0.5 mg of parthenolide b.i.d.
- ***Zingiber officinale* (ginger):** although evidence for ginger's effectiveness against migraine is in the form of case reports rather than full clinical trials, ginger has been shown in numerous studies to exert significant effects against inflammation and platelet aggregation:
  - a typical example was reported in 1990 of a 42-year-old woman with a long history of recurrent migraine. She discontinued all medications for 3 months, then took 500–600 mg of dried ginger mixed with water at the onset of the migraine and repeated that dosage every 4 hours for 4 days. Improvement was evident in 30 min, and there were no side effects. She then began to use uncooked fresh ginger in her daily diet. Migraines became less frequent, and when they did occur, were significantly less severe.
  - the active components of ginger are found in fresh preparations and the oil.
  - dosage: choose one of the following forms:
    - fresh ginger: approximately 6 mm slice (10 g) q.d.
    - dried ginger: 500 mg q.i.d.
    - extract: standardized to contain 20% gingerol and shogaol, 100–200 mg t.i.d. for prevention. Up to 200 mg every 2 hours, up to six times a day, in the treatment of acute migraine.

Drug–herb interaction cautions

- ***Zingiber officinale* (ginger):**
  - plus *oral drugs*: in rats, ginger increases absorption of oral drugs, such as extract with sulphaguanidine, in the small intestine.

Physical medicine

Several forms of physical medicine have been shown to be effective in shortening the duration and decreasing the intensity of a migraine attack, but they do not appear to reduce the frequency of attacks of true migraine.

- **Chiropractic manipulation:** in a 6-month trial of 85 patients in Australia, manipulation of the cervical spine by a chiropractor found no difference in frequency of recurrence, duration or disability, but patients reported greater reduction in pain associated with migraine attacks.

- **Temporomandibular joint (TMJ) dysfunction syndrome:** correction of dysfunction in the TMJ, the jaw joint, may be of help in treating migraines, although it has been shown to be more likely and of more importance in muscle tension headaches.
- **Transcutaneous electrical nerve stimulation (TENS):** TENS involves stimulation of muscles with very low levels of electricity to cause them to contract and then relax:
  - TENS has been shown to be effective in both migraine and muscle tension headaches (55% of patients responded to TENS versus an 18% response to placebo).
  - home TENS units are available through doctors.
- **Acupuncture:** sufficient positive studies exist to suggest that acupuncture may be successful in reducing the frequency of migraine attacks:
  - in one study, 40% of subjects experienced a 50–100% reduction in severity and frequency, although the patients were only followed for 2 months.
  - in another study, five treatments over a period of 1 month decreased recurrence in 45% of patients over a period of 6 months.
  - acupuncture appears to relieve pain by normalizing serotonin levels; however, it was ineffective in those patients with very low levels of serotonin.
- **Biofeedback and relaxation therapy:** the effectiveness of biofeedback and relaxation training on reducing frequency and severity of migraines has been the subject of more than 35 clinical studies. The results showed that these non-drug approaches are as effective as the beta-blocking drug Inderal (propranolol), but unlike the drug, these mind–body therapies have no negative side effects:
  - thermal biofeedback utilizes a feedback gauge to monitor the temperature of the hands. The patient learns how to raise (or lower) hand temperature, with the device providing feedback as to what is effective.
  - relaxation training involves teaching patients how to produce the "relaxation response", a physiological state that is the opposite of the stress response.

Multiple sclerosis

DESCRIPTION

Multiple sclerosis (MS) is a syndrome of chronic nerve disturbances due to a process called *demyelination*, a gradual loss of the myelin sheath surrounding each nerve cell. The myelin sheath plays an essential role in transmission of the nerve impulse. Without the myelin sheath, nerve transmission cannot occur, so nerve function is lost. Symptoms correspond to this loss of function in the affected nerves.

Incidence of MS follows a geographic distribution with areas of highest frequency all located in the higher latitudes, in both the northern and southern hemispheres (50–100 cases per 100,000 in higher latitudes versus 5–10 cases per 100,000 in the tropics). High-risk areas include the northern US, Canada, Great Britain, Scandinavia, northern Europe, New Zealand, and Tasmania. It also appears that the initiating event in MS may occur early in life since people who move from a low-risk to a high-risk area before the age of 15 have a higher risk of developing MS, while those who make the same move after age 15 retain their lower risk.

In about two-thirds of cases, onset is between the ages of 20–40 years, and women are more frequently affected than men – incidence is 60% female to 40% male. The rate of progression varies considerably in MS. One-third of patients have mild, non-progressive disease; one-third worsen slowly; and one-third worsen rapidly.

FREQUENT SIGNS AND SYMPTOMS

Initial symptoms may occur alone or in combination. Typically, symptoms develop over a few days or weeks, recede, then recur.

Early stages
Sudden transient motor and sensory disturbances including:
- intermittent blurred or double vision, fogginess, haziness, eyeball pain or other vague eye problems
- muscle weakness
- feeling of heaviness, leg dragging, stiffness
- tendency to drop things, clumsiness
- dizziness, light-headedness, feeling of spinning, sensation of drunkenness, nausea, vomiting
- difficulty with walking or balance
- vague loss of sensation
- tingling "pins and needles" sensation, numbness, band-like tightness, electrical sensations

Laboratory findings
- Elevated IgG antibodies in cerebrospinal fluid: found in 80–90% of patients with MS, although also present in other neurological conditions
- Nerve function assessment (evoked-potential studies): abnormalities found in 94% of patients with established MS, and 67% of patients with suspected MS
- Magnetic resonance imaging (MRI) showing demyelination in the nervous system
- Excessive platelet adhesiveness (stickiness)
- Decreased levels of omega-3 essential fatty acids in the serum, erythrocytes, and cerebrospinal fluid

Late stages
- Marked muscular weakness and tremor
- Difficulty speaking
- Loss of bladder sensation, bladder or bowel control
- Extreme mood swings
- Sexual impotence in men

CAUSES

The cause(s) of MS remain to be identified conclusively. Numerous causative factors have been proposed including the following.
- **Viral infection:** viruses are known to cause several demyelinating diseases similar to MS in humans and animals, and studies have demonstrated that viruses can cause demyelination either by directly damaging the myelin-producing cells or by prompting an immune response in which antibodies are formed that attack the myelin:
  - a number of viruses have been identified in patients with MS including rabies virus, herpes simplex virus, scrapie virus, parainfluenza virus, subacute myelo-opticoneuropathy virus, coronavirus, and measles virus.
  - measles is the most suspicious potential cause of MS, although recent studies have shown that the

measles-specific antibody in MS patients accounts for only a small percentage of their total antibody level.

■ the cerebrospinal fluid (the fluid surrounding the brain and spinal cord) of most MS patients contains an elevated level of IgG antibodies (proteins made by the immune system's white blood cells that bind to alien molecules such as bacteria, viruses, and cancer cells) in a pattern characteristic of an immune response to an infectious process.

■ at present, however, available data do not suggest a common virus is the cause for these increased IgG antibody levels; they are thought to result from an autoimmune reaction.

■ **Autoimmune reaction:** the lesions in the nerve cells of MS patients are similar to those produced in animals after injecting them with myelin:

■ the autoimmune disease produced in animals (*experimental allergic encephalomyelitis*) is the result of the animals' reaction to a single antigen (myelin basic protein).

■ humans with MS show no evidence of an increase in antibody levels to myelin basic protein. Considerable evidence suggests that MS is an autoimmune disease, but it must be due to some other antigen.

■ **Excessive lipid peroxidation:** patients with MS frequently are found to have reduced levels or activity of a very important antioxidant enzyme called *glutathione peroxidase*:

■ glutathione peroxidase (GSH-Px) is critical for the protection of cells from free radicals. Decreased levels or activity of GSH-Px render the myelin sheath much more susceptible to damage. The myelin sheath is largely composed of fats (lipids), so when it is damaged (oxidized) by free radicals, lipid peroxides are formed.

■ GSH-Px is found in two enzymatic forms: selenium dependent and non-selenium dependent.

● decreased levels of selenium-dependent GSH-Px are most probably the result of inadequate amounts of selenium in the diet. Areas in which selenium levels in the soil are low often overlap areas in which incidence of MS is high.

● reduced activity of GSH-Px in MS patients is most likely the result of genetic factors: MS incidence is higher in individuals with a form of GSH-Px with low activity (GSH-PxL), compared to individuals genetically endowed with a form of GSH-Px with high activity (GSH-PxH).

■ **Pro-inflammatory diet:** a higher prevalence of MS has been correlated with diets high in animal and dairy products, especially when compared to diets high in cold-water fish:

■ inland farming communities in Norway, in which animal products comprise a large portion of the diet, have a higher incidence of MS than areas near the coastline where fish is a primary protein source.

■ in Japan, despite its northern latitude, MS incidence is quite low, and the traditional Japanese diet is also high in seafood, along with seeds and soyfoods.

■ domestically grown animal and dairy products contain high amounts of arachidonic acid, while fish, seeds and soyfoods are abundant in the omega-3 oils (alpha-linolenic, eicosapentaenoic, and docosahexanoic acids):

● arachidonic acid is metabolized in the body to produce series 2 prostaglandins, which promote inflammation.

● omega-3 fats are metabolized in the body to produce series 1 and 3 prostaglandins, both of which are anti-inflammatory.

● deficiencies of these omega-3 oils interfere with the elongation of fats that compose nerve cell membranes and permanently impair formation of normal myelin.

● the epidemiological data suggest that disease results when consumption of animal fats, our primary source of pro-inflammatory arachidonic acid, is not balanced by comparable consumption of the anti-inflammatory omega-3 fats found in fish, seeds, and soyfoods.

■ a diet low in omega-3 fats may be a significant factor in patients with MS:

● normal myelin is largely composed of omega-3 fats.

● omega-3 fats decrease both the platelet aggregation (clumping together) seen in atherosclerosis as well as MS, and the autoimmune response in which the immune system attacks the myelin sheath.

● excessive platelet aggregation and very small clumps of platelets (microemboli) are thought to damage the blood-brain barrier, and cause alterations in the microcirculation of the central nervous system, and reduced blood flow to the brain seen in MS.

● damage to the blood–brain barrier allows passage of blood components toxic to myelin (bacteria, viruses, antibodies, toxic chemicals) into the cerebrospinal fluid.

● reduced blood flow to the brain promotes cellular death via the release of self-destructing enzymes, which can also destroy myelin.

■ **Food allergy:** consumption of two common allergens – gluten (found in wheat and other grains) and cow's milk – has been implicated in MS:

- diets high in gluten and milk are much more common in areas in which prevalence of MS is high.
- intestinal biopsy of MS patients has shown increased frequency of significant damage to the intestinal lining similar to that which occurs in celiac disease and food allergies.

RISK INCREASES WITH

- Children and adolescents raised in northern latitudes.
- High intake of animal products, particularly when comparable intake of fish, seeds and soyfoods is lacking.
- Inadequate intake of selenium results in low levels of GSH-Px.
- Family history of MS: genetic susceptibility; low activity of GSH-Px.
- Food allergy, especially to gluten and milk.
- Use of non-steroidal anti-inflammatory drugs (NSAIDs) such as aspirin, ibuprofen, indometacin, etc.:
  - NSAIDs inhibit the synthesis of prostaglandins from essential fatty acids. The prostaglandins formed from omega-3 fats reduce the autoimmune response, thus lessening the destruction of myelin.
  - individuals with or at risk for MS should avoid NSAIDs.

PREVENTIVE MEASURES

- **Ensure adequate intake of selenium:**
  - in addition to being needed for the selenium-dependent form of GSH-Px, selenium helps disarm free radicals formed from the arachidonic acid cascade and from a defensive tactic of the immune system (the phagocytic respiratory burst).
  - best sources of selenium are seafood and meats. Meat consumption should, however, be minimized since meat is also the primary source of arachidonic acid.
  - best plant sources of selenium include wheat germ, Brazil nuts, apple cider vinegar, red Swiss chard, and oats:
    - the soil content of selenium will determine the amount found in plant sources. Plants grown in low-selenium areas cannot, therefore, be relied upon to supply standard amounts.
  - recommended daily allowances (q.d.) for selenium are:
    - children: 1–6 years, 20 µg; 7–10 years, 30 µg.
    - males: 11–14 years, 40 µg; 15–18 years, 50 µg; 19+ years, 70 µg.
    - females: 11–14 years, 45 µg; 15–18 years, 50 µg; 19+ years, 65 µg.
- **Identify and eliminate food allergens:** wheat and dairy should be prime suspects.
- **Ensure adequate intake of omega-3 oils** by increasing intake of the foods richest in these oils: cold-water fish, nuts (especially walnuts) and seeds (especially flaxseed, discussed below).
- **Increase intake of soyfoods:** a good source of protein that compares favorably with beef, but without the high levels of fat found in most animal foods, soy also contains antioxidant phytochemicals, fiber, and polyunsaturated fats, including omega-3 oils.

Expected outcomes

- Individuals with minimal disability respond better than those with severe disability.
- Treatment including diet, lifestyle modification and supplementation should begin as soon as possible since the earlier in the disease process that treatment is initiated, the better the results.
- Normalization of red blood cell fatty acid levels requires a minimum of 2 years of supplementation. Since myelin-producing cells have a much longer half-life than red blood cells, it could take several years before the total benefits of treatment will be observed.
- Once MS has progressed to significant disability, it is unlikely to be greatly affected by the natural therapies recommended below. Regardless of the progression of MS, these measures will, at the very least, provide the benefit of decreasing risk for atherosclerosis and other degenerative diseases.

TREATMENT

Lifestyle
Avoid excessive fatigue, emotional stress, and marked temperature changes.

Diet
- The Swank diet: Dr Roy Swank, Professor of Neurology at the University of Oregon Medical School, who began successfully treating MS patients with a low animal fat diet in 1948, has provided convincing evidence that such a diet, maintained over a long period of time, reduces the number of attacks and retards the progression of MS.
- Swank's diet effectively reduces the intake of arachidonic acid while increasing intake of essential fatty acids, particularly the omega-3 fats, which prevent platelet aggregation and are required for normal myelin composition (see Causes above).

- The Swank diet recommends:
  - an intake of saturated fat of no more than 10 g q.d.
  - daily intake of 40–50 g of polyunsaturated oils q.d.
  - no margarine, shortening or hydrogenated oils
  - at least 1 tsp of cod liver oil q.d.
  - normal allowance of protein:
    - a diet low in saturated fats significantly restricts animal protein.
    - protein should be primarily derived from fish, legumes, grains, and vegetables.
    - cold-water fish are preferred because of their excellent omega-3 as well as protein content and should be eaten three or more times per week.
- Food allergens should be identified and eliminated from the diet: wheat and dairy products are the most common allergens in patients with MS.
- Fresh whole foods should be emphasized and consumption of animal foods (with the exception of cold-water fish) should be reduced, if not completely eliminated.

Nutritional supplements
- **A high-potency multiple vitamin and mineral supplement:** a daily multiple providing all of the known vitamins and minerals serves as a foundation upon which to build an individualized health-promotion program. Any good multiple should include 400 µg of folic acid, 400 µg of vitamin B_{12}, and 50–100 mg of vitamin B_6. (Folic acid supplementation should always be accompanied by vitamin B_{12} supplementation to prevent folic acid from masking a vitamin B_{12} deficiency.)
- **Flaxseed oil:** flaxseed oil contains both linoleic (an omega-6 essential fatty acid) and alpha-linolenic acid (an omega-3 essential fatty acid):
  - linoleic acid has been shown to greatly inhibit the progression of less severe forms of an autoimmune disease (experimental allergic encephalomyelitis) induced in animals by immunization with myelin.
  - in several double-blind trials in patients with MS, similar beneficial effects have been seen. Supplementation with linoleic acid has resulted in a smaller increase in disability, and reduced severity and duration of relapses, compared with controls.
  - as in animals, individuals with minimal disability respond better than those with severe disability.
  - dosage: 1 tbsp q.d. Flaxseed oil, which is highly susceptible to oxidation, should be refrigerated and never heated. It should taste slightly sweet and nutty. If bitter or off-flavored, it is rancid and should not be consumed.
- **Selenium:** one form of the critically important antioxidant glutathione peroxidase (GSH-Px, discussed

above) is selenium dependent:
  - GSH-Px protects lipids (fats) from oxidation by free radicals.
  - the membranes of cells, including nerve cells, are primarily composed of fats, as is the myelin sheath.
  - dosage: 200–400 µg q.d. (including the amount found in the multiple).
- **Vitamin E:** a fat-soluble antioxidant, vitamin E, which works with selenium, provides the body's primary defense against oxidative damage to all its lipid-rich constituents, including the cell membranes and myelin sheath of nerve cells:
  - one study reported that supplementation of 18 MS patients with high dosages of selenium, vitamin E and vitamin C for 5 weeks increased GSH-Px levels fivefold.
  - dosage: 400–800 IU (mixed tocopherols) q.d.
- **Vitamin B_{12}:** both inborn errors of metabolism involving B_{12} and acquired B_{12} deficiency are well-known causes of demyelination of nerve fibers in the central nervous system (CNS):
  - in MS patients, vitamin B_{12} levels have been found to be low in serum, red blood cells and the CNS.
  - a B_{12} deficiency may aggravate MS or promote another cause of progressive demyelination.
  - in one recent study, researchers found that although the level of B_{12} in the serum of MS patients was normal, B_{12} was not getting into their cells, indicating a defect in the transport of the vitamin into cells:
    - oral administration of 60 mg q.d. of B_{12} in the form of *methylcobalamin* – the main and most active form of B_{12} in the body, and the form directly related to the function of B_{12} in methylation reactions – improved both sight and hearing by nearly 30%.
    - motor function did not improve, indicating that pathways to the brain benefit from B_{12}, while those from the brain do not.
    - these results are equivalent to those produced by cyclophosphamide (a very potent immune-suppressing drug) plus steroids – a combination associated with profound immune suppression and toxicity.
    - no toxic side effects have been attributed to high doses of B_{12}.
  - dosage: B_{12} (in its methylcobalamin form): 2 mg q.d. in the case of B_{12} deficiency; up to 60 mg q.d. when used as therapy.
- **Pancreatin:** in MS, as in other autoimmune diseases, levels of circulating immune complexes (antigens bound by antibodies) are abnormally high. Protein-digesting enzyme preparations (e.g., pancreatic

extracts, bromelain, papain) have been shown to reduce these high levels:

- in MS, pancreatic enzyme preparations have been found to produce good effects in reducing severity and frequency of symptom flare-ups including visual disturbances, sensory disturbances, and urinary, bladder and intestinal malfunction. Little effect, however, has been noted on spasticity, dizziness, or tremor.
- many individuals with MS have some degree of malabsorption:
  - in one study, 42% of MS patients had fat malabsorption, 42% had protein malabsorption, 27% had abnormal sugar absorption, and 12% had abnormal B_{12} absorption.
  - pancreatic enzymes may also improve absorption.
- dosage (10×potency): 350–700 mg t.i.d., taken between meals on an empty stomach.

Botanical medicines

- *Ginkgo biloba* **extract (GBE)**: in MS, increased levels of lipid peroxides and other indicators of free radical damage in the central nervous system suggest the need for antioxidant support:
  - in numerous studies, GBE has demonstrated impressive antioxidant effects, and also lessens platelet aggregation, improves blood flow to the brain and nervous system, and enhances nerve cell function.
- dosage: standardized extract containing 24% ginkgo flavonglycosides: 40–80 mg t.i.d.

Drug–herb interaction cautions
- *Ginkgo biloba*:
  - plus *aspirin*: may induce spontaneous bleeding when combined with chronic use of aspirin. Increased bleeding potential reported after *Ginkgo biloba* usage in a chronic user (2 years) of aspirin.
  - as noted above, however, individuals with MS should avoid the use of aspirin and other NSAIDs since these drugs inhibit the synthesis of myelin-protective anti-inflammatory prostaglandins obtained from omega-3 fats.

Physical medicine
- Avoid excessive fatigue and marked temperature changes.
- Exercise is physically and psychologically helpful:
  - in one study, MS patients were assigned to either an exercise or non-exercise group for 15 weeks. Aerobic training consisted of three 40 min sessions per week on a stationary bike that also had arm handles. The exercise group improved on all measures of physical function, social interaction, emotional behavior, home management, total sickness impact profile score, and recreation.
  - for spastic or severely weakened limbs, assisted movement and massage will improve circulation and may offer emotional and social benefits.

Nausea and vomiting of pregnancy

DESCRIPTION

Mild to severe nausea with or without vomiting is not uncommon during the first trimester of pregnancy. Approximately 50% of women experience these symptoms at some time during pregnancy. Nausea may occur at any time of the day but is most common in the morning, thus the term "morning sickness". Considering the many hormonal and metabolic changes that take place to permit normal growth of the fetus, plus the emotional adjustment to incipient motherhood, the occurrence of these symptoms is not surprising. Nausea almost always stops after the first 12–14 weeks of pregnancy.

Mild symptoms of nausea and vomiting during the first trimester are linked to the numerous hormone changes that occur during pregnancy and are a positive indicator of a healthy pregnancy. If nausea and vomiting are quite severe or last longer than the first trimester, emotional stress may also be a factor.

FREQUENT SIGNS AND SYMPTOMS

- Mild to severe nausea with or without vomiting, usually during the first 3–4 months of pregnancy.
- Nausea occurs most frequently in the morning (morning sickness), but may occur at any time.
- Nausea almost always stops after the first trimester but, although rarely, may continue throughout the pregnancy.

CAUSES

- **Numerous metabolic and hormonal changes that occur during pregnancy:**
  - levels of both progesterone and other hormones rise during pregnancy.
  - progesterone causes involuntary muscles to relax, which also slows the movement of food through the stomach and intestines.
  - changes in hormone levels may also affect the area in the brain that induces vomiting.
  - in many women, blood sugar is lower during early pregnancy, which contributes to gastrointestinal upset.

- **Emotional stress:** physiologically, pregnancy is hard work. The addition of negative psychological factors has been shown to increase susceptibility to and duration of nausea and vomiting:
  - in a study of 86 women, a significant increase in nausea and vomiting during the first trimester was noted in those women whose pregnancies were unplanned or undesired.
  - those women whose problems continued into the third trimester were also significantly more negative in their assessment of their relationships with their own mothers.

RISK INCREASES WITH

- Emotional stress
- Large meals
- Skipping meals
- Certain odors (perfumes, gasoline, cooking odors) or foods may be particularly upsetting.
- Cigarette smoke is a very common trigger of nausea and vomiting during pregnancy.

PREVENTIVE MEASURES

- **Ask for help.** Women, particularly those who are having an unplanned or undesired pregnancy, or who have a poor relationship with their own mother should ask for help. It is quite reasonable to ask for help from family and friends. Consulting with a qualified counselor for assistance in resolving any conflicts is also recommended.
- **Eat small, frequent meals** (see Diet below).
- **Try to identify any odors or foods that aggravate nausea and avoid them.**
- **Don't smoke cigarettes** and ask your family not to smoke around you.

Expected outcomes

Nausea and vomiting should lessen significantly within 2–3 hours and should cease within a few days.

TREATMENT

Diet

■ Place a small, easily digested snack, such as a whole-grain cracker or piece of dry wholegrain toast at the bedside. Eat immediately after waking, before getting up in the morning.

■ Eat a small snack at bedtime and another if waking to use the bathroom during the night.

■ During the day, eat a healthful snack as often as every hour or two:
  ▪ think of snacks as a mini-meal that is balanced with a small portion of a high-protein food along with some fruit, vegetable and/or whole grain.
  ▪ choose organically grown food whenever possible.
  ▪ snack examples: 1–2 tsp of nut butter on apple slices or celery; a small handful of unsalted nuts such as almonds, walnuts or cashews mixed with raisins; a quarter-sandwich; a small piece of cheese or $1/2$ cup cottage cheese and a piece of fruit; a cup of plain yogurt topped with a spoonful of granola and/or some fruit; a cup of split pea soup topped with wholegrain croutons.

■ Avoid processed foods as they are typically high in fat, salt, sugar, and chemicals, and low in fiber, vitamins and minerals.

Nutritional supplements

■ **Vitamin B$_6$**: vitamin B$_6$ is extremely important in breaking down and eliminating excessive amounts of pregnancy-related hormones:
  ▪ in a recent double-blind study, 342 women less than 17 weeks pregnant were given either 30 mg of B$_6$ or placebo. After 5 days of treatment, nausea and vomiting were significantly reduced in almost two-thirds of those receiving B$_6$. However, more than one-third taking B$_6$ still experienced nausea and vomiting. A better recommendation may be a larger dose of B$_6$ and its use in combination with ginger (discussed below).
  ▪ dosage: 25 mg b.i.d.–t.i.d.

■ **Vitamins K and C:** when used together, these two vitamins have shown considerable clinical effectiveness. In one study, 91% of patients experienced no further nausea or vomiting within 72 hours; dosage: vitamin K: 5 mg q.d.; Vitamin C: 250 mg t.i.d.

Botanical Medicines

■ *Zingiber officinale* **(ginger):** ginger has a long history of being very useful in alleviating symptoms of gastrointestinal distress, including the nausea and vomiting of pregnancy.

■ compounds in ginger called *gingerol, shogaol,* and *galanolactone* are the source of ginger's antinausea effects on the digestive tract, which have been demonstrated to be even more effective than Dramamine (dimenhydrinate).

■ in the digestive tract, gingerol and galanolactone block receptor sites for 5-HT$_3$, a precursor of serotonin, which causes smooth muscle contraction.

■ a clinical study has found ginger to be effective against the most severe form of pregnancy-related nausea and vomiting, *hyperemesis gravidarum*:
  ● the dosage used in this double-blind cross-over trial was four 250 mg capsules of ginger root powder q.d. for 4 days.
  ● of the 27 women with hyperemesis gravidarum in early pregnancy (less than 20 weeks) who participated in this study, 19 experienced significant relief.

■ ginger is not only effective but the small dose required is extremely safe, in contrast to antiemetic drugs used in pregnancy, which may cause severe birth defects.

■ most research studies have used 1 g of dry powdered ginger root – a relatively small dose compared to the dietary consumption of ginger in India at a daily dose of 8–10 g.

■ fresh or freeze-dried ginger root or extracts standardized to contain 20% gingerol and shogaol may be even more effective.

■ dosage: choose one of the following forms and take the recommended dosage q.d.:
  ● dry powdered ginger: 1–2 g
  ● standardized ginger extract containing 20% gingerol and shogaol, 100–200 mg.

Drug–herb interaction cautions

■ *Zingiber officinale* **(ginger):**
  ▪ plus *oral drugs*: in rats, ginger increases absorption of oral drugs, such as extract with sulphaguanidine, in the small intestine.

Physical medicine

■ **Acupressure:** acupressure, the application of pressure to acupuncture points, has been shown to help relieve the nausea and vomiting of pregnancy:
  ▪ in one study of 16 pregnant women with morning sickness, the use of acupressure wristbands (elastic wristbands with hardened plastic balls applied to acupuncture sites on the wrist) for 5 days relieved morning sickness for 12 of the 16 women.
  ▪ acupuncture wristbands are available at most drugstores.

Obesity

DESCRIPTION

Obesity is more accurately defined as an excessive percentage of body fat rather than simply an excess amount of body weight relative to height. A muscular athlete, or any individual with the solid, heavier build characteristic of the *mesomorph* body type, may have a higher than normal weight in relation to height, yet have a very low percentage of body fat. Obesity is therefore defined as a percentage of body fat greater than 30% for women and 25% for men.

The most accurate methods of determining body composition are underwater weighing, and caliper measurements of skin-fold thickness at multiple body sites. Bioelectrical impedance testing is also reasonably accurate and increasingly used since convenient digital scales, similar to regular bathroom scales, are now available.

Obesity is divided into two categories – *hyperplastic* and *hypertrophic* – based on the size and number of fat cells as well as how the fat is distributed (i.e., in the abdomen versus on the hips).

Hyperplastic obesity denotes an increased number of fat cells throughout the body (hyper = increased, plastic = cells). The number of fat cells an individual has depends primarily on the mother's diet while the person was still in the womb, as well as on early infant nutrition. An excess of calories during these early stages can lead to the formation of an increased number of fat cells that become part of the individual's constitution for the rest of his or her life. Fortunately, hyperplastic obesity is typically associated with fewer serious health effects compared to hypertrophic obesity.

Hypertrophic obesity refers to an increase in the size of each individual fat cell and is the form primarily linked to diabetes, heart disease, high blood pressure, cancer, and other serious metabolic disturbances. In hypertrophic obesity, fat is distributed around the waist, a placement referred to as *male-pattern* or *android* since it is typically seen in the obese male. If the waist is larger than the hips (apple-shaped), the person is said to have *android obesity*; if the hips are larger than the waist (pear-shaped), then the person is said to have *female-pattern* or *gynecoid obesity*.

Data gathered in The National Health and Nutrition Examination Survey III show that one in three adults in the US is now obese. Even more alarming is the fact that the number of obese children doubled between 1960 and 1991; currently, roughly one in five children in the US is obese. If these children enter their teenage years as obese, the odds are 4 : 1 against their ever being of normal weight as adults; if they end their teenage years as obese, the odds are 28 : 1.

Obesity is not merely a cosmetic problem. Cardiovascular disease is the leading cause of mortality in both women and men, and, in the obese individual, the risk of cardiovascular disease is increased 7.7 times. According to the National Institutes of Health (NIH) and the US Surgeon General, most of "the top ten causes of death due to disease are attributable to health risks associated with excess body fat." The official position of the NIH is: "Obesity is a leading cause of heart disease, hypertension, stroke, diabetes, and even cancer."

The good news is that studies which show even slight reductions in weight (5–10%) can produce significant health benefits, providing this weight loss is maintained. Significant economic benefits have also been linked to weight loss. Individuals who lose 10% of their total body weight, and keep the weight off, can expect to save about $5,200 in medical costs over the course of their lifespan, including the costs of treating hypertension, diabetes, and heart disease.

FREQUENT SIGNS AND SYMPTOMS

- **A body-fat percentage** greater than 30% for women and 25% for men.
- **Weighing more than 20% above the average desirable weight** for men and women of a given height – a less accurate sign in athletes and persons who have a mesomorph body type:
  - the weights given in the following table are for adults aged 25–59 years, based on lowest mortality. Weight is in pounds according to frame size in indoor clothing (5 lb for men and 3 lb for women). (Height and weight can be converted to metric measurements using standard conversion tables.)

1983 Metropolitan life height and weight table

Height	Small frame	Medium frame	Large frame
Men			
5′2″	128–134	131–141	138–150
5′3″	130–136	133–143	140–153
5′4″	132–138	135–145	142–156
5′5″	134–140	137–148	144–160
5′6″	136–142	139–151	146–164
5′7″	138–145	142–154	149–168
5′8″	140–148	145–157	152–172
5′9″	142–151	148–160	155–176
5′10″	144–154	151–163	158–180
5′11″	146–157	154–166	161–184
6′0″	149–160	157–170	164–188
6′1″	152–164	160–174	168–192
6′2″	155–168	164–178	172–197
6′3″	158–172	167–182	176–202
6′4″	162–176	171–187	181–207
Women			
4′10″	102–111	109–121	118–131
4′11″	103–113	111–123	120–134
5′0″	104–115	113–126	122–137
5′1″	106–118	115–129	125–140
5′2″	108–121	118–132	128–143
5′3″	111–124	121–135	131–147
5′4″	114–127	124–138	134–151
5′5″	117–130	127–141	137–155
5′6″	120–133	130–144	140–159
5′7″	123–136	133–147	143–163
5′8″	126–139	136–150	146–167
5′9″	129–142	139–153	149–170
5′10″	132–145	142–156	152–173
5′11″	135–148	145–159	155–176
6′0″	138–151	148–162	158–179

- **Poor exercise tolerance:** excess weight increases the heart's work.
- **Emotional problems:** poor self-image, lack of social contacts with opposite sex, possible job discrimination.

CAUSES

Physiological factors
- **Excessive calorie consumption** by an individual's mother while the person was still in the womb and/or during infancy (hyperplastic obesity).
- **Obesity-promoting diet:** the body's ability to turn food into muscle and energy rather than fat is directly related to the quality of the foods routinely ingested. A diet based on processed foods, with little consumption of fresh vegetables, legumes, fruits, nuts and seeds, whole grains, and cold-water fish is:
  - low in the factors necessary for cellular energy metabolism – antioxidants, vitamin and mineral cofactors, essential fatty acids, magnesium and potassium
  - high in factors that disrupt the body's sensitivity to insulin, and thus its ability to use food to produce energy rather than fat – refined carbohydrates, sugars, saturated and *trans* fats (also called partially hydrogenated oils).
- **Inadequate exercise:** television watching has been linked to obesity, in part because of reduced physical activity in people who watch a lot of TV, and due to an actual lowering of resting (basal) metabolic rate while watching TV to a level similar to that experienced during trance-like states.
- **Low-serotonin:** brain serotonin levels significantly influence eating behavior, specifically, low serotonin levels produce "carbohydrate cravings" and play a major role in the development of obesity:
  - studies have demonstrated that when animals and humans are fed diets deficient in the amino acid *tryptophan*, appetite is substantially increased, resulting in binge eating of carbohydrates.
  - a diet low in tryptophan leads to low brain serotonin levels, which signal the brain that it is starving, triggering forceful stimulation of the appetite control centers.
  - this stimulation results in a craving for carbohydrates since carbohydrate facilitates the absorption and delivery of tryptophan to the brain, resulting in the manufacture of more serotonin.
  - further support for this theory comes from its ability to explain why most diets do not work – the fact that blood levels of tryptophan, and subsequent brain serotonin levels plummet when a person is dieting. In response to this drop in serotonin, the brain puts out a strong message to eat.
  - cravings for carbohydrate (as well as fat) as a result of low serotonin levels can range from very mild to quite severe. One theory suggests that obese individuals are extremely sensitive to internal triggers such as low brain serotonin levels, so their cravings are heightened and harder to resist.
- **Set-point theory:** the set point is the weight the body tries to maintain by regulating the amount of food and calories consumed:
  - one theory postulates that individual fat cells control this set point, and when they become smaller (when the individual consumes fewer calories), the fat cells send a powerful signal to the brain to eat.
  - since obese individuals often have more and larger fat cells, when they diet, the urge to eat as sent by

their fat cells can be overpowering, resulting in rebound overeating, weight gain, and an even higher set point – a situation described as the "ratchet effect" or "yo-yo dieting".

■ the set point is related to fat-cell insulin sensitivity:
  ● obesity leads to insensitivity to insulin – a hormone produced by the beta-cells of the pancreas that increases the rate at which blood sugar is taken up by cells and used to produce energy – from which two factors emerge: (1) both obesity and diabetes are strongly linked to the standard Western diet because it contains high amounts of saturated fats and refined carbohydrates, and (2) excessive consumption of saturated fats and refined carbohydrates disrupts the internal mechanisms that control blood sugar, thus leading to insulin insensitivity.
  ● when cells become insensitive to insulin, not only is transport of blood sugar into cells impaired (a condition which leads to diabetes), but also the burning of stored fat for energy is impaired.
  ● in response to insulin insensitivity, the body secretes more insulin to get the job done. This is particularly problematic in an overweight individual, because when fat cells are already filled with fat, insulin triggers the production of additional fat cells, which then signal the brain to urge the person to eat more, so these new fat cells can also be filled with fat.
  ● the key to lowering the fat cell's set point is by increasing its sensitivity to insulin – a feat which can be accomplished by a combination of exercise, a diet specially designed to improve insulin sensitivity, and several nutritional supplements (discussed below).

■ **Diet-induced thermogenesis:** a certain amount of the food we eat is immediately used to produce heat (thermo = heat, genesis = production). In lean individuals, a meal may stimulate up to a 40% increase in thermogenesis. In overweight individuals, heat production only increases about 10%, and the rest of the food's energy is stored. Causes of decreased thermogenesis include:
■ insulin insensitivity
■ impaired sympathetic nervous system activity:
  ● the sympathetic nervous system controls the body's metabolic rate. Many overweight individuals have a "slow metabolism" due to a lack of stimulation by the sympathetic nervous system.
  ● several natural plant stimulants (discussed below) can activate the sympathetic nervous system, thus increasing metabolism and thermogenesis.

■ the amount of brown fat an individual has:
  ● most fat in the body is white fat, which consists of an energy reserve of fat stored as *triglycerides* and housed in white fat cells in one large droplet.
  ● brown fat cells are composed of multiple smaller triglyceride-containing droplets surrounding numerous energy-producing organelles called *mitochondria*, which burn fat.
  ● in other tissues of the body, including white fat cells, energy is produced efficiently, and very little is lost as heat. In brown fat cells, however, energy production is inefficient, and much is wasted as heat.
  ● while the amount of brown fat in modern humans is extremely small (estimates are 0.5–5% of total body weight), because of its profound effect on diet-induced thermogenesis, even as little as 25 g (1 oz) of brown fat can make the difference between maintaining body weight and gaining 4.5 kg (10 lb) per year.
■ people predisposed to obesity because of decreased diet-induced thermogenesis tend to be much more likely to gain weight when consuming a high-fat diet than lean individuals. In addition, they tend to consume much more dietary fat and to exercise less than lean individuals.

Psychological factors

One theory suggests that overweight individuals are insensitive to internal signals for hunger and satiety, while being extremely sensitive to external stimuli (sight, smell, taste) that can increase appetite.

Television watching is one source of external stimuli that has been shown to be associated with obesity, and the effect is dose related (i.e., the more TV one watches, the greater the degree of obesity).

RISK INCREASES WITH

■ Obese parents, particularly if the mother was obese during pregnancy.
■ Watching television 3 or more hours per day.
■ Lack of regular exercise.
■ Consumption of the Western diet, which, due to its high levels of saturated fats, sugar and refined carbohydrates, promotes insulin insensitivity.
■ Hypothyroidism: the thyroid gland regulates the body's metabolic rate. Low thyroid function results in a lowered metabolic rate.
■ Non-insulin dependent diabetes (type II diabetes): insulin insensitivity is the primary malfunction in NIDDM.

PREVENTIVE MEASURES

■ **Regular exercise:** a minimum of 30 min, at least five times per week:
  ▪ *strength training*, which increases muscle mass, is recommended twice a week. Even when resting, muscles burn calories, thus an increase in muscle mass translates into an increase in basal (resting) metabolic rate.
  ▪ *aerobic exercise*, which immediately burns calories and conditions the cardiovascular system, is recommended at least three times a week.
■ **A health-promoting diet:** a balanced diet composed of whole, unprocessed, preferably organic foods, especially plant foods (fruits, vegetables, whole grains, beans [especially soybeans], nuts [especially walnuts], and seeds), organically raised eggs, and cold-water fish (see Diet below).

Expected outcomes
Adoption of long-term dietary and lifestyle modifications will result in gradual, but lasting, weight reduction of up to 450 g (1 lb) per week.

TREATMENT

The successful program for the treatment of obesity must include the following.
■ **A positive mental attitude:**
  ▪ become aware of self-talk. Replace negative self-talk with positive self-talk by asking helpful questions, employing positive affirmations, and setting positive goals.
  ▪ instead of asking why (Why me? Why this situation?), ask what (What am I grateful for today? What must I do today to achieve my long-term goal?).
  ▪ use positive affirmations to create a healthy self-image (My life is filled with blessings. I am so thankful I have the courage, knowledge, and strength to accomplish my goals. Yes I can!). The guidelines that follow can create positive affirmations:
    ● always phrase an affirmation in the present tense and imagine it has already come to pass.
    ● always phrase an affirmation as a positive statement. Do not use the words "not" or "never".
    ● do your best to deeply feel the positive feelings generated by the affirmation.
    ● keep the affirmation short and simple, but personal and full of meaning.
  ▪ set positive goals by:
    ● stating the goal in positive terms, e.g., "I enjoy taking care of myself by exercising and eating delicious, health-promoting foods", rather than "I will not eat cookies, chips, French fries, ice cream and other fattening foods".
    ● making some goals quickly attainable for immediate positive feedback, e.g., "I will enjoy a half hour walk today".
    ● be specific and clearly define what you want to achieve, e.g., "I am losing one pound this week", "I am attaining a healthy body fat percentage of 25% (women), 20% (men)".
    ● state your goal in the present tense and believe you have already achieved it, and success will be yours.
    ● get in the habit of asking yourself each morning and evening, "What must I do today to achieve my long-term goal?".
■ **A healthy lifestyle** (regular exercise, adequate sleep, minimal consumption of alcohol or other drugs, no smoking).
■ **A health-promoting diet** and supplementary measures (described below).

Diet
In order for an individual to lose weight, energy intake must be less than energy expenditure. This goal can be achieved by decreasing caloric intake (dieting) or by increasing the rate at which calories are burned (exercising).

To lose 450 g (1 lb) per week, an individual must take in 500 calories less than he or she expends each day.

Most individuals will lose weight if they decrease caloric intake below 1,500 calories per day and do aerobic exercise for 15–20 min three to four times per week.

The dietary goal is to eat a balanced whole foods diet that will optimize insulin sensitivity. Such a diet includes the following.
■ **Protein:** average minimum requirement for women is 60–70 g q.d.; men need 70–80 g q.d. Spread the protein intake throughout the day, consuming some protein at every meal:
  ▪ whenever possible buy hormone-free, antibiotic-free, range-fed meat and poultry, and eggs from chickens fed a diet rich in omega-3 essential fatty acids (DHA).
  ▪ at least three times each week, choose deep-sea, cold-water fish such as salmon, mackerel, herring, and halibut. In addition to protein, these fish are excellent sources of omega-3 fats. Omega-3 fats increase insulin sensitivity and are protective against cardiovascular disease and diabetcs.

■ **Fats:** *real* fats are necessary for health and do not disrupt insulin sensitivity. Do not be afraid to eat real organic fats in moderation, including butter, and cold or pure pressed oils (heat processes used to extract oils damage the fats, making them harmful), especially flaxseed oil (high in essential fatty acids) and extra virgin olive oil (a very stable monounsaturated fat that is the best choice for cooking):

- in animals, toxins are concentrated in fat stores, so choose organic butter whenever possible.
- do not eat damaged fats. Fats used in deep-frying, oils derived by heat processing, and hydrogenated or *trans* fats are damaging to your health. Hydrogenated fats are mutated into abnormal chemical structures the body cannot use for normal metabolic functions. Fats subjected to the high temperatures of deep-frying and oils derived via processing at high heat are both mutated and oxidized, which turns them into free radicals.
- all fats should be refrigerated to prevent oxidation.
- when purchasing oils, look for cold-pressed oils sold in opaque containers that lessen oxidation caused by exposure to light.
- saturated (butter) and monounsaturated (olive oil) fats are more resistant to damage from heat, so are best used for cooking. Even better, sauté or stir fry with a little herb-seasoned broth, then, after cooking, add a little fat for flavoring.
- all proteins (meat, poultry, eggs, fish) should be cooked at low, even temperatures to avoid damaging the fats they contain.

■ **Non-starchy vegetables:** non-starchy vegetables contain no more than 5 g of carbohydrate per ¹/₂ cup serving:

- eat as many non-starchy vegetables as desired. Try to consume at least 6–8 servings of non-starchy vegetables daily.
- commonly eaten non-starchy vegetables include: asparagus, bell peppers, broccoli, Brussels sprouts, cabbage, carrots (raw), cauliflower, celery, cucumber, eggplant, green beans, greens (beet greens, chicory greens, dandelion green, mustard greens, etc.), jicama (raw), jalapeno peppers, kale, lettuce, mushrooms, onions, parsley, radishes, snap beans, snow peas, spinach, spaghetti squash, summer squash (crookneck, scallop, zucchini), Swiss chard, tomatoes, watercress.
- non-starchy vegetables (along with fruits, discussed next) provide vitamins, minerals, and fiber. The vitamins and minerals are used as coenzymes in virtually all the chemical reactions involved in metabolism. Fiber slows down the digestive process, lowering the *glycemic index* of the entire meal, and is essential for a healthy digestive system.

- the glycemic index of a food is a measure of how fast insulin rises after the food has been eaten. The faster a food is digested, the faster its sugars arrive, and the higher the food's glycemic index:
  - in general, proteins, fats, and non-starchy vegetables have a low glycemic index; complex carbohydrates have a higher glycemic index, and refined carbohydrates have a high glycemic index.
  - consuming high glycemic index foods throughout the day translates into frequent exposure to abnormally high levels of insulin, which leads to insulin insensitivity.
- when a balanced meal composed of protein, fat, non-starchy vegetables and complex carbohydrates is consumed, not only does the body receive each of the types of nutrients it needs to function properly, but the glycemic index of the meal will also be balanced, so insulin levels will not rise excessively.

■ **Carbohydrates:** carbohydrates should never be eaten alone and should be thought of as fuel. Since the goal is to use stored fat as fuel, fewer carbohydrates should be consumed:

- to increase insulin sensitivity, begin construction of a balanced whole foods diet by eating each day:
  - three balanced meals containing protein, fat, non-starchy vegetables, and a carbohydrate selection containing 15 g of carbohydrate
  - plus two balanced snacks containing protein, fat, non-starchy vegetables, and a carbohydrate selection containing 7.5 g of carbohydrate.
- always eat carbohydrates with protein and fat.
- if already depressed and becoming more depressed, add 7.5 g more carbohydrate to each meal and snack (and/or take 5-HTP, described below under Nutritional supplements). This small additional carbohydrate will raise insulin levels slightly. Insulin assists in the transfer of tryptophan from the circulatory system into the brain, where it is used to make serotonin (see Causes above).
- do not eat refined carbohydrates, examples of which include:
  - *products made from refined grains* such as wheat flour or white rice, e.g., bagels, cold cereal, noodles, pancakes, pasta, pizza dough, pie crust, spaghetti, waffles, white bread, English muffins, hamburger buns, white rice.
  - *sugar*: check labels for sucrose, fructose, maltose, dextrose, polydextrose, corn syrup, maple syrup, molasses, sorbitol, maltodextrin.
  - *desserts*: flavored yogurts, fruit leathers, granola and other snack bars, as well as cakes, candy, cookies, ice cream, etc.

- *processed snack foods* including corn chips, pork skins, potato chips, pretzels, tortilla chips, trail mix.
- *condiments* containing sugar and chemicals including barbecue sauces, fish sauces, Hoisin sauce, ketchup, relishes, sweet pickles, Worcestershire.

■ best carbohydrate choices include:
- *starchy vegetables*: e.g., acorn and butternut squash, artichokes, beets, cooked carrots, corn, green peas, lima beans, potatoes, rutabagas, yams, turnips
- *legumes*: e.g., black beans, garbanzo beans, kidney beans, lentils, navy beans, pinto beans, soybeans (see below), split peas
- *fruits*: choose fresh or frozen fruits without added sugar. Examples of fruit servings include: 1 small apple, $1/2$ medium banana, $3/4$ cup blueberries, 1 cup (with pits) cherries, $1/2$ large grapefruit, 15 grapes, 1 large kiwi, $1/2$ medium cantaloupe, $11/2$ cups diced honeydew, 1 medium orange, 1 medium peach, $1/2$ large pear, $3/4$ cup pineapple, 2 tbsp raisins, 1 cup raspberries, $11/2$ cups strawberries, 2 small tangerines, 1 medium tomato, $11/4$ cups diced watermelon.
- *whole grains and products made from whole grain flours*: whole grains are preferable to products made from their flours as whole grains are more slowly digested. Examples of whole grains include: brown rice, wild rice, buckwheat kasha, bulgur (tabouli), corn grits, couscous farina, millet, oats, polenta, popcorn, quinoa, rye, wheat berries. A $1/3$-cup serving of most grains contains approximately 15 g of carbohydrate. Examples of products made from whole grains include: wholewheat bread or crackers, sprouted wheat bread (Essene bread), whole rye bread, corn tortilla, wholegrain crackers). A slice of bread, a corn tortilla, $1/2$ English muffin, 2 brown rice cakes, 2 rye wafers, or 4 small wholewheat crackers contains approximately 15 g of carbohydrate.

■ **Protein foods which contain carbohydrates:**
- ▪ nuts, nut butters and seeds are good sources of healthful fats and protein. An average serving of most nuts (25 g [1 oz] of nuts or 2 tbsp of nut butter) and seeds contains approximately 6 g of carbohydrate.
- ▪ soy products are excellent sources of high quality protein. A typical serving of soy products (1 cup soy milk, 1 cup tofu, 38 g [1.5 oz] soy protein) contains approximately 15 g of carbohydrate.
- ▪ organic whole milk yogurt (whole milk is preferable because the fat content lowers the glycemic index of

this healthful food) contains approximately 15 g of carbohydrate.

For additional information, see Appendix 1 and follow the recommendations given for the 1,500 calorie diet.

Nutritional supplements

■ **5-Hydroxytryptophan (5-HTP):** 5-HTP has been shown to significantly reduce excessive food consumption and promote weight loss in overweight individuals:
- ▪ 5-HTP is the immediate precursor to serotonin, a neurotransmitter involved in the brain's transmission of the message to stop eating.
- ▪ serotonin is manufactured in the body from the amino acid tryptophan by an enzyme that first converts tryptophan into 5-HTP.
- ▪ individuals with a low level of activity of the enzyme that starts the manufacture of serotonin from tryptophan are predisposed to obesity because they don't get the message of fullness until they have consumed too much food for their metabolic needs.
- ▪ when 5-HTP is provided, this genetic defect is bypassed, and more serotonin is manufactured, naturally turning off hunger.
- ▪ three human clinical trials of overweight women, conducted at the University of Rome, have all shown that 5-HTP reduced caloric intake and promoted weight loss, even when the women made no conscious effort to lose weight:
  - best study results occurred, however, when participants were placed on a 1,200 calorie per day diet along with the 5-HTP (300 mg t.i.d.): 100% of those receiving 5-HTP reported early satiety, and these women lost an average of 2 kg (4.39 lb) at 6 weeks and 5.3 kg (11.63 lb) at 12 weeks.
  - in contrast, those in the placebo group had trouble staying on the diet and lost an average of 0.3 kg (0.62 lb) at 6 weeks and 0.8 kg (1.87 lb) at 12 weeks.
  - during the first 6 weeks of the study, mild nausea was reported by many of the women receiving 5-HTP (300 mg t.i.d.), but the symptom was never severe enough for any of the women to drop out of the study, and no other side effects were reported.
- ▪ dosage: 50–100 mg taken 20 min before meals for the first 2 weeks; then double the dosage if weight loss is less than 450 g (1 lb) per week. The dosage may be raised to 300 mg t.i.d. after 3 weeks. This dosage has been associated with mild nausea, but gradually increasing the dosage may avoid this symptom; if not, it disappears after 6 weeks of use.

■ **Conjugated linoleic acid (CLA):** a fatty acid produced by cows that eat natural grass and found in their meat and milk, CLA:

- transports dietary fat into cells, where it is used to produce energy.
- optimizes function of cell membranes, which are composed primarily of fats:
  - when the membranes of the cell and its mitochondria (the cell's energy production factories) are composed of fats such as CLA and the omega-3 fats (EPA and DHA, which are highest in cold-water fish, see Diet recommendations), the transport of nutrients into the cell and its mitochondria is enhanced.
- improves insulin sensitivity by activating certain enzymes and enhancing glucose transport into cells, thus lowering blood sugar levels and normalizing insulin levels.
- has demonstrated a wide range of benefits in animal studies, including antioxidant, anticancer, and immune-enhancing effects, in addition to increasing lean muscle mass.
- has been found in human clinical trials to lower the body fat percentage even in subjects of normal weight. In one 3-month study involving 20 healthy volunteers, half were given six 500 mg CLA capsules q.d. while the others received placebo. Although the subjects did not alter their diet or lifestyle, those in the CLA group experienced a 15–20% reduction in body fat (from 21.3 to 17%), while in the placebo group, body fat increased slightly (from 22 to 22.4%).
- is highly likely to be deficient in the US. In 1963, the CLA percentage in milk was as high as 2.81%; by 1992, the CLA percentage rarely exceeded 1%. This drop is due to changes in feeding patterns of cattle from natural grass to modern artificial livestock feeding methods.
- dosage: three 1,000 mg capsules standardized to contain 70% CLA, taken in the morning on an empty stomach.

■ **Fiber supplements:** in addition to consuming a high fiber diet, supplementing with additional fiber will help promote weight loss:

- fiber sources such as psyllium, chitin, guar gum, glucomannan, gum karaya, and pectin are recommended because they are rich in water-soluble fibers:
  - when taken with water before meals, these fibers bind to water in the stomach to form a gelatinous mass that provides a feeling of fullness, thus making overeating less likely.
  - in addition, supplements of these fibers have been shown to enhance blood sugar control and

insulin sensitivity and to actually reduce the number of calories absorbed by the body from 30–180 calories q.d.

- avoid water-soluble fiber products that contain sugar or other sweeteners and be sure to drink adequate amounts of water when taking any fiber supplement, especially if it is in pill form.
- guar gum, a water-soluble fiber derived from the Indian cluster bean (*Cyamopsis tetragonoloba*), has achieved the most impressive weight-loss results. In one study, nine women who weighed between 72 and 109 kg (160 and 242 lb) were given 10 g of guar gum immediately before lunch and dinner, and were told not to alter their eating habits. After 2 months, the women reported an average weight loss of 4.3 kg (9.4 lb) – over 450 g (1 lb) a week. Reductions in cholesterol and triglyceride levels were also noted.
- studies show that the higher the dosage, the greater the weight loss and cholesterol–lowering effects.
- dosage: to avoid gas (flatulence) and abdominal discomfort, start with a small dosage of between 1 and 2 g before meals and at bedtime, and increase gradually to 5 g before meals and at bedtime.

■ **Chromium:** this trace mineral is essential for insulin sensitivity:

- chromium is the major component in glucose tolerance factor (GTF), which helps insulin bind to receptors in the cellular membrane. Without chromium, insulin cannot bind, so its action is blocked, blood sugar levels are elevated, and thermogenesis is inhibited.
- evidence suggests that marginal chromium deficiency is common in the US.
- chromium supplementation has been shown to lower body weight yet increase lean body mass. Since muscle cells burn fat even at rest, greater muscle mass means more fat-burning potential.
- in studies involving subjects with diabetes and hypoglycemia, chromium supplementation has not only improved blood sugar control and increased the number of insulin receptors on red blood cells, but has also lowered cholesterol and triglyceride levels.
- dosage: 200–400 µg q.d.:
  - chromium in the form of chromium picolinate may be more effective as, in one small study, those given chromium picolinate increased their muscle mass three times as much as those who were given chromium polynicotinate.

■ **Medium-chain triglycerides:** MCTs are special types of saturated fats separated out from coconut oil that are used by the body differently from long-chain triglycerides (LCTs), the most abundant fats found in nature:

- while LCTs, which are larger and therefore harder to metabolize, are stored as fat deposits, MCTs are rapidly burned as energy and actually promote weight loss by also increasing the burning of LCTs.
- in one study, the thermogenic effect of a diet containing 40% MCTs was compared to a diet containing 40% LCTs. The thermogenic effect (calories wasted 6 hours after a meal) of the MCT-rich diet was almost twice as great as that of the LCTs: 120 vs. 66 calories.
- a follow-up study demonstrated that MCT oil given over a 6-day period can increase diet-induced thermogenesis by 50%.
- in another study, LCTs were found to elevate blood fat levels by 68% while MCTs had no effect on blood fat level.
- to gain benefit from MCTs, the diet must remain low in LCTs. MCTs can be used as an oil for salad dressing, a bread spread, or simply taken as a supplement.
- **warning:** diabetics and individuals with liver disease must be monitored very closely when using MCTs, as they may develop ketoacidosis.
- dosage: 1–2 tbsp q.d. Products containing MCTs are available in health food stores.

- **Hydroxycitrate:** a natural substance isolated from the fruit of the Malabar tamarind (*Garcinia cambogia*), hydroxycitrate has been shown in animal studies to be a powerful inhibitor of fat production:
  - when using hydroxycitrate, a low-fat diet is critical since hydroxycitrate only inhibits the conversion of carbohydrates into fat, so will have no effect if a high-fat diet is consumed.
  - hydroxycitrate may be taken by itself or taken in formulations in which it is combined with thermogenic plant stimulants (see Botanical medicines below), which, in addition to inhibiting fat production, increase fat burning.
  - dosage: 500 mg t.i.d.
- **Coenzyme Q_{10}:** CoQ_{10} is essential for the proper transport and breakdown of fat into energy.
  - in one study, CoQ_{10} levels were low in 52% of overweight subjects tested (14 of 27). After 9 weeks of supplementation with CoQ_{10} along with a low-calorie diet, mean weight loss in the CoQ_{10}-deficient group was 13.5 kg (29.7 lb) compared with 5.8 kg (12.76 lb) in those with initially normal levels of CoQ_{10}.
  - dosage: 100–300 mg q.d.

Botanical medicines

Thermogenic formulas, such as combinations of an ephedrine source – for example *Ephedra sinica* – with a methylxanthine (caffeine) source, such as coffee (*Coffea arabica*), tea (*Camellia sinensis*), cola nut (*Cola nitida*) and/or guarana (*Paullinea cupana*), may be helpful for overweight individuals with impaired sympathetic nervous system activity.

- When properly combined, plant stimulants such as ephedrine and caffeine can activate the sympathetic nervous system, thereby increasing metabolic rate and diet-induced thermogenesis.
- A key benefit of thermogenic formulas containing ephedrine and caffeine is their ability to promote fat breakdown, but not loss of lean muscle mass during weight-reduction diets:
  - in one study, 16 obese women placed on a weight-reduction diet were given either a combination of ephedrine (20 mg) and caffeine (200 mg) twice daily or placebo. Those given the ephedrine–caffeine combination lost 4.5 kg (9.9 lb) more body fat and 2.8 kg (6.16 lb) less lean body mass than those given placebo.
  - in addition, the ephedrine–caffeine combination increased energy levels, thus enabling more calorie-burning activity in the subjects who took the thermogenic formula.
- Thermogenic formulas are, however, not for everyone, and if tolerated, should be used carefully and not abused:
  - tremendous variation exists in people's response to ephedrine and caffeine. Some can tolerate high levels easily, while others are extremely sensitive to the central nervous system stimulating effects:
    - the Federal Drug Administration Advisory Review Panel on non-prescription drugs recommended that ephedrine not be taken by patients taking antihypertensive or antidepressant drugs, or patients with heart disease, high blood pressure, thyroid disease, diabetes, or difficulty in urination due to enlarged prostate.
  - side effects reported at week 4 in 60% of subjects in studies using a daily dosage of 60 mg of ephedrine and 600 mg of caffeine included dizziness, headache, insomnia, heart palpitations, and headache.
  - by week 8, however, the rate of side effects was substantially reduced and was no higher than that of the placebo group.
  - in addition, systolic and diastolic blood pressure decreased, indicating that the weight lost more than compensated for any increase in blood pressure caused by the ephedrine–caffeine formula. Blood glucose, triglyceride, and cholesterol levels also decreased with weight loss and were not affected by ephedrine and caffeine.

although recent studies have used a daily dosage of 60 mg ephedrine and 600 mg caffeine, these high dosages may not be necessary. In one study, a daily dosage of 22 mg ephedrine, 30 mg of caffeine, and 50 mg of theophylline greatly increased basal metabolic rate and diet-induced thermogenesis.

- Dosage: a formula that provides 20–30 mg of ephedrine and 80–100 mg of methylxanthines q.d. divided into two dosages, morning and noon.

Drug–herb interaction cautions

- *Ephedra sinica* (Ma huang):
  - plus *monoamine oxidase inhibitors*: ephedrine can induce toxicity with MAO inhibitors due to dangerous elevations in blood pressure from increased vasoconstriction and release of nor-adrenaline. Ephedrine should be avoided for 2 weeks after stopping MAO inhibitors.
  - plus *diabetes drugs*: monitor for hyperglycemia while using *Ephedra* as it may diminish insulin response.
  - plus *dexamethasone*: ephedrine increases the clearance and thereby reduces the effect of this corticosteroid.

Physical medicine

- **Regular exercise:** see Preventive Measures above.

Osteoarthritis

DESCRIPTION

Osteoarthritis, a degenerative disease of the joints, is primarily characterized by the loss of joint cartilage – a gel-like substance that covers the ends of the bones forming the joint and acts like a shock absorber. The highly movable joints of the hands and the weight-bearing joints – the knees, hips, and spine – are the areas most often affected since these joints are under the most stress from weight and use. Osteoarthritis is classified as either primary or secondary.

Primary osteoarthritis, the more common form, typically occurs after the fifth or sixth decade of life and is thought to be largely due to "wear and tear". The cumulative stress of decades of use eventually damages the *collagen matrix*, the support structure of cartilage. Damage to the collagen matrix triggers the release of enzymes that, in their attempt to clean up the debris, destroy cartilage. In our youth, the body quickly synthesizes new cartilage structures to replace the damaged cartilage, but as we age, our ability to generate new cartilage decreases, so damage outpaces repair. Loss of cartilage results in increasing stress on the underlying bones, which start to thicken, eventually forming bone spurs. If cartilage continues to be lost, pain, swelling, deformation and reduced range of motion will occur.

The same scenario occurs in secondary osteoarthritis, except that some predisposing factor, not just cumulative wear and tear, initiates the degenerative joint changes. Predisposing factors include: inherited abnormalities in joint structure or function; trauma (fractures along joint surfaces, surgery, etc.); presence of abnormal cartilage; and previous inflammatory joint disease (rheumatoid arthritis, gout, septic arthritis, etc.).

Onset of osteoarthritis can be subtle. Mild morning joint stiffness is often the first symptom. As the disease progresses, motion of the involved joint causes pain that is made worse by continued activity and relieved by rest. Symptoms vary depending on the joint involved. In the hands, osteoarthritis leads to local pain and limitation of use. In the knee, pain, swelling, and instability result. Osteoarthritis of the hip causes local pain and a limp. Spinal osteoarthritis, which is very common, can result in compression of nerves and blood vessels, causing pain and inadequate blood flow to affected areas. Surprisingly, the severity of osteoarthritis (as determined by degenerative changes seen on X-ray) does not correlate with the degree of pain felt. In some cases, although the joint appears normal, the pain can be quite severe, while in other cases, tremendous deformity can be present with little or no pain. In fact, about 40% of those with the worst X-ray findings for osteoarthritis are pain free. Although the exact cause of pain in osteoarthritis is not yet well defined, depression and anxiety do appear to increase the experience of pain in this disease.

Over 40 million Americans have osteoarthritis, including 80% of Americans over the age of 50. Under the age of 45, osteoarthritis is much more common in men; after 45, women have a slightly higher rate of incidence. The good news is that repair of the collagen matrix, and regeneration of cartilage, can be enhanced using natural therapies. Osteoarthritis can be halted and even reversed.

FREQUENT SIGNS AND SYMPTOMS

Clinical symptoms
- Morning joint stiffness – may be quite mild initially
- Pain on motion of the involved joint that worsens with continued activity and is relieved by rest
- Stiffness following periods of rest
- Backache
- Weather changes may increase aching
- Cracking or grating sounds with joint movement (sometimes)
- Usually no signs of inflammation (redness, heat, fever)
- Loss of joint function

Clinical signs
- Local tenderness
- Soft tissue swelling, especially in finger joints
- Joint grating
- Bony swelling (Heberden's nodes – nodes on the finger joints closest to the hand; less commonly, Bouchard's nodes – nodes on the finger joints furthest from the hand)
- Restricted mobility

X-ray findings
- Narrowed joint space
- Cartilage erosion
- Sclerosis (hardening) of cartilage
- Bone spurs
- Swelling around the joint capsule
- Soft tissue swelling

CAUSES

- **Age-related slowing** of collagen-matrix repair mechanisms.
- **Genetic predisposition:** some individuals' unique biochemistry renders them less able to regenerate cartilage.
- **Frequent use of non-steroidal anti-inflammatory drugs (NSAIDs)**, e.g., aspirin, ibuprofen (Advil, Motrin, Nuprin) piroxicam (Feldene), diclofenac (Voltaren), fenoprofen (Nalfon), indometacin (Indocin), naproxen (Naprosyn), tolmetin (Tolectin), and sulindac (Clinoril):
  - in addition to causing gastrointestinal upset, ulcer formation, headaches and dizziness, NSAIDs inhibit cartilage synthesis and accelerate cartilage destruction. Thus, although NSAIDs suppress the symptoms of osteoarthritis, these drugs accelerate the progression of the disease.
- **Fractures and mechanical damage**
- **Hormonal factors:**
  - *excessive estrogen*:
    - after the age of 45, osteoarthritis is more prevalent among women.
    - estradiol (one of the estrogens) worsens osteoarthritis, while tamoxifen (an antiestrogen drug) relieves it by decreasing cartilage erosion.
    - botanicals commonly used in the treatment of osteoarthritis contain compounds with very weak estrogenic activity. These phytoestrogens bind to estrogen receptors, thus blocking estrogen from binding and thereby decreasing estrogenic activity.
    - good food sources of phytoestrogens include soy, fennel, celery, parsley, nuts, whole grains, and apples.
  - *growth hormone*: excessive levels of growth hormone can have detrimental effects on bone and joint structures.
  - *hypothyroidism*: patients with hypothyroidism have an increased risk of osteoarthritis compared with age- and sex-matched population samples:
    - thyroid hormones control the body's metabolic rate; a lessening in thyroid activity thus slows

down all bodily functions, including cartilage repair.
- **Hypermobility/joint instability:** loosened ligaments resulting from, for example, an athletic injury can render a joint unstable or misaligned, increasing stress and trauma.
- **Inflammatory joint disease (rheumatoid arthritis, gout):** in these diseases, the synovial membrane, which lines the joint space, becomes inflamed and damaged. In a healthy joint, this membrane secretes synovial fluid, which not only lubricates the area between the cartilage-covered bones forming the joint, but also provides the cartilage, which contains no blood vessels, with the majority of its nutrients (some are supplied by the bone). Damage to the synovial membrane deprives cartilage of nutrients needed for maintenance and repair.
- **Bacterial endotoxins:**
  - the human gastrointestinal tract contains a complex ecosystem of more than 400 species of bacteria that significantly affect our health:
    - many of these organisms have a symbiotic relationship with their human host, and their metabolic by-products provide nourishment for intestinal cells.
    - other organisms are either neutral or frankly pathogenic. When unfriendly flora are allowed to colonize the gastrointestinal tract, they not only supplant helpful bacteria, but their metabolic by-products (*bacterial endotoxins*) are also absorbed into the bloodstream and travel to the joints where they have been shown to depress the manufacture of cartilage.
  - a vegetarian diet, most likely because of its high fiber content, has been shown to significantly improve the numbers of friendly bacteria (which consume indigestible fiber as their preferred food) while lowering numbers of unfriendly organisms in the gastrointestinal tract.

RISK INCREASES WITH

- **Aging:** cumulative wear and tear coupled with slower regeneration of damaged cartilage.
- **Excess weight:** this causes increased stress on the weight-bearing joints.
- **Occupations that stress joints**, e.g., dancers, carpet layers, instrumental musicians, football players.
- **Extreme sports**, e.g., running marathons, dirt bike racing, bungee jumping, skateboarding, etc.
- **Broken bones:** healing may result in a less than ideal joint alignment; ligaments may be loosened resulting in joint instability.

- **Inappropriate exercise:** poor alignment and/or excessive stress can result in bad joint mechanics, thus damaging cartilage.
- **Athletic or other injury:** ligaments may be strained or loosened, resulting in joint instability/hypermobility.
- **Rheumatoid arthritis, gout:** these inflammatory joint diseases are characterized by damage to the synovial membrane that lines the joint capsule and provides nutrients for the maintenance and repair of cartilage.
- **Conditions associated with excessive estrogen:**
  - excessive estrogen is a primary cause of the unpleasant symptoms in premenstrual syndrome.
  - in perimenopause and menopause, estrogen levels fluctuate widely, often spiking to high levels.
- **Estrogen replacement:** may raise and keep estrogen at high levels.
- **Liver dysfunction:** estrogen is detoxified and readied for excretion in the liver.
- **Hypothyroidism:** this results in a slowing down of all metabolic functions, including cartilage repair.

PREVENTIVE MEASURES

- Maintain normal weight.
- Minimize use of NSAIDs.
- Correct any underlying endocrine imbalance (excessive estrogen, growth hormone levels, hypothyroidism) or liver dysfunction.
- Increase consumption of phytoestrogen-containing foods: soy, fennel, celery, parsley, nuts, whole grains, and apples.
- Avoid or lessen frequency and/or duration of activities with a high risk of joint injury, especially after age 40. Stretch regularly. Warm up before exercising; cool down afterwards.
- Ensure proper body alignment, especially when lifting heavy objects or weight training. If you work in an office, be sure your desk chair and the height of your desk support proper body alignment.
- Minimize consumption of foods from the genus Solanaceae – the nightshade family – including tomatoes, potatoes, peppers, eggplant, and tobacco (see Diet below).

Expected outcomes

Symptoms should gradually improve as repair of the collagen matrix and regeneration by the connective-tissue cells are enhanced.

- In studies in which researchers have sought to determine the "natural course" of osteoarthritis (what happens when no medical treatment is given), they have found that gradual and even complete recovery occurs over time.
- At the beginning of a 10-year study of osteoarthritis of the hip, X-rays showed changes indicating advanced osteoarthritis in all subjects, yet over time, X-rays confirmed marked clinical improvements, including complete recovery in 14 of 31 hips.
- Since conventional treatment of osteoarthritis relies on NSAIDs, giving no medical treatment actually contributed to healing. Clinical studies have shown that NSAID use increases joint destruction, accelerating the progression of osteoarthritis.

TREATMENT

Diet

- Achieve normal body weight. If weight loss is necessary, see the chapter on obesity.
- Eliminate consumption of foods from the genus Solanaceae (the nightshade family) including tomatoes, potatoes, peppers, eggplant, and tobacco:
  - nightshade family foods contain alkaloids that may, in genetically susceptible individuals, inhibit normal collagen repair in the joints or promote inflammatory degeneration of the joint.
  - Norman Childers, a horticulturist, popularized this dietary treatment after elimination of nightshade family foods cured his own osteoarthritis, and some patients have responded very well to a nightshade-free diet.
- Consume a whole foods, plant-based diet: due in part to its high fiber content, a vegetarian diet has been shown to significantly improve the numbers of friendly bacteria, which rely on fiber for their food, while lowering numbers of unfriendly organisms in the gastrointestinal tract:
  - unfriendly intestinal bacteria produce *endotoxins* that are absorbed into the bloodstream and travel to the joints where they inhibit the manufacture of cartilage.
- After removing nightshade family foods, choose a balanced diet composed of whole, unprocessed, preferably organic foods, emphasizing plant foods (fruits, vegetables, whole grains, beans, nuts [especially walnuts], and seeds), and cold-water fish:
  - avoid all simple, processed, and concentrated carbohydrates. Eliminate hydrogenated fats and minimize consumption of saturated fats.
  - for more detailed information, see Appendix 1.
- Consume a minimum of 1 cup of flavonoid-rich berries daily: flavonoids, plant pigments responsible for the colors of many fruits and flowers, are extremely

effective in reducing inflammation and stabilizing collagen structures. Flavonoids help maintain healthy collagen by:

- decreasing blood vessel permeability, and thus the influx of inflammatory mediators into areas of damage
- preventing free radical damage via their potent antioxidant properties
- inhibiting enzymes that break down collagen
- inhibiting the release of inflammatory chemicals
- reinforcing the natural crosslinking of collagen fibers, making them stronger.

Nutritional supplements

- **Glucosamine sulfate:** loss of the ability to manufacture sufficient glucosamine, which occurs in many people as they age, may be the primary factor leading to osteoarthritis. Glucosamine, a simple molecule composed of glucose and an amine, stimulates cartilage cells (*chondrocytes*) to manufacture *glycosaminoglycans* (GAGs) and also promotes the incorporation of sulfur into cartilage:
  - GAGs are a type of protein that absorbs and holds on to water, making cartilage a gel-like cushion that is resilient to the shocks incurred in movement.
  - cartilage is composed of GAGs mixed in with collagen, the protein that gives cartilage its structure and strength. Collagen is also dependent upon GAGs, without which it dries out and is easily worn away, leading to joint inflammation and possibly pain.
  - head-to-head double-blind studies have shown that glucosamine sulfate produces better long-term results than NSAIDs:
    - NSAIDs offer only symptomatic relief while actually promoting the disease process. Glucosamine sulfate promotes cartilage synthesis, thus not only relieving symptoms, including pain, but also helping the body repair damaged joints.
  - in comparative studies of glucosamine and NSAIDs, pain scores initially decrease more quickly in the NSAID group (within 1–2 weeks), but by the end of another week or two, those taking glucosamine sulfate have improved more than those taking NSAIDs:
    - side effects from taking glucosamine are mild and affect only a small number of subjects (e.g., 6% in a typical study), while NSAIDs produce significant side effects and much more frequently (35% of subjects in the same study).
    - in another study in which glucosamine sulfate was compared to the NSAID piroxicam, not only was glucosamine sulfate strikingly more effective than piroxicam alone or when given in combination with piroxicam, but the patients taking

glucosamine sulfate had fewer side effects than those in the control (placebo) group!

- obesity, peptic ulcers and diuretic use may reduce the effectiveness of glucosamine sulfate:
  - in an open trial in Portugal involving 252 doctors and 1,506 patients, although 95% of patients achieved benefit from glucosamine sulfate, obesity, peptic ulcers and diuretic use was associated with a shift from "good" to "sufficient" benefit.
  - *obesity*: Higher dosages may be required or oral glucosamine may not be enough to counteract the stress of obesity on the joints.
  - *peptic ulcers*: individuals with peptic ulcers should take glucosamine sulfate with foods.
  - *diuretics*: increase the dosage to compensate for increased excretion.
- glucosamine may need to be taken for long periods of time or in repeated short-term courses:
  - improvements noted with glucosamine treatment in these studies lasted for a period of 6–12 weeks after treatment was discontinued.
  - given the safety and excellent tolerability of glucosamine, it is suitable for long-term or even continuous use.
- dosage: glucosamine sulfate 500 mg t.i.d.
- **Chondroitin sulfate:** although popularized as a source of GAGs (glycosaminoglycans), chondroitin sulfate is much less effective in promoting cartilage repair than glucosamine sulfate and is therefore not recommended:
  - chondroitin is not effective because of its much larger molecular size and resulting poor absorption rate; this ranges from 0–13%, while that of glucosamine sulfate ranges from 90–98%.
  - while glucosamine sulfate's small size allows it to penetrate the joint cartilage and be delivered to the chondrocyte to stimulate GAG synthesis, the GAG molecules contained in chondroitin sulfate, which are 50 to 300 times larger than glucosamine sulfate, cannot be absorbed intact, and even if partially digested and absorbed, are still too large to be delivered to cartilage cells.
- **Niacinamide:** among its numerous functions, niacinamide plays a role as an antioxidant, thus helping to limit inflammatory processes:
  - in the 1940s and 1950s, Drs William Kaufman and Abram Hoffer reported very good clinical results using high-dose niacinamide in the treatment of hundreds of patients with rheumatoid and osteoarthritis.
  - a recent well-designed double-blind, placebo-controlled trial of 72 patients with osteoarthritis

confirmed earlier results. In this trial, niacinamide produced a 29% improvement in all symptoms and signs, compared to a 10% worsening in the placebo group.

- ▥ dosage: 500 mg t.i.d. (with meals to avoid possible mild gastrointestinal discomfort).
- ▥ **caution:** niacinamide at this high dose can result in significant side effects in some individuals (e.g., glucose intolerance and liver damage), and therefore requires strict supervision, i.e., a blood measurement to check liver enzymes taken every 3 months.

- ■ **S-adenosylmethionine (SAM):** a deficiency of SAM in joint tissue, like a deficiency of glucosamine, leads to loss of the gel-like nature and shock-absorption ability of cartilage:
  - ▥ in published clinical trials involving 21,524 patients, SAM has been shown to increase cartilage formation, as measured by magnetic resonance imaging, in patients with osteoarthritis of the hands, and has also demonstrated reductions in pain scores and clinical symptoms comparable to NSAIDs.
  - ▥ dosage: 400 mg t.i.d.

- ■ **Vitamin E:** because of its antioxidant and cell membrane stabilizing actions, vitamin E helps to inhibit the breakdown of cartilage and stimulate the formation of new cartilage components:
  - ▥ a clinical trial using 600 IU of vitamin E to treat patients with osteoarthritis demonstrated significant benefit.
  - ▥ dosage: 400–800 IU (mixed tocopherols) q.d.

- ■ **Vitamin C:** like vitamin E, with which it works synergistically, vitamin C protects cartilage and promotes cartilage formation by enhancing the stability of GAGs, the water-absorbing proteins that give cartilage its gel-like consistency and resilience:
  - ▥ deficient intake of vitamin C is common among the elderly, resulting in compromised synthesis and repair of cartilage.
  - ▥ dosage: 1,000–3,000 mg q.d.

- ■ **Pantothenic acid (vitamin B$_5$):** in rat studies, acute deficiency of B$_5$ causes a failure of cartilage growth that eventually results in lesions similar to those seen in osteoarthritis. In human clinical trials, administration of as little as 12.5 mg of B$_5$ q.d. has produced relief from osteoarthritis symptoms within 7–14 days; dosage: 12.5 mg q.d.

- ■ **Vitamins A and B$_6$, and the trace minerals, zinc, copper, and boron:**
  - ▥ along with the other nutrients described above, these vitamins and trace minerals are required for the manufacture and maintenance of cartilage

structures. A deficiency of any of these nutrients will allow accelerated joint degeneration, while supplementation at appropriate levels may promote cartilage repair and synthesis.

- ▥ dosages q.d.:
  - ● vitamin A: 5,000 IU
  - ● vitamin B$_6$: 50 mg
  - ● zinc: 30–45 mg
  - ● copper: 1–2 mg
  - ● boron: 6 mg.

Botanical medicines

When inflammation is present, curcumin, ginger, and bromelain are recommended.

- ■ *Curcuma longa* **(curcumin):**
  - ▥ the yellow pigment of *Curcuma longa* (turmeric), curcumin is an excellent anti-inflammatory and antioxidant agent:
    - ● in models of acute inflammation, curcumin has been found to be as effective as either cortisone or the potent anti-inflammatory drug phenylbutazone – but unlike these drugs, which are associated with significant toxicity, curcumin is without side effects.
  - ▥ curcumin directly inhibits the formation of the major chemical mediators of inflammation (thromboxanes and leukotrienes).
  - ▥ curcumin also works indirectly by enhancing the body's own anti-inflammatory mechanisms including:
    - ● stimulating the release of adrenal corticosteroids
    - ● sensitizing or priming cortisone receptor sites, thus improving the action of the body's own cortisone
    - ● preventing the breakdown of cortisone.
  - ▥ dosage: 400 mg t.i.d.

- ■ *Zingiber officinale* **(ginger):**
  - ▥ ginger inhibits the formation of inflammatory mediators (e.g., prostaglandins, thromboxanes, leukotrienes), exerts powerful antioxidant actions, and contains a protease compound that breaks down *fibrin*.
    - ● fibrin promotes swelling by forming a matrix that walls off the inflamed area, blocking blood vessels and preventing tissue drainage.
  - ▥ in clinical studies, ginger has demonstrated anti-inflammatory efficacy, even in treating rheumatoid arthritis patients who had not been helped by conventional drugs. Patients reported substantial improvement including pain relief, joint mobility and a decrease in swelling and morning stiffness.
  - ▥ although most scientific studies have used powdered ginger root, fresh ginger root at an equivalent dosage

may yield better results since it contains higher levels of two pharmacologically active components in ginger – *gingerol* and the protease compound.

- dosage: incorporate 8–10 g of fresh ginger, roughly a 2.5 cm (1″) slice, into the diet each day. This amount could easily be added as an ingredient in fresh fruit and vegetable juices. Or use ginger extracts standardized to contain 20% gingerol and shogaol, 100–200 mg t.i.d.:
  - average daily dietary consumption of ginger in India is 8–10 g; no side effects have been noted using ginger at these doses.

- **Bromelain:**
  - bromelain is a mixture of enzymes found in pineapple whose effectiveness in reducing inflammation is well documented.
  - bromelain's beneficial effects are primarily due to compounds that break down fibrin (see Ginger above).
  - bromelain also blocks the production of *kinins* – compounds produced during inflammation that increase swelling and cause pain.
  - dosage: 250–750 mg (1,800–2,000 MCU) taken between meals t.i.d.

Botanicals that promote cartilage regeneration
- **Yucca:**
  - yucca contains saponins that decrease bacterial endotoxin absorption, thus preventing their inhibition of cartilage manufacture.
  - dosage: yucca leaves, 2–4 g t.i.d.
- ***Harpagophytum procumbens* (Devil's claw):**
  - in several animal studies of inflammation, Devil's claw has produced anti-inflammatory and pain-relieving effects comparable to those of the potent drug phenylbutazone. Other studies, however, have indicated little if any anti-inflammatory activity from Devil's claw.
  - since saponins are the main active components in Devil's claw, its beneficial effects on osteoarthritis may be the result of the same mechanism of action seen in yucca – prevention of bacterial endotoxin absorption.
  - dosage: choose one of the following forms and take the recommended dosage t.i.d.:
    - dried powdered root: 1–2 g
    - tincture (1 : 5): 4–5 ml
    - dry solid extract (3 : 1): 400 mg
- ***Boswellia serrata*:**
  - a large branching tree native to India, *Boswellia* yields a gum resin that has been used for centuries in the treatment of osteoarthritis.

- extracts of the resin's active components, boswellic acids, have demonstrated good results in both rheumatoid and osteoarthritis in clinical studies, and no side effects have been reported.
- mechanisms of action include inhibition of inflammatory mediators, prevention of decreased cartilage synthesis, and improved blood supply to joint tissues.
- dosage: 400 mg of boswellic acids t.i.d.

Drug–herb interaction cautions
None.

Topical medicine
Topical application of preparations containing menthol (e.g., Tiger Balm, Ben-Gay, etc.) or *capsaicin*, the pungent and irritating compound from cayenne pepper, may prove helpful.

- Capsaicin, when applied to the skin, depletes the small diameter nerve fibers of the neurotransmitter *substance P*. Substance P is the principal chemical responsible for the transmission of pain impulses and has also been shown to activate inflammatory mediators in joint tissues in both rheumatoid and osteoarthritis.
- Apply menthol-based creams or creams containing 0.025–0.075% capsaicin to affected areas up to four times a day.

Physical medicine
- Avoid any physical activity that overly strains the joint.
- Chiropractic and other techniques that aid in normalization of posture, as well as orthopedic correction of structural abnormalities are recommended to limit joint strain.
- Daily non-traumatic exercise (isometrics, swimming) is recommended to increase circulation to the joint and strengthen surrounding muscles.
- Studies indicate that short-wave diathermy (a method of administering deep heat) is beneficial, most likely as a result of improving blood perfusion and hydration within the joint capsule:
  - hydrotherapy and other physical therapy modalities that improve joint perfusion are also recommended.
  - these therapies are most effective when combined with periodic ice massage, rest, isometrics and/or swimming.
- In patients with osteoarthritis of the knee, regular walking has been shown to improve functional status and relieve pain.

Osteoporosis

DESCRIPTION

Osteoporosis, which literally means "porous bone", is a progressive reduction in normal bone mineral density, mass, and strength resulting in marked bone thinning and vulnerability to fracture. Although bone mass normally declines 1.5–2% per year in both sexes after age 40, women are at greater risk for osteoporosis since their peak bone mass is naturally less than that of men due to their smaller size and muscle mass. Osteoporosis is very uncommon in men and is typically due to some underlying cause such as long-term use of anticonvulsive or corticosteroid drugs, alcoholism or hyperthyroidism. In women, osteoporosis is quite common, occurring in approximately one in four women after menopause, and is due, in part, to the perimenopausal decrease in progesterone and postmenopausal drop in estrogen, both of which play important roles in maintaining bone mass.

Bone is dynamic, living tissue that is constantly being broken down and rebuilt, even in adults. Although insufficient dietary calcium and the postmenopausal drop in estrogen have been singled out as the only issues, osteoporosis involves much more than simply a lack of these factors. Normal bone metabolism is an intricate interplay among over two dozen nutrients including the vitamins D, K, B_6, B_{12}, and folic acid, and the minerals boron, magnesium, and phosphorus as well as calcium. While estrogen regulates the action of *osteoclasts*, specialized bone cells that remove dead portions of demineralized bone, progesterone is required by the *osteoblasts*, the bone-forming cells that pull calcium, magnesium, and phosphorus from the blood to build new bone mass. All these factors are discussed below.

Osteoporosis may affect the entire skeleton, but bone loss is usually greatest in the spine, hips, and ribs, which, since they bear a great deal of weight, are susceptible to pain, deformity or fracture. Twenty million Americans may have osteoporosis or be at significant risk for it. Osteoporosis is responsible for at least 1.5 million fractures each year, including 250,000 hip fractures. Nearly one-third of all women and one-sixth of all men will fracture their hips in their lifetime. The most catastrophic of fractures, hip fracture leads to death in 12–20% of cases and long-term nursing home care for 50% of those who survive.

FREQUENT SIGNS AND SYMPTOMS

Early symptoms
- Usually none
- Backache
- Bone density tests showing demineralization of the spine and pelvis, e.g., dual energy X-ray absorptiometry (DEXA) test. Currently the most reliable measurement of bone density, the DEXA test also produces less radiation exposure than other X-ray procedures for evaluating bone density.
- Osteomark-NXT test is a urine test that measures levels of a compound linked to bone breakdown (crosslinked N-telopeptide of type I collagen). The Osteomark-NXT can be used to monitor the rate of bone loss and thus the success (or failure) of therapy.

Late symptoms
- Loss of height
- Deformed spinal column with humps
- Fractures, especially of the hip, arm or wrist, occurring with minor injury
- Severe backache
- Sudden back pain with a cracking sound indicating vertebral (spinal bone) fracture
- Hip fracture

CAUSES

Men
- Long-term use of corticosteroid or anticonvulsant drugs
- Hyperthyroidism
- Increased parathyroid hormone levels
- Alcoholism
- Crohn's disease
- Cystic fibrosis
- Hormonal deficiencies

Women
- **Inadequate stomach acid:** in order for calcium to be absorbed in the intestines, it must first be made soluble and ionized by stomach acid. Studies have found that about 40% of postmenopausal women are severely

deficient in stomach acid:

- patients with inadequate stomach acid absorb only about 4% of an oral dose of calcium carbonate.
- calcium carbonate, although it is the most widely utilized form of calcium for nutritional supplementation, is neither soluble nor ionized. Even persons with normal stomach acid absorb only 22% of an oral dose of calcium carbonate.
- ionized, soluble forms of calcium are much more effectively absorbed and are discussed below under Nutritional supplements.

- **Inability to convert vitamin D to its most active form:** the active form of vitamin D – the form that stimulates the absorption of calcium – is manufactured inside the body:
  - first, sunlight changes a compound in the skin that the body manufactures from cholesterol (*7-dehydrocholesterol*) into vitamin D_3 (*cholecalciferol*).
  - vitamin D_3 is then transported to the liver where it is converted by an enzyme into 25-$(OH)D_3$ (*25-hydroxycholcalciferol*) – a compound that is five times more potent than vitamin D_3.
  - finally, 25-$(OH)D_3$ is sent to the kidneys where it is converted by an enzyme into 1,25-$(OH)_2D_3$ (*1,25-dihydroxycholcalciferol*) – a compound ten times more potent than D_3.
  - many patients with osteoporosis have high levels of the intermediate form of vitamin D_3 (25-$(OH)D_3$) and very low levels of the most active form (1,25-$(OH)_2D_3$). This means the enzyme in their kidneys is not making the conversion:
    - since this enzyme is affected by estrogen, magnesium and boron, a deficiency of any of these nutrients will inhibit the conversion.

- **Low levels of estrogen and progesterone after menopause:**
  - when estrogen levels drop during the 3–5 year period around menopause, the *osteoclasts* (the cells that remove dead portions of demineralized bone) become more sensitive to parathyroid hormone. Parathyroid hormone signals osteoclasts to increase their activity.
  - in addition, the drop in estrogen that occurs during menopause triggers the production of the inflammatory mediator *interleukin-6*, which stimulates the growth of additional osteoclasts, thus also increasing bone loss:
    - lack of estrogen causing increased bone loss is most noticeable during the 5 years immediately following menopause. After this period, bone loss has been found to proceed at the same rate in women receiving estrogen as in those not on estrogen.

- progesterone stimulates the osteoblasts, the cells that pull calcium, magnesium, and phosphorus from the blood to build bone mass.
- supplementation with transdermal natural progesterone has been shown to result in osteoblast-mediated new bone formation of up to a 15% increase in bone mineral density within a 3-year period.

- **Lifestyle factors:**
  - *coffee, alcohol, smoking:* all cause a *negative calcium balance* – more calcium being lost than taken in.
  - *lack of exercise:* exercise, especially weight bearing exercise, stimulates osteoblasts, the cells responsible for bone formation. In contrast, immobilization doubles the rate of urinary and fecal calcium excretion, resulting in significant negative calcium balance.
  - *lack of sun exposure:* exposure to sunlight is the first step in the body's production of the active form of vitamin D, which controls calcium absorption.

- **Dietary factors:**
  - *high protein diet:* a slightly alkaline body chemistry is required for good bone health. A diet high in animal protein results in an acidic body chemistry, which the body attempts to buffer by withdrawing alkaline minerals, i.e., calcium, from bone:
    - raising daily protein intake from 47 to 142 g doubles the excretion of calcium in the urine; a diet this high in protein is common in the US.
  - *soft drinks:* soft drinks contain large amounts of phosphates and virtually no calcium. When phosphate levels are high, and calcium levels are low, calcium is pulled out of the bones to restore balance.
  - *refined sugar:* promotes acidic body chemistry. Following sugar intake, the urinary excretion of calcium increases. The average American consumes 150 g of sucrose each day, plus processed foods containing other refined simple sugars, plus carbonated beverages high in sugar and phosphates.
  - *inadequate consumption of green leafy vegetables:* green leafy vegetables provide a broad range of vitamins and minerals necessary for bone health including calcium, vitamin K_1, and boron:
    - vitamin K_1, the form of vitamin K found in plants, converts inactive *osteocalcin* to its active form. Osteocalcin, the major noncollagen protein in bone, anchors calcium molecules and holds them in place within the bone. Low vitamin K_1 therefore leads to impaired mineralization of bone as a result of inadequate osteocalcin levels.
    - boron is required for the conversion of estrogen to 17-beta-estradiol, its most active form, and is

also involved in the reaction in the kidneys which converts vitamin D to its most active form ($1,25$-$(OH)_2D_3$).

■ *inadequate consumption of magnesium*: when magnesium levels are insufficient, a decrease occurs in the serum concentration of the most active form of vitamin D ($1,25$-$(OH)_2D_3$). In addition, magnesium mediates the secretion of *parathyroid hormone* and *calcitonin* – the two hormones responsible for maintaining the proper concentration of calcium within the blood:

● when calcium levels are too low, *parathyroid hormone* stimulates osteoclasts to break down bone, thus increasing blood calcium levels.

● when calcium levels are too high, *calcitonin* suppresses osteoclastic activity.

■ *inadequate consumption of vitamins B_6, B_{12} and folic acid*: these three vitamins are involved in the conversion of the amino acid methionine to cysteine. If a person is deficient in these vitamins or if an individual has a genetic defect in the enzymes responsible for this conversion, levels of an intermediate product called *homocysteine* will build up:

● increased homocysteine concentrations, which have been demonstrated in postmenopausal women, interfere with collagen crosslinking, leading to a defective bone matrix.

■ *inadequate consumption of vitamin C*: vitamin C is necessary for the secretion of intercellular substances by all cells, including the formation of *osteoid* (a cartilage-like material in which calcium is deposited) by the osteoblasts.

RISK INCREASES WITH

■ **Family history of osteoporosis**

■ **Gastric or small bowel resection:** reduces absorptive surface of the intestines thus lessening the body's ability to absorb the nutrients needed to maintain and form healthy bone.

■ **Disorders of the liver or kidneys:** vitamin D is converted into its most active form in two stages, the first of which occurs in the liver, the second in the kidneys.

■ **Hyperparathyroidism:** excessive parathyroid activity. Parathyroid hormone increases activity of the osteoclasts (the cells that break down bone).

■ **Hyperthyroidism:** normally, when blood levels of calcium increase as a result of parathyroid hormone's upregulation of osteoclast activity, the thyroid secretes the hormone calcitonin, which downregulates the osteoclasts. In hyperthyroidism, this balancing activity is disrupted.

■ **Inactivity:** weight-bearing activity is necessary for the stimulation of the osteoblasts, the cells responsible for bone formation. At least 30 min four to five times per week of weight-bearing exercise (walk briskly, jog, aerobics, hard physical labor) is recommended.

■ **Seldom getting outside into the sunlight:** the process of manufacturing vitamin D begins with the action of sunlight on 7-dehydrocholesterol (a compound the body makes from cholesterol) in the skin.

■ **Leanness:** osteoblasts are stimulated by weight-bearing movement against resistance. In normal daily activities, weight-bearing is simply movement of the body against the resistance offered by gravity. A lean individual has less weight to move, so provides osteoblasts with less stimulation during normal activities.

■ **Long-term use of anticonvulsants:** barbiturates such as phenobarbital or primidone (Mysoline) alter the metabolism of vitamin D. Phenytoin (Dilantin) interferes with vitamin D, and may also cause deficiency of folic acid or vitamin B_6 or a reduction in blood levels of vitamin K.

■ **Frequent use of antacids:** for calcium to be absorbed, it must first be made soluble and ionized by stomach acid.

■ **Long-term use of cortisone drugs:** cortisone drugs, e.g., prednisone (prednisolone), deplete the body of vitamin D_3, thus interfering with normal calcium metabolism and absorption.

■ **Smoking:** nicotine causes the body to produce cortisol, the body's own cortisone. Excessive production of cortisol interferes with vitamin D metabolism.

■ **Heavy alcohol use:** more than three glasses of alcohol per week:

■ alcohol disrupts liver function; the liver is involved in the conversion of vitamin D to its active form.

■ alcohol suppresses the bone-forming activity of osteoblasts.

■ heavy alcohol use is associated with numerous nutritional deficiencies, including deficiencies of vitamin B_6 and folic acid. Low levels of these B vitamins results in an increase in homocysteine levels. Homocysteine interferes with collagen crosslinking, leading to a defective bone matrix.

■ **Dietary factors:**

■ *consuming more than two cups of coffee per day*: coffee has a diuretic effect and has been shown to cause a short-term increase in urinary calcium loss. This temporary increase may be significant in older individuals with low calcium intakes, especially if they do not consume milk with their coffee.

■ *consuming more than 110 g (4 oz) of meat on a daily basis*: a high protein diet promotes an acid body chemistry. Calcium, an alkaline mineral, will be pulled from the bones to restore the slightly alkaline chemistry necessary for the majority of chemical reactions that occur in normal metabolism.

- *drinking soft drinks regularly*: to balance the phosphates in soft drinks, the body leaches calcium from the bones, which is then excreted in the urine.
- *consuming less than three servings of vegetables* including at least 1 cup of green leafy vegetables daily: these vegetables contain vitamins and minerals necessary for bone formation.
- *high salt intake*: when sodium is excreted, it causes an increase in the kidney's excretion of calcium. At the high levels of sodium intake typical in the US, over 90% of ingested sodium is excreted. For each 500 mg of sodium excreted, 10 mg of calcium are also lost in the urine.
- *high intake of refined sugar*: increases urinary excretion of calcium.

- **Postmenopause:** studies have found that for approximately 7 years following menopause while the body is acclimating to the drop in estrogen, the lower estrogen levels render the osteoclasts more sensitive to parathyroid hormone, the hormone that stimulates osteoclasts to break down bone.
- **Premature menopause:** estrogen levels drop.
- **Nulliparity (not having given birth to a child):** in addition to the positive hormonal effects on bone during pregnancy, the increased weight experienced during child bearing is thought to help strengthen the bones.
- **Short stature and small bones:** less bone reserve.
- **Caucasian or Asian race:** typically have smaller, lighter bones.

PREVENTIVE MEASURES

- Regular, weight-bearing exercise: at least 30 min of jogging, aerobics, tennis, weight lifting, dancing, brisk walking or other weight-bearing exercise daily.
- Don't smoke.
- Limit alcohol consumption to less than three servings per week. One serving equals 350 ml (12 US fl oz) of beer, 140 ml (4–5 US fl oz) of wine, or 45 ml (1.5 US fl oz) of distilled spirits.
- Don't consume soft drinks.
- Don't drink more than two cups of coffee per day. Even better, have a latté made with cow's milk or soymilk fortified with calcium and vitamin D.
- Enjoy some sunshine. To ensure vitamin D production, a 40-year-old woman should spend 10–15 min, twice

each week in direct sunlight. After age 65, sun exposure should be increased to 30–60 min, two to three times a week.
- Avoid processed foods. Their high salt and sugar content makes them a bad choice for bone health.
- Consume a nutrient-dense, primarily vegetarian diet rich in whole, unprocessed, preferably organic foods, especially plant foods (green leafy and other vegetables, fruits, beans, whole grains, seeds and nuts), and cold-water fish (for more detailed information, see Appendix 1).

Expected outcomes

The primary goal in treating osteoporosis is prevention. Results will vary, but most women should expect a stabilization of bone turnover or, at the very least, a slowing down of bone resorption.

Improvements in laboratory tests of bone resorption are generally noted within 3–6 months. Improvements in the DEXA usually take longer to manifest, i.e., 1–2 years.

Biochemical tests of bone resorption should be run every 3 months until a normal reading is obtained, every 6 months in high-risk patients, and every year for normal-risk individuals. DEXA scans should be done at yearly intervals in high-risk patients, and every other year in normal-risk individuals.

In severe cases, the physician may recommend combining the recommendations given here with allopathic prescription drugs such as alendronic acid (Fosamax), etidronate (Didronel), calcitonin (Miacalcic), and raloxifene (Evista):

- **Fosamax and Didronel** are bisphosphonate drugs that destroy osteoclasts, thus preventing them from breaking down bone, and lessening bone loss – although bone is generally resorbed because it has become old and brittle:
  - Fosamax, the more effective of the two, must be taken exactly according to instructions or ulceration of the esophagus may result.
- **Miacalcic** is a synthetic version of calcitonin, the thyroid hormone that inhibits the osteoclast's resorption of bone tissue; its ability to affect bone density appears to be minimal, and possible side effects include nausea, vomiting, rashes, and flushing sensations.
- **Evista** is a selective estrogen receptor modulator (SERM), a new class of drugs that have estrogen-like effects in some parts of the body but not in others. SERMs have been shown to prevent bone loss in the spine and hip; possible side effects include hot flashes and blood clot formation in the veins.

TREATMENT

Natural HRT

- **Natural progesterone:** 3% cream applied at bedtime daily, 21 days a month if postmenopausal, or the 2 weeks before menses if not menopausal. The physician will specify the amount to apply, but typical usage is 25–50 g a month. Dose may be reduced depending on follow-up bone mineral density test results.
- **Natural estrogen (estriol):** if not medically contra-indicated, a low dose (0.3–0.625 mg q.d.) of estriol for 3 weeks per month may be suggested, then discontinued when follow-up bone mineral density tests show increased bone mass.

Diet

- Limit dietary factors that promote calcium excretion: salt, sugar, animal protein, soft drinks, alcohol, and coffee.
- Follow the dietary recommendations for a whole foods, primarily vegetarian diet given in Appendix 1, with special emphasis on increasing consumption of:
  - *green leafy vegetables*: kale, collard greens, parsley, and lettuce (except iceberg) are particularly rich sources of calcium, vitamin K_1 and boron.
  - *foods rich in vitamin K_1*: the richest sources of vitamin K_1 are dark green leafy vegetables (broccoli, lettuce, cabbage, spinach), and green tea. Other good sources include asparagus, oats, whole wheat, and fresh green peas.
  - *calcium-rich foods*: in addition to dairy products, good non-dairy sources of calcium include kelp, bok choy, spinach, greens (collard, mustard, turnip), nuts and seeds (sesame seeds, almonds, chestnuts, walnuts), and beans (garbanzo, soy, tofu). Cabbage family plants (kale, collards) have very absorbable calcium:
    - when eating spinach, to eliminate its oxalic acid, a compound that reduces calcium absorption, immerse in water and cook first, then drain.
  - *magnesium-rich foods*: kelp, wheat bran, wheat germ, almonds, cashews, blackstrap molasses, Brewer's yeast, buckwheat, English walnuts, rye, tofu, beet greens, soybeans, spinach, brown rice.
- If the soil contains adequate levels of boron, most fruits and vegetables will contain it. Since soil levels vary, however, supplementation may be advisable, especially for menopausal women.

Nutritional supplements

- **Calcium:** a number of studies have shown that calcium supplementation improves bone density in peri-menopausal women and slows the rate of bone loss in postmenopausal women by 30–50%, significantly reducing the risk of hip fracture:
  - avoid calcium derived from oyster shells (i.e., calcium carbonate), dolomite or bone meal; studies have indicated that these calcium supplements may contain substantial amounts of lead, a toxic metal that primarily affects the brain, kidney and manufacture of red blood cells:
    - lead toxicity, which is especially harmful in children, is a significant problem in industrialized countries including the US and has been directly linked to a lowered IQ and criminal behavior.
  - calcium hydroxyapatite, which is basically a purified bone meal, should also be avoided. Not only is it derived from bone meal (a high lead source of calcium), but comparison studies have also shown that it is not as well absorbed (only 20% absorption) as either calcium carbonate or calcium citrate (both of which had a 30% absorption rate).
  - calcium bound to citrate (or other Krebs cycle intermediate such as fumarate, malate, succinate or aspartate) is recommended. These forms, which are already ionized and soluble, are both well absorbed and non-toxic:
    - the Krebs cycle, part of the energy production process in the mitochondria (the energy factories in every cell), utilizes these intermediate compounds to produce energy, with the remainder being excreted in the urine where they act to prevent stone formation.
    - Krebs cycle intermediates are easily ionized, almost completely degraded, have virtually no toxicity, and have been shown to increase the absorption of calcium and other minerals.
    - using calcium bound to a Krebs cycle intermediate is especially important for persons with reduced stomach acid because (1) the body's ability to secrete stomach acid frequently lessens with age, and (2) about 45% of the calcium is absorbed from an oral dose of calcium citrate in patients with reduced stomach acid, compared to 4% absorption for calcium carbonate.
  - dosage: calcium citrate (or calcium bound to another Krebs cycle intermediate) taken immediately before or at the beginning of meals. Age 25–35: 800 mg; age 36–50: 1,000 mg; age 51–65+: 1,500 mg (1,200 mg if on HRT).
- **Vitamin D:** a variety of studies on postmenopausal women have shown that vitamin D, especially in its most active form (D_3), stimulates the absorption of calcium, thus increasing bone mineral density and reducing the risk of hip fracture:
  - vitamin D can be especially helpful for older people who don't get sufficient sun exposure, e.g., those

who live in nursing homes or farther away from the equator or who don't regularly get outside.

- dosage: 400 IU of vitamin D_3 q.d. (Taking higher doses offers no significant benefit and may adversely affect magnesium levels.)

- **Magnesium:** women with osteoporosis have been found to have lower bone magnesium content and other indicators of magnesium deficiency than women without osteoporosis:
  - a 2-year study of magnesium supplementation in postmenopausal women found that those receiving magnesium had a slight improvement in bone density while those receiving placebo experienced a slight decrease in bone density.
  - in human magnesium deficiency, serum concentration of the most active form of vitamin D $(1,25\text{-}(OH)_2D_3)$ is lowered because the enzyme responsible for the conversion of $1,25\text{-}(OH)_2D_3$ is dependent upon magnesium.
  - magnesium also mediates the secretion of parathyroid hormone and calcitonin – the two hormones that maintain proper calcium concentration in the blood.
  - dosage: 400–800 mg q.d.

- **Boron:** a trace mineral required for the activation of both estrogen and vitamin D, boron has been shown to be a protective factor against osteoporosis:
  - when estrogen levels are low, as is the case after menopause, osteoclasts become more sensitive to parathyroid hormone, the hormone that directs them to break down bone:
    - boron has been shown to dramatically increase levels of 17-beta-estradiol, the most biologically active estrogen, and to mimic some of the positive effects of estrogen therapy in postmenopausal women.
  - vitamin D is converted to its most active form $(1,25\text{-}(OH)_2D_3)$ in the kidney, and this conversion reaction requires boron:
    - in one study of postmenopausal women, supplementation with 3 mg of boron q.d. reduced urinary calcium excretion by 44%.
  - fruits and vegetables are the main dietary sources of boron, so diets low in these foods are likely to be deficient:
    - the US Second National Health and Nutrition Examination survey found that fewer than 10% of Americans meet the minimum recommendation of two fruit and three vegetable servings per day, and 51% of Americans eat only one serving of vegetables per day.
    - the boron content of fruits and vegetables depends upon the boron content of the soil in

which they were grown, which may vary. To ensure consistent, adequate levels of boron, supplementation is recommended.
  - dosage: boron (as sodium tetrahydroborate) 3–5 mg q.d.

- **Ipriflavone:** a semisynthetic flavonoid similar in structure to soy isoflavonoids, ipriflavone is approved in Japan, Hungary, and Italy as a drug for the treatment and prevention of osteoporosis:
  - the mechanism of action appears to be enhancement of calcitonin's effects on calcium metabolism. Calcitonin, the hormone secreted by the thyroid when calcium levels in the blood rise, shuts down the activity of osteoclasts, the cells responsible for breaking down old bone, thus releasing calcium into the bloodstream.
  - ipriflavone has shown impressive results in a number of studies:
    - in one study of 100 women with osteoporosis, ipriflavone (200 mg t.i.d.) increased bone density measurements by 2% after 6 months and 5.8% after 12 months.
    - in another 1-year study of women with osteoporosis, ipriflavone (600 mg q.d.) produced a 6% increase in bone density while the placebo group lost 0.3% in bone density.
  - dosage: 600 mg q.d.

- **Silicon:** silicon is responsible for crosslinking collagen strands, thus greatly contributing to the strength and integrity of the connective tissue matrix of bone. Silicon is more concentrated at calcification sites in growing bone, suggesting that bone remodeling may depend on adequate levels of silicon:
  - in patients with osteoporosis, silicon requirements may be increased, so supplementation may be appropriate.
  - dosage: no recommended daily allowance currently exists for silicon. It is generally regarded that the daily requirement is in the range of 5–20 mg. Daily dosages should not exceed this range until more is learned about the role and need for silicon.

- **Vitamin B_6, folic acid, and vitamin B_{12}:** these three B vitamins are all involved in the conversion of the amino acid methionine to cysteine. If a person is deficient in any of these vitamins or if the enzymes responsible for the conversion are defective, levels of an intermediate compound, homocysteine, will rise:
  - homocysteine interferes with collagen crosslinking, thus leading to a defective bone matrix and osteoporosis.
  - low levels of B_6, folic acid and B_{12} are very common in the elderly population.

- increased levels of homocysteine have been found in postmenopausal women.
- although all three vitamins work together, even supplementation with folic acid alone has been shown to reduce homocysteine levels in post-menopausal women, despite the fact that according to standard laboratory criteria, none was deficient in folic acid.
- dosage: 400 μg folic acid, 400 μg vitamin B_{12}, and 25–100 mg vitamin B_6 q.d.
- **caution** for individuals taking barbiturate anticon-vulsant drugs: either folic acid or B_6 can reduce levels of barbiturate anticonvulsants, potentially leading to seizures. If supplementation is needed, it should be carefully monitored.

Physical medicine

- **Regular weight-bearing exercise:** weight-bearing exercise (jogging, aerobics, brisk walking, weight training, dancing) stimulates osteoblasts and can help reverse or at least slow bone loss in postmenopausal women:
  - in one study, a group of previously inactive post-menopausal women increased their bone density by 5.2% in 9 months by engaging in 50–60 min of weight-bearing exercise three times a week.
  - after 22 months, their bone density was up 6.1%, while a control group of women who did not exer-cise lost an average of 1.1% in bone density.

Otitis media

DESCRIPTION

Otitis media is a condition in which inflammation, swelling or infection in the middle ear – the space in which nerves and small bones connect to the eardrum on one side and the *Eustachian tube* on the other – results in an earache (the Eustachian tube is the passageway that connects the middle ear with the throat). Middle ear infections may be either acute or chronic. *Acute otitis media* is usually preceded by an upper respiratory infection or allergy. *Chronic otitis media* (also called *serous, secretory,* or *non-suppurative otitis media; chronic otitis media with effusion;* or *glue ear*) refers to a constant swelling of the middle ear and is typically related to allergy. Most studies show that 85–93% of children with chronic otitis media have allergies.

Ear infections are the most common diagnosis in children, accounting for over 50% of all visits to pediatricians. In the United States, two-thirds of children have had an acute ear infection by age 2, and chronic ear infections affect two-thirds of children under the age of 6. Obviously, the standard medical approach to otitis media in children – antibiotics, analgesics (e.g., acetaminophen), and/or antihistamines – does not prevent recurrence. In the most recent analysis of antibiotic use (an extensive review of the scientific literature on the value of antibiotics in treating otitis media over the past 30 years, published in 1997 in the *British Medical Journal*), a group of eight international experts from the US, Britain, and the Netherlands reported that antibiotics are not recommended for treating otitis media in most cases. In some studies, children who did not receive antibiotics had fewer recurrences of earache than those given antibiotics. This most likely reflects the fact that antibiotics suppress immune function and depopulate the normal protective flora of the upper respiratory tract, thus increasing susceptibility to colonization by viruses or unfriendly bacteria.

If the ear infection is chronic and unresponsive to drugs, a surgical procedure (*myringotomy*) is performed in which a tiny plastic tube is inserted into the eardrum, where it remains to drain fluid into the throat via the Eustachian tube. Not only is this *not* curative, but children with myringotomy tubes in their ears have also been found to be even *more* likely to experience further ear infections than those who have not undergone this procedure. Despite this fact, myringotomies are performed on nearly one million American children each year.

A number of well-designed studies have demonstrated no differences in the clinical course of acute otitis media when conventional treatments, including antibiotics, ear tubes, or ear tubes with antibiotics, were compared with a placebo. In fact, 80% of children with acute otitis media respond to a placebo within 48 hours.

Doctors scare patients into believing drugs and ear tubes are necessary to reduce the risk of the infection spreading to the mastoid (the area of bone behind and under the ear) and brain. No evidence exists, however, that either antibiotics or myringotomy prevent this. This fact, coupled with the risks and failures associated with antibiotics and the high rate of recurrent ear infections following the insertion of ear tubes, supports first using the natural, non-invasive therapies outlined below before resorting to drugs or surgery. **Caveat:** although standard antibiotic and surgical procedures may not be statistically effective, because otitis media is a potentially dangerous disease, each child must be evaluated by a physician before a decision not to use these procedures is considered, and treatment should be supervised by a physician.

FREQUENT SIGNS AND SYMPTOMS

Acute otitis media
- Irritability
- Pulling at the ear (small children)
- Earache
- History of recent upper respiratory tract infection or allergy
- Red, opaque, bulging eardrum with loss of the normal features
- Feeling of fullness in the ear
- Hearing loss
- Fever, chills
- Dizziness
- Discharge or leakage from the ear
- Diarrhea, vomiting (sometimes)

Chronic otitis media
- Painless hearing loss
- Dull, immobile eardrum (*tympanic* membrane)

Otitis externa (infection or inflammation of the external ear canal)
- Itching, discharge, or burning pain

CAUSES

- **Abnormal Eustachian tube function:** the Eustachian tube regulates gas pressure in the middle ear, protects the middle ear from nose and throat secretions and bacteria, and clears fluids from the middle ear. Swallowing causes active opening of the Eustachian tube due to the action of surrounding muscles:
  - infants and small children are more susceptible to Eustachian tube problems since theirs are smaller in diameter and more horizontal.
  - obstruction of the Eustachian tube results in fluid buildup and then, if bacteria start to grow, bacterial infection:
    - the organisms most commonly cultured from middle-ear fluid during acute otitis media are the bacteria *Streptococcus pneumoniae* (40%) and *Haemophilus influenzae* (25%).
  - obstruction may be caused by:
    - blockage with mucus in response to allergy or irritation
    - viral or bacterial infection in the nose or throat that spreads to the Eustachian tube
    - collapse of the tube (due to weak tissues holding the tube in place and/or an abnormal opening mechanism).
- **Food allergy:** numerous medical studies have found that 85–93% of children with chronic otitis media have food allergies: 16% to inhalants, 14% to food, and 70% to both:
  - the allergic reaction causes blockage of the Eustachian tube by two mechanisms:
    - inflammatory swelling of the tube
    - inflammatory swelling of the nose that causes the *Toynbee phenomenon* (swallowing when both mouth and nose are closed, forcing air and secretions into the middle ear).
  - several studies of children with chronic otitis media have demonstrated that allergy elimination diets successfully prevent recurrence (in 78–92% of patients) and that the reintroduction of offending foods provokes recurrence (in 94% of patients).
  - allergenic foods linked to chronic otitis media include (in descending order of frequency): cow's milk, wheat, egg white, peanut, soy, corn, tomato, chicken, and apple.
- children with chronic otitis media are typically allergic to several foods:
  - in a study of 104 children with chronic otitis media, ranging in age from 1.5–9 years; 13.6% were allergic to one food, 81.5% were allergic to two to four foods, 3.7% were allergic to five to seven foods, and 1.3% were allergic to eight to 10 foods.

RISK INCREASES WITH

- **Respiratory infection**
- **Recurrent infections, even very mild colds:** recurrent illness signals a weakened immune system that is unable to effectively prevent infection.
- **Day care attendance:** increased exposure to infectious agents.
- **Wood-burning stoves:** the particulate matter emitted by these stoves is a significant respiratory tract irritant.
- **Crowded, unsanitary living conditions:** increased exposure to respiratory tract irritants and infectious agents.
- **Parental smoking** (or exposure to other second-hand smoke): cigarette smoke contains more than 4,000 chemicals. Not only are most respiratory irritants, more than 50 have been identified as carcinogens.
- **Not being breast-fed:** breast-feeding for a minimum of 4 months is protective:
  - human breast milk contains high amounts of antibodies protective against infectious agents commonly found in acute otitis media, whether bacterial (*Streptococcus pneumoniae* or *Haemophilus influenzae*) or viral (*respiratory syncytial virus* or *Influenza A*).
  - the thymus gland (the major organ of the immune system) in breast-fed infants is roughly 20 times larger than that of formula-fed infants.
  - breast milk is typically free of food allergens:
    - particularly if the mother avoids eating foods to which she is allergic during pregnancy and lactation.
    - formulas are frequently based on cow's milk, the most common allergen, or soy protein, another common allergen.
- **Bottle-feeding while a child is lying on his or her back:** this leads to regurgitation of the bottle's contents into the middle ear.
- **Frequent consumption of fruit juice:** even in an adult, consuming 75 g (3 oz) of sugar in one sitting in

any form (sucrose, honey, approximately 240–300 ml [8–10 US fl oz] of fruit juice) depresses white (immune) cell activity by 50% for 1–5 hours.
■ **Changes in altitude** (e.g., flying, driving up mountains) increase pressure in the middle ear.

PREVENTIVE MEASURES

■ Breast-feeding for a minimum of 4 months, although 9 months is recommended.
■ If the mother has any food allergies, she should avoid these foods during pregnancy and lactation.
■ If either or both parents have food allergies, special care may reduce and/or prevent the development of food allergies in the infant:
  ▪ during the first 3 months, a breast-feeding mother should avoid consuming common food allergens.
  ▪ she should introduce potentially allergenic foods to her diet one food at a time, and carefully watch her infant for any reaction for 2 days before introducing another new food.
■ Breast- or bottle-feed infants in a sitting position with the head up, never lying down.
■ Even if the parents do not have food allergies, during the infant's first 9 months we recommend excluding common food allergens – dairy, wheat, egg, and fowl – from the child's diet.
■ When beginning to introduce the baby to foods (around 6–8 months), give new foods one at a time, carefully watching for any reaction for 2 days before introducing another food.
■ Minimize consumption of processed, sugar-laden foods. Too much sugar in the diet leads to lowered white blood cell activity. Children may also react to chemical additives used in food processing.
■ Supplement with a good children's multiple vitamin and mineral formula: even marginal deficiency of any nutrient can profoundly impair the immune system.
■ Avoid use of wood-burning stoves.
■ Do not smoke in the house or allow a child to be exposed to second-hand smoke.
■ If possible, minimize plane travel. If traveling by plane, breast-feeding during take-off and landing is recommended, as this will induce frequent swallowing, relieving pressure and clearing fluid from the middle ear.

Expected outcomes
Complete resolution of acute ear infection within 2–3 days; elimination of chronic ear infections within 2 weeks.

TREATMENT

Diet

Infants
■ Breast-feeding for at least the first 4, preferably 9 months.
■ During pregnancy and while breast-feeding, the mother should avoid any foods to which she is allergic.
■ When beginning to introduce foods, exclude wheat, egg, fowl, and dairy – the foods to which children are most commonly allergic – during the first 9 months, then introduce these foods one at a time. Watch carefully for any reaction for 2 days before introducing a new food.
■ Avoid too frequent consumption of any food.

Children
■ **Eliminate suspected food allergens:** since it is usually not possible to determine the exact allergen(s) during an acute attack, all the most common allergenic foods should be eliminated from the diet: milk and dairy products, eggs, wheat, corn, oranges, and peanut butter.
■ **Avoid frequent consumption of any food:** in susceptible individuals, excessive exposure to any food increases the possibility of developing a sensitivity to that food.
■ **Eliminate concentrated simple carbohydrates:** sugar, honey, dried fruit, undiluted fruit juice, soda, baked goods, sweetened cereals, candy, etc. Consumption of 75 g (3 oz) of sugar in one sitting depresses immune function by 50% for up to 5 hours.
■ **A health-promoting diet:** after identifying and removing allergenic foods, consume a health-promoting diet rich in whole, unprocessed, preferably organic foods, especially plant foods (fruits, vegetables, beans, seeds and nuts, and whole grains) and cold-water fish, and low in processed and sugar-laden foods (for more detailed information, see Appendix 1).

Nutritional supplements
■ **Vitamin A:** known as the "anti-infective vitamin", vitamin A plays an essential role in immune function by:
  ▪ maintaining the surfaces of the skin, respiratory tract, and gastrointestinal tract and their secretions – all of which constitute a barrier that is the body's first line of defense against micro-organisms
  ▪ stimulating and/or enhancing numerous immune processes including white blood cell function and antibody response
  ▪ direct antiviral activity

- preventing immune suppression resulting from stress-induced adrenal hormones, severe burns and surgery
- some of these latter effects are most likely a result of vitamin A's ability to prevent stress-induced shrinkage of the thymus gland and to promote thymus growth
- dosage: 50,000 IU q.d. for up to 2 days in children under 6 years of age; up to 4 days in children over 6 years of age.

- **Beta-carotene:** called "pro-vitamin A" since it can be converted into vitamin A, beta-carotene is a more powerful antioxidant than vitamin A and exerts additional immune-stimulating effects, including enhancing thymus function:
  - specifically, beta-carotene has been shown to increase the production of helper/inducer T cells by 30% after 7 days and all T cells after 14 days.
  - dosage: multiply age in years by 10,000 IU q.d. (up to 100,000 IU q.d.). For example, dosage for a 6-year-old child would be 6 × 10,000 IU = 60,000 IU).

- **Vitamin C:** directly antiviral and antibacterial, vitamin C has numerous immune-enhancing effects including:
  - improving white blood cell response and function
  - increasing levels of interferon (a special chemical factor that fights viral infection and cancer)
  - increasing secretion of hormones from the thymus gland
  - dosage: multiply age in years by 50 mg every 2 hours.

- **Bioflavonoids:** a group of plant pigments largely responsible for the colors of fruits and flowers, flavonoids are powerful antioxidants in their own right, and, when taken with vitamin C, significantly enhance its absorption and effectiveness; dosage: multiply age in years by 50 mg every 2 hours.

- **Zinc:** a critical mineral for immune function, zinc plays many protective roles including:
  - promoting the destruction of foreign particles and micro-organisms
  - protecting against free radical damage
  - acting synergistically with vitamin A
  - being required for proper white cell function
  - being necessary for the activation of serum thymic factor – a thymus hormone with profound immune-enhancing actions
  - inhibiting replication of several viruses, including those of the common cold
  - dosage: multiply age in years by 2.5 mg q.d. (up to 30 mg).

- **Thymus extract:** thymus gland extracts have been shown to enhance immune function by improving thymus function. The thymus gland secretes a family of hormones that act on white cells to ensure their proper development and function:
  - in children, studies using calf thymus extracts given orally have demonstrated impressive clinical results in improving immune function, decreasing food allergies, and improving resistance to chronic respiratory infections.
  - dosage: equivalent of 120 mg of pure polypeptides with molecular weights less than 10,000, or roughly 500 mg of the crude polypeptide fraction, q.d.

Botanical medicines

- ***Echinacea* spp.:** the two most widely used species are *Echinacea angustifolia* and *Echinacea purpurea*, both of which have numerous immune-enhancing effects:
  - one of *Echinacea*'s most important immune-stimulating components is *inulin*, a large polysaccharide that activates the *alternative complement pathway*, part of the immune system's first line of defense, and increases the production of immune chemicals that activate *macrophages* (immune cells that gobble up invaders). The result is increased activity of many key immune parameters: production of T cells, macrophage phagocytosis, antibody binding, natural killer cell activity, and levels of circulating neutrophils.
  - in addition to immune support, echinacea is directly antiviral and helps prevent bacterial infection by inhibiting the bacterial enzyme *hyaluronidase*. Bacteria secrete hyaluronidase to break through the body's first line of defense – its protective membranes such as the skin or mucous membranes – so the bacteria can enter the body.
  - dosage: *Echinacea* spp. are very safe for children. For children under 6, use one-half the adult dosage. The adult dosage (given below) is appropriate for children over age 6. Choose one of the following forms. All dosages listed here can safely be given t.i.d.:
    - dried root (or as tea): 0.5–1 g
    - freeze-dried plant: 325–650 mg
    - juice of aerial portion of *E. purpurea* stabilized in 22% ethanol: 2–3 ml
    - tincture (1 : 5): 2–4 ml
    - fluid extract (1 : 1): 2–4 ml
    - solid (dry powdered) extract (6.5 : 1 or 3.5% echinacoside): 150–300 mg.

Drug–herb interaction cautions
None.

Topical medicine
- **Humidifier:** animal studies have shown that low humidity (10–12%) significantly increases fluid in the

Eustachian tubes:

- low humidity may induce nasal swelling and reduced ventilation of the Eustachian tube or it may dry the Eustachian tube lining, which could lead to increased secretions and an inability to clear fluid.
- mast cells, a type of white blood cell, which reside in the lining of the Eustachian tubes, may also be triggered to release histamine, an inflammatory chemical that promotes swelling.

- **Locally applied heat** can help to reduce pressure in the middle ear and promote fluid drainage, thus greatly reducing discomfort:
  - apply heat as a hot pack with warm oil (especially mullein oil), or by blowing hot air into the ear with the aid of a straw and a hair dryer.

Pelvic inflammatory disease

DESCRIPTION

Pelvic inflammatory disease (PID) is an infection of the female reproductive organs that occurs when infectious organisms, usually bacteria such as *Neisseria gonorrhea* or *Chlamydia trachomatis*, enter the uterus and spread, infecting the fallopian tubes, cervix, uterus, ovaries, and/ or urinary bladder. PID is most often caused by a sexually transmitted bacterium, although a pelvic infection can develop after miscarriage, induced abortion or other invasive medical procedure. An estimated 2.5 million women see physicians for PID each year. PID is most common in sexually active women in their late teens and early 20s, and in women who have been fitted with intrauterine devices (IUDs) for contraception, but rarely occurs in women who have passed menopause.

Any suspicion that a sexually transmitted disease or other type of genital infection has been contracted should be evaluated promptly. Appropriate, well-timed treatment can prevent complications such as PID from developing. Infection in the ovaries or fallopian tubes can result in scarring that can lead to infertility. In addition to aggressive care of acute PID, learning how to prevent recurrence is of the utmost importance. All women who have had PID are at risk for recurrence, and one-fourth will suffer serious long-term consequences. The risk for ectopic pregnancy increases sixfold after a single episode of PID. Risk for infertility increases 13% after one infection, and 70% after three.

FREQUENT SIGNS AND SYMPTOMS

Early stages (up to 1 week)
- Foul-smelling vaginal discharge
- Pain with intercourse
- Pain and tenderness in the lower pelvic area (abdomen) on one or both sides
- Backache
- General ill feeling
- Low fever
- Frequent, painful urination
- Abnormal bleeding
- Menstrual periods may arrive early, pain may increase during menstrual periods, and menstrual flow may be heavy

- Onset of menses may correspond with onset of PID

Later symptoms (1–3 weeks later)
- Severe pain and tenderness in the lower abdomen
- High fever
- Heavy, foul-smelling vaginal discharge

CAUSES

- Bacterial infection with *Neisseria gonorrhea* (40–60% of cases), *Chlamydia trachomatis* (30% of cases):
  - other bacteria, including *Mycoplasma hominis*, streptococci, and *Haemophilus influenzae*, while not the primary agents, are often also found as contributors to the bacterial milieu in PID.
  - infection is most often transmitted by an infected sexual partner.
  - infection may be transmitted via invasive medical procedures including:
    - childbirth
    - abortion
    - curettage (scraping out of the uterus)
    - pelvic surgery
    - insertion of an IUD.

RISK INCREASES WITH

- **Multiple sexual partners:** women with multiple partners have 4.6 times greater risk than women in monogamous relationships.
- **Use or history of use of an IUD**
- **Previous PID or cervicitis** (inflammation of the cervix).
- **Early "sexual debut":** the risk in sexually active 15-year-olds is 1 in 8, while in the average 24-year-old, risk drops to 1 in 80.
- **Use of oral contraceptives:** increases susceptibility to infection with *Chlamydia*.
- **Invasive medical procedures** that may introduce bacteria including:
  - cervical dilation
  - abortion
  - curettage: scraping of the uterus to remove growths, obtain specimens for diagnosis, or perform abortion

- tubal insufflation: blowing air into the fallopian tubes to take an X-ray
- hysterosalpingography: injection of dye into the uterus to take an X-ray.
- **Smoking:** in a study of 197 women hospitalized with their first episode of PID, cigarette smokers had 1.7 times the risk of PID compared to women who had never smoked. Former smokers had an elevated risk of 2.3. Other studies have found similar results.
- **Frequent douching:** frequent douching disturbs normal vaginal flora, increasing susceptibility to infection. A study of 100 patients hospitalized with PID found that women who douched three or more times per month were 3.6 times more likely to get PID than those who douched less than once per month.

PREVENTIVE MEASURES

- **Use barrier methods of birth control**, preferably rubber condoms:
  - rubber condoms are excellent choices for the prevention of PID.
  - condoms are preferred over diaphragms, cervical caps, spermicidal creams or sponges since, when condoms are used, sperm rarely reach the vagina.
- **Avoid intercourse during menstruation** unless a rubber condom is used since the risk of infection is increased during menstruation:
  - during menses, the protective cervical mucus plug is lost; blood, a medium in which gonococci thrive, is present.
  - the uterine lining, which is thought to offer protection against local bacterial invasion, is sloughed off.
- **Don't smoke:** smokers, even former smokers, have been found to have an increased risk for PID.
- **Do not use an IUD:**
  - numerous studies show a significant increase in PID when an IUD is present.
  - an IUD allows colonization of bacteria on its surface while simultaneously reducing local immune responsiveness.
- **Avoid haphazard or frequent douching:** by altering normal vaginal flora, frequent douching may increase susceptibility to infection
  - **exception:** if a woman believes she has had intercourse with an infected partner, a douche with a water-soluble chlorophyll solution may be a protective measure.
- **Do not use oral contraceptives:** women who use oral contraceptives have a higher risk of infection by *Chlamydia*. In animal studies, those receiving estrogen have a higher number of infected cervical cells and a longer lasting infection.

Expected outcomes

Response to antibiotic therapy should be noted within 1–2 days. By following the comprehensive protocol outlined below, which combines the prescribed herbal or pharmaceutical antibiotic with appropriate natural non-toxic therapies, complete resolution of pelvic inflammatory disease should occur within 2 weeks.

TREATMENT

Although standard medical treatment depends on antibiotics, antibiotic therapy is not itself curative: 15% of women with PID fail to respond, 20% have at least one recurrence, and 15% are rendered infertile. Reliance on antibiotics fails because PID typically involves more than one infectious organism, and drugs effective against gonococci do not affect *Chlamydia*. In addition, many organisms have developed strains that are resistant to antibiotics – a trend that is increasing.

A more effective approach is to use antibiotics, whether herbal or pharmaceutical, as part of a comprehensive plan in conjunction with natural non-toxic therapies, described below, that support immune resistance and heal damaged genitourinary tissues.

Diet

- Minimize consumption of sugars, alcohol, and refined foods, all of which inhibit immune function:
  - consuming 75 g (3 oz) of sugar in one sitting in any form (sucrose, honey, fruit juice) depresses white (immune) cell activity by 50% for up to 5 hours.
  - alcohol increases insulin secretion, and high levels of insulin suppress immune function.
  - refined foods, which are primarily composed of simple carbohydrates, are rapidly digested into sugar.
- Consume a nutrient-dense diet rich in whole, unprocessed, preferably organic foods, especially plant foods (fruits, vegetables, beans, seeds and nuts, and whole grains) and cold-water fish, and low in animal products and processed foods (for more detailed information, see Appendix 1).

Nutritional supplements

- **A high-potency multiple vitamin and mineral supplement:** this should include 400 µg of folic acid, 400 µg of vitamin B_{12}, and 50–100 mg of vitamin B_6. (Folic acid supplementation should always be accompanied by vitamin B_{12} supplementation to prevent folic acid from masking a vitamin B_{12} deficiency.) A daily multiple providing all of the known vitamins and minerals is recommended since a deficiency of virtually any nutrient can render the body more susceptible to infection.

- **Vitamin A**: the "anti-infective vitamin", plays an essential role in immune function by:
  - maintaining the surfaces of the skin, respiratory tract, and gastrointestinal tract and their secretions – all of which constitute a barrier that is the body's first line of defense against micro-organisms.
  - stimulating and/or enhancing numerous immune processes including white blood cell function and antibody response.
  - direct antiviral activity.
  - preventing immune suppression resulting from stress-induced adrenal hormones, severe burns and surgery.
  - some of these latter effects are most likely a result of vitamin A's ability to prevent stress-induced shrinkage and promote the growth of the thymus gland, the master gland of the immune system.
  - dosage: 50,000 IU q.d. for up to 1 week.
  - **caution**: sexually active women of child-bearing age should **not** use vitamin A unless effective birth control is being used because of possible birth defects at high dosages.
- **Beta-carotene**: called "pro-vitamin A" since it can be converted into vitamin A, beta-carotene is a more powerful antioxidant than vitamin A and exerts additional immune-stimulating effects, including enhancing thymus function:
  - beta-carotene has been shown to enhance thymus function by increasing the production of helper/inducer T cells by 30% after 7 days and all T cells after 14 days:
  - beta-carotene is highly concentrated in the ovary where it plays a variety of defensive roles:
    - an antioxidant, beta-carotene protects against cell damage caused by inflammation.
    - an immune-enhancer, beta-carotene increases the activity of interferon (a special chemical that fights viral infection and cancer), increases antibody levels, and increases the activity of white blood cells (which attack infectious agents).
  - dosage: 100,000 IU q.d. for 2+ months.
- **Vitamin C**: directly antiviral and antibacterial, vitamin C has numerous immune-enhancing effects including:
  - improving white blood cell response and function
  - increasing levels of interferon
  - increasing secretion of hormones from the thymus gland
  - dosage: 500 mg q.i.d. for the first week of treatment, then decrease over 3 days to 250 mg t.i.d.
- **Bioflavonoids**: a group of plant pigments largely responsible for the colors of fruits and flowers, bioflavonoids are powerful antioxidants in their own right, and, when taken with vitamin C, significantly enhance its absorption and effectiveness; dosage: 1,000 mg q.d.
- **Zinc:** a critical mineral for immune function, zinc is necessary for the activation of serum thymic factor – a thymus hormone with profound immune-enhancing actions. In addition, zinc is required for proper white cell function, promotes the destruction of foreign particles and micro-organisms, acts synergistically with vitamin A, and inhibits the replication of several viruses; dosage: 30 mg q.d.
- **Thymus extract:** substantial clinical data demonstrate that thymus extracts restore and enhance immune system function by improving the activity of the thymus gland:
  - the thymus gland secretes a family of hormones that act on white cells to ensure their proper development and function. A low level of these hormones is associated with depressed immunity and increases susceptibility to infection.
  - T cells, thymus-derived immune cells, orchestrate many immune functions and are the major components of cell-mediated immunity, which is extremely important in resistance to infection by bacteria and viruses.
  - dosage: consume the equivalent of 120 mg pure polypeptides with molecular weights less than 10,000, or roughly 500 mg of the crude polypeptide fraction q.d.

Botanical medicines

- **Chlorophyll:** chlorophyll contains cell-stimulating agents that aid in the regeneration of tissues; specifically, by breaking down carbon dioxide and releasing oxygen, chlorophyll is thought to increase the cells' resistance to invading bacteria, which are *anaerobic* (do not live in oxygen); dosage: 10 mg of fat/oil soluble chlorophyll q.i.d. for 1 month.
- **Bromelain:** during the acute stage of PID, tissue irritation can be severe, resulting in the formation of abscesses and adhesions in the fallopian tubes that can lead to scarring and tubal blockage. Bromelain, a group of sulfur-containing, proteolytic (protein-digesting) enzymes obtained from the pineapple plant, inhibits a wide variety of inflammatory agents, thus greatly reducing the tissue damage seen in PID. The rapid decrease in inflammation results in a faster recovery with much less risk of scarring. Bromelain has also demonstrated antimicrobial properties, and an Italian study shows it penetrates the fallopian tubes:
  - to maximize its anti-inflammatory effects, bromelain should be taken between meals to ensure its enzymes are not used in digesting food.

- dosage: 250 mg (1,800 MCU) taken between meals q.i.d. for the first week, then t.i.d. for 6 weeks.
- ***Hydrastis canadensis* (goldenseal):** goldenseal is a remarkably safe and effective natural antibiotic. Its most active alkaloid constituent, berberine sulfate, exhibits a broad range of antibiotic action against a wide variety of bacteria (including *Chlamydia* and streptococci), protozoa and fungi. Its action against some of these pathogens is actually stronger than that of commonly used antibiotics, but unlike antibiotic drugs, goldenseal does not destroy the protective bacteria (lactobacilli) in the vagina and intestines:
  - berberine is a more effective antimicrobial agent in an alkaline environment. Alkalinity can be increased by consuming fewer animal products and more plant foods, especially fruits. Although most fruits are acidic, digestion uses up their acid components leaving behind an alkaline residue.
  - dosage: solid (dry powdered) extract (4 : 1 or 8–12% alkaloid content): 400 mg t.i.d. during the acute phase, then 200 mg t.i.d. during recovery. (The dosage should be based on berberine content, and standardized extracts are recommended.)
- ***Symphytum officinale* (comfrey):** comfrey's common names, which include boneset and bruisewort, indicate its wound-healing abilities. A demulcent (agent whose actions soothe mucous membranes), comfrey contains astringent tannins, which help contract wounded tissues, along with mucilages (which form a thick, protective adhesive liquid), and *allantoin*, a plant chemical that promotes the growth of new cells. Allantoin is very highly diffusible, reaching deep tissues even when externally applied:
  - dosage: after the acute phase, choose one of the following forms. Take either 500 mg of freeze-dried herb t.i.d. or use a 1 : 1 fluid extract, and take 30 drops b.i.d. during recovery.
  - caution: while topical use of comfrey is safe, comfrey should not be taken internally without direct supervision by a physician. Individuals using comfrey internally must be carefully monitored by their physicians since an alkaloid in comfrey has been linked to liver disease.

Drug–herb interaction cautions
None.

Topical medicine
- **Chlorophyll douche:** careful vaginal douching with chlorophyll will diminish the population of anerobic organisms and encourage cervical and possibly upper tract healing, thus reducing the risk of infertility or ectopic pregnancy:
  - dosage: prepare a douche solution containing 1 tbsp of water-soluble chlorophyll for each cup of water used. After the acute phase, use chlorophyll douches every other day, alternating with vaginal depletion packs, for 3 weeks.
- **Vaginal depletion pack:** promotes drainage from damaged tissues. Essentially, a vaginal depletion pack is a cotton tampon containing a formula composed of several botanical medicines and minerals that promotes a cleansing drainage and tissue healing. If this procedure is suggested, a vaginal depletion pack will be prepared and inserted by a physician, who will provide full instructions at that time. After insertion, the pack is left in for 24 hours, then removed by pulling on the string. A chlorophyll douche should be performed after the vaginal depletion pack has been removed.

Physical medicine
- **Diathermy:** pulsed high-frequency diathermy (the use of pulsing electric energy for a short duration (65 μs every 1600 μs) at high intensity has been shown to enhance local tissue recovery and increase gammaglobulins (a type of immune system antibody that protects mucosal surfaces from invasion by bacteria and viruses) in PID; dosage: 2–3 sessions of approximately 30 min each per week during the acute phase.
- **Contrasting sitz baths:** these dramatically increase pelvic circulation and drainage, and improve the tone of the smooth muscles in the pelvic area:
  - contrast sitz baths involve partial immersion up to the top of the pelvic region in first hot, then cold water. The hot bath, which also has pain-relieving effects, is taken first for 3 min at 105–115°F. The cold bath is taken immediately following at a temperature of 55–75°F and lasts for 30 sec.
  - the water level of the hot bath should be at least 2.5 cm (1") inch above the level of the cold water; this ensures adequate warming of the area, thereby preventing chilling.
  - friction rubs to the hips during the cold sitz bath promote an increased reaction.
  - contrast sitz baths are given in groups of three, in other words, three alterations of hot to cold, finishing with the cold. Two separate tubs are necessary. While few of us have two adjacent bathtubs, this feat can be accomplished by employing a bathtub for the hot sitz bath and a large plastic tub for the cold sitz bath.
  - dosage: once or twice a day throughout the acute phase.

Peptic ulcer

DESCRIPTION

Peptic ulcers (an ulcer is an erosion in the mucous membranes that produces a crater-like lesion) can occur anywhere in the digestive tract, but are most common in the lower half of the stomach (*gastric ulcer*) or in the upper part of the duodenum, the first 30 cm (12") of the small intestine directly below the stomach (*duodenal ulcer*). Duodenal ulcers are four to five times more common than gastric ulcers, and are four times more common in men than in women. While duodenal ulcers are almost always benign, gastric ulcers may become malignant. Ulcers can affect all ages, and about 1 in 10 Americans develops a peptic ulcer at some period in his or her lifetime.

Despite their different locations, both types of ulcer are the result of excessive damage to the mucosal cells that line the stomach and duodenum. To protect the stomach and small intestine from the corrosive gastric juices secreted to digest food (hydrochloric acid and pepsin), these cells produce a layer of *mucin*, a thick slippery mucus, along with other factors that neutralize any acid that manages to come into contact with the stomach or intestinal lining. Mucosal cells lining the stomach and intestines are constantly renewed, with normal turnover occurring every 72 hours, so any damaged cells are quickly replaced. These protective mechanisms are normally quite effective; only when the mucosal cells are overwhelmed can an ulcer form.

Contrary to popular opinion, excessive secretion of gastric acid is rarely the problem. In fact, patients with gastric ulcers tend to secrete normal or even reduced levels of gastric acid. About half of patients with duodenal ulcers do have a higher than normal gastric acid output, because as a group, duodenal ulcer patients have twice as many acid-producing cells (*parietal cells*) in their stomachs as people without ulcers. Even with this increase in parietal cells, however, the protection offered by the mucosal cells lining the stomach and small intestine is normally more than adequate to prevent ulcer formation. Problems only arise when normal mucosal cell function is disrupted by factors such as *Helicobacter pylori* infection, aspirin and other non-steroidal anti-inflammatory drugs (NSAIDs), alcohol, nutrient deficiencies, stress, and other factors (discussed below).

FREQUENT SIGNS AND SYMPTOMS

- Burning, gnawing, cramp-like or aching pain or "heartburn" that occurs shortly before a meal, 45–60 min after eating, or hours later, during the night.
- Pain may be severe enough to cause wakening from a sound sleep.
- Pain typically lasts 30 min to 3 hours.
- Pain is often interpreted as heartburn, indigestion or hunger.
- Pain is usually in the upper abdomen, but may also be below the breastbone or in the back.
- Pain is usually greatly relieved by eating, drinking milk, or taking antacids.
- Pain can be relieved by vomiting (some people).
- Nausea, loss of appetite, with resulting weight loss.
- Weight gain due to eating more to ease discomfort.
- Pain is comes and goes. Weeks of intermittent pain may alternate with short pain-free periods.
- Pain may follow a predictable pattern, increasing in frequency during periods of stress.
- Ulcer crater or deformity in the stomach or upper small intestine is visible on X-ray or fiberoptic (endoscopic) examination.
- Positive test for blood in the stool.
- Anemia.

Warning: individuals experiencing any peptic ulcer symptoms must be monitored by a physician, even if following the natural approaches outlined below. Peptic ulcer complications such as hemorrhage, perforation, and obstruction are medical emergencies that require immediate hospitalization.

CAUSES

- ***Helicobacter pylori* infection:** in some people *H. pylori* infection increases gastric acidity, leading to ulcer formation:
  - infection with the bacterium *H. pylori* is found in 90–100% of duodenal ulcer patients, and 70% of gastric ulcer patients.
  - approximately 50% of people over age 50 test positive for *H. pylori*, which does not always cause ulcers, but is now thought to be a factor in other stomach disorders (e.g., gastritis, esophagitis, acid indigestion, stomach cancer).

- tests to determine the presence of *H. pylori* include:
  - measuring the level of antibodies to *H. pylori* in the blood or saliva
  - a breath test that measures the level of a gas produced by *H. pylori* as a metabolic by-product
  - culturing material collected during an *endoscopy* (an examination of the stomach or duodenum using a fiberoptic tube with a lens attached to it).
- predisposing factors for *H. pylori* infection are:
  - *low* gastric acid levels: (1) In addition to its use in digesting food, gastric acid destroys invading pathogens; low gastric acid secretion therefore provides a hospitable environment for colonization by *H. pylori*. (2) The ability to secrete stomach acid decreases with age; studies have found low stomach acidity in more than half of those over age 60. (3) Low acidity may also result from the use of antacids and H_2 blockers (e.g., Pepcid, Tagamet, Zantac).
  - low levels of vitamin C, E, and other antioxidants in the gastrointestinal lining: *H. pylori* damages the stomach and intestinal lining by producing oxidants (a type of free radical), which may explain why not everyone with *H. pylori* develops ulcers; those whose diets are high in antioxidants are afforded protection.
- **Non-steroidal anti-inflammatory drugs (NSAIDs):** NSAIDs relieve pain and inflammation by blocking the enzyme cyclo-oxygenase (COX):
  - COX comes in two forms, one of which (COX-2) triggers the synthesis of inflammatory compounds, while the other (COX-1) balances this action by causing the production of factors that protect the gastrointestinal mucosal cells and limit gastric acid output.
  - NSAIDs block both COX-1 and COX-2, thus significantly increasing the risk of ulcer formation.
  - studies have shown that the risk for gastrointestinal bleeding because of peptic ulcers is increased not only in individuals using higher doses of NSAIDs to treat arthritis and headaches, but also in those using the lower doses (300 mg, 150 mg, 75 mg) commonly recommended to prevent heart attacks and strokes:
    - risk is dose dependent – a dosage of 75 mg q.d. is associated with 30% less bleeding than 150 mg q.d., and 40% less bleeding than 400 mg q.d.
  - combining NSAID use with smoking is especially harmful; NSAID use causes an ulcer, and smoking stimulates gastric acid output, worsening ulcer symptoms and severity.
- **Smoking:** smoking causes increased frequency of ulcer formation, decreased response to peptic ulcer therapy,

and increased mortality as a result of peptic ulcers:
- smoking increases occurrence and severity of peptic ulcers by:
  - increasing the backflow (*reflux*) of bile salts into the stomach. Bile salts are extremely irritating to the stomach and initial portions of the duodenum
  - decreasing the secretion of bicarbonate (an important neutralizer of gastric acid) by the pancreas
  - accelerating the passage of food from the stomach into the duodenum.
- the chronic anxiety and psychological stress associated with smoking appear to worsen ulcer activity.
- **Stress and emotions:** a large study of 4,000 persons found that while the number of stressful events did not correlate with ulcer risk, those individuals who perceived their lives as stressful were at increased risk of developing peptic ulcer. These data suggest that the person's response, not the amount of stress, is the significant causative factor. As a group, ulcer patients tend to repress emotions.
- **Food allergy:** clinical and experimental evidence shows food allergy is a primary factor in many cases of peptic ulcer:
  - in one study, 98% of patients with X-ray evidence of peptic ulcer also had food allergies. In another study of 43 allergic children with X-ray-diagnosed peptic ulcer, 25 had food allergies.
  - milk, in particular, may be a causative factor since it is not only a highly allergenic food but also significantly increases the production of gastric juices.

RISK INCREASES WITH

- *Helicobacter pylori* infection.
- NSAID use (e.g., aspirin, ibuprofen, acetaminophen)
- Frequent use of antacids or drugs such as Pepcid, Tagamet, Zantac: a low acid environment increases susceptibility to *H. pylori* infection and contributes to nutrient deficiencies and food allergies since food cannot be properly digested without sufficient hydrochloric acid. Taken regularly, antacids can also lead to bowel irregularities, kidney stones and other side effects.
- Male sex: peptic ulcers are roughly twice as common in men as in women; duodenal ulcers are four times more common in men than in women.
- Smoking.
- Food allergy.
- Type O blood group (for duodenal ulcers): persons with this blood type typically secrete more stomach acid than those with the other blood types.

- Excessive stress, especially when coupled with a tendency to repress emotions.
- Disease-promoting diet: a diet based on animal products and processed foods, with little consumption of fresh vegetables, legumes, fruits, nuts and seeds, and whole grains is low in protective factors – fiber, flavonoids, and antioxidants.

PREVENTIVE MEASURES

- **Avoid frequent use of NSAIDs:** work with a physician to discover and heal the underlying causes of pain and inflammation. Effective natural anti-inflammatory agents exist that provide the temporary relief needed during healing without damaging the lining of the gastrointestinal tract.
- **Don't smoke**
- **Avoid frequent use of antacids:** antacids are relatively safe when used occasionally according to label instructions, but avoid antacids that contain aluminum. For gas (flatulence) and bloating, activated charcoal is an effective natural remedy that, unlike antacids, will not disrupt proper digestion.
- **Avoid excessive stress** as best you can by avoiding excessive work hours, poor nutrition, and inadequate rest.
- **Identify and eliminate** any allergenic foods from your diet.
- **Follow a health-promoting diet:** consume a nutrient-dense diet rich in whole, unprocessed, preferably organic foods, especially plant foods (fruits, vegetables, beans, seeds and nuts), and cold-water fish, and low in animal products (for more detailed information, see Appendix 1).
- **Don't repress feelings:** be assertive, expressing thoughts and feelings in a kind way, as one would wish to be treated, to help improve relationships at work and at home.
- **Build long-term health:** take time to build long-term health by discovering enjoyable outlets of self-expression, getting regular exercise, and performing stress-reduction techniques and calming, deep-breathing exercises.

Expected outcomes
Complete healing of peptic ulcers within 2–4 weeks.

TREATMENT

Diet
- Identify and eliminate allergenic foods, especially milk, from your diet.

- Identify and eliminate foods that irritate your stomach lining or cause additional secretion of stomach acid. Common food irritants include coffee, alcohol, citrus juices, sugar, and hot and spicy foods.
- Eat a diet rich in high-fiber plant foods: a fiber-rich diet is associated with a reduced rate of ulcers. Therapeutic use of a high-fiber diet in patients with duodenal ulcers decreases the recurrence rate by 50%. Consuming fiber-rich fruits and vegetables is preferable to the use of fiber supplements (pectin, guar gum, psyllium) since plant foods also contain a wide variety of protective flavonoids and antioxidants.
- Increase consumption of steamed green vegetables, leafy greens and alfalfa sprouts: all are good sources of vitamin K, which promotes healing of the mucosal lining and prevents bleeding.
- Consume fresh cabbage juice and other vegetable juices daily: raw cabbage juice is well documented as producing remarkable recovery from peptic ulcers. In one study, 1 L of fresh cabbage juice q.d., taken in divided doses, resulted in total ulcer healing in an average of 10 days. The cabbage should be juiced, and the juice taken immediately after preparation. Cabbage juice's high glutamine content is likely a primary reason for its effectiveness. (Glutamine is also recommended as a nutritional supplement, see below.)
- Eat five mini-meals a day: by consuming frequent small meals, triggering excessive digestive acid production is avoided and will ensure that any acid present has something to digest other than the stomach lining.
- Try a cup of chamomile tea with meals: chamomile is an antispasmodic, eases abdominal gas, has a mild anti-inflammatory effect on the lining of the digestive tract, and also has antimicrobial properties.

Nutritional supplements
- **Vitamin A:** all mucosal tissues rely on vitamin A. When vitamin A status is inadequate, keratin is secreted in these tissues, transforming them from their normally pliable, moist condition into stiff dry tissue that is unable to carry out its normal functions, and leading to breaches in integrity that significantly increase susceptibility to infection, food allergy, and peptic ulcer formation:
  - in rats, vitamin A has been shown to inhibit the development of stress ulcers.
  - dosage: 5,000 IU q.d.
  - **caution:** doses up to 20,000 IU q.d. may be recommended by the physician but doses higher than 5,000 IU q.d. should not be taken without physician supervision due to possible toxicity.
- **Vitamin E:** a powerful antioxidant, vitamin E protects fat-soluble components of the body, such as mucosal

cell membranes, from damage by free radicals:

- vitamin E, like vitamin A, has been shown to inhibit development of stress ulcers in rats.
- in addition, vitamin E protects vitamin A and increases its storage.
- dosage: 100 IU t.i.d.

- **Vitamin C:** an essential antioxidant found in all water-soluble body compartments, vitamin C strengthens and maintains normal mucosal integrity, improves ulcer healing, and enhances immune function. In addition, vitamin C regenerates vitamin E after it has used up its antioxidant potential; dosage: 500 mg t.i.d.

- **Flavonoids:** a group of plant pigments largely responsible for the colors of fruits and flowers, flavonoids exert significant antiulcer activity by:
  - counteracting both the production and secretion of histamine, an inflammatory chemical that stimulates the release of gastric acid:
    - studies on guinea pigs and rats have demonstrated that the flavonoid, *catechin*, provides significant antiulcer protection.
    - in human studies, catechin reduced histamine levels in gastric tissue in both normal patients and those with gastric and duodenal ulcers.
  - several flavonoids have also been shown to inhibit *H. pylori*, plus, unlike antibiotics, the flavonoids also augmented natural defense factors that prevent ulcer formation.
  - dosage: 500 mg t.i.d.

- **Glutamine:** an amino acid, glutamine is a critical nutrient for the growth and function of intestinal cells, playing an important role in the manufacture of compounds that line and protect the stomach and small intestine:
  - the high glutamine content of cabbage juice is thought to be largely responsible for its effectiveness in treating peptic ulcers.
  - dosage: 500 mg t.i.d.

- **Bismuth subcitrate:** a naturally occurring mineral, bismuth acts as an antacid and exerts activity against *H. pylori*:
  - although Pepto-Bismol, which is bismuth subsalicylate, is the best known bismuth preparation, another form of bismuth, bismuth subcitrate, has produced better results against *H. pylori*.
  - dosage: bismuth subcitrate 240 mg b.i.d. before meals. In the US, bismuth subcitrate is primarily available through compounding pharmacies:
    - if bismuth subsalycilate is used, the dosage is 500 mg q.i.d.
    - **warning:** bismuth subsalycilate should not be taken by children recovering from the flu,

chicken pox, or other viral infection as it may mask nausea and vomiting associated with Reye's syndrome, a rare but serious illness.

- **Zinc:** zinc increases mucin production and has been shown to have a protective effect against peptic ulcers in animals and a curative effect in humans:
  - in addition to its effect on mucin production, zinc protects against free radical damage, acts synergistically with vitamin A, and is involved in wound healing, immune system activity, inflammation control, and tissue regeneration.
  - dosage: 20–30 mg q.d.

Botanical medicines

- **Deglycyrrhizinated licorice (DGL):** a form of licorice from which the compound glycyrrhetinic acid has been removed (it causes elevations in blood pressure in some cases), DGL is a very effective antiulcer agent with no known side effects:
  - DGL stimulates and/or accelerates the factors that protect against ulcer formation, and is composed of several flavonoids that have been shown to inhibit *H. pylori*.
  - DGL may promote the release of salivary compounds that stimulate the growth and regeneration of stomach and intestinal cells. DGL is therefore given as a chewable tablet, so it can promote and mix with saliva.
  - DGL has been shown to reduce the gastric bleeding caused by aspirin and is recommended for prevention of gastric ulcers in patients who require long-term treatment with ulcer-causing drugs, such as aspirin, other NSAIDs, or corticosteroids.
  - DGL is also very effective in treating duodenal ulcers. In a study of 40 patients with duodenal ulcers of 4–12 years' duration, all of whom had been referred for surgery, initially half of the patients, then the other half were given DGL. All 40 showed substantial improvement, usually within 5–7 days of beginning DGL, and none required surgery during the 1-year follow-up.
  - in several head-to-head comparison studies, DGL has been shown to be more effective than Tagamet, Zantac, or antacids in both short-term and maintenance treatment of peptic ulcers:
    - in addition, these drugs, which work by neutralizing or suppressing gastric acid, have significant side effects, while DGL is extremely safe and at $15 for a month's supply, costs only a fraction as much as Tagamet or Zantac for which a month's supply costs well over $100.
  - dosage: DGL is given in chewable tablets since, in order to be effective in healing peptic ulcers,

DGL must mix with saliva:

- in acute cases, the standard dosage is two to four 380 mg chewable tablets between or 20 min before meals.
- in more mild or chronic cases, or for maintenance, the dosage is one to two 380 mg tablets between or 20 min before meals. (Taking DGL with meals is associated with poor results.)

■ **Aloe vera and rhubarb:** in over 90% of 312 cases of active intestinal bleeding, alcohol-extracted tablets of rhubarb (*Rheum* species) stopped active bleeding in under 60 hours:

- both aloe vera and rhubarb contain similar flavonoids that act as astringents (i.e., drying agents), but aloe vera juice is recommended since it is more accessible.
- dosage: when active bleeding of an ulcer is present, drink 1 L q.d. of aloe vera juice.

Drug–herb interaction cautions
None.

Psychological medicine
■ **Develop an effective stress-reduction program:** eliminate or control stressors and design a regular relaxation plan.

Periodontal disease

DESCRIPTION

Periodontal disease is an inclusive term that refers to inflammatory conditions of the *periodontium*, the tissues that surround and support the teeth, including the jawbone. Periodontal disease can progress from *gingivitis*, an inflammatory condition of the gums, to *periodontitis* (also called *pyorrhea*) in which the supporting bone also becomes inflamed and eroded.

Periodontal disease is best treated with the combined expertise of a dentist or periodontist and a nutritionally minded physician. Meticulous oral hygiene, while essential in treating and preventing periodontal disease is not, by itself, sufficient; the patient's immune system and other defense mechanisms must also be normalized to prevent disease progression and restore oral health.

Periodontal disease is extremely common; an estimated 75% of Americans over the age of 35 have some degree of periodontal disease. Incidence of periodontal disease increases with age from 15% of children at age 10, to 38% of individuals at age 20, 46% of individuals at age 35, and 54% of individuals at age 50. Men have a higher prevalence and severity of periodontal disease than women.

FREQUENT SIGNS AND SYMPTOMS

Gingivitis
- Unpleasant taste in the mouth
- Bad breath
- Red, inflamed gums (gums are typically swollen, sore, and tender)
- Bleeding gums (especially when the teeth are brushed)

Periodontitis
- Localized pain
- Loosening of teeth in their sockets
- Aching teeth and gums (especially when eating hot, cold or sweet food)
- Redness, swelling, and/or signs of infection
- Dental pockets
- An abscess (will be accompanied by tenderness, swelling, pain, and fever)
- X-ray may reveal erosion of the *alveolar bone* (the bone that supports the teeth)

CAUSES

- **Bacterial infection:** plaque, the sticky film of mucus and bacteria that adheres to teeth, particularly along the gum line, promotes infection:
  - poor dental hygiene results in the accumulation of plaque.
  - bacteria in plaque produce and secrete numerous compounds detrimental to immune defenses including endotoxins and exotoxins; free radicals and collagen-destroying enzymes; leukotoxins; and bacterial antigens, waste products, and toxic compounds.
  - although periodontal disease usually begins as a bacterial infection that thrives in the *gingival sulcus* (the hard to cleanse area between the gums and the tooth), the presence of bacteria is, in itself, insufficient to cause periodontal disease. Experts have concluded that a variety of immune and other host defense factors (discussed below) must be depressed to allow bacterial infection to develop and progress.
- **The gingival sulcus:** the gingival sulcus – the V-shaped crevice that surrounds each tooth and bound by the surface of the tooth on one side and the lining of cells (*epithelium*) of the gums (*gingiva*) on the other – provides an ideal environment for the growth of bacteria:
  - the crevice is resistant to the washing, cleansing action of saliva.
  - the fluid in the gingival sulcus provides a rich source of nutrients for micro-organisms.
- **Defects in neutrophil function:** abnormalities in neutrophil function are catastrophic for the periodontium (the gums and support structures of the teeth):
  - neutrophils, white blood cells that constitute the immune system's first line of defense against microbial overgrowth, are critical for the protection of the periodontium:
    - neutrophil function is depressed in the geriatric population as a whole, and in patients with diabetes, Crohn's disease, Chediak-Higashi syndrome, Down's syndrome, and juvenile periodontitis. Individuals with these conditions are at significant risk for developing rapidly progressing periodontal disease.

- consuming 75 g (3 oz) of sugar in one sitting in any form (sucrose, honey, fruit juice) depresses neutrophil activity by 50% for 1–5 hours.
- the average American consumes an excess of 150 g (5 oz) of sucrose and other refined carbohydrates per day. Neutrophil function is therefore chronically depressed in most Americans.

■ excessive activation of the immune response is, however, also harmful. In addition, neutrophils play a major role in tissue destruction by releasing inflammatory compounds, a compound that stimulates alveolar bone destruction, and numerous free radicals that break down collagen – all of which, if excessively produced, contribute to periodontal disease.

■ temporary depression of neutrophil function may be responsible for periods of ebb and flow noted in periodontal disease.

■ **Sugar consumption:** sugar significantly increases plaque accumulation while decreasing neutrophil function.

■ **Complement activation:** the complement system is composed of at least 22 proteins that circulate in the blood and, when activated, deploy in a cascade fashion. Like neutrophils, the complement system can be a double-edged sword:

■ complement plays a critical role in resistance to infection but is also a major factor in the tissue destruction seen in periodontal disease.

■ the net effect of complement activation is an increase in gingival permeability, which results in increased penetration by bacteria and harmful bacterial by-products – a situation that sets up a vicious feed-forward cycle.

■ **Mast cells and IgE:** mast cells are white blood cells that reside in tissues and contain histamine and other inflammatory compounds in packets called *granules*. Mast cell *degranulation* (the release of the contents of these packets) is another major factor in the progression of periodontal disease:

■ mast cells degranulate when stimulated by IgE complexes (IgE is an antibody formed in response to allergens), complement components, mechanical trauma, endotoxins, and/or free radicals.

■ increased levels of IgE (the allergy antibody) are found in the gums of patients with periodontal disease, suggesting allergic reactions may be a factor.

■ **Atrophy of the collagen matrix:** collagen is the primary protein in dental tissue. The collagen matrix serves as the anchor to the alveolar bone and dissipates the tremendous pressure exerted during chewing:

■ poor integrity in the collagen matrix of the periodontium (gums and supportive structures of the teeth) results in increased permeability to inflammatory

mediators, bacteria and their by-products, and destructive enzymes from the mouth.

■ as a result of the high rate of protein turnover in periodontal collagen, the collagen matrix in this area is extremely vulnerable to atrophy when the necessary nutrient cofactors for collagen synthesis are deficient:

- cofactors for collagen synthesis (which include protein, zinc, copper, vitamins C, B_6, and A) are discussed under Nutritional supplements below.

■ **Amalgam restorations:** silver fillings contain the toxic metal, mercury, which depletes the body's protective antioxidant enzymes (glutathione peroxidase, superoxide dismutase, and catalase). The support structures of the teeth, which are particularly sensitive to free radical damage, are thus deprived of their defenses.

■ **Other local factors:** a variety of local factors can contribute to the progression of periodontal disease including:

■ *smoking*: tobacco smoke is loaded with free radicals that damage the epithelial cells lining the mouth, and smoking greatly reduces vitamin C levels, thus enhancing free radical damage.

■ *faulty dental work*: overhanging margins from a poorly done filling or crown provide an ideal location for plaque accumulation and bacterial growth. Poorly fitting dental appliances or improperly shaped dental fillings are a common cause of gingival inflammation and periodontal destruction.

■ *food impaction*: food retained around teeth provides nutrients for bacteria and increases plaque formation.

■ *malocclusion*: misaligned teeth significantly increase stress and trauma of the teeth and their support structures.

■ *missing teeth*: if not replaced, contribute to malocclusion.

■ *tongue thrusting*: promotes malocclusion.

■ *bruxism*: teeth grinding traumatizes teeth and their support structures.

■ *excessive or improper tooth brushing* can damage gingival tissue.

■ *mouth breathing*: dries out protective saliva, increasing gingival tissue susceptibility to bacterial invasion.

■ **Systemic disease:** periodontal disease may be a manifestation of a systemic condition such as diabetes mellitus, collagen diseases, anemia, vitamin deficiency, hardening of the arteries, or leukemia or other disorders of leukocyte (a type of white blood cell) function.

■ **Non-inflammatory alveolar bone loss:** significant loss of alveolar bone (the bone that supports teeth) and resulting tooth loss can occur with little inflammation as a result of osteoporosis, the use of certain drugs, or endocrine imbalances (such as the hormonal changes of pregnancy) rather than periodontal disease. When inflammation is not present, the focus should be on identifying and treating the underlying condition.

RISK INCREASES WITH

- Poor dental hygiene
- Faulty dental work
- Malocclusion (misaligned teeth)
- Missing teeth
- Teeth grinding
- Mouth breathing
- Excessive or improper tooth brushing
- Smoking
- Frequent consumption of foods high in sugar, especially foods with a sticky texture
- Inadequate consumption of nutrients necessary for periodontal collagen synthesis (discussed below under Nutritional supplements)
- Pregnancy, use of birth control pills, chemotherapy agents, epilepsy drugs, and drugs used in both Crohn's disease and ulcerative colitis all interfere with folic acid absorption (see Nutritional supplements below).

PREVENTIVE MEASURES

- Meticulous oral hygiene, including daily brushing, flossing, and regular dental visits for teeth cleaning and scaling to remove plaque:
    - use a soft brush, which is less likely to damage teeth and gums than a hard one.
    - brush teeth carefully after eating, and floss thoroughly at least once a day to remove bacteria from between gums and teeth.
    - to verify that you are using the best brushing and flossing technique, ask the dentist or dental hygienist to demonstrate.
- Buy a new toothbrush every 2 weeks until gums have completely regained their health:
    - bacteria can cling to your toothbrush, resulting in reinfection.
    - disinfect your toothbrush between brushings by immersing it in hydrogen peroxide or a citrus seed extract solution. Be sure to rinse it thoroughly with running water before using again.
- Use a rotary electric or battery-powered toothbrush (these have been shown to remove up to 95% of plaque compared with 48% for hand brushing).
- Don't smoke.

- Avoid sugary foods, especially foods with a sticky texture.
- Eat a high-fiber diet rich in fresh, raw vegetables and whole grains. Chew thoroughly to stimulate saliva secretion.

Expected outcomes

The progression of periodontal disease can be halted almost immediately.

Reversal of tissue damage can be expected to manifest within the first month of therapy; however, the degree of restoration of normal tooth pocket depths will often depend upon the severity of the disease when treatment is initiated and the length of time the disease process has progressed.

TREATMENT

Diet

- Avoid sugar and all refined carbohydrates, which are found in processed foods.
- Increase consumption of foods rich in fiber, e.g., raw vegetables and fruits, and whole grains.
- Identify and remove any allergenic foods from the diet.
- To promote consumption of both fiber and the nutrients necessary for periodontal collagen synthesis, base the diet on whole, unprocessed plant foods (fruits, vegetables, beans, seeds and nuts, and whole grains), and cold-water fish (for more detailed information, see the Appendix 1).

Nutritional supplements

- **Vitamin C**: the classical symptom of gingivitis seen in *scurvy* (severe vitamin C deficiency) illustrates vitamin C's pivotal role in maintaining the integrity and immune defenses of the collagen matrix and periodontal membrane:
    - deficiency of vitamin C results in defective formation and maintenance of collagen, ground substance and intercellular cement substances.
    - decreased levels of vitamin C are also associated with delayed wound healing and increased permeability of oral tissues to endotoxin and bacterial by-products, as well as impaired white blood cell (particularly neutrophil) function.
    - supplementation with vitamin C has been shown to increase neutrophil function even in individuals with Chediak-Higashi syndrome, an inherited disorder in which white blood cell function is compromised, leading to extremely rapidly progressing periodontal disease.
    - vitamin C also possesses significant antioxidant and anti-inflammatory actions.
    - dosage: 3–5 g q.d. in divided doses.

- **Vitamin A:** vitamin A is necessary for collagen synthesis, wound healing, and enhancing a wide variety of immune functions:
  - deficiency of vitamin A is associated with abnormal cell structures in the periodontium, inflammatory infiltration and degeneration, periodontal pocket formation, plaque formation, increased susceptibility to infection, and abnormal alveolar bone formation.
  - dosage: 5,000 IU q.d.
  - **caution:** no more than 5,000 IU q.d. of vitamin A should be taken by sexually active women of childbearing age. Higher doses may be toxic. Early warning signs of impending toxicity: chapped lips and dry skin. Signs of vitamin A toxicity: headache followed by fatigue, emotional instability, and muscle and joint pain. Women of childbearing age should use effective birth control during vitamin A treatment and for at least 1 month after discontinuation.
- **Beta-carotene:** also known as "pro-vitamin A" since it can be converted to vitamin A within the body, beta-carotene is a powerful antioxidant essential to epithelial health and is recommended instead of vitamin A because of its similar effects and greater safety; dosage: 250,000 IU q.d. (higher doses if indicated) for up to 6 months.
- **Zinc:** zinc is critically important for the treatment of periodontal disease for a wide variety of reasons:
  - zinc functions synergistically with vitamin A in many body processes.
  - functions of zinc in the gingiva and periodontium include stabilization of membranes, antioxidant activity, collagen synthesis, inhibition of plaque growth, and inhibition of mast cell degranulation. Zinc is an essential cofactor in numerous immune defense activities and is also known to significantly reduce wound healing time.
  - severity of periodontal disease is positively associated with decreased zinc levels. Marginal zinc deficiency is widespread in the US, especially among the elderly.
  - plaque growth can be inhibited by regular, twice-daily use of a mouthwash containing a 5% zinc solution.
  - dosage: 30 mg zinc picolinate q.d. (60 mg q.d. if any other form is used); or wash mouth with 15 ml of a 5% zinc solution b.i.d.
- **Vitamin E:** supplementation with vitamin E is associated with decreased wound healing time:
  - as an antioxidant, vitamin E works synergistically with the trace mineral selenium to lessen the destructive effects of free radicals on gums.
  - vitamin E's antioxidant effects are particularly important if silver fillings (mercury amalgams) are

present. Mercury depletes the tissues of the antioxidant enzymes superoxide dismutase, glutathione peroxidase, and catalase. In animal studies, vitamin E supplementation has been shown to prevent this toxic effect.
  - dosage: Vitamin E 400–800 IU mixed tocopherols q.d. along with selenium 400 µg q.d.
- **Folic acid:** the use of folic acid, either as a mouthwash or pill, has produced significant reductions in gum inflammation, swelling and bleeding in double-blind studies:
  - folic acid binds to plaque-derived toxins, and folic acid mouthwash has been demonstrated to be significantly more effective than pill form, suggesting a local mechanism of action.
  - the blood and white blood cells of pregnant women and oral contraceptive users contain a macromolecule that binds folic acid resulting in a deficiency of this nutrient in the cells of the oral cavity (and the cervix).
  - chemotherapy agents, epilepsy drugs, and drugs used in Crohn's disease and ulcerative colitis also interfere with folic acid absorption.
  - folic acid, which is involved in the synthesis of nucleic acids (components of DNA and RNA), is essential to all rapidly dividing cells.
  - folic acid also plays an indirect role in the formation of the antioxidant enzyme glutathione peroxidase since the synthesis of one of glutathione's components (cysteine) depends upon adequate folic acid.
  - dosage: 2 mg q.d.; or wash mouth with 15 ml of a 0.1% solution of folic acid b.i.d.
  - **caution:** folic acid supplementation should always be accompanied by vitamin B_{12} supplementation (400 µg q.d.) to prevent folic acid from masking a vitamin B_{12} deficiency.
- **Quercetin:** quercetin is one of the more biologically active flavonoids, plant compounds that are extremely effective in reducing inflammation and stabilizing collagen structures:
  - flavonoids support collagen structure integrity by: decreasing membrane permeability, and thus the load of inflammatory mediators and bacterial products; preventing free radical damage via their potent antioxidant properties; inhibiting mast cell degranulation; and crosslinking directly with collagen fibers.
  - dosage: 500 mg t.i.d.
- **Coenzyme Q_{10}:** through its role in energy production in the mitochondria (the cell's energy factories), CoQ_{10} increases the supply of healing oxygen to tissues. CoQ_{10} is also an effective antioxidant:
  - CoQ_{10} is widely used in Japan to treat a variety of conditions including periodontal disease. A review

of seven Japanese studies that used CoQ_{10} found that 70% of 332 patients with periodontal disease benefited significantly from supplementation.

- dosage: 150–300 mg q.d.

Botanical medicines

- **High flavonoid content extracts:** like quercetin (described above), the biologically active flavonoids listed below are extremely effective against periodontal disease due to their antioxidant, anti-inflammatory, and collagen stabilizing effects.
  - dosage: 150–300 mg q.d. of a high flavonoid extract, such as one from bilberry (*Vaccinium myrtillus*), hawthorn (*Crataegus* spp.), or grape seed (*Vitis vinifera*).
  - green tea (*Camellia sinensis*) may be liberally consumed as a beverage, or a green tea extract with a 50% polyphenol content may be taken at a dosage of 200–300 mg b.i.d.

- ***Sanguinaria canadensis* (bloodroot):** one of the alkaloids in bloodroot, *sanguinarine*, has broad antimicrobial activity and anti-inflammatory properties, and prevents dental plaque formation by inhibiting bacterial adherence. Electron microscope studies demonstrate that when bacteria are exposed to sanguinarine, they aggregate and become morphologically irregular. Dosage: sanguinarine is available in commercial toothpastes and mouth rinses. Use a toothpaste containing this extract.

- ***Centella asiatica* (gotu kola)** triterpenoids: an extract containing gotu kola triterpenoids has been shown to be quite helpful in speeding healing after laser surgery for severe periodontal disease; dosage: 30 mg b.i.d. of pure triterpenoids.

Drug–herb interaction cautions
None.

Pneumonia

DESCRIPTION

Pneumonia (viral, bacterial, mycoplasmal) is a serious infection of the lungs, in which the *alveoli* (the tiny air sacs in lung tissue) become inflamed and filled with fluid, mucus and pus. A number of different infectious agents including viruses, bacteria, protozoa, and fungi can cause pneumonia, and antimicrobial treatment varies depending upon the causative agent. Although pneumonia may appear in healthy individuals, it is typically an opportunistic disease that gains a foothold when the immune system is compromised, as it is in individuals with chronic lung disease or other debilitating illness, individuals using respiratory therapy or immunosuppressive drugs, or drug and/or alcohol abusers.

Normally, the airway below the larynx (voicebox) is sterile as a result of several protective mechanisms. The cough reflex in the lower respiratory tract causes ejection of foreign matter and mucus. Respiratory secretions contain the antiviral and antibacterial *immunoglobulins* (protective immune proteins) IgA and IgG, and the alveoli are protected by *macrophages* (large immune defense cells that gobble up invaders), a rich blood supply capable of delivering additional immune support, and an efficient lymphatic drainage network. Therefore, in healthy individuals, pneumonia most often follows an insult to host defense mechanisms such as viral infection (especially influenza), cigarette smoke and other noxious fumes, hospitalization, or loss of consciousness (which depresses the gag reflex, allowing foreign material or fluid to be sucked into the airways).

About 2 million cases of pneumonia are diagnosed in the US every year, and 40,000–70,000 deaths result. Acute pneumonia, which is still the fifth leading cause of death in the US, is particularly dangerous in the elderly. Depending upon the infectious agent, treatment for pneumonia may take from 2–6 weeks. Weakness may persist for an additional 4–8 weeks after the acute phase of the infection has resolved, and a cough can sometimes hang on for up to 2 months after the infection is gone.

FREQUENT SIGNS AND SYMPTOMS

Viral pneumonia
- 20% of pneumonias are viral, with 3% occurring as a result of influenza
- Often begins as an upper respiratory infection, e.g., influenza
- Contagious
- Can affect all ages but is most severe in infants and adults over age 60
- Flu-like symptoms of fever, chills, muscle aches, headache, fatigue
- Can progress suddenly or gradually
- Cough, can be mild or severe, usually without sputum until later stages
- Sore throat
- Rapid, labored (sometimes) breathing
- Chest pain
- Loss of appetite, upset stomach
- Enlarged lymph glands in the neck
- Bluish nails and skin
- Low-grade fever (temperature generally less than 102°F)

Bacterial pneumonia
- 12% of pneumonias are bacterial; 6% are bacterial superimposed on viral
- Comes on suddenly, often as a complication of other illnesses
- Not usually contagious, but the most serious form of pneumonia
- Can affect all ages but is most severe in young children and adults over age 60
- High fever (over 102°F)
- Sudden onset of shaking, chills, fever, chest pain
- Difficulty breathing (shortness of breath, rapid breathing)
- Lethargy
- Cough with sputum that may be blood-specked or pinkish at first, becoming rusty at the height of infection, and finally yellow during resolution
- Chest pain that worsens with inhalations

- Initially, rattling sounds (*rales*) heard on inhalation that change to crackling sounds (*crepitant rales*) after the acute phase
- Abdominal pain
- May be pale and sweaty
- Bluish lips and nails (severe cases)

Mycoplasmal and chlamydial pneumonia

- Between 10 and 20% of pneumonias are mycoplasmal, and approximately 10% are chlamydial
- Can affect all ages but is most common in persons under the age of 35, especially children aged 1–12
- Contagious
- Sore throat
- Dry cough that gradually increases and produces sputum, which may contain blood
- All-over achy sick feeling
- Fever
- Labored breathing
- Chest pain
- Abdominal pain (infrequent)
- Bluish skin (severe cases)

A chest X-ray to determine which part of the lungs is involved will likely be performed as well as a blood test and/or a sputum sample to determine what type of infectious agent is responsible.

CAUSES

Pneumonia is an opportunistic disease that occurs when the host's immune system is compromised allowing an infectious agent to gain entry and multiply. Agents that are typically involved include the following:

- **Viral pneumonia:** viral infection including influenza, chickenpox, respiratory viruses (especially respiratory syncytial virus [RSV] in adults), measles, and cytomegalovirus (especially in infants).
- **Bacterial pneumonia:** bacterial infection with agents such as *Streptococcus pneumoniae*, pneumococci, *Haemophilus influenzae* or staphylococci:
  - *Streptococcus pneumoniae* is the most common bacterial pneumonia and the most common cause of pneumonia requiring hospitalization.
  - a blood culture is a more accurate method of diagnosis than a sputum culture since the *nasopharynx* (the end of the nasal passage and upper portion of the throat) is the natural habitat of pneumococcus.
- **Mycoplasmal pneumonia:** previous infection in the nose, throat, or bronchial tubes with *Mycoplasma pneumoniae*, a type of bacteria that lack cell walls.

RISK INCREASES WITH

- **Lifestyle practices that weaken immune function:**
  - alcohol consumption
  - smoking
  - drug abuse
  - a diet high in saturated and *trans* fats, sugars, and refined foods
  - low intake of green vegetables
  - nutrient deficiency: an overwhelming number of clinical and experimental studies show that a deficiency of any nutrient can profoundly impair the immune system:
    - marginal (subclinical) nutrient deficiency is widespread in the US.
    - numerous studies have shown that most elderly Americans are deficient in at least one nutrient.
  - irregular meals
  - less than 7 hours sleep per night
  - lack of regular exercise
  - obesity is associated with decreased immune function:
    - levels of various lipids (fats), including cholesterol, free fatty acids and triglycerides are usually elevated in obese individuals. When lipid levels are high, various immune functions are inhibited including the ability of white cells to divide, move to areas of infection, and destroy micro-organisms.
    - in experimental studies, the white blood cells of overweight individuals were less able to destroy bacteria.
  - crowded or unsanitary living conditions
  - excessive stress: stress leads to immune suppression by:
    - increasing levels of adrenal gland hormones, including adrenaline and corticosteroids, which inhibit white blood cell formation and cause the thymus gland (the master gland of the immune system) to shrink.
    - stimulating the *sympathetic nervous system* (the part of the autonomic nervous system responsible for the fight-or-flight response). The immune system functions better under the *parasympathetic nervous system* (the other arm of the autonomic nervous system), which is responsible for bodily functions during periods of rest, relaxation, meditation and sleep.
- **Age:** newborns and infants, and adults over 60.
- **Exposure to cold, harsh weather**
- **Exposure to persons ill with respiratory infections**
- **Acute or chronic illness that has lowered resistance:** influenza, common cold, heart disease, congestive heart failure, diabetes, cancer

- **Chronic lung disease** such as asthma, cystic fibrosis, emphysema
- **Hospitalization**
- **Immunosuppressive drugs**
- **Respiratory therapy:** increased risk of inhalation of a foreign body into the lung
- **Impairment of consciousness:** the use of drugs or anesthesia depresses the gag reflex, a primary initial defense against inhalation of a foreign body.

PREVENTIVE MEASURES

- Get at least 7–8 hours of sleep each night. During the deepest levels of sleep, potent immune-enhancing compounds are released, and many immune functions are greatly increased.
- Don't smoke.
- Minimize consumption of sugar, saturated and *trans* fats, and refined foods.
- Increase consumption of vegetables, especially green vegetables, which are excellent sources of numerous immune-building phytonutrients, vitamins and minerals.
- Eat regular, small, balanced meals.
- Ensure adequate intake of lean protein.
- A high-potency multiple vitamin and mineral supplement: a deficiency of any single nutrient can impair immune function. A daily multiple providing all of the known vitamins and minerals serves as the foundation of an immune-support program. Any good multiple should include 400 µg of folic acid, 400 µg of vitamin B_{12}, and 50–100 mg of vitamin B_6. (Folic acid supplementation should always be accompanied by vitamin B_{12} supplementation to prevent folic acid from masking a vitamin B_{12} deficiency.)
- Exercise regularly: at least 30 min four to five times each week.
- Avoid exposure to individuals with respiratory infections.
- Wear protective clothing and try not to get chilled or wet in cold weather.
- Maintain a healthy weight.

Expected outcomes
The acute phase should resolve within 7–10 days.
- **Viral pneumonia:** viral infection is usually curable within a few days to a week, although postviral fatigue is common.
- **Bacterial pneumonia:** treatment with the correct antibiotic will lead to substantial improvement within a few days.
- **Mycoplasmal pneumonia:** slow recovery is the general rule, but the course is quite variable.

Regardless which infectious agent is the cause, weakness and fatigue typically persist for 6–8 weeks after the acute phase of the infection has resolved.

TREATMENT

- Rest is essential to recovery. Bed rest is necessary until any fever subsides, then plenty of rest should continue to be a priority, and normal activities should be resumed only gradually.
- The general approach to all pneumonias is a protocol (described below) that enhances general immune function and respiratory tract drainage in conjunction with cause-specific antimicrobial medications:
  - *viral pneumonia*: antibiotics are not effective against viruses. Treatment will be aimed at easing discomfort and preventing a secondary bacterial infection from taking hold. If herpes or varicella (chickenpox) is the infectious agent, aciclovir may be prescribed. For RSV or severe influenza, aerosolized ribavirin may be prescribed.
  - *bacterial pneumonia*: this is a serious infection that requires aggressive treatment with either oral or IV antibiotics, typically penicillin.
  - *mycoplasmal pneumonia*: an antibiotic, typically an erythromycin or tetracycline, may reduce the length of time symptoms such as fever, cough and general discomfort are present, but will not actually kill the mycoplasma responsible for the infection.

Diet
- **Drink at least one full glass of fluid every waking hour:** liquids prevent dehydration and help thin lung secretions, so they are easier to cough out:
  - try to take lots of soups, diluted fresh juices, herb teas, and purified water spiked with fresh lemon juice.
  - fruit juices, and the juices of beets and carrots, which are high in sugars, should be diluted at least half and half with water and/or green vegetable juices or herb tea.
- **Eliminate concentrated simple carbohydrates:** sugar, honey, dried fruit, undiluted fruit juice, soda, baked goods, sweetened cereals, candy, etc. Consumption of 75 g (3 oz) of sugar in one sitting depresses immune function by 50% for up to 5 hours.
- **Eliminate alcohol:** alcohol increases susceptibility to infections, and alcoholics are known to be more susceptible to pneumonia:
  - immediately after alcohol is consumed, the rate of mobilization of human white blood cells (the body's

primary defense mechanism against infection) drops profoundly.

- the more alcohol consumed, the greater the impairment in white blood cell motility.

■ **Avoid dairy products:** dairy products may increase mucus production.

■ **Consume a health-promoting diet:** eat small, frequent, nutrient-dense meals composed of whole, unprocessed, preferably organic foods, especially plant foods (fruits, vegetables, beans, seeds and nuts, and whole grains) and cold-water fish (more detailed information can be found in Appendix 1).

■ **Adequate protein** is essential for optimal immune function. To ensure sufficient protein, please follow the recommendations given for protein intake in Appendix 1. If loss of appetite is a problem, smoothies made with a high-quality protein powder supplement may be helpful.

■ **Choose lean protein:** increased levels of cholesterol, free fatty acids, and bile acids – all of which increase when foods high in fat are eaten – inhibit various immune functions, including the ability of white blood cells to divide, move to areas of infection, and destroy micro-organisms.

Nutritional supplements

■ *Lactobacillus acidophilus* and *Bifidobacterium bifidum*: antibiotics destroy not only pathogenic bacteria but also these important friendly bacteria, which are necessary for intestinal (and in women, vaginal) health. Whenever antibiotics are used, it is important to reseed the gastrointestinal tract with these friendly bacteria:

- dosage: 1–2 billion live organisms q.d. both while antibiotics are being taken and for at least 10 days following the cessation of antibiotic use. Do not take at the same time of day as the antibiotics.

■ **Vitamin A:** people deficient in vitamin A are more susceptible to infectious diseases in general, but especially to viral infections; during infection, vitamin A stores plummet:

- known as the "anti-infective vitamin", vitamin A maintains the surfaces of the respiratory tract and its secretions, which constitute a barrier that is the respiratory system's first line of defense against micro-organisms.
- vitamin A is directly antiviral and stimulates a number of immune processes including white blood cell function and antibody response.
- vitamin A also promotes the growth of the thymus, the master gland of the immune system.

- supplementation with vitamin A is strongly recommended in children with pneumonia as a complication of measles, a condition known to decrease vitamin A levels:
  - in a study of 189 South African children with measles (average age 10 months), vitamin A supplementation reduced the death rate by 50% and the duration of pneumonia, diarrhea and hospital stay by 33%.
- dosage: 50,000 IU q.d. for 1 week or beta-carotene 200,000 IU q.d.
- **caution:** vitamin A should not be used by sexually active menstruating women. Doses higher than 5,000 IU q.d. may cause birth defects. Menstruating women should use beta-carotene (discussed below) instead of vitamin A.

■ **Beta-carotene:** beta-carotene is recommended for menstruating women because of its similar effects to vitamin A and greater safety:

- called "pro-vitamin A", since it can be converted into vitamin A, beta-carotene is a more powerful antioxidant than vitamin A and also exerts a number of immune-stimulating effects, including enhancing the thymus gland's production T cells. (T cells are part of the immune system's initial strike force, which immediately attack invaders and either prevent their entry into the body or quickly destroy them.)
- dosage: 200,000 IU q.d.

■ **Vitamin C:** if started on the first or second day of infection, large doses of vitamin C have been shown to halt the progression of pneumonia. If administered later, vitamin C lessens the severity of the disease:

- researchers have demonstrated that, during pneumonia, white cells take up large amounts of vitamin C, and that elderly patients hospitalized for pneumonia fare significantly better when given vitamin C.
- in addition to directly killing many bacteria and viruses, vitamin C significantly enhances immune function by:
  - stimulating white cells to fight infection
  - increasing levels of *interferon* (a special chemical factor that fights viral infection and cancer)
  - increasing the secretion of thymus gland hormones that stimulate the maturation and activation of immune cells
  - improving the integrity of the linings of mucous membranes
  - acting as a water-soluble antioxidant and regenerating the fat-soluble antioxidant, vitamin E, after it has been inactivated by disarming free radicals.
- dosage: 500 mg every 2 hours.

- **Bioflavonoids:** a group of plant pigments largely responsible for the colors of fruits and flowers, flavonoids are powerful antioxidants in their own right, and, when taken with vitamin C, significantly enhance its absorption and effectiveness; dosage: 1,000 mg q.d.
- **Vitamin E:** vitamin E is the primary antioxidant protecting all fat-containing structures such as cell membranes and also boosts both types of immune defense: non-specific or cell-mediated immunity and specific or humoral immunity. Cell-mediated immunity is the body's primary mode of protection against bacteria and viruses:
  - patients with pneumonia that develops after influenza, especially those who are seriously ill, have been found to experience a sharp rise in *lipid peroxidation products* (fats damaged by free radicals). Administration of vitamin E results in a significant decrease in free radical damage and an improved clinical response.
  - vitamin E has been shown to significantly boost immune function in the elderly. In a study of 88 patients over age 65, supplementation with 200 IU q.d. of vitamin E for 235 days increased T-cell function by 58%.
  - dosage: 200 IU mixed tocopherols q.d.
- **Zinc:** the most important mineral for immune function, zinc inhibits the growth of several viruses, promotes the destruction of foreign particles and micro-organisms, protects against free radical damage, acts synergistically with vitamin A, is required for proper white blood cell function, and is necessary for the activation of serum thymic factor – a thymus hormone with profound immune-enhancing properties:
  - in elderly subjects, zinc supplementation has been shown to result in increased numbers of T cells and enhanced cell-mediated immune responses.
  - dosage: 30 mg q.d.; zinc picolinate is recommended as this form is better absorbed.
- **Thymus extract:** the thymus gland secretes a family of hormones that act on white cells to ensure their proper development and function:
  - in double-blind studies, orally administered thymus extracts have been shown to not only eliminate respiratory infection, but in children with recurrent respiratory infection, continued thymus extract supplementation over the course of a year also reduced the number of respiratory infections and significantly improved immune function.
  - dosage: equivalent of 120 mg of pure polypeptides with molecular weights less than 10,000, or roughly 500 mg of the crude polypeptide fraction q.d.

- **Bromelain:** bromelain is a mixture of enzymes found in pineapple whose effectiveness in reducing inflammation is well documented:
  - bromelain is particularly effective in pneumonia as a result of its ability to dissolve mucus, increase tissue drainage, and enhance antibiotic absorption.
  - dosage: 250–750 mg (1,800–2,000 MCU) taken between meals t.i.d.

Botanical medicines

For all types of pneumonia
- ***Lobelia inflata* (Indian tobacco):** lobelia is an effective expectorant and also relaxes the airways:
  - dosage: choose one of the following forms and take the recommended dosage t.i.d.:
    - dried herb: 0.2–0.6 g
    - tincture: 15–30 drops
    - fluid extract: 8–10 drops
- ***Echinacea* species:** the two most widely used species are *Echinacea angustifolia* and *Echinacea purpurea*, both of which exert numerous immune-enhancing effects:
  - one of *Echinacea*'s most important immune-stimulating components is *inulin*, a large polysaccharide that activates the *alternative complement pathway*, part of the immune system's first line of defense, and increases the production of immune chemicals that activate macrophages. The result is increased activity of many key immune parameters: production of T cells, macrophage phagocytosis, antibody binding, natural killer cell activity, and levels of circulating neutrophils.
  - in addition to immune support, echinacea is directly antiviral and helps prevent bacterial infection by inhibiting the bacterial enzyme *hyaluronidase*. Bacteria secrete hyaluronidase to break through the body's first line of defense – its protective membranes such as the skin or mucous membranes – so the bacteria can enter the body.
  - choose one of the following forms and take the recommended dosage t.i.d.:
    - dried root or as tea: 0.5–1 g
    - freeze-dried plant: 325–650 mg
    - juice of aerial portion of *E. purpurea* stabilized in 22% ethanol: 2–3 ml
    - tincture (1 : 5): 2–4 ml
    - fluid extract (1 : 1): 2–4 ml
    - solid (dry powdered) extract (6.5 : 1 or 3.5% echinacoside): 150–300 mg.

For streptococcal pneumonia
- ***Hydrastis canadensis* (goldenseal):** goldenseal is a remarkably safe and effective natural antibiotic.

Its most active alkaloid constituent, berberine sulfate, exhibits a broad range of antibiotic action against a wide variety of bacteria (including streptococci), protozoa and fungi. Its action against some of these pathogens is actually stronger than that of commonly used antibiotics, but unlike antibiotic drugs, goldenseal does not destroy the friendly protective bacteria in the intestines:

■ berberine is a more effective antimicrobial agent in an alkaline environment. Alkalinity can be increased by consuming fewer animal products and more plant foods, especially fruits. Although most fruits are acidic, digestion uses up their acid components leaving behind an alkaline residue.

■ choose one of the following forms and take the recommended dosage t.i.d. (the dosage should be based on berberine content, and standardized extracts are recommended):
  ● dried root or as infusion (tea): 2–4 g
  ● tincture (1 : 5): 6–12 ml (1.5–3 tsp)
  ● fluid extract (1 : 1): 2–4 ml (0.5–1 tsp)
  ● solid (dry powdered) extract (4 : 1 or 8–12% alkaloid content): 250–500 mg.

For viral pneumonia

■ ***Glycyrrhiza glabra* (licorice root):** licorice is antiviral, anti-inflammatory, and an effective expectorant. Glycyrrhiza can, however, also lessen coughing. If the cough is productive, use lobelia (discussed above) instead:
  ■ dosage: choose one of the following forms and take the recommended dosage t.i.d.:
    ● powdered root: 1–2 g
    ● fluid extract (1 : 1): 2–4 ml
    ● solid (dry powdered) extract (4 : 1): 250–500 mg.

Drug–herb interaction cautions
■ ***Glycyrrhiza glabra* (licorice):**
  ■ plus *digoxin, digitalis*: due to a reduction of potassium in the blood, licorice enhances the toxicity of cardiac glycosides. Interaction with these cardiac glycoside drugs could lead to arrhythmias and cardiac arrest.
  ■ plus *stimulant laxatives or diuretics* (thiazides, spironolactone or amiloride): licorice should not be used with these drugs because of the additive increase of potassium loss to potentially dangerous levels.

Premenstrual syndrome

DESCRIPTION

Premenstrual syndrome (PMS) is a recurrent condition in menstruating women, characterized by a wide range of troublesome physical and emotional symptoms that arise during the week or two before menstruation, but usually cease when the menstrual flow begins. Common physical symptoms include tender, swollen breasts; headache; backache; abdominal bloating; fluid retention causing puffiness in ankles, fingers and face; decreased energy level; acne outbreaks; and higher incidence of minor infections such as colds. Common emotional symptoms include irritability, nervousness, depression, mood swings, and altered (decreased or increased) sex drive.

Between 30 and 40% of menstruating women are affected by PMS, primarily during their 30s and 40s. Most experience only mild symptoms, but for about 10%, symptoms can be severe enough to affect work and social relationships.

All PMS symptoms stem from some abnormality in the complex hormonal changes that occur in a woman's body during the menstrual cycle. Each month during a woman's reproductive years, various hormones are secreted to ensure that only a single egg is released by the ovaries that month, and to prepare the *endometrium* (the lining of the uterus) for implantation of the fertilized egg. The hormonal secretions that occur to achieve these goals are controlled by complex interactions between the hypothalamus, pituitary, and ovaries. The hypothalamus, a region of the brain in the middle of the head just behind the eyes, controls the female hormonal system by releasing hormones – such as gonadotropin-releasing hormone (GnRH) and follicle-stimulating hormone-releasing hormone (FSH-RH) – which stimulate the release of pituitary hormones. In response to the hormones secreted by the hypothalamus, the pituitary gland then releases follicle-stimulating hormone (FSH) and luteinizing hormone (LH).

FSH, the hormone released by the pituitary during the first phase of the menstrual cycle, is primarily responsible for the maturation of an egg (*ovum*). Follicle-stimulating hormone is so named because each egg is housed inside an individual follicle within the ovary. As the follicle grows, estrogen levels increase, triggering the secretion of LH, the hormone responsible for initiating *ovulation* – the release of the fully developed egg. After ovulation, the now eggless follicle is transformed into the *corpus luteum*, which secretes progesterone and estrogen to help a fertilized egg become well established in the uterine lining. If fertilization does not occur, the corpus luteum recedes, hormone production decreases, and, approximately 2 weeks later, the lining is shed in the menstrual flow, and the entire process begins anew.

The normal menstrual cycle, which is completed in about 1 month, is divided into three phases, in order of occurrence: follicular, ovulatory, and luteal. The follicular phase lasts 10–14 days, the ovulatory phase when the egg is released lasts about 36 hours, and the luteal phase lasts for about 14 days.

Because of the complex interrelationships among the components of the *endocrine system* (a group of glands that secrete hormones, including the adrenals, thyroid, parathyroid and pancreas as well as the hypothalamus, pituitary, and ovaries), a disorder in any of these glands can affect hormone secretion and lead to menstrual abnormalities and/or PMS. For example, *hypothyroidism* (low thyroid function) and elevated *cortisol* (an adrenal hormone) are common in PMS. Elevated levels of *prolactin* (another hormone produced by the pituitary that regulates the development of the mammary gland and milk secretion during and after pregnancy) also play a role in PMS and infertility. In *non-lactating* women (women who are not producing milk), prolactin can inhibit maturation of the follicles in the ovaries and has been linked to PMS, menstrual abnormalities, absence of ovulation, ovarian cysts, and breast tenderness. Common hormonal patterns have been found in women with PMS that differ from those of women with no PMS symptoms.

The primary hormonal abnormality is that estrogen levels are elevated and plasma progesterone levels are reduced during the luteal phase of the menstrual cycle, 5–10 days before menses, or the ratio of estrogen to progesterone is increased.

Many researchers theorize that PMS reflects corpus luteum insufficiency. In addition to PMS, corpus luteum insufficiency has been linked to abnormal menstruation (excessive blood loss; absent, persistent, or more frequent menstruation), elevations in prolactin level, and low thyroid function. Corpus luteum insufficiency is usually diagnosed by measuring the level of progesterone in the blood 3 weeks after the onset of menstruation. If the level is below 10–12 ng/mg, corpus luteum insufficiency is a strong possibility.

Hypothyroidism and/or elevated prolactin levels are also common, FSH levels are typically elevated 6–9 days prior to the onset of menses, and *aldosterone* (a hormone produced by the adrenal glands that leads to sodium and water retention) levels are marginally elevated 2–8 days prior to the onset of menses.

In an attempt to bring some order to the clinical complexities of PMS, it has been classified into four distinct subgroups, each of which is linked to predominant symptoms, hormonal patterns, and metabolic abnormalities. However, women rarely fit into only one subgroup, and instead, usually experience symptoms related to two or more of the following subgroups:

- **PMS-A (A = anxiety):** the most common symptom category, PMS-A is associated with excessive estrogen and deficient progesterone levels during the premenstrual phase. Common symptoms are anxiety, irritability, and emotional instability.
- **PMS-C (C = carbohydrate cravings):** PMS-C is associated with increased appetite, craving for sweets, headache, fatigue, fainting spells, and heart palpitations. Glucose tolerance tests (GTT) performed during the 5–10 days before menses show a flattening of the early part of the curve (which usually implies excessive secretion of insulin in response to sugar consumption). This increased binding capacity for insulin appears to be hormonally regulated, but other factors including high salt intake, decreased levels of magnesium or hormone-like compounds called *prostaglandins* may also be involved.
- **PMS-D (D = depression):** the least common type, PMS-D is associated with depression, occasional crying fits, forgetfulness, mild mental confusion, and episodes of insomnia. Depression, the key symptom, is usually associated with low levels of neurotransmitters in the central nervous system, which may, in turn, be due to increased neurotransmitter breakdown as a result of decreased output of estrogen by the ovaries (in contrast to PMS-A, which shows the opposite results). The decrease in ovarian estrogen output has been attributed to a stress-induced increase in adrenal androgen and/or progesterone secretion.
- **PMS-H (H = hyperhydration):** PMS-H is characterized by weight gain (greater than 1.3 kg [3 lb]), abdominal bloating and discomfort, breast tenderness and congestion, and occasional swelling of the face, hands, and ankles. Symptoms are the result of an excess of the hormone aldosterone, which causes increased fluid retention. Aldosterone excess may be caused by stress, estrogen excess, magnesium deficiency, or excess salt intake.

By analyzing the symptoms and relating them to their probable subgroup(s) and cause(s) an effective treatment plan tailored to specific needs can be developed with physician guidance.

FREQUENT SIGNS AND SYMPTOMS

Use the menstrual symptom questionnaire on the next page as a diary to help clarify the symptom pattern and document improvements.

CAUSES

Excess estrogen
One of the most common findings in women with PMS is an elevated estrogen-to-progesterone ratio, typically, mild estrogen excess combined with mild progesterone deficiency. This derangement contributes to PMS by leading to the following impairments:

- **Impaired liver function:** the liver is responsible for detoxifying estrogen and excreting it in the bile. When bile flow is diminished, a condition medically labeled *cholestasis*, estrogen detoxification and clearance are reduced. Since excess estrogen itself causes cholestasis, a vicious cycle is induced. In addition to estrogen excess, the following also cause cholestasis and can therefore promote estrogen excess:
  - alcohol
  - anabolic steroids
  - endotoxins (internally produced toxic by-products of metabolism)
  - birth control pills
  - hereditary disorders, such as *Gilbert's syndrome* (a thyroid disorder)
  - pregnancy
  - presence of gallstones
  - various chemicals or drugs.
- **Reduced neurotransmitter synthesis:** *neurotransmitters* are compounds that transmit nerve impulses. An increase in the estrogen-to-progesterone ratio results in the impairment of neurotransmitter manufacture, contributing to depression and insomnia:
  - one group of neurotransmitters, the *monoamines*, includes *serotonin*, a lack of which negatively affects mood, and *melatonin*, which is integral to sleep.

Menstrual symptom questionnaire/diary

Date: _____

Grading of symptoms
1. None
2. Mild – present but does not interfere with activities
3. Moderate – present and interferes with activities but not disabling
4. Severe – disabling (unable to function)

Grade your symptoms for last menstrual cycle only.

Subgroup	Symptoms	Week after period	Week before period
PMS-A	Nervous tension	_____	_____
	Mood swings	_____	_____
	Irritability	_____	_____
	Anxiety	_____	_____
	Total:	_____	_____
PMS-C	Headache	_____	_____
	Craving for sweets	_____	_____
	Increased appetite	_____	_____
	Heart pounding	_____	_____
	Fatigue	_____	_____
	Dizziness or fainting	_____	_____
	Total:	_____	_____
PMS-D	Depression	_____	_____
	Forgetfulness	_____	_____
	Crying	_____	_____
	Confusion	_____	_____
	Insomnia	_____	_____
	Total:	_____	_____
PMS-H	Weight gain	_____	_____
	Swelling of extremities	_____	_____
	Breast tenderness	_____	_____
	Abdominal bloating	_____	_____
	Total:	_____	_____
	Total MSQ score:	_____	_____
Other symptoms	Oily skin	_____	_____
	Acne	_____	_____
During first 2 days of period	Menstrual cramps	_____	_____
	Menstrual backache	_____	_____

- the majority of the more than 12 million patients on Prozac (an antidepressant drug that increases serotonin levels in the brain, but has numerous, potentially dangerous side effects) are women between the ages of 25 and 50 – the same population that has a high frequency of PMS.

- in women with PMS, the use of natural therapies to normalize the estrogen-to-progesterone ratio (which, unlike Prozac, have only beneficial effects) may resolve the monoamine imbalances conventionally treated with antidepressant drugs.

- **Reduced endorphin levels:** *endorphins* are the body's own mood-elevating and pain-relieving substances. When the estrogen-to-progesterone ratio increases, endorphin levels decline:

  - low endorphin levels during the luteal phase are common in women with PMS.
  - endorphin levels are lowered by stress and raised by exercise.

■ **Decreased action of vitamin B$_6$:** the negative impact of estrogen excess on neurotransmitter and endorphin levels during the luteal phase may be secondary to estrogen's impairment of vitamin B$_6$ action:

- estrogens negatively affect vitamin B$_6$ function.
- vitamin B$_6$ – which is involved in the formation of red blood cells, hormone-like compounds called prostaglandins, neurotransmitters and endorphins – is critical to maintaining hormonal balance.
- vitamin B$_6$ levels are typically quite low in depressed patients, particularly women taking estrogens (birth control pills or Premarin).
- supplementation with vitamin B$_6$ has been shown to improve all PMS symptoms, especially depression, by reducing mid-luteal estrogen levels while increasing mid-luteal progesterone levels.

■ **Hypothyroidism:** another component of the interactive endocrine system, the thyroid gland secretes hormones that regulate metabolic rate. The hormone primarily secreted by the thyroid, T$_4$, is inactive until it is converted, largely in the liver, to its active form, T$_3$:

- excess estrogens, both internally produced and ingested (as birth control pills, Premarin, hormone residues in meat and dairy products, or estrogenic pesticide residues in foods) can impair liver function, thus decreasing conversion of T$_4$ to T$_3$.
- several studies have shown that a large percentage of women with PMS have low thyroid function, and many women with both PMS and confirmed hypothyroidism have experienced complete relief of symptoms when given thyroid hormone.
- hypothyroidism, depression, and PMS are metabolically linked:
  - a recent study indicates that both T$_3$ and L-tryptophan (the dietary amino acid that the body uses to produce serotonin, a neurotransmitter that is important for feelings of well-being) are taken up by red blood cells using the same carrier.
  - since vitamin B$_6$ is needed for the formation of red blood cells, when B$_6$ levels are low, neither T$_3$ nor L-tryptophan will be adequately circulated.

■ **Increased aldosterone secretion:** estrogen excess increases secretion of aldosterone, a hormone produced by the adrenal glands that leads to retention of sodium and water:

- in many cases of PMS, aldosterone levels are elevated 2–8 days prior to onset of menses.

■ **Increased prolactin secretion:** estrogens, both internally produced and ingested (as birth control pills or Premarin, hormone residues in meat and dairy products, or estrogenic pesticide residues in foods),

increase prolactin secretion by the pituitary gland:

- in women with breast pain or fibrocystic breast disease, elevated levels of prolactin are specifically implicated.
- prolactin levels also tend to be elevated in cases of low thyroid function.

Progesterone deficiency

Although the adrenal cortex makes some progesterone, it is mainly used as a precursor in the production of *corticosteroid hormones* (see Stress and adrenal dysfunction immediately below). The body's supply of progesterone is primarily derived from the corpus luteum, which is produced after ovulation from the empty follicle. If ovulation does not occur, no corpus luteum will develop to secrete progesterone, thus leading to an imbalance in the estrogen-to-progesterone ratio.

■ Ovulation is triggered as a result of complex interactions between the hypothalamus, pituitary, and ovaries. Any disruption in this hormonal symphony from, for example, stress, illness, intense physical activity, emotional or psychological difficulties, can prevent ovulation.

■ Ovulation naturally begins to decline when a woman reaches her 30s, and by the mid-30s, *anovulatory* (without ovulation) cycles are common. Since no corpus luteum is formed, no progesterone is secreted, and estrogen, essentially unopposed, dominates the hormonal environment.

■ In addition to the corpus luteum, over 5000 plants have been identified as producing sterols with progestogenic effects, but when foods are processed or consumed days after being picked – as is typical of the food supply in the US – their sterol levels drop precipitously. The result is that our diets do not provide sufficient progestogenic substances to help offset the natural decline in progesterone that accompanies aging.

Stress and adrenal dysfunction

Progesterone is a major precursor of corticosteroid hormones made by the adrenal glands. These hormones are responsible for mineral balance, sugar control, and our capacity to respond to all types of stressors including emotional stress, inflammation, and trauma. A lack of corticosteroids can lead to fatigue, immune dysfunction, hypoglycemia, allergies, and arthritis.

■ Constant stress increases the demand for corticosteroid production, exhausting the adrenal glands and using all the progesterone they produce to make corticosteroids.

■ Eventually, the overworked adrenal glands become so depleted they cannot even make enough progesterone to keep up with the demand for corticosteroids. Should ovulation occur, since the body places a higher premium on immediate survival needs than reproduction, much of the progesterone produced will be also shunted into corticosteroid production. The outcome is a hormonal imbalance in which lack of sufficient progesterone results in estrogen dominance.

Depression

Elevations in the level of the corticosteroid hormone cortisol are typical in depression and reflect a disturbance in the control mechanisms for adrenal function that reside in the hypothalamus and pituitary glands.

As explained under Stress and adrenal dysfunction (immediately above), excessive cortisol production depletes progesterone, thus promoting estrogen dominance and PMS.

Macronutrient excesses and micronutrient deficiency

Women who suffer from PMS typically have a low-fiber, high-fat, high-sugar diet that is even worse than the Standard American Diet (SAD).

- Compared to symptom-free women, PMS patients consume: 62% more refined carbohydrates, 275% more refined sugar, 79% more dairy products, 78% more sodium, 53% less manganese, and 52% less zinc.
- A low-fiber diet contributes to estrogen retention and recirculation:
  - fiber promotes the excretion of estrogens both directly, by binding to estrogens prepared for excretion, and indirectly, because fiber is the preferred food of beneficial bacteria in the gut. These friendly bacteria produce only a tiny amount of the enzyme *beta-glucuronidase* that recycles estrogen, in contrast to unfriendly bacteria, which produce a lot of beta-glucuronidase.
  - beta-glucuronidase breaks the bond between estrogen and *glucuronic acid* – a carrier that is attached to estrogen in the liver to prepare it for excretion via the bile, which is then secreted into the small intestine.
  - when friendly bacteria, which depend on fiber as their food source, colonize the intestines, they supplant the unfriendly bacteria that produce beta-glucuronidase.
  - supplementation with friendly bacteria (see Nutritional supplements below) along with a high-fiber diet can reduce beta-glucuronidase activity.
- A diet high in fat, particularly saturated fat, and/or sugar has been shown to significantly increase levels

of circulating estrogens:
  - foods high in simple sugars not only impair estrogen metabolism, but also stress blood sugar control and, particularly when combined with caffeine, have a detrimental effect on mood in women with PMS.
  - in one study, when 17 women switched from the SAD diet (40% of calories as fat, 12 g of fiber q.d.) to a low-fat, high-fiber diet (25% of calories as fat, 40 g of fiber), their blood estrogen levels dropped 36% in 8–10 weeks.
- Excessive salt consumption, especially when coupled with low intake of foods rich in potassium (fresh fruits and vegetables, whole grains, and beans), greatly stresses the kidneys' ability to maintain proper fluid volume, resulting in fluid retention.
- The micronutrients most important in PMS are discussed below under Nutritional supplements.

RISK INCREASES WITH

- **Stress:** increases cortisol production, further depleting progesterone.
- **Lack of exercise:** exercise decreases cortisol levels and increases endorphin levels.
- **SAD (Standard American Diet):** the SAD is high in refined carbohydrates, sugar, salt, fat, and caffeine – factors that impair estrogen metabolism, leading to an increase in circulating estrogen levels; have detrimental effects on mood; and promote water retention. In addition, the SAD is low in vegetables, fruits, whole grains, nuts and seeds, and legumes – the sources of the fiber, essential fatty acids, vitamins and minerals necessary for proper hormone metabolism.
- **Depression:** elevations in the stress-induced hormone cortisol are typical, and since progesterone is used to produce cortisol, an increase in cortisol production results in a decrease in progesterone.
- **Perimenopause:** during the years preceding menopause, anovulatory cycles increase and estrogen levels may fluctuate widely, further stressing a woman's physical and emotional equilibrium.
- **Hypothyroidism:** PMS and hypothyroidism can result from the same metabolic dysfunctions, e.g., cholestasis (impaired liver function) promotes estrogen retention and recirculation and lessens the conversion of T_4 to T_3, the active form of thyroid hormone.
- **Gilbert's syndrome:** a type of hypothyroidism.
- **Gallstones:** indicate cholestasis.
- **Alcohol consumption:** alcohol dehydrates the body and leads to fluctuations in blood sugar levels that aggravate many premenstrual problems.

- **Birth control pills:** increase estrogen levels.
- **Smoking:** among its many harmful effects, cigarette smoke contains numerous toxic chemicals that place a significant burden on the liver.
- **Caffeine:** particularly in sensitive individuals, caffeine causes fluctuations in blood sugar levels, increasing adrenal stress and carbohydrate cravings.
- **Frequent digestive disturbances:** frequent bloating and/or gas suggests that unfriendly bacteria, which promote the reabsorption of estrogen from the intestines, are present in the digestive tract.
- **Constipation:** increases the time during which estrogen can be reabsorbed.

PREVENTIVE MEASURES

- Exercise regularly.
- Don't smoke.
- Minimize consumption of caffeine: if anxiety or depression, or breast tenderness or fibrocystic breast disease are major symptoms, avoid all sources of caffeine, including coffee, tea, chocolate, and caffeinated sodas.
- Minimize consumption of alcohol: alcohol should be consumed no more than three times per week in the amount of no more than 350 ml (12 US fl oz) of beer, 140 ml (4–5 US fl oz) of wine, or 45 ml (1.5 US fl oz) of distilled spirits.
- Avoid salt.
- Consume a nutrient-dense fiber-rich diet based on whole, minimally processed, preferably organic foods, especially plant foods (fruits, vegetables, beans [particularly soybeans], seeds and nuts [particularly flaxseed and walnuts], and whole grains) and cold-water fish, and low in animal products and refined foods (for more detailed information, see Appendix 1).
- Take a high-potency daily multiple vitamin and mineral supplement to ensure basic micronutrient needs are met. This should include 400 µg of folic acid, 400 µg of vitamin B_{12}, and 50–100 mg of vitamin B_6. Folic acid supplementation should always be accompanied by vitamin B_{12} supplementation to prevent folic acid from masking a vitamin B_{12} deficiency (for more information on what a good daily multiple should contain, see Appendix 2).
- If using birth control pills, discuss alternative methods of contraception with a health care provider.

Expected outcomes

Significant improvement should be noted within two to three menstrual cycles.

The first month may be devoted to clarifying which PMS subset(s) match the characteristics of the symptoms while following the general recommendations outlined in Preventive Measures.

During the second month, an individualized program targeted at the underlying causes should result in a lessening of symptoms.

By the third menstrual cycle, the hormonal and nutritional imbalances identified as contributing to the PMS symptoms should resolve.

TREATMENT

- Evaluate PMS symptoms by completing the symptom diary above.
- Rule out hypothyroidism: determine basal body temperature (discussed in the chapter on Hypothyroidism). If this is below 97.8°F, or if suffering from other symptoms associated with PMS, consult with a physician for complete thyroid function testing.
- Rule out depression: review the symptoms discussed in the chapter on Affective disorders: depression. If four or more of the eight symptoms listed have been present for a month or more, follow the recommendations given in that chapter.
- Follow the dietary recommendations given below.
- Select the appropriate herbal support.
- Get regular exercise.
- Avoid excessive stress as much as possible by avoiding excessive work hours, poor nutrition, and inadequate rest.

Diet
- **Follow a vegetarian or predominantly vegetarian diet:** vegetarian women have been shown to excrete two to three times more estrogen in their feces and have 50% lower levels of estrogen in their blood than omnivorous women:
  - these differences are thought to result from the lower fat and higher fiber intake of a vegetarian diet and may also explain the lower incidence of breast cancer, heart disease and menopausal symptoms in vegetarian women.
- **Increase consumption of soy foods:** soy foods contain *phytoestrogens* (plant estrogens) whose estrogenic effect is only 2% as strong as that of human estrogens. When these phytoestrogens bind to estrogen receptors, they prevent human estrogens from doing so, thus decreasing overall estrogenic effects.
- **Eat less saturated fat and cholesterol** by reducing or eliminating meat and dairy products. Avoid the hydrogenated or *trans* fats in margarine and many

processed foods:

- a diet low in fat, especially saturated fat, has been shown to dramatically reduce circulating estrogen levels – changing from a diet composed of 40% of calories as fat and only 12 g of fiber to a diet consisting of 25% of calories as fat and 40 g of fiber daily resulted in a 36% reduction in blood estrogen levels in 8–10 weeks.
- a low-fat diet has also been shown to relieve PMS symptoms.
- saturated and *trans* fats are used to produce the types of prostaglandins that promote inflammation and pain.

■ **Limit consumption of animal protein sources** to 110–175 g (4–6 oz) q.d.:

- eliminate red meat, which promotes the absorption of estrogen from the intestines.
- choose wild-caught cold-water fish, such as salmon, several times a week. In addition to protein, cold-water fish contain anti-inflammatory omega-3 fats. Wild-caught is preferred over farm-raised since wild fish contain higher amounts of omega-3 fats.
- if eating chicken, remove the skin, preferably before cooking.

■ **Increase consumption of fiber-rich plant foods** (fruits, vegetables, grains, legumes): a higher intake of dietary fiber promotes the excretion of estrogens both directly and indirectly by nourishing the friendly intestinal bacteria that produce lower levels of beta-glucuronidase (the enzyme that frees estrogen bound for excretion and sends it back into circulation).

■ **Eliminate high-sugar foods:**

- when high-sugar foods are eaten alone, blood sugar levels rise quickly, producing a strain on blood sugar control.
- sugar, especially when combined with caffeine, has a detrimental effect on PMS and mood. The most significant symptom-producing food in PMS appears to be chocolate, which contains sugar, saturated fat and caffeine.
- a high intake of sugar impairs estrogen metabolism and is associated with higher estrogen levels and higher frequency of PMS.
- read food labels carefully. Sugar can appear as sucrose, glucose, maltose, lactose, fructose, corn syrup, or white grape juice concentrate.

■ **Eliminate caffeine:** especially if anxiety or depression, or breast tenderness and fibrocystic breast disease are major symptoms. Considerable evidence shows that caffeine consumption is strongly related to the presence and severity of PMS (caffeine is found in sodas, chocolate, and tea, as well as coffee).

■ **Monitor salt and potassium consumption:** keep salt intake below 1,800 mg and increase intake of foods high in potassium. Excessive salt consumption, especially when coupled with diminished dietary potassium, stresses the kidneys' ability to maintain proper fluid volume, leading to fluid retention and, in sensitive individuals, high blood pressure:

- if water retention is a problem, consuming potassium-rich foods can have a beneficial diuretic effect.
- potassium is found in fresh fruits, vegetables (especially green leafy vegetables), whole grains, and beans.
- salt (as sodium) is found in most processed foods.

■ **Reduce exposure to environmental estrogens in food:** a variety of toxic pesticides including DDT, DDE, PCB, PCP, dieldrin, and chlordane are known to mimic estrogen in the body and are thought to be a major factor in the growing epidemics of estrogen-related health problems including PMS, breast cancer and low sperm counts:

- these chemicals are hard to break down and are stored in fat cells – another reason to avoid meat, cheese, whole milk, and eggs.
- whenever possible, choose organically grown foods. Even in conventionally grown produce, however, the presence of pesticides in fruits and vegetables is much lower than levels found in animal products, plus the various antioxidant compounds of fruits and vegetables help the body deal with the pesticides.
- for additional information on lowering dietary pesticide levels see Appendix 1.

■ **Eat small meals** at regular intervals throughout the day to keep blood sugar on an even keel.

Nutritional supplements

■ **A high-potency multiple vitamin and mineral supplement:** this should include 400 μg of folic acid, 400 μg of vitamin B_{12}, and 50–100 mg of vitamin B_6. (folic acid supplementation should always be accompanied by vitamin B_{12} supplementation to prevent folic acid from masking a vitamin B_{12} deficiency):

- many PMS symptoms are caused by deficiencies of the nutrients needed for normal hormonal regulation. A daily multiple providing all of the known vitamins and minerals provides a foundation upon which to build an individualized PMS treatment program.

■ **Vitamin B_6:** in the early 1970s, vitamin B_6 was successfully used to treat depression caused by birth control pills, and since then, the effectiveness of vitamin B_6 in relieving PMS has been studied in at least a dozen double-blind clinical trials:

- although vitamin B_6 supplementation alone was found to benefit most PMS patients, some did not improve. These negative results may result from the inability of some women to convert B_6 to its active form (pyridoxal-5-phosphate) because of a deficiency in another nutrient needed for the conversion (e.g., riboflavin or magnesium) that was not supplemented.
- to overcome this potential conversion problem, supplementation with a multiple vitamin and mineral as described above is recommended. In addition, vitamin B_6 can be supplemented in its active form (pyridoxal-5-phosphate).
- **caution:** one-time doses of greater than 2,000 mg q.d. can produce symptoms of nerve toxicity in some individuals:
  - chronic intake of more than 500 mg of B_6 q.d. can be toxic over many months or years.
  - although quite rare, toxicity has been reported at chronic long-term dosages as low as 150 mg q.d.
  - toxicity is thought to result from supplemental pyridoxine overwhelming the liver's ability to add a phosphate group to produce the active form of vitamin B_6 (pyridoxal-5-phosphate).
- dosage ranges: to err on the side of safety, limit doses of pyridoxine to no more than 50 mg at a time; if more than 50 mg q.d. is desired, spread doses throughout the day.

- **Magnesium:** magnesium plays such an integral part in normal cellular function that magnesium deficiency alone can account for many of the symptoms attributed to PMS, and red blood cell magnesium levels have been shown to be significantly lower in PMS patients than normal subjects:
  - estrogen increases the uptake of magnesium in bone and soft tissues (which helps to explain why estrogen protects young women against osteoporosis and heart disease, as well as women's increased risk of these diseases during and after menopause when estrogen levels drop). However, when estrogen levels are too high, as they frequently are in PMS, too much magnesium is transferred into bone and soft tissue, leaving too little available for many types of cells to function normally.
  - magnesium stabilizes cellular membranes, activates more than 300 cellular enzymes, and is involved in the production of ATP, the energy currency of the body.
  - magnesium interacts extensively with vitamin B_6 in many enzyme systems and is also dependent upon B_6 to gain entry into cells. One of the primary ways

in which vitamin B_6 relieves symptoms of PMS is by increasing levels of magnesium within cells.
- a low magnesium state triggers cells to release stress hormones and other substances that promote inflammation and pain, and can impair circulation.
- four independent studies have now confirmed that intracellular magnesium is chronically depleted in women with PMS and that it is a major predisposing factor to luteal-phase emotional instability, excessive nervous sensitivity, generalized aches and pains, and a lower premenstrual pain threshold.
- supplementation with magnesium alone has been shown to dramatically reduce PMS-related mood changes, nervousness, breast tenderness and weight gain.
- in several studies, when PMS patients were given a multivitamin and mineral containing high doses of both magnesium and vitamin B_6, they experienced a tremendous reduction in PMS symptoms.
- dosage: 12 mg/kg (2.2 lb) body weight (for example, a 110-lb woman would take 600 mg since 110 divided by $2.2 = 50 \times 12 = 600$):
  - magnesium bound to aspartate or one of the Krebs cycle intermediates (malate, succinate, fumarate, or citrate) is preferred since these forms are better absorbed and have fewer laxative side effects.
  - for best results, magnesium should be taken with vitamin B_6.

- **Calcium:** women with PMS frequently have reduced bone mineral density, and studies have shown improvements in mood, concentration, and lowered water retention with supplementation of calcium and manganese (1,336 mg and 5.6 mg, respectively):
  - animal research suggests that calcium improves altered hormonal patterns, neurotransmitter levels, and smooth muscle responsiveness in PMS.
  - **caution:** high calcium intake due to high milk consumption is a possible causative factor of PMS via the amalgamation of calcium with vitamin D and phosphorous in milk since this combination reduces the absorption of magnesium.
  - dosage: 1,000–1,336 mg q.d. Calcium bound to citrate (or other Krebs cycle intermediate such as fumarate, malate, succinate or aspartate) is recommended. These forms, which are already ionized and soluble, are therefore much better absorbed than calcium carbonate:
    - avoid calcium derived from oyster shells, dolomite or bone meal; studies have indicated that these calcium supplements may contain substantial amounts of lead, a toxic metal that

primarily affects the brain, kidney and manufacture of red blood cells.

- calcium hydroxyapatite, which is basically a purified bone meal, should also be avoided. Not only is it derived from bone meal (a high lead source of calcium), but comparison studies have also shown that it is not as well absorbed (only 20% absorption) as either calcium carbonate or calcium citrate (both of which have a 30% absorption rate).

■ **Zinc:** in women with PMS, zinc levels have been shown to be low:
  ▨ zinc is involved in the control of hormone secretion and is required for the proper action of many hormones, including sex hormones:
    - specifically, zinc is one of the control factors for prolactin secretion – low zinc levels promote prolactin release; high zinc levels inhibit prolactin release.
    - high prolactin levels have been correlated with PMS symptoms.
  ▨ zinc is particularly helpful in lessening premenstrual acne.
  ▨ dosage: for general health, 15 mg of zinc picolinate (a well-absorbed form) q.d. If prolactin levels are elevated, take 30–45 mg of zinc picolinate q.d.:
    - take zinc with food to prevent stomach upset.
    - if taking more than 30 mg q.d. for more than 1 month, also take 1–2 mg of copper q.d. to maintain proper mineral balance. (This amount of copper should be present in the daily multiple.)

■ **Vitamin E:** double-blind studies have demonstrated significant reductions in breast tenderness, weight gain, anxiety, headaches, cravings for sweets, depression, insomnia, and fatigue with vitamin E supplementation. Higher energy levels have also been noted:
  ▨ dosage: 400 IU q.d. of natural mixed tocopherols.
  ▨ **caution:** avoid D-alpha-tocopherol, which is synthetic vitamin E.

■ **Flaxseed oil:** women with PMS frequently exhibit essential fatty acid and prostaglandin abnormalities. The abnormality most often reported is a decrease in gamma-linolenic acid (GLA):
  ▨ GLA is derived from linoleic acid in a conversion that requires adequate vitamin B_6, magnesium, and zinc levels, as these nutrients are all necessary components of delta-6-desaturase, the key enzyme responsible for the conversion.
  ▨ studies using GLA supplements in the forms of evening primrose oil, blackcurrant, and borage oil have, however, failed to show benefits. A better approach is to provide the nutrients necessary for proper essential fatty acid metabolism along with

an excellent source of essential fatty acids, such as flaxseed oil.
  ▨ dosage: 1 tbsp q.d. Flaxseed oil, which is highly perishable, should be packaged in an opaque container, always be refrigerated, and never heated. A delicious, nutty-tasting oil, flaxseed can be enjoyed in place of other oils as a salad dressing, drizzled over bread or vegetables, or added to smoothies.

Botanical medicines

■ *Angelica sinensis* **(dong quai):** angelica, a uterine tonic with beneficial phytoestrogenic effects, is particularly helpful in, in addition to PMS, women who experience painful menstruation (dysmenorrhea). The pre-eminent female remedy in Asia, *Angelica* is used to treat menopausal symptoms (especially hot flashes); painful, abnormal or lack of menstruation; and to assure a healthy pregnancy and delivery:
  ▨ to treat PMS, begin taking *Angelica* on day 14 and continue until menstruation begins.
  ▨ if dysmenorrhea is experienced, continue taking *Angelica* until the menstrual flow has stopped.
  ▨ dosage: choose one of the following forms and take the recommended dosage t.i.d.:
    - powdered root or as tea: 1–2 g
    - tincture (1 : 5): 4 ml (1 tsp)
    - fluid extract: 1 ml (0.25 tsp).

■ *Glycyrrhiza glabra* **(licorice root):** particularly useful in treating water retention associated with PMS, licorice blocks the effects of aldosterone, the adrenal hormone that reduces sodium excretion, thus causing water retention (edema). In addition, licorice lowers estrogen levels, while raising progesterone levels by inhibiting the enzyme responsible for breaking down progesterone:
  ▨ licorice lessens the effects of aldosterone in much the same way that it impacts estrogen, via its chief component, glycyrrhetinic acid, which binds to aldosterone receptors, but its activity is only about one-fourth as strong as aldosterone. The result in cases of high aldosterone (as often occur in PMS) is a lessening of aldosterone's effect.
  ▨ **caution:** if aldosterone levels are normal, chronic ingestion of licorice in large doses can result in symptoms of aldosterone excess – high blood pressure due to sodium and water retention. Prevention of this potential side effect may be possible by following a high-potassium, low-sodium diet (the diet recommended above for PMS). Patients who normally consume high-potassium foods and restrict sodium intake, even those who have high blood pressure and angina,

have been reported to be free of the aldosterone-like side effects of glycyrrhizin:

- to err on the side of safety, licorice should probably not be used by patients with a history of hypertension, renal failure, or who are currently using digitalis preparations.

■ dosage: begin taking licorice on day 14 of the cycle and continue until menstruation begins. Choose one of the following forms and take the recommended dosage t.i.d.:

- powdered root or as tea: 1–2 g
- fluid extract (1 : 1): 4 ml (1 tsp)
- solid (dry powdered) extract (4 : 1): 250–500 mg.

■ ***Cimicifuga racemosa* (black cohosh):** a special extract of *Cimicifuga* standardized to contain 1 mg of triterpenes calculated as 27-deoxyactein per tablet (trade name: Remifemin) has been used in Germany for over 40 years and has been found to be a safe and effective natural alternative to HRT, as well as offering benefits in PMS:

■ in one study of 135 women, Remifemin "performed very well" in reducing feelings of depression, anxiety, tension, and mood swings.

■ black cohosh is also recommended for patients with uterine fibroids.

■ dosage: one tablet containing 4 mg of 27-deoxyactein q.d.–b.i.d.

■ ***Vitex agnus-castus* (chasteberry):** the most popular herbal used in treating PMS in Germany, chasteberry has been evaluated in studies involving more than 1,500 women. One-third of the women experienced complete resolution of their symptoms; another 57% reported significant improvement; 90% reported symptom improvement or resolution:

■ chasteberry, which affects the function of the hypothalamus and pituitary, is able to normalize the secretion of hormones; for example, it reduces the secretion of prolactin and lowers the estrogen-to-progesterone ratio, making it especially useful in cases of prolactin excess or corpus luteum insufficiency.

■ chasteberry is particularly recommended if there is PMS-associated breast pain, infrequent periods, or a history of ovarian cysts.

■ chasteberry may resolve amenorrhea (lack of menstruation) resulting from prolactin excess, but it takes about 3 months for chasteberry to lower prolactin levels.

■ dosage: chasteberry extract (standardized to contain 0.5% agnuside) in tablet or capsule form – 175–225 mg q.d.; as a liquid extract – 2 ml q.d.

Drug–herb interaction cautions

■ ***Glycyrrhiza glabra* (licorice):**

■ plus *digoxin, digitalis*: due to a reduction of potassium in the blood, licorice enhances the toxicity of cardiac glycosides. Interaction with these cardiac glycoside drugs could lead to arrhythmias and cardiac arrest.

■ plus *stimulant laxatives or diuretics* (thiazides, spironolactone or amiloride): licorice should not be used with these drugs because of the additive increase of potassium loss to potentially dangerous levels.

■ ***Vitex agnus-castus* (chasteberry):**

■ plus *birth control pills*: might interfere with efficacy of birth control pills because of its hormone-regulative actions.

Psoriasis

DESCRIPTION

Psoriasis is an extremely common, chronic skin disorder characterized by sharply bordered, thick patches of reddened skin covered with overlapping silvery scales. Although any area of the body may be affected, psoriasis characteristically appears on the scalp, backside of the wrists, elbows, knees, buttocks, ankles, and back; and sites of repeated trauma. In the United States, psoriasis affects an estimated 2–4% of the population, mainly Caucasians. Among Black Americans, psoriasis affects few in tropical zones, but is more common in temperate zones. Psoriasis is common among Japanese Americans, but is rare in American Indians. Psoriasis affects men and women equally, typically first appearing between the ages of 15 and 25 (although onset can occur as early as age 2), and following a pattern of acute flare-ups followed by periods of healing.

In addition to affecting the skin, psoriasis can cause an inflammatory form of arthritis (psoriatic arthritis) and affect the nails, which develop thimble-like indents referred to as "oil drop" stippling.

FREQUENT SIGNS AND SYMPTOMS

- Sharply bordered reddened rash or plaques covered with overlapping silvery scales
- Characteristic locations: the scalp, backside of the wrists, elbows, knees, buttocks, and ankles; and sites of repeated trauma
- Nail involvement results in characteristic "oil drop" stippling (thimble-like appearance)
- Possible arthritis

CAUSES

Abnormally high rate of skin cell replication
Psoriasis is the result of a pile-up of skin cells that have replicated too rapidly for normal shedding to occur.
- In psoriasis, the rate at which skin cells divide is 1,000 times greater than in normal skin.
- Excessive replication is the result of an imbalance in the ratio between two internal compounds that

control the rate at which skin cells divide: cyclic adenosine monophosphate (cAMP) and cyclic guanidine monophosphate (cGMP):
- increased levels of cGMP are associated with increased cell proliferation, while increased levels of cAMP are associated with enhanced cell maturation and decreased cell replication.
- both increased cGMP and decreased cAMP have been measured in the skin of individuals with psoriasis.

cGMP : cAMP ratio
The imbalance in the cGMP : cAMP ratio may be caused by the following.
- **A genetic error** in the control of how skin cells divide.
- **Incomplete protein digestion:**
  - when protein is not properly digested and absorbed, the undigested amino acids and polypeptides are metabolized by bowel bacteria into toxic compounds that unbalance the cGMP : cAMP ratio.
  - the toxic metabolites formed from the amino acids arginine and ornithine are called polyamines (examples include putrescine, cadaverine, spermidine).
  - polyamines inhibit the formation of cAMP, the compound associated with cell maturation and decreased cell replication, thus promoting excessive cell division.
  - in individuals with psoriasis, levels of polyamines are increased. Lowered skin and urinary levels of polyamines are associated with clinical improvement in psoriasis patients.
  - excessive formation of polyamines can be prevented by:
    - improving digestive function (for more information on common causes and natural treatments to improve digestive function, see the chapter on Intestinal dysbiosis)
    - a number of natural compounds, including vitamin A and goldenseal (discussed below), inhibit the formation of polyamines.
- **Bowel toxemia:** gut-derived toxins can cause increases in cGMP levels within skin cells, thereby significantly increasing their rate of proliferation:
  - these toxins include endotoxins (cell wall components of bacteria), *Candida albicans* (a type of yeast), yeast compounds, and immune complexes.

- in particular, overgrowth of *C. albicans* in the intestines can play a major role in psoriasis (see the chapter on Chronic candidiasis for further information).
- a diet low in fiber is associated with increased levels of gut-derived toxins since fiber components bind bowel toxins and promote their excretion in the feces.

■ **Impaired liver function:**
  - psoriasis has been linked to the presence of several microbial by-products in the blood.
  - the liver filters and detoxifies the blood. If the liver is overwhelmed by excessive levels of microbial toxins in the blood or if the liver's detoxification ability is impaired, the level of toxins in the blood will increase, worsening psoriasis.

■ **Alcohol consumption:** alcohol consumption significantly worsens psoriasis since alcohol increases the absorption of toxins from the gut and impairs liver function.

■ **Excessive consumption of animal products** (meat, animal fats, and dairy products):
  - animal products contain arachidonic acid, a fatty acid that the body converts into potent inflammatory agents called leukotrienes.
  - leukotrienes promote increased cGMP levels.
  - leukotriene production is many times greater than normal in the skin of individuals with psoriasis.

■ **Inadequate amounts of certain nutritional factors:** decreased levels of several nutritional factors critical for skin health are common in individuals with psoriasis, and supplementation with these factors (discussed below) has resulted in complete healing of the skin.

■ **Stress:**
  - when levels of stress hormones, e.g., cortisol, increase in the circulation, immune system defenses, many of which involve inflammatory chemicals, are upregulated.
  - a few case histories in the medical literature have documented successful treatment of psoriasis with hypnosis and biofeedback alone.

RISK INCREASES WITH

■ **Family history of psoriasis:** 36% of psoriasis patients have one or more family members with psoriasis, which suggests a genetic link.

■ **Rheumatoid arthritis:** also a chronic inflammatory condition, rheumatoid arthritis shares a number of underlying causative factors with psoriasis.

■ **Repeated local injury:** the injury/repair process involves both inflammation and a more rapid than normal generation of new cells.

■ **Viral or bacterial infections elsewhere in the body:** the immune response involves inflammatory chemicals. Viruses and bacteria produce toxins, increasing the load that circulates in the bloodstream.

■ **Intestinal dysbiosis:** the overgrowth of potentially pathogenic organisms such as *Candida albicans* in the intestinal tract results in the production of high levels of polyamines, which inhibit formation of cAMP (for more information see the chapter on Intestinal dysbiosis).

■ **Consumption of the Standard American Diet (SAD):** based on animal products and processed foods, with little consumption of fresh vegetables, legumes, fruits, nuts and seeds, and whole grains, the SAD is low in protective factors – fiber, vitamin A, vitamin E, omega-3 essential fatty acids, chromium, selenium, and zinc – and high in factors that promote inflammation and an imbalance in the cAMP : cGMP ratio – animal fats, meat, dairy products, sugars and refined carbohydrates.

■ **Alcohol consumption:** increases absorption of toxins from the gut and impairs liver function.

■ **Stress:** 39% of patients who have psoriasis report that a specific stressful event occurred within 1 month prior to their initial episode.

■ **Cold climate:** skin tends to become dry in cold weather, further increasing susceptibility to damage.

■ **Prolonged antibiotic use:** antibiotics suppress the immune system and kill off not only their targets, but also the friendly intestinal bacteria that prevent colonization by pathogenic microbes and yeast overgrowth.

PREVENTIVE MEASURES

■ **Consume a nutrient-dense diet** rich in whole, unprocessed, preferably organic foods, especially plant foods (fruits, vegetables, beans, seeds and nuts, and whole grains) and cold-water fish, and low in animal products and processed foods (for more detailed information, see Appendix 1).

■ **A high-potency multiple vitamin and mineral supplement:** a daily multiple providing all of the known vitamins and minerals serves as a foundation upon which to build an individualized health-promotion program. Any good multiple should include 400 µg of folic acid, 400 µg of vitamin B_{12}, and 50–100 mg of vitamin B_6. (Folic acid supplementation should always be accompanied by vitamin B_{12} supplementation to prevent folic acid from masking a vitamin B_{12} deficiency.)

■ **Avoid situations likely to result in skin injury**, including traumatic sports activities, exposure to severe cold, or harsh scrubbing.

■ **Cope with stress constructively:** meditate, pray, learn stress reduction techniques such as biofeedback or self-hypnosis, exercise, seek assistance from a religious or psychological counselor. Taking the time to discover which practices help and to integrate them into a lifestyle will significantly benefit not just skin health, but will improve overall health, joy in living, and longevity.

Expected outcomes

Improvements are generally noted within 6–8 weeks. If the treatment protocol below is fully adopted, complete resolution is possible after 2–3 months; however, don't be discouraged if flare-ups occur. Consistent adherence to treatment will promote faster resolution of flare-ups.

TREATMENT

Diet

■ **Limit consumption of sugar, meat, animal fats, and alcohol**
■ **Increase consumption of fiber-rich fruits, vegetables, whole grains, and legumes**
■ **Increase consumption of wild-caught, cold-water fish**, such as salmon, which are high in anti-inflammatory omega-3 essential fatty acids:
  ■ studies in which fish oils were given as supplements to the diet (1.8 g EPA and 1.2 g DHA q.d.) have demonstrated significant improvement in psoriasis.
  ■ fish oil supplementation is not, however, recommended since most commercially available fish oils contain very high levels of damaged fats (lipid peroxides), which greatly stress antioxidant defenses.
  ■ consumption of 150 g (5 oz) of wild-caught salmon, mackerel or herring will provide the amount of EPA and DHA used in studies.
  ■ farm-raised fish, which are largely fed on grains, contain significantly less omega-3 fats.
■ **Consume 1 tbsp of flaxseed oil q.d.:** flaxseed oil, the best plant source of omega-3 fatty acids, is highly perishable and should be packaged in an opaque container, refrigerated, and never heated. Add flaxseed oil to smoothies, drizzle over steamed vegetables, or use as a dipping oil for bread or as the oil in a favorite salad dressing.
■ **Eliminate wheat and other sources of gluten:** psoriasis is a chronic inflammatory disease in which gut-derived toxins and polyamines play a significant causative role. In psoriatic patients, gluten, the major protein component in wheat, may significantly increase blood levels of these toxins:
  ■ partially digested gluten is perceived by the immune system as an invader that must be destroyed. In the process of attempting to eliminate gluten, the immune system, which uses inflammatory chemicals as defensive agents, may damage surrounding intestinal tissue. Once intestinal integrity is breached, microbial toxins can more easily gain access to the bloodstream.
  ■ gluten is also found in rye, barley, triticale, and oats.
  ■ rice and corn do not contain gluten. Breads, crackers and cereals made from rice and/or corn may be substituted for wheat products.
  ■ in studies, psoriatic patients have significantly benefited from gluten-free and elimination diets (for more information see the chapter on Food allergy).

Nutritional supplements

■ **A high-potency multiple vitamin and mineral supplement:** see Preventive Measures above.
■ **Omega-3 fatty acids:** most commercially available fish oils contain very high levels of damaged fats (lipid peroxides), which greatly deplete antioxidant defenses. Fish oil supplements are therefore not recommended. See the diet recommendations above for flaxseed oil and cold-water fish, two excellent food sources of omega-3s.
■ **Vitamin A:** the two most critical nutrients for skin health are vitamin A and zinc (discussed immediately below). All epithelial surfaces including the skin and the lining of the gastrointestinal tract rely upon vitamin A. When vitamin A status is inadequate, keratin is secreted in epithelial tissues, transforming them from their normally pliable, moist condition into stiff dry tissue that is unable to carry out its normal functions:
  ■ decreased levels of vitamin A are common in psoriasis patients.
  ■ vitamin A (and components in goldenseal, discussed below) inhibits bacterial decarboxylase, the enzyme that converts undigested amino acids into polyamines.
  ■ in the intestinal tract, lack of vitamin A promotes breaches in epithelial integrity that significantly increase absorption of gut-derived toxins and polyamines.
  ■ in the skin, lack of vitamin A significantly contributes to the development of the scaly plaques typical of psoriasis.
  ■ dosage: 50,000 IU q.d.
  ■ **caution:** at high doses, vitamin A has been linked to birth defects. Sexually active women of childbearing age should not use vitamin A at doses higher than 5,000 IU q.d. without effective birth control.
■ **Zinc:** adequate levels of zinc are critical for vitamin A function, wound healing, immune system activity,

inflammation control, and tissue regeneration; dosage: 30 mg q.d. of zinc picolinate (a well-absorbed form).

- **Chromium:** chromium is the mineral component in glucose tolerance factor, a molecule that helps cells respond appropriately to insulin:
  - marginal chromium deficiency is common in the United States, and individuals with psoriasis are typically found to have increased serum levels of both insulin and glucose.
  - chromium levels are depleted by lack of exercise and by consuming foods containing refined sugars and white flour.
  - dosage: 400 µg q.d.
- **Selenium and vitamin E:** selenium is a trace mineral integral to a very important antioxidant enzyme called glutathione peroxidase:
  - levels of glutathione peroxidase are typically low in psoriasis patients, possibly because excessive loss of skin cells robs the body of key nutrients.
  - factors such as alcohol abuse and nutrient deficiency may also contribute to the depressed levels of glutathione peroxidase seen in psoriasis.
  - glutathione levels will normalize with oral selenium and vitamin E supplementation.
  - in the treatment of psoriasis, vitamin E also plays an important role as an antioxidant that protects vitamin A and increases its storage.
  - dosage: selenium – 200 µg q.d.; vitamin E – 400 IU mixed tocopherols q.d.
- **Active vitamin D:** the active form of vitamin D (1,25-dihydroxycholecalciferol) plays a role in controlling cellular processes involved with replication:
  - patients with severe psoriasis have been found to have significantly low serum levels of active vitamin D, which normalized after oral supplementation.
  - studies have shown that both topical application (2–5 weeks) and oral supplementation (1–3 months) of active vitamin D resulted in definite to total improvement in all patients.
  - dosage: oral dose used was 1.0 µg of 1-alpha (OH)D$_3$.
- **Fumaric acid:** oral intake of dimethylfumaric acid (240 mg q.d.) or monoethylfumaric acid (720 mg q.d.) and the topical application of 1–3% monoethylfumaric acid has become increasingly popular in Western Europe for treatment of psoriasis as clinical studies have confirmed its usefulness:
  - because of the potential side effects of fumaric acid therapy (flushing of the skin, nausea, diarrhea, general malaise, gastric pain, and mild liver and kidney disturbances), we recommend using fumaric acid only if other natural therapies have proven ineffective.

Botanical medicines

- ***Hydrastis canadensis* (goldenseal):** the alkaloids in goldenseal, such as berberine, inhibit the enzyme bacterial decarboxylase, which converts undigested amino acids into polyamines:
  - berberine also has a broad spectrum of antibiotic activity against disease-causing bacteria, protozoa, fungi, and yeast, particularly *Candida albicans*. Since berberine inhibits both pathogenic bacteria and Candida, it prevents the yeast overgrowth that is a common side effect of antibiotic use and may contribute significantly to psoriasis.
  - dosage: since dosage should be based on berberine content, standardized extracts are preferred. Choose one of the following forms and take the recommended dosage t.i.d.:
    - dried root or as infusion (tea): 2–4 g
    - fluid extract (1 : 1): 2–4 ml (0.5–1 tsp)
    - solid (dry powdered) extract (4 : 1 or 8–12% alkaloid content): 250–500 mg.
- ***Silybum marianum* (milk thistle):** silymarin, the flavonoid component of milk thistle, improves liver function, inhibits inflammation, and reduces excessive cellular proliferation. Silymarin has been found to be a valuable component of psoriasis treatment; dosage: silymarin 70–210 mg t.i.d.
- ***Smilax sarsaparilla*:** components in sarsaparilla bind to and promote the excretion of bacterial endotoxins:
  - in a controlled study of 92 psoriasis patients, sarsaparilla provided significant benefits for 80% of subjects, greatly relieving psoriasis in 62% and providing complete clearance in another 18%.
  - dosage: choose one of the following forms of sarsaparilla species and take the recommended dosage t.i.d.:
    - dried root or by decoction: 1–4 g
    - liquid extract (1 : 1): 8–16 ml (2–4 tsp)
    - solid (dry powdered) extract (4 : 1): 250–500 mg.

Drug–herb interaction cautions
None.

Topical medicine
Preparations containing glycyrrhetinic acid from licorice (*Glycyrrhiza glabra*), extracts from chamomile (*Matricaria chamomilla*), and capsaicin, the active component from cayenne pepper (*Capsicum frutescens*), have been shown to provide symptomatic relief comparable or superior to topical hydrocortisone.

- **Glycyrrhetinic acid** has been shown to be more effective in treating both psoriasis and eczema than topical cortisone in several studies:
  - glycyrrhetinic acid can also be used to improve the effectiveness of topically applied hydrocortisone

since glycyrrhetinic acid inhibits the enzyme (11-beta-hydroxysteroid dehydrogenase) that catalyses the conversion of hydrocortisone into an inactive form.

- **Chamomile** contains flavonoid and essential oil components with significant anti-inflammatory and antiallergy activity.
- **Capsaicin**, when topically applied, stimulates and then blocks small-diameter pain fibers by depleting them of neurotransmitter substance P:
  - substance P is the principal chemical mediator of pain impulses from the periphery and has also been shown to activate inflammatory mediators in psoriasis.
  - in one study of 98 psoriasis patients treated with 0.025-capsaicin cream applied q.i.d. for 6 weeks, those given capsaicin cream demonstrated significantly greater improvement than those given placebo in reduction of psoriasis symptoms including itching, scaling, thickness, and redness.

- **Dosage:** using the amount recommended on the product label, apply preparations containing one or more of these ingredients to affected skin areas b.i.d.–t.i.d.

Physical medicine

- **Ultrasound:** localized elevation of temperature to 108°F (42–45°C) in the affected area by ultrasound and heating pads has been shown to be an effective treatment for psoriasis; dosage: 20 min three times a week.
- **UVB:** sunlight (ultraviolet light) is extremely beneficial for individuals with psoriasis. UVB exposure alone leads to inhibition of cell proliferation and has been shown to be as effective as standard medical PUVA therapy (treatment with the drug psoralen and ultraviolet A) with fewer side effects; dosage: 295–305 nm, 2 mW/cm^2 for 3 min three times a week.

Rheumatoid arthritis

DESCRIPTION

Rheumatoid arthritis (RA) is an autoimmune disease – a disease in which the body mistakenly attacks itself. In RA, the result is chronic inflammation that affects the entire body, but especially the joints.

Joints are held together by a joint capsule designed to facilitate smooth movement between the adjacent bones. In the highly movable joints (the joints commonly affected by RA) the bone ends are covered by cartilage, and the joint space is enclosed by a thin *synovial membrane*. In a healthy joint, this membrane secretes synovial fluid, which lubricates the area between the cartilage-covered bones forming the joint. The cartilage, a gel-like substance, acts like a shock absorber, further ensuring smooth and easy movement in the joint. The cartilage covering bone ends contains no blood vessels or nerves and receives its nutrients by diffusion from the synovial fluid and from the bone.

In RA, the body mistakenly attacks the joint's synovial membrane causing chronic inflammation and thickening of the synovial lining, with resulting destruction of both the synovium and cartilage of the joints.

RA affects 3% of the population, striking women three times as often as men. Although RA may begin at any age, onset typically occurs between the ages of 20 and 40 years. Onset may be sudden, but usually happens gradually with fatigue, low-grade fever, weakness, joint stiffness, and vague joint pain preceding the appearance of painful, swollen joints by several weeks. In about one-third of persons with RA, only one or a few joints are affected initially, often in a symmetrical fashion, e.g., both wrists, hands or feet. Involved joints are quite warm, tender and swollen, and the skin covering the joint takes on a ruddy purplish hue. As RA progresses, deformities frequently develop in the joints of the hands and feet.

FREQUENT SIGNS AND SYMPTOMS

Slow or sudden onset of:
- fatigue
- low-grade fever
- weakness
- weight loss

- joint stiffness
- redness, pain, warmth, tenderness in any or all active joints of the hands, wrists, elbows, shoulders, feet, and ankles
- morning stiffness
- nodules under the skin or over bony prominences on joints (sometimes).

Medical findings include:
- history of swelling (soft tissue thickening or fluid, not bony overgrowth alone) in at least one joint
- tenderness or pain on motion with a history of recurrence or persistence:
  - possible RA – at least 3 weeks' duration of symptoms
  - probable RA – at least 6 weeks' duration of symptoms
- X-ray changes typical of RA, including bony decalcification localized to or most marked adjacent to the involved joints, and not just degenerative changes
- positive demonstration of "rheumatoid factor" by an acceptable method
- signs of inflammation on examination of joint fluid
- elevated sedimentation rate (a blood test that provides a rough estimate of inflammation)
- characteristic biopsy results.

CAUSES

RA is an autoimmune disease – a disease in which the immune system attacks body tissues as if they were foreign invaders. In RA, the immune system develops antibodies against the synovial lining and cartilage of the joints. RA is a multifactorial disease in which both genetic and environmental factors contribute to the initiation of the autoimmune reaction and perpetuation of the disease process.

Genetic factors
- Susceptibility to RA has a genetic component:
  - about 70% of patients with RA have a specific genetic marker (HLA-DRw$_4$) compared to only 28% of persons who do not have RA.
  - severe RA is found at four times greater frequency in the offspring of parents with RA.
- Although these genetic associations are strong, the good news is that in studies of identical twins, rarely

do both get RA. If RA were a purely genetic disease, both twins would be affected every time. The fact that they are not means that environmental factors are necessary for the development of the disease.

Abnormal bowel permeability

- Individuals with RA have increased intestinal permeability (also called a "leaky gut"), which allows dietary and bacterial components (*antigens*) to leak into the bloodstream:
  - the immune system perceives these antigens as invaders and forms antibodies against them.
  - the antibodies attach to the antigens, creating the high levels of antibody–antigen complexes (also called *immune complexes*) characteristic of RA.
- Immune complexes deposit in the synovial lining of the joints, triggering the release of inflammatory *cytokines* (immune defense chemicals) that damage the synovium:
  - the immune system's response to the presence of damaged synovial tissue is to produce more antibodies to clear it out.
  - if this process happens frequently or long enough, the immune system eventually develops antibodies to the synovial tissue itself – initiating the autoimmune response characteristic of RA.
- Food allergies:
  - in response to food allergens (antigens), antibodies are produced and form immune complexes in the gut wall.
  - the reaction that occurs when these immune complexes are formed damages the intestinal lining, thus increasing intestinal permeability.
  - increased intestinal permeability results in more antigens leaking into the bloodstream, provoking the formation of more antibodies and immune complexes.
- Non-steroidal anti-inflammatory drugs (NSAIDs):
  - NSAIDs, such as aspirin and ibuprofen, are known to cause increased intestinal permeability.
  - NSAIDs lessen pain and inflammation by inhibiting the production of the enzyme cyclo-oxygenase (COX).
  - COX has two forms, COX-1, which is necessary for the production of substances that protect the intestinal lining and limit gastric acid output, and COX-2, which causes inflammation.
  - NSAIDs block both COX-1 and COX-2.
  - the use of NSAIDs to treat RA not only greatly increases the already excessive intestinal permeability seen in RA, but is a significant cause of serious gastrointestinal tract disturbances, including ulcers, hemorrhage, and perforation.

- in individuals with RA, NSAID use causes approximately 20,000 hospitalizations and 2,600 deaths each year.
- Increased gut permeability results in increased absorption of microbial antigens similar to proteins found in joint tissues. The antibodies formed against these microbial antigens may also mistakenly attack joint proteins:
  - antibodies to several bacteria (e.g., *Campylobacter*, *Salmonella*, *Shigella*) have been shown to cross-react with collagen (the main protein in joint tissue).
  - antibodies to other bacteria (*Klebsiella pneumoniae*, *Proteus vulgaris*, *Yersinia enterocolitica*) have been shown to cross-react with other protein components of joint tissues.

Small-intestinal bacterial overgrowth

- Many patients with RA have an overgrowth of bacteria in the small intestine – (the upper portion of the intestine), which is supposed to be mostly free of bacteria.
- When numerous bacteria are present in the small intestine, they compete with their host for incoming food. If bacteria get to the food first, many problems result:
  - bacteria ferment carbohydrates, producing excessive gas, bloating and abdominal distension.
  - bacteria break down protein via the process of putrefaction, producing compounds called *vasoactive amines*.
  - in the intestinal tract, vasoactive amines cause abdominal pain, altered gut motility and increased gut permeability.
- A 1993 study demonstrated that the severity of RA symptoms correlates with the severity of small-intestinal bacterial overgrowth.

Alterations in gastrointestinal tract flora

- Human intestinal flora comprise a complex ecosystem including over 400 species and play a major role in health:
  - many of these organisms have developed a symbiotic relationship with their human host. In metabolizing the foods on which they thrive, they supply by-products that provide intestinal cells with a variety of nourishing, protective factors.
  - in addition, these *probiotic* (pro-life) organisms prevent the growth of large populations of other organisms that are classified as neutral, neutral but potentially pathogenic, or pathogenic.
- The total surface area of the gastrointestinal system is quite large – 300–400 m² – and only a single layer of

cells separates the bloodstream from enormous amounts of dietary and microbial antigens that continuously pass through the digestive tract:

- when unfriendly flora flourish in the gastrointestinal tract, their metabolic by-products damage the intestinal lining, allowing them to leak into the bloodstream where they are perceived as antigens and trigger the formation of antibodies and immune complexes.
- A vegetarian diet has been shown to significantly improve the numbers of probiotic flora while lowering numbers of unfriendly organisms in the gastrointestinal tract (see Diet below).

Deficiency of digestive factors

- Many individuals with RA are deficient in hydrochloric acid and pancreatic enzymes, both of which are necessary for digestion.
- When breakdown and assimilation of food is inadequate, not only are nutritional needs not met, but also incompletely digested food molecules can be inappropriately absorbed, resulting in the formation of antibodies and immune complexes.

Abnormal antibodies and immune complexes

- The serum and joint fluid of nearly all individuals with RA contain the *rheumatoid factor* – a number of antibodies that attack a fragment (the Fc fragment) on the immune system's own IgG antibody. In other words, in RA, abnormal antibodies are being formed against the body's normal antibodies.
- As noted earlier, individuals with RA have large amounts of circulating immune complexes. These complexes, which form when antibodies join to antigens, are capable of stimulating immune cells to release inflammatory cytokines, which then damage joint tissues.

Microbial hypotheses

- While no one microbe has been consistently found in RA patients, several (e.g., Epstein–Barr virus, measles virus, amoebic organisms, mycoplasma) have been suggested as causative factors in RA.
- All microbes are seen by the immune system as antigens and provoke the production of antibodies, which then join with the antigens to form circulating immune complexes.

Decreased DHEA levels

- Defective manufacture of androgens (male hormones such as testosterone and dehydroepiandrosterone [DHEA]) has been proposed as a predisposing factor for RA.

- DHEA-S (the main form of DHEA in the blood) levels have been found to be below normal in patients with RA.
- Supplemental DHEA has shown therapeutic benefits in patients with systemic lupus erythematosus, another autoimmune disease that shares common features with RA.
- If DHEA is used, the dosage should be determined in collaboration with a physician and may be above 50 mg q.d., a level that may cause mild to severe acne in women.

RISK INCREASES WITH

- Family history of RA or other autoimmune disorders
- Native American ethnicity (prevalence is higher in this group)
- Female age 20–50 years
- Food allergies
- Excessive intestinal permeability (leaky gut)
- Small-intestinal bacterial overgrowth
- Frequent use of NSAIDs: aspirin, ibuprofen (Advil, Motrin, Nuprin), piroxicam (Feldene), diclofenac (Voltaren [Voltarol]), fenoprofen (Nalfon), indometacin (Indocin), naproxen (Naprosyn), tolmetin (Tolectin), sulindac (Clinoril).
- Use of antibiotics: antibiotics kill friendly as well as pathogenic organisms, thus disrupting normal gut ecology and increasing susceptibility to invasion by unfriendly microbes, yeast or bacterial overgrowth.
- Emotional stress may trigger flare-ups: prolonged stress can exhaust the adrenal gland's reserves of *glucocorticoid* hormones (*cortisol, corticosterone, cortisone*) which play a critical role in the body's ability to utilize blood sugar, reduce inflammation and prevent allergic reactions.

PREVENTIVE MEASURES

- Evaluate for possible food allergies and eliminate food allergens from the diet (for more information see the chapter on Food allergy).
- After removing allergenic foods, consume a nutrient-dense diet centered around whole foods, vegetables and fiber. Minimize intake of sugar, meat, refined carbohydrates, and animal fats.
- Increase consumption of foods rich in anti-inflammatory omega-3 fatty acids and flavonoids (discussed under Diet below).
- Minimize use of NSAIDs and antibiotics.

Expected outcomes

Improvements should be noticeable within several weeks. Over several months, progressive improvement should be seen, eventually resulting in elimination of all or nearly all symptoms.

TREATMENT

A multifactorial condition, RA requires a comprehensive therapeutic approach that reduces the factors known to be involved in the disease process (gut permeability, circulating immune complexes, free radicals, immune dysfunction), while controlling inflammation and promoting joint regeneration.

Diet

■ **A primarily vegetarian, whole foods diet is recommended:**
  ▣ in population studies, RA is not found in areas where people eat a more "primitive" diet rich in whole foods, vegetables and fiber. In contrast, RA is found at a relatively high rate in places where people consume the so-called "Western" diet, which is high in meat, and refined carbohydrates, sugars and fats.
  ▣ altered gastrointestinal tract flora have been linked to RA and other autoimmune diseases, and studies have demonstrated that improvements in gut flora are associated with clinical improvements in RA:
    ● in two recent clinical studies, significant positive alteration in fecal flora was observed when patients with RA changed from an omnivorous to a vegetarian diet, and these positive changes correlated with improvements in RA.

■ **Eliminate allergenic foods:**
  ▣ virtually any food can aggravate RA, but the most common offenders are wheat, corn, milk and other dairy products, beef, nightshade-family foods (tomato, potato, eggplant, peppers, and tobacco).
  ▣ beef and dairy products, in addition to being potential allergens, are the primary sources of *arachidonic acid*, a fatty acid used in the body to produce pro-inflammatory prostaglandins.

■ **Consider beginning a therapeutic diet with a 7–10 day modified fast**, then gradually reintroducing foods to identify and eliminate those that aggravate RA symptoms:
  ▣ fasting decreases absorption of allergenic food components and reduces levels of inflammatory mediators.
  ▣ this approach was very successful in a well-designed 13-month study, in which a control group ate as they wished while the treatment group fasted

for 7–10 days, then gradually reintroduced foods consistent with a vegetarian diet.
  ▣ during the fast, the treatment group consumed only herbal teas, garlic, vegetable broth, a decoction of potatoes and parsley, and juices of carrots, beets, and celery. No fruit juices were allowed.
  ▣ after the fast, foods were reintroduced one at a time, every second day:
    ● if an increase in pain, stiffness or joint swelling occurred within 2–48 hours, the reintroduced food was omitted from the diet for at least 7 days, then reintroduced a second time.
    ● if the food again caused worsening of symptoms, it was omitted permanently from the diet.
  ▣ in the 1-year-follow-up, all patients who responded to the diet still followed the diet.
  ▣ the majority of these patients remained in complete remission or were significantly better.

■ **Decrease intake of arachidonic acid** by decreasing consumption of animal foods (meat and dairy products):
  ▣ arachidonic acid is an omega-6 fatty acid that is found only in animal foods. In the body, arachidonic acid is used to produce pro-inflammatory prostaglandins and leukotrienes.

■ **Increase intake of anti-inflammatory EPA** (eicosapentaenoic acid) by increasing consumption of wild-caught cold-water fish such as mackerel, herring, sardines, and salmon:
  ▣ EPA is an omega-3 fatty acid that is used in the body to produce anti-inflammatory prostaglandins that reduce the allergenic–inflammatory response so harmful in RA.
  ▣ wild-caught (but not farm-raised) cold-water fish are rich in EPA:
    ● wild fish such as salmon dine on smaller wild fish, which contain EPA, thus building up their stores of this omega-3 fat.
    ● farm-raised fish are fed on grains and other foods lacking high levels of EPA. As a result, their levels of EPA are significantly lower.
  ▣ since most commercially available fish oils contain very high levels of *lipid peroxides* (damaged fats) and greatly stress antioxidant defense mechanisms, at this time it is best to rely on cold-water fish and flaxseed oil (discussed next) as sources of omega-3 oils.
  ▣ fish should be baked or broiled, and eaten at least twice, and preferably three or more times a week:
    ● in a population-based study of 324 women with RA and 1,245 women without RA living in the Seattle area, consumption of broiled or baked (but not fried) fish was associated with a decreased risk of RA.

- consuming more than two servings of fish per week offered greater protection than one serving per week.
- **Consume at least 1 tbsp of flaxseed oil q.d.:**
  - flaxseed oil contains *alpha-linolenic acid*, which is converted in the body to EPA and another anti-inflammatory omega-3 fatty acid, DHA:
    - for these conversions to occur, adequate zinc must also be present since zinc is a component of *delta-6 desaturase*, the enzyme that converts alpha-linolenic acid to EPA (see discussion of zinc under Nutritional supplements).
  - for vegetarians, flaxseed oil can provide an alternative to fish as a source of EPA:
    - when used in conjunction with a diet low in omega-6 oils (achieved by restricting corn, safflower, sunflower and soy oils and animal products), flaxseed oil has been shown to raise tissue EPA levels comparably to fish oil supplementation.
    - several human and animal studies have demonstrated that flaxseed oil (1 tbsp q.d.) can inhibit the autoimmune reaction as effectively as EPA.
  - flaxseed oil is highly perishable, so it should always be refrigerated and never heated:
    - use flaxseed oil instead of butter on bread, in salad dressings, add to smoothies, or drizzle over already cooked vegetables or grains.
- **Increase consumption of fresh fruits and vegetables**, especially flavonoid-rich berries (cherries, hawthorn berries, blueberries, blackberries, etc.):
  - flavonoids, the components in plants that provide their colors, not only neutralize inflammation, but also support the collagen structures of the joints.
  - fresh fruits and vegetables are the best sources of dietary antioxidants including vitamin C, beta-carotene, vitamin A, vitamin E, selenium, and zinc – all of which play important roles in neutralizing free radicals involved in the inflammatory process. Several studies have shown that risk of RA is highest in persons with the lowest levels of these antioxidants.

Nutritional supplements

- **Betaine HCl:** many patients with RA are deficient in HCl (hydrochloric acid), which is necessary for digestion, particularly of protein. When foods are not well digested, the resulting large molecules are much more likely to be perceived as antigens:
  - hydrochloric acid in supplement form is always paired with a carrier molecule such as betaine to make it more portable and safer for teeth.
  - **caution:** never take HCl at the same time as any NSAID or corticosteroid drug (e.g., prednisone

[prednisolone]). These drugs can by themselves cause stomach bleeding and ulcers; taking them with HCl increases this risk.
  - how to take betaine HCl:
    - begin by taking 1 tablet or capsule, containing 10 grains (600 mg) of hydrochloric acid, at the next large meal. If this does not aggravate RA symptoms, at every subsequent meal of the same size, take one more tablet or capsule (1 at the next meal, 2 at the meal after that, then 3 at the next meal). When taking a number of tablets or capsules, do not take them all at once. Space them throughout the meal.
    - continue to increase the dose up to 7 tablets or until a feeling of warmth in the stomach is experienced, whichever occurs first. A warm feeling in the stomach means that too many tablets have been taken for that meal, and that one less tablet should be taken for a meal of that size. It is a good idea, however, to try the larger dose again at another meal to make sure that the HCl was what caused the warmth, and not something else.
    - after identifying the largest dose that can be taken at large meals without feeling any stomach warmth, maintain that dose at all meals of a similar size. Take less at smaller meals.
    - as the stomach begins to regain the ability to produce the amount of HCl needed to digest food properly, the warm feeling will be noticed again and the dose level should be cut down.
  - dosage: 10–70 grains with meals.
- **Pancreatic enzymes:** many individuals with RA are deficient in these digestive enzymes. In addition to their role in digestion, pancreatic enzymes, specifically the protein-digesting enzymes, have been shown to reduce levels of circulating immune complexes:
  - use a non-enteric-coated enzyme product. Enzyme products are often *enteric*-coated to prevent digestion in the stomach, so the enzymes will be liberated in the small intestine. However, numerous studies have shown that non-enteric-coated enzyme preparations actually outperform enteric-coated products if they are taken prior to a meal.
  - bromelain (discussed under Botanical medicines) may be used instead.
  - dosage: pancreatin (10×USP), 350–750 mg between meals t.i.d.
- **Selenium and vitamin E:**
  - free radicals, oxidants, inflammatory prostaglandins and leukotrienes cause much of the tissue damage in RA.
  - selenium is both a powerful antioxidant and is the mineral cofactor in the free radical scavenging

enzyme, glutathione peroxidase, which plays a critical role in reducing the production of inflammatory prostaglandins and leukotrienes.
- levels of selenium are frequently low in patients with RA.
- clinical studies have not yet demonstrated that selenium alone relieves RA, but one study found that selenium combined with vitamin E had a positive effect.
- dosage: selenium 200 µg q.d.; vitamin E (mixed tocopherols) 400–800 IU q.d.

■ **Zinc:**
- zinc is a cofactor in one form of the important antioxidant enzyme superoxide dismutase (copper–zinc SOD).
- zinc levels are typically reduced in patients with RA.
- foods rich in zinc include oysters, whole grains, nuts and seeds.
- several studies using zinc sulfate in the treatment of RA have shown some therapeutic benefit, despite the fact that zinc sulfate is not as well absorbed as zinc picolinate, zinc monomethionine, or zinc citrate. Better results might be realized by using one of these forms of zinc.
- dosage: 45 mg q.d.

■ **Manganese:**
- manganese functions in a different form of superoxide dismutase (manganese SOD).
- levels of manganese-containing SOD are deficient in patients with RA, and the injectable form of this enzyme (available in Europe) has been shown to be effective in the treatment of RA.
- orally administered SOD would not be as effective since most of it would be dismantled by digestive secretions in the intestinal tract.
- manganese supplementation has, however, been shown to increase antioxidant SOD activity.
- good dietary sources of manganese include nuts, whole grains, dried fruits, and green leafy vegetables.
- dosage: 15 mg q.d.

■ **Vitamin C:**
- supplementation with vitamin C increases SOD activity and decreases levels of histamine (an allergy-related inflammatory chemical). The body's primary water-soluble antioxidant, vitamin C also provides anti-inflammatory action by neutralizing free radicals.
- in RA patients, white blood cell and plasma concentrations of vitamin C are significantly decreased.
- foods rich in vitamin C include broccoli, Brussels sprouts, cabbage, citrus fruits, tomatoes, and berries.
- dosage: 1–3 g q.d. in divided doses.

■ **Pantothenic acid:**
- pantothenic acid (vitamin B$_5$) participates in numerous reactions involved in energy production and cell repair.
- whole-blood pantothenic acid levels have been reported to be lower in RA patients than in normal controls, and the severity of RA symptoms was inversely correlated with pantothenic acid levels.
- in a double-blind study, correction of low pantothenic acid levels resulted in improvements in duration of morning stiffness, degree of disability, and severity of pain.
- good dietary sources of pantothenic acid are whole grains and legumes.
- dosage: 500 mg q.i.d.

■ **Copper:**
- copper is a component, along with zinc, of one form of the important antioxidant enzyme SOD, which may be the reason for the long-time folk remedy for RA of wearing copper bracelets.
- **caution:** *excess* intake of copper may be detrimental since copper can combine with peroxides and damage joint tissues.
- copper aspirinate is a form of aspirin that yields better results in reducing pain and inflammation than standard aspirin. Should aspirin be used, this copper-containing form may be more beneficial for individuals with RA.
- dosage: 1 mg q.d.

■ **Sulfur:**
- the sulfur content of the fingernails of arthritis sufferers is lower than that of healthy controls. Normalizing the nails' sulfur content by using injectable sulfur was reported to alleviate pain and swelling, according to clinical data from the 1930s.
- dosage: increase consumption of sulfur-rich foods such as legumes, garlic, onions, Brussels sprouts, and cabbage.

■ **Niacinamide:**
- Drs William Kaufman and Abram Hoffer have reported very good clinical results using high-dose niacinamide in the treatment of hundreds of patients with osteoarthritis and RA. These promising results have been confirmed in osteoarthritis but have never been fully evaluated in detailed clinical studies of RA patients.
- among its numerous functions, niacinamide plays a role as an antioxidant and has been shown to inhibit the autoimmune process in insulin-dependent (type I or juvenile) diabetes mellitus, both of which suggest it may be quite useful in RA.
- **caution:** long-term supplementation – more than 3 months – must be monitored by a physician

because of the possibility of niacinamide harming the liver.
- dosage: 500 mg q.i.d. (check liver enzyme values in the blood every 3 months).

Botanical medicines

The following botanicals may be used alone or in combination.

Individuals with a history of corticosteroid use (e.g., prednisone [prednisolone]) and those being weaned off corticosteroids should take adrenal-supportive herbs (discussed below) such as *Bupleuri falcatum* (Chinese thoroughwax), *Glycyrrhiza glabra* (licorice), and Panax ginseng. These herbs help to prevent or reverse the adrenal atrophy (shrinkage) induced by corticosteroid drugs.

- **Curcuma longa (curcumin):**
  - the yellow pigment of *Curcuma longa* (turmeric), curcumin is an excellent anti-inflammatory and antioxidant agent:
    - in models of acute inflammation, curcumin is as effective as either cortisone or the potent anti-inflammatory drug phenylbutazone – but unlike these drugs, which are associated with significant toxicity, curcumin is without side effects.
  - curcumin directly inhibits the formation of the major chemical mediators of inflammation (thromboxanes and leukotrienes).
  - curcumin also works indirectly by enhancing the body's own anti-inflammatory mechanisms including:
    - stimulating the release of adrenal corticosteroids
    - sensitizing or priming cortisone receptor sites, thus improving the action of the body's own cortisone
    - preventing the breakdown of cortisone.
  - dosage: 400 mg t.i.d.
- **Zingiber officinale (ginger):**
  - ginger inhibits the formation of inflammatory mediators (e.g., prostaglandins, thromboxanes, leukotrienes), exerts powerful antioxidant actions, and contains a protease compound that breaks down *fibrin*:
    - fibrin promotes swelling by forming a matrix that walls off the inflamed area, blocking blood vessels and preventing tissue drainage.
  - in clinical studies, ginger has demonstrated efficacy, even in treating patients with RA who had not been helped by conventional drugs. Patients reported substantial improvement including pain relief, joint mobility and a decrease in swelling and morning stiffness.
  - although most scientific studies have used powdered ginger root, fresh ginger root at an equivalent

dosage may yield better results since it contains higher levels of two pharmacologically active components in ginger – *gingerol* and the protease compound.
- dosage: incorporate 8–10 g of fresh ginger, roughly a 2.5 cm (1″) slice, into the diet each day. This amount could easily be added as an ingredient in fresh fruit and vegetable juices. Or use ginger extracts standardized to contain 20% gingerol and shogaol, 100–200 mg t.i.d.:
  - the average daily dietary consumption of ginger in India is 8–10 g; no side effects have been noted using ginger at these doses.
- **Bromelain:**
  - bromelain is a mixture of enzymes found in pineapple whose effectiveness in reducing inflammation in RA is well documented.
  - bromelain's beneficial effects are primarily due to compounds that break down fibrin (see Ginger above).
  - bromelain also blocks the production of *kinins* – compounds produced during inflammation that increase swelling and cause pain.
  - vegetarians who do not wish to use pancreatic enzymes may substitute bromelain, although best results will most likely be seen using both types of enzymes.
  - dosage: 250–750 mg (1,800–2,000 MCU) taken between meals t.i.d.
- **Bupleuri falcatum (Chinese thoroughwax):**
  - steroid-like components (*saikosaponins*) in Chinese thoroughwax exert significant anti-inflammatory action by increasing the adrenal gland's release of cortisone and other hormones and enhancing their effects.
  - saikosaponins have also been shown to prevent the adrenal gland atrophy caused by corticosteroids, and have therefore been used in conjunction with corticosteroid drugs such as prednisone (prednisolone).
  - dosages: choose one of the following forms and take the recommended dosage t.i.d.:
    - dried root: 2–4 g
    - tincture (1 : 5): 5–10 ml
    - fluid extract (1 : 1): 2–4 ml
    - solid extract (4 : 1): 200–400 mg.
- **Glycyrrhiza glabra (licorice) and Panax ginseng:**
  - both licorice and Panax ginseng enhance the action of Chinese thoroughwax, and the three botanicals are almost always used together in Chinese herbal formulas. Both licorice root and Panax ginseng contain components with anti-inflammatory activity, and both herbs have also been shown to improve adrenal gland function.

- Chinese thoroughwax promotes secretion of corticosteroids by the adrenals, and licorice inhibits the breakdown of these hormones by the liver. When the two are used together, the result is an increase in circulating corticosteroid levels.
- licorice dosages: choose one of the following forms and take the recommended dosage t.i.d.:
  - dried root: 2–4 g
  - tincture (1 : 5): 10–20 ml
  - fluid extract (1 : 1): 4–6 ml
  - solid extract (4 : 1): 250–500 mg.
- Panax ginseng safeguards the adrenal glands during both short- and long-term stress. Ginseng appears to tune up the adrenal cortex so that adrenal response to short-term stress is quicker, and when stress decreases, corticosteroid levels fall more rapidly to normal. During prolonged stress, ginseng exerts a sparing effect on the adrenal glands by increasing adrenal capacity while lowering glucocorticoid production.
- Panax ginseng dosages: choose one of the following forms and take the recommended dosage t.i.d.:
  - crude herb: 4.5–6 g
  - standardized extract (5% ginsenosides): 500 mg.

Drug–herb interaction cautions

- *Glycyrrhiza glabra* (licorice):
  - plus *digoxin, digitalis*: due to a reduction of potassium in the blood, licorice enhances the toxicity of cardiac glycosides. Interaction with these cardiac glycoside drugs could lead to arrhythmias and cardiac arrest.
  - plus *stimulant laxatives or diuretics* (thiazides, spironolactone or amiloride): licorice should not be used with these drugs because of the additive increase of potassium loss to potentially dangerous levels.
- **Panax ginseng:**
  - plus *monoamine oxidase inhibitor, phenelzine*: may produce manic-like symptoms.
  - plus *caffeine*: long-term use (13 weeks) of large amounts (3 g q.d. on average) of ginseng may lead to hypertension in one person out of six.
  - plus *insulin*: dosage may need adjusting because of ginseng's hypoglycemic effects in diabetic patients.
  - plus *warfarin*: anticoagulant activity may be reduced.

Physical medicine

Physical therapy, while not curative, can significantly lessen discomfort and preserve joint and muscle function.

- **Heat** is typically used to help relieve stiffness and pain, relax muscles, and increase range of motion:
  - moist heat (e.g., moist packs, hot baths) is more effective than dry heat (e.g., sauna, heating pad).
  - mineral salts (*balneotherapy*) may be helpful.
  - 20–30 min q.d.–t.i.d.
- **Balneotherapy**, the therapeutic use of mineral baths and mud packs, is often used in Europe to treat RA:
  - a study conducted in Israel at the Ein Gedi Spa on the western shore of the Dead Sea provides evidence of a statistically significant improvement lasting up to 3 months after treatment. Improvements were noted in morning stiffness, 15 m walk time, grip strength, activities of daily living, and patient's assessment of disease activity.
  - improvements may be due to the trace mineral content of the Dead Sea:
    - trace minerals such as zinc and copper (key components of the antioxidant enzyme SOD), as well as boron, selenium, rubidium and other minerals may be absorbed through the skin.
    - below-normal levels of several trace minerals have been reported in patients with RA.
- **Paraffin (wax) baths** can be applied if frequent immersion in hot water causes skin irritation.
- **Active (or in severe cases, passive) range of motion exercises** improve and maintain range of motion:
  - patients with advanced disease or significant inflammation should begin with passive exercise, switching to active exercise as inflammation lessens.
- **Isometric exercises** (in which muscle tension is increased without movement, e.g., progressive relaxation techniques) help to maintain and improve muscle strength:
  - 3–10 repetitions, several times per day, with generous periods of rest between sessions.
- **Isotonic exercises** (in which the muscle shortens against a constant load, e.g., weight lifting) should be added as the joints improve:
  - 3–10 repetitions several times per day.
- **Massage:** by improving circulation, massage helps to provide muscles and joints with nutrients while aiding in the removal of waste products:
  - once per week.

Rosacea

DESCRIPTION

Rosacea is a common chronic inflammatory skin disorder in which the skin of the nose and cheeks is abnormally red and may be covered with bumps and pimples similar to those seen in acne. In addition, the small blood vessels beneath the skin may dilate, resulting in reddish blotches known as *telangiectasias*. If untreated, rosacea can lead to permanent thickening and redness of the affected skin, particularly the nose, a condition called *rhinophyma*. Although rosacea may occur in children as young as 10, it typically appears in adults between the ages of 30 and 50. Rosacea is more common in persons with lighter rather than darker complexions, and in women, who are affected three times as often as men, although rosacea is more severe in men.

FREQUENT SIGNS AND SYMPTOMS

- Chronic acne-like eruption on the nose and cheeks
- Affected areas appear red and flushed
- Excessive flow of *sebum* – the mixture of oils and waxes that lubricates the skin and prevents water loss
- Reddish blotches (telangiectasias) resulting from the dilation of small blood vessels beneath the skin

CAUSES

Although the exact causes of rosacea have not yet been determined, the following are suspected causal factors:

- **Gastrointestinal disorders**, including hypochlorhydria and pancreatic enzyme insufficiency:
  - *hypochlorhydria* (a deficiency of hydrochloric acid):
    - hydrochloric acid is secreted by the stomach to digest food. When hydrochloric acid secretion is inadequate, food digestion is incomplete and subclinical nutrient deficiencies can develop.
    - in addition, since hydrochloric acid also destroys pathogenic organisms ingested with food, hypochlorhydria results in a hospitable environment for pathogens such as *Helicobacter pylori*, the bacterium responsible for most ulcers.

- incidence of *H. pylori* infection is high in rosacea patients.
- *H. pylori* damages the lining of the stomach, further disrupting digestive function and increasing the likelihood that dietary protein will leak into the bloodstream, thereby provoking food allergies – another common finding in individuals with rosacea.
- in addition to increasing the absorption of potentially allergenic proteins, a damaged gut lining allows *vasoactive amines* to enter the circulation. Vasoactive amines are chemicals in certain foods, such as aged cheese and red wine, which affect blood vessel tone and can trigger dilation and flushing.
- our ability to secrete hydrochloric acid lessens with age and can also be disrupted by stress.
  - *insufficient pancreatic enzymes*: rosacea patients have frequently been found to have decreased secretion of *lipase*, the pancreatic enzyme that digests fat.
- **Seborrhea (excessive flow of sebum):** sebum is a mixture of oils and waxes that lubricate the skin and prevent it from dehydration. When sebum production is excessive, the skin's pores can become congested and blocked, resulting in the bumps and pimples of rosacea, which are similar to those seen in acne (for a detailed explanation of the causes and treatment of seborrhea, see the chapter on Acne).
- **B vitamin deficiencies**, especially of vitamin B_2 (riboflavin): administration of large doses of B vitamins (excluding niacin, which may cause flushing) has been shown to be quite effective in treating rosacea:
  - this may be due, at least in part, to riboflavin's protective effect against a small organism – the skin mite *Demodex folliculorum* – which has been considered a causative factor in rosacea. Researchers were able to infect the skin of riboflavin-deficient rats with Demodex, but not the skin of normal rats.
- **Excessive alcohol consumption** (more than one glass of wine or 30 ml (1 US fl oz) distilled spirits q.d.) exacerbates rosacea through several harmful mechanisms:
  - alcohol also damages the gut lining, thus increasing the absorption of vasoactive amines (chemicals that

affect blood vessel tone and can trigger dilation), potential allergens, and other toxins from the gut.

- alcohol impairs liver function (the liver is responsible for filtering toxins from the blood).
- excessive alcohol consumption is known to result in numerous nutrient deficiencies.

■ **Menopausal flushing (hot flashes):** in menstruating women, the brain's hypothalamus signals the pituitary to tell the ovaries to ovulate. During perimenopause, as levels of estrogen and progesterone fall, the ovaries stop responding, which causes the hypothalamus and pituitary to send stronger signals:

- this signaling overactivity can trigger the vasomotor center, specifically the arcuate nucleus of the hypothalamus, which controls capillary dilation, resulting in menopausal flushing or hot flashes.

■ **Local infection:** the hallmarks of an immune response to local infection are inflammation, redness and swelling:

- a key part of the immune system's response to infection is the deployment of specialized cells that use inflammatory chemicals as weapons against the invader.
- the redness is largely the result of blood vessel dilation, which is the body's attempt to rapidly increase the flow of defenders to the area.
- swelling results from the body's walling off of the area to prevent the spread of infection.

RISK INCREASES WITH

■ **Reflex flushing:** frequent consumption of coffee, alcohol, hot beverages, and/or spicy foods that cause flushing.
■ **Migraine headaches:** migraines, which have also been linked to hyperreactive blood vessels, are three times more common in individuals with rosacea than in age- and sex-matched controls:

- vasoactive amines, which can cause blood vessels to dilate abruptly, are a well-known migraine trigger.

■ **Alcohol consumption:** see Causes above.
■ **Stress:** stress disrupts digestive secretions. Psychological factors such as worry, depression, or other stress often reduce gastric acidity. In addition, when levels of stress hormones, i.e., cortisol, increase in the circulation, immune system defenses, many of which involve inflammatory chemicals, are upregulated.
■ **Disease-promoting diet:** a diet based on animal products and processed foods, with little consumption of fresh vegetables, legumes, fruits, nuts and seeds, and whole grains, is low in factors that promote gut health, blood vessel stability and normal sebum

production – fiber, vitamins and minerals, and essential fatty acids – and high in damaging factors – meat, saturated fat, *trans* fats (also called partially hydrogenated oils), sugars, and refined carbohydrates.
■ **Antibiotic use:** antibiotics kill not only unfriendly but also the friendly microflora that inhabit the gut, leaving the intestinal tract wide open to colonization by pathogens such as *Helicobacter pylori*.
■ **Drug therapy:** in addition to antibiotics, numerous drugs damage the intestinal lining, including over-the-counter non-steroidal anti-inflammatory drugs such as aspirin and ibuprofen.

PREVENTIVE MEASURES

■ Follow the dietary recommendations given below.
■ Take a high-potency daily multiple vitamin and mineral supplement: a daily multiple providing all of the known vitamins and minerals serves as a foundation upon which to build an individualized health-promotion program. Any good multiple should include 400 µg of folic acid, 400 µg of vitamin B_{12}, and 50–100 mg of vitamin B_6. (Folic acid supplementation should always be accompanied by vitamin B_{12} supplementation to prevent folic acid from masking a vitamin B_{12} deficiency.)
■ Learn to cope with stress constructively. Meditate, pray, learn stress reduction techniques such as biofeedback or self-hypnosis, exercise, seek assistance from a religious or psychological counselor. Taking the time to discover which practices help and to integrate them into a lifestyle will significantly benefit not just skin health, but will improve overall health, joy in living, and longevity.
■ Avoid the use of greasy creams or cosmetics.
■ Wash pillowcases every 2–3 days in hypoallergenic laundry soap containing no added colors or fragrances.

Expected outcomes

Improvements are generally noted within the first month of therapy.

If the treatment protocol below is fully adopted, complete resolution is possible after 2–3 months; however, don't be discouraged if flare-ups occur. Consistent adherence to treatment will promote faster resolution of flare-ups.

TREATMENT

Diet

■ Avoid coffee, alcohol, hot beverages, spicy foods, and any other food or drink that causes flushing of facial skin.

- Consume a nutrient-dense diet rich in whole, unprocessed, preferably organic foods, especially plant foods (fruits, vegetables, beans, seeds and nuts) and cold-water fish, and low in animal products (for more detailed information, see Appendix 1).
- Increase consumption of wild-caught, cold-water fish such as salmon, mackerel, herring, halibut, and sardines. These fish are excellent sources of anti-inflammatory omega-3 essential fatty acids:
  - farm-raised fish, which are largely fed on grains, have significantly lower levels of omega-3 fats.
- Consume 1 tbsp of flaxseed oil daily: flaxseed oil is the best plant source of omega-3 fatty acids:
  - flaxseed oil is highly perishable and should be packaged in an opaque container, refrigerated, and never heated. Add flaxseed oil to smoothies, drizzle over steamed vegetables, use as a dipping oil for bread, or as the oil in a favorite homemade salad dressing.
- Reduce consumption of meat and other animal products. Animal products contain arachidonic acid, a fatty acid converted in the body to inflammatory prostaglandins (hormone-like messenger molecules).
- Eliminate all refined and/or concentrated simple sugars from the diet. Rosacea involves acne-like lesions. The skin cells of acne patients have been found to be insulin insensitive and to utilize sugar so poorly that one researcher has referred to acne as "skin diabetes".
- Limit intake of high-fat foods and eliminate foods containing *trans*-fatty acids (margarine, shortening, and other synthetically hydrogenated oils). Since most fried foods are cooked in hydrogenated oils, and the heat of frying further damages (oxidizes) these *trans* fats, fried foods should be eliminated from the diet.
- Consumption of cow's milk and milk products should also be limited to avoid the *trans* fats and high hormone content present in cow's milk.
- Drink at least eight 240 ml (8 US fl oz) glasses of pure, clean water daily.
- In some people, iodine causes an inflammatory reaction. Those who are iodine sensitive should eliminate foods high in iodine and foods with a high salt content as most salt is iodized:
  - sea salt does not have much iodine and can be used sparingly.
  - iodine is especially high in clams, shrimp, haddock, and sea vegetables – all of which are healthful foods for those who are not iodine sensitive.

Nutritional supplements
- **A high-potency daily multiple vitamin and mineral supplement:** as described in Preventive Measures above.

- **B-complex vitamins:** often called the antistress vitamins, the B-complex vitamins play a wide variety of critical roles, many of which are essential for a healthy nervous system. Administration of large doses of B vitamins (excluding niacin, which often causes flushing at high doses) has been shown to be quite effective in treating rosacea:
  - the beneficial effects of supplemental B vitamins may be due, in part, to a protective effect of the B vitamin riboflavin against infection by the skin mite *Demodex folliculorum*, which is considered a potential causative factor in rosacea.
  - dosage: B-complex (without niacin) 100 mg q.d.
- **Hydrochloric acid supplementation:** insufficient production of stomach acid is common in patients with rosacea and is considered a causative factor. Use the following protocol to determine the appropriate dosage:
  - begin by taking 1 tablet or capsule, containing 10 grains (600 mg) of hydrochloric acid, at the next large meal. If this does not aggravate rosacea symptoms, at every subsequent meal of the same size, take one more tablet or capsule (1 at the next meal, 2 at the meal after that, then 3 at the next meal). When taking a number of tablets or capsules, do not take them all at once. Space them throughout the meal.
  - continue to increase the dose up to 7 tablets or until a feeling of warmth in the stomach is experienced, whichever occurs first. A warm feeling in the stomach means that too many tablets have been taken for that meal, and that one less tablet should be taken for a meal of that size. It is a good idea, however, to try the larger dose again at another meal to make sure that the HCl was what caused the warmth, and not something else.
  - after identifying the largest dose that can be taken at large meals without feeling any stomach warmth, maintain that dose at all meals of a similar size. Take less at smaller meals.
  - as the stomach begins to regain the ability to produce the amount of HCl needed to digest food properly, the warm feeling will be noticed again and the dose level should be cut down.
- **Pancreatic enzymes:** lack of adequate pancreatic enzymes, especially lipase, is another common finding in rosacea patients:
  - dosage: use a $10 \times$ USP pancreatic enzyme product and take 350–1,000 mg t.i.d. immediately before meals.
  - use a non-enteric-coated enzyme product. (Enzyme products are often *enteric*-coated to prevent digestion in the stomach, so the enzymes will be liberated

in the small intestine. However, numerous studies have shown that non-enteric-coated enzyme preparations actually outperform enteric-coated products if they are taken prior to a meal.)

■ for vegetarians, *bromelain* and *papain* (protein-digesting enzymes from pineapple and papaya, respectively) can substitute for pancreatic enzymes in the treatment of pancreatic insufficiency. However, best results are obtained if they are used in combination with pancreatin and ox bile.

■ **Probiotics:** friendly intestinal flora are needed to repopulate the intestines, both for their numerous beneficial effects on gut health and also to compete with, and thereby prevent colonization by, unfriendly organisms such as *Helicobacter pylori*:

■ dosage: 1–10 billion viable *Lactobacillus acidophilus* and *Bifidobacterium bifidum* cells q.d.

Seborrheic dermatitis

DESCRIPTION

A common skin disorder that may be associated with excessive oiliness (seborrhea) and dandruff, seborrheic dermatitis is characterized by scaly patches on the scalp, face, and skin folds (the armpits, groin, and neck). The scale may be greasy or dry, somewhat red or yellowish, and may or may not be itchy. Scaly bumps may coalesce to form large plaques or patches. Seborrheic dermatitis may occur in infancy (usually between 2 and 12 weeks of age) or in adulthood. "Cradle cap" and dandruff are both forms of seborrheic dermatitis, which, although not contagious, has a tendency to recur intermittently for life and to worsen with advancing age.

FREQUENT SIGNS AND SYMPTOMS

- Superficial reddened small bumps and flaking, white scaly patches on the scalp, eyebrows, forehead, cheeks, behind the ears, over the breastbone (sternum), and/or skin folds (around the nose, the armpit, groin, and neck)
- Scales anchor to hair shafts
- Usually does not itch
- Usually painless unless complicated by infection
- Worsened by dry climates and cold weather
- Symptoms tend to be worse in persons infected with HIV

CAUSES

The cause is unknown, but the following have all been implicated as contributing factors.
- **Genetic predisposition:** seborrheic dermatitis usually begins in infancy as "cradle cap" and, although not primarily an allergic disease, has been strongly associated with food allergy – 67% of infants who get cradle cap develop some form of allergy by age 10. If food allergies are suspected, see the chapter on Food allergy, for further information.
- **Emotional stress**
- **Nutrient deficiencies:** the B vitamins – biotin, pyridoxine, pantothenic acid, niacin, and thiamin – and the lipotropics (nutritional factors that promote the flow of fat to and from the liver, such as choline, methionine, and inositol) are vital for proper skin metabolism:
  - a biotin deficiency is the most frequent cause of "cradle cap".
  - in adults, treatment with biotin alone is usually of no value; it must be used in conjunction with the other B-complex vitamins.
  - treatment with high doses of B vitamins, both as oral supplements and as a topically applied ointment, has been shown to be effective.
- **Drugs or other factors that can block vitamin B_6 function:** taking a drug that causes vitamin B_6 deficiency (e.g., a hydralazine-containing drug) has been shown to cause lesions that are indistinguishable from seborrheic dermatitis. Similar lesions have been produced experimentally in rats by placing them on a B_6-deficient diet:
  - use of a water-soluble ointment containing B_6 resulted in complete clearance of a form of seborrheic dermatitis called the *sicca variant* within 10 days, although other types of seborrheic dermatitis did not respond to this therapy.
  - drugs that interfere with B_6 function include isoniazid (Laniazid, INH), hydralazine (Apresoline), penicillamine (Cuprimine, Depen), dopamine, and oral contraceptives. Individuals taking these drugs need to supplement with vitamin B_6 at the dosages recommended below.
  - the hydrazine dyes (FD&C yellow #5) and excessive protein intake also block B_6.
- **Hormones:** estrogens negatively affect vitamin B_6 function, and vitamin B_6 levels are typically quite low in women taking estrogens (birth control pills or Premarin):
  - when B_6 levels drop, so do the levels of magnesium within cells. Magnesium interacts extensively with vitamin B_6 in many enzyme systems and is also dependent upon B_6 to gain entry into cells. A low magnesium state within cells triggers the release of stress hormones and other substances that promote inflammation.
- **Infection with yeast-like organisms**

RISK INCREASES WITH

- **AIDS:** seborrheic dermatitis is now recognized as one of the most common manifestations of AIDS, affecting as many as 83% of individuals with AIDS. This recent observation has given credence to the infection theory of seborrheic dermatitis.
- **Stress:** when levels of stress hormones, i.e., cortisol, increase in the circulation, immune system defenses, many of which involve inflammatory chemicals, are upregulated.
- **Winter:** Seborrheic dermatitis worsens in dry, cold weather
- **Other skin disorders**, such as acne, rosacea, or psoriasis.
- **Oily skin**
- **Infrequent shampoos**
- **Irritants:** use of irritating soaps, harsh scrubbing, and drying lotions that contain alcohol.

PREVENTIVE MEASURES

- A high-potency multiple vitamin and mineral supplement including 400 μg of folic acid, 400 μg of vitamin B_{12}, and 50–100 mg of vitamin B_6. (Folic acid supplementation should always be accompanied by vitamin B_{12} supplementation to prevent folic acid from masking a vitamin B_{12} deficiency.) A daily multiple providing all of the known vitamins and minerals serves as a foundation upon which to build an individualized health-promotion program.
- Especially during the winter, when cold weather and indoor heating increase the need for hydration, drink at least eight 240 ml (8 US fl oz) glasses of pure, clean water daily.
- Cleanse the skin daily and shampoo frequently using gentle, hypoallergenic products. Soaps and shampoos containing rosemary, calendula and/or chamomile are recommended.

Expected outcomes

Improvements are generally noted within the first month of therapy with most patients experiencing complete resolution.

TREATMENT

Diet

- **For infants**, control of food allergies is key:
  - if the child is nursing, the mother should avoid any foods to which she is allergic as well as common food allergens (milk, corn, wheat, citrus, peanuts, and eggs).
  - if the child is being given formula, this should be based on hydrolyzed protein. Hydrolyzed protein has been broken down or predigested and is therefore hypoallergenic.
- **For adults**, after identifying and removing allergenic foods from the diet, choose a health-promoting diet rich in whole, unprocessed, preferably organic foods, especially plant foods (fruits, vegetables, whole grains, beans, nuts [especially walnuts], and seeds), and cold-water fish:
  - wild-caught cold-water fish are recommended over farm-raised fish since wild-caught fish contain much higher levels of beneficial anti-inflammatory omega-3 fats.
  - for more detailed information, see Appendix 1.

Nutritional supplements

For infants

- **Biotin:** for breast-fed infants, biotin can be given to the mother (see dosage under recommendations for adults below). For infants given formula, 50 μg of biotin can be added q.d.

For adults

- **Biotin:** 3 mg b.i.d.
- **B-complex vitamins:** perhaps the best way to take the following amounts of the B-complex vitamins is in a high-potency multiple vitamin and mineral supplement. Any good multiple should include the B-complex vitamins in the following amounts:

Vitamin	Amount
Vitamin B1 (thiamin)	10–100 mg
Vitamin B2 (riboflavin)	10–50 mg
Niacin	10–100 mg
Niacinamide	10–30 mg
Vitamin B6 (pyridoxine)	25–100 mg
Biotin	100–300 μg
Pantothenic acid	25–100 mg
Folic acid	400 μg
Vitamin B12	400 μg
Choline	10–100 mg
Inositol	10–100 mg

- **Zinc:** a cofactor in numerous enzymatic reactions, zinc is required to create the enzyme delta-6 desaturase, which is responsible for converting the omega-6 fat linoleic acid into gamma-linolenic acid (GLA). The body uses GLA to produce a type of anti-inflammatory prostaglandin:
  - when zinc levels are inadequate, linoleic acid is converted into arachidonic acid, which is used to

produce pro-inflammatory prostaglandins and leukotrienes.

- low zinc levels are a contributing factor not only in seborrheic dermatitis, but also in numerous inflammatory skin disorders including acne, eczema, and psoriasis.
- dosage: 20–30 mg q.d. of zinc picolinate (a well-absorbed form)

■ **Flaxseed oil:** flaxseed oil is the best plant source of anti-inflammatory omega-3 fatty acids:

- flaxseed oil is highly perishable and should be packaged in an opaque container, refrigerated, and never heated. Add flaxseed oil to smoothies, drizzle over steamed vegetables, or use as a dipping oil for bread or as the oil in a favorite salad dressing.
- dosage: 1 tbsp of flaxseed oil q.d.

Topical medicine

■ **Pyridoxine ointment:** in one study, all patients with a form of seborrheic dermatitis called the sicca variant, which involves only the scalp (dandruff), brow, nose and bearded area, experienced complete resolution within 10 days by locally applying a water-soluble ointment containing 50 mg of pyridoxine (vitamin B_6) per gram of ointment:

- improvement may have been the result of correcting a vitamin B_6 deficiency or may have been due to reduction in sebaceous secretion caused by the ointment.
- other forms of seborrheic dermatitis did not respond to this therapy.
- pyridoxine ointment can be obtained from a compounding pharmacist. To locate a compounding pharmacist in your area, call the International Academy of Compounding Pharmacists (1-800-927-4227).

Senile cataracts

DESCRIPTION

Cataracts are white, opaque blemishes on the normally transparent lens of the eye. This lens, a tiny structure located just behind the pupil, is responsible for focusing incoming light (via changes in shape), so it forms clear images on the retina. The lens, which is convex on both sides, is composed of tightly packed, transparent cells. When damaged, the protein structures in the cells turn milky white – much like the clear protein of eggs turns to egg "white" when eggs are cooked.

With normal aging, the lens progressively increases in size, weight, and density, and the majority of people over the age of 60 display some degree of cataract formation; however, although cataracts are common, impaired vision due to significant cataract formation should not be considered an inescapable part of aging. A variety of factors may contribute to cataract formation, but all share the same underlying means of inflicting injury: excessive, unchecked free radical damage that overwhelms normal protective mechanisms.

The lens, like many other tissues of the body, is dependent upon adequate levels of the antioxidant enzymes superoxide dismutase (SOD), catalase, and glutathione (GSH); the vitamin and mineral antioxidants, especially the vitamins E and C, and the mineral selenium; and accessory nutrients, i.e., the carotenes. Individuals with higher dietary intakes of these protective compounds (discussed below) have a much lower risk of developing cataracts. Cataracts evolve gradually, usually over many years. During the early stages, preventive treatment can stop and even reverse cataract formation. Once cataracts are well developed, surgery to remove the lens and implant a plastic intraocular lens may be the only alternative. Fortunately, if the eye is otherwise healthy, this common surgery is successful in 90–95% of cases.

Cataracts are the leading cause of impaired vision in the United States; approximately 4 million people have some degree of vision-impairing cataract, and at least 40,000 are blind as a result of cataracts.

FREQUENT SIGNS AND SYMPTOMS

- Loss of visual clarity and detail, and possibly some blurring
- Difficulty night driving: lights may seem to scatter or have halos
- Blurred vision, especially in bright light
- Double vision (occasionally)
- Opaque, milky-white pupil (advanced cases only)

CAUSES

- **Natural aging:** with normal aging, the transparency of the lens decreases as its size, weight, and density increase.
- **Injury to the eye**
- **Surgery**
- **Ocular disease**, e.g., *uveitis*, an inflammation of the iris.
- **Drugs:** especially cortisone and its derivatives.
- **Heavy metals:** a number of heavy metals have been found in increased concentrations in both the aging lens and lenses with a cataract. All heavy metals promote free radical formation. For example, concentration of cadmium is two to three times higher than normal in lenses containing cataracts. Cadmium prevents zinc from binding in important protective antioxidant enzymes, thus compromising free radical quenching and other protective mechanisms.
- **Exposure to** X-rays, microwaves, infrared radiation, ultraviolet and near-ultraviolet light.
- **Hereditary disease**, e.g., the effect of German measles (rubella) on an unborn child of a mother who contracts this disease early in pregnancy.
- **Illnesses associated with high blood sugar:** diabetes mellitus; *galactosemia* (an inherited disease in which infants cannot digest milk sugar). High blood sugar promotes free radical production and glycation, a process in which sugar molecules bind to and distort protein molecules, rendering them useless.

RISK INCREASES WITH

- Aging
- Exposure to direct sunlight and bright light
- Exposure to X-rays, microwaves, infrared radiation
- Smoking or exposure to second-hand smoke
- Diabetes mellitus
- Drug use, particularly cortisone

■ Standard American Diet: based on animal products and processed foods, with little consumption of fresh vegetables, legumes, fruits, nuts and seeds, and whole grains, the Standard American Diet is low in protective antioxidants, and high in saturated fat, *trans* fats (also called partially hydrogenated oils), sugars and refined carbohydrates, all of which promote inflammation and free radical formation, and increase the risk for obesity, cardiovascular disease, and diabetes, as well as cataracts.

PREVENTIVE MEASURES

■ Avoid direct sunlight and bright light in general.

■ Wear sunglasses with UV protection when outdoors.

■ A high-potency multiple vitamin and mineral supplement including 400 µg of folic acid, 400 µg of vitamin B_{12}, and 50–100 mg of vitamin B_6. (Folic acid supplementation should always be accompanied by vitamin B_{12} supplementation to prevent folic acid from masking a vitamin B_{12} deficiency.) A daily multiple providing all of the known vitamins and minerals serves as a foundation upon which to build an individualized health-promotion program.

■ Consume a nutrient-dense diet rich in whole, unprocessed, preferably organic foods, especially plant foods (fruits, vegetables, beans, seeds and nuts, and whole grains) and cold-water fish, and low in animal products and processed foods (for more detailed information, see Appendix 1).

Expected outcomes

Progression of age-related cataract formation can be stopped, and early cataracts can be reversed. Improvements should be noted within 6 months.

TREATMENT

Diet

■ Follow the dietary recommendations given in Preventive measures.

■ Avoid fried foods, rancid foods, charred meats, and other sources of free radicals.

■ Avoid hydrogenated fats (also called *trans* fats). These chemically altered fats are produced under extreme heat, which promotes free radical formation.

■ Refrigerate all fats (oils, butter) to minimize oxidation and free radical formation.

■ Since exposure to heat causes oxidation (free radical formation) of fats, instead of cooking with fats, cook foods in flavored broths and, if desired, add fats after cooking for flavor.

■ Rely on olive oil, a stable monounsaturated fat, or flaxseed oil, an excellent source of anti-inflammatory omega-3 essential fatty acids, as the fats to add to cooked foods and for salad dressings.

■ Consume both fat and salt judiciously. Excessive consumption of either fat or salt has been linked to increased risk of cataract formation.

■ Increase consumption of legumes. Legumes are high in the sulfur-containing amino acids that are necessary for the proper formation of proteins in the cells of the lens.

■ Increase consumption of vegetables high in carotenes. All yellow-orange vegetables including yams and carrots are high in carotenes, as are leafy greens and broccoli.

■ Increase consumption of whole grains, nuts (especially almonds), and seeds (especially sunflower seeds), which are high in vitamin E.

■ Increase consumption of fresh vegetables (particularly red and green sweet peppers, kale, broccoli, and parsley) and fruits (particularly strawberries, papaya, and oranges), all of which are good sources of vitamin C.

■ Increase consumption of green leafy plants, legumes, and Brewer's yeast. These are the best sources of folic acid. In the body, folic acid is converted into its active form, *tetrahydrobiopterin*, which is believed to play a protective role against cataract formation via prevention of damage caused by ultraviolet light.

Nutritional supplements

■ **Vitamin C:** a water-soluble antioxidant, vitamin C is the body's first line of defense, covering the aqueous environments in the body, both inside and outside cells, and working with vitamin E and carotenes (its fat-soluble partners), as well as with antioxidant enzymes such as glutathione peroxidase, catalase, and superoxide dismutase. In addition, vitamin C regenerates oxidized vitamin E, enabling it to resume its antioxidant defense activities:

  ■ several clinical studies, including one in which cataract patients were followed for 11 years, have demonstrated that vitamin C supplementation at 1 g q.d. can halt cataract progression and, in some cases, significantly improve vision.

  ■ the lens of the eye, as well as other active tissues in the body, requires higher concentrations of vitamin C. While the level of vitamin C is 0.5 mg/dl in the blood, in the lens of the eye, vitamin C is concentrated by at least a factor of 20 times that amount.

  ■ to maintain this concentration, the body must work against the laws of physics, in which elements naturally flow from a higher to a lower concentration. Maintaining the high levels of vitamin C needed for lens health therefore requires a tremendous amount of energy.

- keeping blood levels of vitamin C elevated reduces this gradient, significantly reducing the effort the body must expend to concentrate vitamin C in the lens.
- dosage: 1 g t.i.d.

■ **Selenium:** the antioxidant enzyme *glutathione peroxidase*, which is a key protective factor found in high concentrations in the healthy lens, requires the trace mineral selenium in order to neutralize free radicals:

- early studies showed that selenium content in a human lens with a cataract is only 15% of normal levels.
- a recent study found that a decreased level of selenium was most pronounced in the aqueous humor (fluid) of the eye in patients with cataracts.
- among its many protective activities, selenium-dependent glutathione peroxidase is responsible for the breakdown of hydrogen peroxide, which is associated with free radical damage and damage to the lens, and is found in the aqueous humor of cataract patients at levels up to 25 times higher than normal.
- glutathione levels will normalize with oral selenium and vitamin E supplementation.
- dosage: selenium: 400 µg q.d.

■ **Vitamin E:** the body's primary fat-soluble antioxidant, vitamin E protects all bodily components that contain fat such as the membranes surrounding every cell, including those of the lens of the eye:

- selenium and vitamin E work together, functioning synergistically.
- dosage: 400–800 IU mixed tocopherols q.d.

■ **Superoxide dismutase (SOD) cofactors:** SOD is another important antioxidant enzyme whose levels have been shown to decrease as cataract formation progresses:

- while taking oral forms of SOD has not been shown to increase SOD activity, supplementation with its trace mineral cofactors – zinc, copper, and manganese – is recommended. Levels of these cofactors are greatly reduced in lenses with cataracts. Copper and zinc levels are reduced by over 90%, and manganese by 50%.
- dosage: a high-potency multiple containing the following dosages of these trace minerals is recommended:
  - copper: 1–2 mg
  - manganese: 5–15 mg
  - zinc: 15–45 mg.

■ **Beta-carotene:** a powerful antioxidant, beta-carotene is thought to act as a filter, protecting against light-induced damage to the fiber portion of the lens.

Low levels of beta-carotene leave the lens very susceptible to free radical damage and cataract formation; dosage: 200,000 IU q.d.

■ **Quercetin:** a bioflavonoid with potent antioxidant activity and vitamin-C sparing action, quercetin is especially helpful in preventing cataract formation since it inhibits the enzyme (*aldose reductase*) that converts blood sugar into sorbitol, a compound strongly implicated in cataract formation:

- the lens of the eye lacks the enzyme (*polyol dehydrogenase*) needed to break down sorbitol, which thus accumulates in the lens. This accumulation causes an osmotic gradient that results in water being drawn into cells. As the water is drawn in, the cell must release small molecules, such as the antioxidants vitamin C and glutathione, to maintain osmotic balance. As antioxidant defenses drop, susceptibility to free radical damage increases, resulting in cataract formation.
- dosage: 500 mg t.i.d.

■ **L-cysteine or N-acetylcysteine:** cysteine is an amino acid that is an integral component of glutathione. Cysteine, along with L-glutamine, and L-glycine, the other amino acid precursors of glutathione, has been shown to be of some aid in cataract treatment. However, cysteine given in the form of N-acetylcysteine is believed to be better utilized than L-cysteine:

- dosages:
  - L-cysteine or N-acetylcysteine: 400 mg q.d.
  - L-glutamine: 200 mg q.d.
  - L-glycine: 200 mg q.d.

■ **Methionine:** an amino acid that is a component of *methionine sulfoxide reductase* (an important antioxidant enzyme in the lens), methionine can also be converted to cysteine; dosage: 250–500 mg q.d.

■ **Riboflavin:** the regeneration of active glutathione in the lens requires the vitamin riboflavin. Riboflavin deficiency is fairly common in the geriatric population (33% of persons over age 65 show evidence of low levels of riboflavin):

- **caution:** cataract patients should not take more than 10 mg of riboflavin q.d. since it is a photosensitizing substance that reacts with sunlight to produce free radicals.
- dosage: keep supplementary intake below 10 mg q.d.

Botanical medicines

■ *Vaccinium myrtillus* (bilberry): rich in flavonoids, especially *anthocyanins*, bilberry extract plus vitamin E stopped progression of cataract formation in 48 of 50 patients with cataracts:

- anthocyanins are potent antioxidants with an affinity for the retina and pupil. Even in healthy subjects, bilberry extract has been shown to significantly improve adaptation to dark and night vision. Improvement was evident 2 hours after treatment with a dose of bilberry extract equivalent to 86 mg anthocyanins.

■ bilberry has also been shown to improve visual perception in individuals with defective vision in bright light.

■ dosage: bilberry extract (25% anthocyanidin content): 40–80 mg t.i.d.

■ **Hachimijiogan formula:** this ancient Chinese formula has been shown to increase the antioxidant level of the lens of the eye. In one study, 60% of subjects given Hachimijiogan noted significant improvement, 20% showed no progression, and only the remaining 20% displayed cataract progression.

■ Hachimijiogan formula contains the following eight herbs per 22 g:

● *Rehmania glutinosa*: 6,000 mg

● *Poria cocos sclerotium*: 3,000 mg

● *Dioscorea opposita*: 3,000 mg

● *Cormus officinalis*: 3,000 mg

● *Epimedium grandiflorum*: 3,000 mg

● *Alisma plantago*: 3,000 mg

● *Astragalus membranaceus*: 2,500 mg

● *Cinnamonum cassia*: 1,000 mg

■ dosage: 150 mg t.i.d.

Drug–herb interaction cautions

■ *Vaccinium myrtillus* **(bilberry):**

■ plus *warfarin and antiplatelet drugs*: very high doses (600–800 mg t.i.d.) should be used with caution in patients with hemorrhagic disorders and those taking warfarin and antiplatelet drugs.

Streptococcal pharyngitis

DESCRIPTION

Streptococcal pharyngitis – commonly called *strep throat* – is a sore throat caused by an inflammation of the *pharynx* (the medical term for the throat) as a result of infection by streptococcal bacteria. Although the majority (over 90%) of sore throats are due to viral infections – against which antibiotics are ineffective and which typically resolve after a few days of bed rest, extra fluids, and basic immune support (discussed below) – in the event of a sore throat developing, consulting with a physician to rule out strep throat, for which antibiotics may be suggested, is a good idea. Only a throat culture can accurately diagnose strep throat, but physicians now have swabs that can immediately test for strep, providing a definitive answer in as little as 15 min.

Even if strep is diagnosed, antibiotics may not be necessary. Strep throat is usually a self-limiting disease, and recent research has shown that clinical recovery is similar in cases given or not given antibiotics. The primary concern with not using antibiotics is the development of rheumatic fever or kidney disease. (Rheumatic fever, which may develop 2–3 weeks after a strep throat, is associated with inflammation of the heart, arthritis, and fever.) Unfortunately, antibiotics do not significantly reduce the frequency of these complications, and, in 20% of patients, antibiotics such as penicillin fail to kill off all the streptococci because other organisms (primarily *Staphylococcus aureus* and *Bacteroides* species) are present that deactivate the penicillin, thus shielding the streptococci. We recommend using antibiotics only for those with a prior history of rheumatic fever or strep-induced kidney disease, those suffering from severe infection, or those who are unresponsive after 1 week of treatment with the natural therapies described below.

FREQUENT SIGNS AND SYMPTOMS

Signs suggestive of sore throat due to strep infection
- Sudden onset
- Very painful sore throat
- Tender, swollen lymph nodes in the neck
- Much difficulty in swallowing

- Appetite loss
- General ill feeling
- Headache, stomach pain, vomiting
- Red swollen tonsils, with white splotches (pus)
- Fever of 102°F or higher

Signs suggestive of sore throat due to viral infection
- Gradual onset from mild scratchy throat to uncomfortable sore throat
- Mild difficulty in swallowing
- Cough
- Headache
- Runny nose
- Hoarseness
- Tonsils may or may not be swollen
- Tonsils may or may not have a white coating
- Throat may be red
- Mild to moderate fever, if any

Caution: if you are recovering from a sore throat and develop fever, joint pain, all-over aches and pain, a rash or muscle spasms, call a physician immediately. These may be signs of rheumatic fever.

CAUSES

Bacterial infection with group A beta-hemolytic *Streptococcus pharyngotonsillitis*.

RISK INCREASES WITH

- **Cold, wet, weather:** sore throats occur more often in late winter and early spring.
- **Illness that has lowered resistance**
- **Fatigue or overwork:** inadequate rest results in depressed immune function. Overwork exacerbates stress.
- **Stress:** stress increases levels of adrenal gland hormones, including adrenaline and corticosteroids, which inhibit white blood cell formation and function, and cause the thymus gland (the master gland of the

immune system) to shrink:

- stress also stimulates the sympathetic nervous system – the part of the autonomic nervous system responsible for the fight-or-flight response.
- the immune system functions better under the other arm of the autonomic nervous system – the parasympathetic nervous system – which assumes control over the body during periods of rest, relaxation, meditation, and sleep.

- **Smoking:** both smoking and exposure to cigarette smoke increase susceptibility to strep throat via several mechanisms:
  - exposure to cigarette smoke depletes the body's vitamin C stores.
  - nicotine causes the body to produce cortisol, a hormone that suppresses the immune system.
  - cigarette smoke is a local irritant, damaging the protective mucous membranes lining the throat.

- **Alcohol consumption:** studies of human blood cells show a profound depression in the rate of mobilization into areas of infection after people consume alcohol.

- **Frequent consumption of sugar, refined foods:** consuming 75 g (3 oz) of sugar in one sitting in any form (sucrose, honey, fruit juice) depresses white (immune) cell activity by 50% for 1–5 hours.

- **Local irritation:** a variety of factors can damage the throat's protective mucosal lining, including: overuse of the *larynx* (the voice box); inhaled environmental pollutants: gasoline fumes, pesticides; chemicals used in the workplace, e.g., copy machines, beauty salon hair and nail products, car cleaning products, painting supplies; cigarette smoke, smoke from burning leaves or wood-burning fireplaces; house cleaning products; dust, or dry winter air.

- **Nutrient deficiency:** an overwhelming number of clinical and experimental studies show that a deficiency of any single nutrient can profoundly impair immune function.

- **Standard American Diet:** immune function is directly related to the quality of foods routinely eaten. The Standard American Diet, which is based on processed foods, is high in fats and sugars (both of which depress immune function), and leads to obesity, which has also been linked to suppressed immune function.

- **Obesity:** in experimental studies, the white blood cells of overweight individuals were less able to destroy bacteria.

- **Less than 7 hours sleep per night:** during the deepest levels of sleep, potent immune-enhancing compounds are released and many immune functions are greatly increased.

- **Food allergy:** the typical upper respiratory tract symptoms of chronic delayed food allergy include chronic sore throat, runny nose, sinusitis, tonsillitis, and laryngitis.

PREVENTIVE MEASURES

- Don't smoke, and avoid exposure to second-hand smoke.
- Minimize consumption of sugars and refined foods.
- Minimize alcohol consumption.
- Consume a nutrient-dense diet rich in whole, unprocessed, preferably organic foods, especially plant foods (fruits, vegetables, beans, seeds and nuts, and whole grains) and cold-water fish, and low in animal products and processed foods (for more detailed information, see Appendix 1).
- A high-potency multiple vitamin and mineral supplement including 400 µg of folic acid, 400 µg of vitamin B_{12}, and 50–100 mg of vitamin B_6. (Folic acid supplementation should always be accompanied by vitamin B_{12} supplementation to prevent folic acid from masking a vitamin B_{12} deficiency.) A daily multiple providing all of the known vitamins and minerals serves as a foundation upon which to build an individualized health-promotion program.
- To prevent reinfection from microbes residing in a toothbrush, wash the toothbrush in the dishwasher at least once a week, and change to a new toothbrush every 2–4 weeks.
- Identify and eliminate food allergens from the diet.

Expected outcomes

Acute infection should resolve within 4–10 days. Failure to respond within this time frame may require antibiotic therapy.

Once all contributing factors have been identified and appropriate measures (described in Preventive Measures and Treatment) have been instituted, chronic sore throats should no longer be a problem.

TREATMENT

Fever is a natural immune defense mechanism and should be supported, rather than suppressed by using drugs – unless the body temperature approaches 104°F, at which point the body's ability to control temperature becomes impaired.

Diet

- **Eliminate all sources of concentrated simple sugars:** sugar, honey, fruit juice, dried fruit, candy, cake, cookies, baked goods, ice cream, popsicles, etc.

- **Eliminate refined carbohydrates**, which are quickly broken down into sugars in the digestive tract. Products made from refined flour (white or wheat – rather than whole wheat – flour) include bread, cereals, crackers, chips, and pasta. Use whole wheat or whole grain versions of these products.
- **Minimize consumption of dairy products:** a common allergen, dairy also increases mucus production in some people.
- **Increase fluid intake** to 240 ml (8 US fl oz) per hour, using filtered water and the herbal teas listed below.
- **Follow food recommendations** given in Preventive Measures.
- **Eliminate all suspected food allergens** from the diet (for additional information see the chapter on Food allergy).

Nutritional supplements

- **Vitamin A:** often called the anti-infective vitamin, vitamin A is essential for the health of the epithelium, including the mucous membranes in the respiratory system. The epithelium, a layer of cells forming the epidermis of the skin and the surface layer of mucous and serous membranes, is the body's first line of defense against invading pathogens. All epithelial surfaces rely upon vitamin A. When vitamin A levels are inadequate, keratin is secreted in these tissues, transforming them from their normally pliable, moist condition into stiff dry tissue that is unable to carry out its functions, and leading to breaches in epithelial integrity that significantly increase susceptibility to the development of infection and allergy:
  - dosage: 50,000 IU q.d. for up to 2 days in infants and up to 1 week in adults, or beta-carotene: 200,000 IU q.d.
  - **caution:** at high doses, vitamin A has been linked to birth defects. Women of childbearing age who are pregnant or at risk for pregnancy should **not** use vitamin A. For these women, beta-carotene, also called pro-vitamin A since it can be converted in the body to vitamin A, is a safe and effective alternative.
- **Vitamin C:** the body's primary water-soluble antioxidant, vitamin C is directly antiviral and antibacterial, but its most potent protective benefits result from its amplification of immune function via numerous mechanisms including: enhancing white blood cell response and function, increasing interferon levels (a special chemical factor that fights viral infection and cancer), increasing the secretion of thymic hormones (the thymus is the master gland of the immune system), and improving the integrity of the lining of

the mucous membranes:
  - both experimental animal research and population surveys have demonstrated a correlation between vitamin C deficiency and the development of rheumatic fever. Findings showed that when vitamin C intake was high, rheumatic fever was virtually nonexistent; 18% of children in high-risk groups had subnormal serum vitamin C levels; supplementation with vitamin C totally prevented the development of rheumatic fever in streptococcal-infected rheumatic-fever-susceptible guinea pigs.
  - dosage: 500 mg every 2 waking hours.
- **Bioflavonoids:** a group of plant pigments largely responsible for the colors of fruits and flowers, bioflavonoids are powerful antioxidants in their own right, and, when taken with vitamin C, significantly enhance both its absorption and effectiveness:
  - dosage: 1,000 mg q.d.
- **Thymus extract:** substantial clinical data demonstrate that thymus extracts restore and enhance immune system function by improving the function of the thymus, the master gland of the immune system. In double-blind studies, thymus extracts have been shown not only to treat current respiratory tract infections but also, over the course of a year, to significantly reduce the number of respiratory infections while improving numerous immune parameters:
  - dosage: the equivalent of 120 mg pure polypeptides with molecular weights less than 10,000, or roughly 500 mg of the crude polypeptide fraction.
- **Zinc:** the most critical mineral for immune function, zinc promotes the destruction of foreign particles and micro-organisms, protects against free radical damage, acts synergistically with vitamin A, is required for proper white cell function, and is necessary for the activation of serum thymic factor – a thymus hormone with profound immune-enhancing actions. Zinc also inhibits replication of several viruses, including those that cause the common cold:
  - dosage: take lozenges that supply 15–25 mg of elemental zinc (use the gluconate form without citrate, mannitol or sorbitol). Dissolve one lozenge in the mouth every 2 waking hours after an initial double dose. Continue for up to 3 days.
- **Probiotics:** if antibiotics are or have been used, a probiotic supplement containing *Lactobacillus acidophilus* and *Bifidobacterium bifidus* are definitely indicated. Probiotic supplementation helps prevent and treat antibiotic-induced diarrhea, Candida overgrowth, and urinary tract infections. Taking *L. acidophilus* products during antibiotic therapy can help prevent reductions in levels of friendly bacteria, and/or a superinfection

with antibiotic-resistant flora:

- dosage: during antibiotic usage, a dosage of at least 15–20 billion organisms q.d. is required and should be taken as far apart in time from the antibiotic as possible. After the course of antibiotics is finished, a dosage of 1–2 billion live organisms q.d. is sufficient.

Botanical medicines

- ***Hydrastis canadensis* (goldenseal):** a berberine alkaloid that is an active component in goldenseal exerts specific antibiotic activity against streptococci:
  - dosage: since dosage should be based on berberine content, standardized extracts are recommended. Choose one of the following forms and take the recommended dosage t.i.d.:
    - dried root or as infusion (tea): 2–4 g
    - tincture (1 : 5): 6–12 ml (1.5–3 tsp)
    - fluid extract (1 : 1): 2–4 ml (0.5–1 tsp)
    - solid (dry powdered) extract (4 : 1 or 8–12% alkaloid content): 250–500 mg.
- ***Echinacea* spp. (*Echinacea angustifolia* and *Echinacea purpurea*):** both of these widely used species of *Echinacea* exert profound immune-enhancing effects that result in increased activity of many key immune functions including: production of T cells, macrophage phagocytosis, antibody binding, natural killer cell activity, and levels of circulating neutrophils:
  - in relation to strep throat, specifically, echinacea prevents bacteria, including streptococci, from initiating an infection. *Echinacea* does this by inhibiting an enzyme secreted by bacteria (*hyaluronidase*) that damages the protective mucous membranes, thus allowing the organism to enter the body.
  - dosage: choose one of the following forms of *Echinacea* spp. and take the recommended dosage t.i.d.:
    - dried root (or as tea): 0.5–1 g
    - freeze-dried plant: 325–650 mg
    - juice of aerial portion of *E. purpurea* stabilized in 22% ethanol: 2–3 ml
    - tincture (1 : 5): 2–4 ml
    - fluid extract (1 : 1): 2–4 ml
    - solid (dry powdered) extract (6.5 : 1 or 3.5% echinacoside): 150–300 mg.

Drug–herb interaction cautions
None.

Topical medicine

- **Gargle with salt water b.i.d.:** 1 tbsp of salt dissolved in 240 ml (8 US fl oz) of warm water.
- ***Zingiber officinale* (ginger) tea:** fresh ginger has analgesic properties, so a strong ginger tea is helpful in relieving throat irritation. To prepare an analgesic tea, dice several thin slices of fresh ginger root, place in a teacup or mug, pour in boiling water, and let steep for 5–10 min.

Trichomoniasis

DESCRIPTION

Trichomoniasis is a very contagious sexually transmitted disease caused by a tiny parasite, *Trichomonas vaginalis*, which lives in the lower genitourinary tract of infected men and women. Although typically sexually transmitted, trichomoniasis can also be contracted from an infected washcloth or towel, and can be transmitted from mother to baby during childbirth. In women, the principal sites of infection are the vagina, urethra and bladder. In men, the urethra, epididymis (a C-shaped structure attached to the upper part of each testicle in which sperm mature), and prostate gland may be involved. *Trichomonas* may live in its host for years without producing symptoms, then, perhaps due to lowered resistance, it can suddenly multiply rapidly, producing the unpleasant symptoms noted below.

Trichomoniasis is the second most prevalent vaginal infection in the US. Approximately 2.5 million women in the US acquire this infection annually, and one in five women will be infected with *T. vaginalis* at some time in her life. Although the incidence is lower in men, and most infected men experience no symptoms, it is estimated that 5–15% of non-gonococcal urethritis is caused by trichomonal infection, and mild cases of urethritis, prostatitis, and epididymitis have been reported.

Although trichomoniasis is not considered a serious infection and is exceedingly common, trichomonal infections should be taken very seriously.

- Trichomoniasis and gonorrhea are common coexisting infections, with up to 40% of women who have trichomoniasis having gonorrhea and vice versa.
- Trichomoniasis is a frequent cause (90%) of cervical erosion and therefore may be a factor in the development of cervical cancer.
- Prostatitis and epididymitis are common in infected men.
- Trichomoniasis increases the incidence of sterility among men and women. In men, the organism's toxic by-products decrease sperm motility. In women, trichomonal infection may result in inflammation with potential scarring of the uterine tube.
- Newborns infected in the birth canal may manifest serious illness, although this is rare.

- Metronidazole (Flagyl), the drug must commonly used to eliminate *Trichomonas*, has been found to be carcinogenic and teratogenic (causing birth defects) in rodents.

Because *Trichomonas* is now known to persist in the male as well as the female reproductive tract, and reinfection of sexually active partners is well documented, treatment of both sexual partners is necessary.

FREQUENT SIGNS AND SYMPTOMS

Women
- Profuse, foul-smelling, white to green-colored vaginal discharge
- Vaginal discharge is most noticeable several days after a menstrual period
- Vaginal itching, burning, irritation, pain
- Painful urination, if the urine touches inflamed tissue
- Redness of the labia (vaginal lips) and vagina
- Prepubescent and postmenopausal women seldom have symptomatic infections
- Laboratory testing: positive culture of the organism grown from a sample of vaginal discharge, swabs taken from the urethra, or PAP smear

Men
- Frequently no symptoms
- Some urethral discomfort
- Head of the penis may be inflamed
- Laboratory testing: trichomonads identified in semen, urethral discharge, urine, and prostatic fluid

CAUSES

Infection with the flagellate protozoan *Trichomonas vaginalis*.

RISK INCREASES WITH

- **Number of sexual partners**
- **Oral contraceptives and/or HRT:** oral contraceptives are estrogens. Conventional HRT (hormone

replacement therapy) typically involves estrogen. Under the stimulation of excess estrogen, the vaginal walls become packed full of glycogen – a storage form of sugar that provides the optimal fuel for *Trichomonas* to flourish and multiply.

- **Antibiotic use:** antibiotics kill off not only their pathogenic target organisms, but also friendly *Lactobacillus acidophilus*. In the vagina, these lactobacilli help to maintain a normal pH of 3.5–4.5. A decrease in the number of these friendly vaginal flora allows the pH to increase. *Trichomonas* thrives in a vaginal pH of 5.5–5.8.
- **Wearing tight jeans, nylon underwear, or pantyhose:** these foster the warm, moist environment in which infections thrive.
- **Depression and anxiety** have been associated with exacerbation of trichomonal infections.

PREVENTIVE MEASURES

- **Ideally:** restrict sexual relations to a monogamous relationship with an uninfected partner.
- **Practice safe sex:** restrict the number of sexual partners, and use a latex (rubber) condom every time you have sexual intercourse.
- **Wear cotton underwear and clothing** made from natural, breathable fabric that is loose enough to allow air to circulate, so moisture can evaporate. Rather than pantyhose, wear a garter belt and stockings or thigh-high stockings, which are held up by an elasticized band around the thigh. If pantyhose are essential, cut a slit in the crotch to improve airflow. (The crotch panel in most pantyhose is reinforced on all four sides, so cutting an opening should not create a run in the stockings.)
- **Standard American Diet:** immune function is directly related to the quality of foods routinely eaten. The Standard American Diet, which is based on processed foods, is high in fats and sugars (both of which depress immune function), and leads to obesity, which has also been linked to suppressed immune function.
- **Nutrient deficiency:** a deficiency of any nutrient can impair the immune system's ability to prevent infection. A high-potency multiple vitamin and mineral supplement is therefore recommended. A good multiple should include $400\,\mu g$ of folic acid, $400\,\mu g$ of vitamin B_{12}, and $50–100\,mg$ of vitamin B_6. (Folic acid supplementation should always be accompanied by vitamin B_{12} supplementation to prevent folic acid from masking a vitamin B_{12} deficiency.)
- **Take action to reduce stress:** get a minimum of 7 hours sleep each night, eat regular meals, exercise regularly, meditate, seek counseling, attend services at the denomination of your choice.

Expected outcomes

Signs and symptoms usually resolve within 4–7 days or even sooner. Nonetheless, it is important to continue treatment for at least 2–4 weeks to ensure complete elimination of the infection.

TREATMENT

Diet

- **Consume a health-promoting diet:** to support the immune system's ability to eradicate infection, consume a nutrient-dense diet rich in natural fiber from fruits, vegetables, beans, and whole grains, and low in fat, sugar and refined carbohydrates from meat and dairy products and processed foods (for more detailed information, see the Appendix 1).
- **Eliminate all sources of concentrated simple sugars:** sugar, honey, fruit juice, dried fruit, candy, cake, cookies, baked goods, ice cream, popsicles, etc.:
  - consuming $75\,g$ ($3\,oz$) of sugar in one sitting in any form (sucrose, honey, fruit juice) depresses white (immune) cell activity by 50% for 1–5 hours.
- **Eliminate refined carbohydrates**, which are quickly broken down into sugars in the digestive tract. Products made from refined flour (white or wheat – rather than whole wheat – flour) include bread, cereals, crackers, chips, and pasta. Use whole wheat or whole grain versions of these products.
- **Decrease consumption of fats:** increased blood levels of fats inhibit various immune functions, including the ability of white blood cells to divide, move to areas of infection, and destroy micro-organisms.
- **Minimize alcohol consumption:** studies have shown that after people consume alcohol, the rate at which immune defenses are mobilized into areas of infection is significantly depressed.

Nutritional supplements

- **Vitamin A:** often called the anti-infective vitamin, vitamin A is essential for the health and integrity of the mucous membranes that line the genitourinary tract. When vitamin A levels are inadequate, keratin is secreted in these mucous membranes, transforming them from their normally pliable, moist condition into stiff dry tissue that is unable to carry out its functions, and leading to breaches in mucosal integrity that significantly increase susceptibility to infectious organisms:
  - dosage: 25,000 IU q.d. or beta-carotene: 200,000 IU q.d.

- **caution:** at high doses, vitamin A has been linked to birth defects. Women of childbearing age who are pregnant or at risk for pregnancy should **not** use high doses of vitamin A. For these women, beta-carotene, also called pro-vitamin A since it can be converted in the body to vitamin A, is a safe and effective alternative.
- **Vitamin C:** vitamin C aids in the migration of phagocytic cells – the immune defenders that engulf and destroy pathogens – to the area of infection. Phagocytic cells use free radicals as weapons to destroy their prey. Once generated, however, the free radicals must themselves be disarmed or they will damage surrounding tissue. Vitamin C preserves the integrity of healthy cells by inactivating these free radicals; dosage: 500–1,000 mg every 4 hours.
- **B-complex vitamins:** the B vitamins pyridoxine, pantothenic acid, vitamin B_{12}, and folate all enhance the activity of neutrophils, B cells and T cells. Neutrophils engulf and destroy bacteria; B cells produce antibodies that bind to bacteria, initiating a sequence of events that leads to their destruction, and T cells orchestrate many immune defense functions including the destruction of infected cells.
- **Zinc:** zinc promotes the destruction of foreign particles and microorganisms including *T. vaginalis*, and also protects against free radical damage, acts synergistically with vitamin A, is required for proper white cell function, and is necessary for the activation of serum thymic factor – a thymus hormone with profound immune-enhancing actions:
  - *for men*: trichomonads are readily killed by zinc at a concentration of 0.042% (6.4 mmol/L) – a concentration that can occur in the prostatic fluid. Persistent trichomonal infections in men may be the result of low-level zinc deficiency.
  - *for women*: in one study of drug-resistant trichomoniasis of 4 months to 4 years' duration, zinc douches in combination with metronidazole cured the infection (see Topical medicine below).
  - dosage: zinc picolinate (a well-absorbed form): 10–15 mg q.d.
- **Vitamin E:** given in doses higher than the minimum requirements, vitamin E has been shown to enhance antibody responses and host resistance, and to accelerate the clearance of dead particulate matter; dosage: 200 IU (mixed tocopherols) q.d.
- **Probiotics:** if antibiotics are or have been used, a probiotic supplement containing *Lactobacillus acidophilus* and *Bifidobacterium bifidus* are definitely indicated. In addition to maintaining a pH that discourages *Trichomonas*, these probiotics help to prevent and treat antibiotic-induced diarrhea, Candida

overgrowth, and urinary tract infections. Taking *L. acidophilus* products during antibiotic therapy can help prevent reductions in levels of friendly bacteria, and/or a superinfection with antibiotic-resistant flora:
- dosage: during antibiotic usage, a dosage of at least 15–20 billion organisms q.d. is required and should be taken as far apart in time from the antibiotic as possible. After the course of antibiotics is finished, a dosage of 1–2 billion live organisms q.d. is sufficient.

Botanical medicines

- ***Hydrastis canadensis* (goldenseal):** a berberine alkaloid that is an active component in goldenseal has been shown *in vitro* (test tube studies) to inhibit the growth of several protozoa including *T. vaginalis*:
  - dosage: since dosage should be based on berberine content, standardized extracts are recommended. Choose one of the following forms and take the recommended dosage t.i.d.:
    - dried root: 0.5–1 g
    - tincture (1 : 10): 6–12 ml (1.5–3 tsp)
    - fluid extract (1 : 1): 1–2 ml (0.5 tsp)
    - solid (dry powdered) extract (4 : 1 or 8–12% alkaloid content): 250 mg.
- ***Echinacea* spp. (*Echinacea purpurea* and *Echinacea angustifolia*):** both of these widely used species of *Echinacea* exert profound immune-enhancing effects that result in increased activity of many key immune functions including: production of T cells, macrophage phagocytosis, antibody binding, natural killer cell activity, and levels of circulating neutrophils:
  - *inulin*, an active constituent of *Echinacea*, activates *complement*, a group of at least 20 immune defense proteins that has been shown to destroy *T. vaginalis* both *in vitro* (test tube) and *in vivo* (in live subjects). In addition, inulin promotes the migration of immune defense cells to the area of infection.
  - dosage: choose one of the following forms of *Echinacea* spp. and take the recommended dosage t.i.d.:
    - dried root (or as tea): 0.5–1 g
    - freeze-dried plant: 325–650 mg
    - juice of aerial portion of *E. purpurea* stabilized in 22% ethanol: 2–3 ml
    - tincture (1 : 5): 2–4 ml
    - fluid extract (1 : 1): 2–4 ml
    - solid (dry powdered) extract (6.5 : 1 or 3.5% echinacoside): 150–300 mg.
- ***Angelica* spp.:** *Angelica* contains coumarin compounds that have been shown to activate complement:
  - dosage: choose one of the following forms of *Angelica* spp. and take the recommended dosage t.i.d.:
    - dried dried root or rhizome: 1–2 g

- tincture (1 : 5): 3–5 ml
- fluid extract (1 : 1): 0.5–2 ml.

Drug–herb interaction cautions
None.

Topical medicine

■ **Zinc sulfate douche:** use a 1% solution of zinc sulfate as a douche b.i.d. for 14 days.

■ **Betadine (povidone-iodine) douche or saturated tampon:** povidone-iodine is well recognized as highly effective in killing a large number of organisms causing vaginitis, including *Trichomonas*. Povidone-iodine is preferred since it does not sting, is water-soluble, and washes out of clothing. A success rate of 98.1% has been reported in patients with intractable trichomonal vaginitis with a 2-week treatment regimen using Betadine preparations. Other studies suggest a 28-day course of Betadine *pessaries* (a *pessary* is a saturated tampon used as a vaginal suppository), particularly if the patient is using oral contraceptives:

  - dosage: b.i.d. for 14 days.

■ ***Melaleuca alternifolia* (tea tree oil):** commonly used as a germicidal agent in Great Britain and Australia, a 40% solution of tea tree oil has been found to be a highly effective treatment for *Trichomonas* infection that produced no irritation, burning, or other side-effects:

  - dosage: swab on affected area b.i.d., or use a douche made from 1 L of a 0.4% solution b.i.d., or if using a vaginal suppository, insert one at night.

■ **Lactobacillus culture yogurt douches:** as described above under Risks and Nutritional supplements, lactobacilli promote a pH that is unfavorable to *T. vaginalis* and, when well established, supplant unfriendly organisms:

  - dosage: daily culture yogurt douches, preferably in the morning.

Urticaria

DESCRIPTION

Urticaria (hives) is an allergic reaction that is characterized by raised, swollen welts with blanched centers, and is limited to the superficial portion of the skin. These welts, also called *wheals* and *flare lesions*, are surrounded with redness and may coalesce to become giant lesions. About 50% of patients with hives develop *angioedema* – a deeper, more serious reaction involving the tissue below the surface of the skin and causing a more diffuse swelling of the affected area.

The proximate cause of hives is the release of *histamine* (an allergic mediator in the skin) and other inflammatory mediators from white blood cells (*mast cells* and *basophils*), which play a key role in allergies. Mast cells are found near small blood vessels throughout the body, but especially in the skin, while basophils circulate in the blood. When these immune cells are activated, they release histamine and other inflammatory compounds. Mast cells and basophils can be triggered as a result of the classic allergic reaction in which complexes of allergic antibodies (IgE) and antigens (foreign molecules) bind to the mast cells and basophils, initiating histamine release; however, a variety of other factors including reactions to drugs, food additives, foods, and infection with Candida yeast (discussed below) appear to be more important in stimulating the release of histamine in hives.

Although hives can disappear in a matter of hours, and most cases spontaneously clear within a few days to a few weeks, in some people, hives can become chronic, lasting for several months or even longer. Recurrent episodes of hives or angioedema of less than 6 weeks' duration are considered "acute", while attacks persisting beyond 6 weeks are designated "chronic".

Hives and angioedema are relatively common: 15–20% of the US population is estimated to have had hives at some time in their lives. Acute or chronic hives may affect any age group, but young adults (post-adolescence through the third decade of life) are those most often affected.

FREQUENT SIGNS AND SYMPTOMS

Urticaria
- Itching, which can be intense, is usually the first symptom, soon followed by the appearance of patches of raised, swollen welts with blanched centers (wheals).
- Wheals measure 1–5 cm in diameter and have clearly defined edges and flat tops.
- Wheals may coalesce to form giant welts or plaques.
- Wheals and plaques may rapidly change shape, resolve, and reappear in minutes or hours.
- Wheals are limited to the superficial portion of the skin.

Angioedema
- Similar eruptions to hives, but with larger swollen areas that involve structures beneath the skin.

CAUSES

Physical conditions
Hives can result from a reaction to various physical conditions. The most common types of urticaria due to physical conditions are as follows:
- **Dermographic urticaria:** hives evolve rapidly when moderate amounts of pressure are applied. Pressure may occur from simple contact with another person, furniture, bracelets, watch bands, towels, or bedding:
  - the most frequent type of physical urticaria; affects 1.5–5% of the population and is found twice as frequently in women than in men, with average age of onset in the 30s.
  - incidence is much higher among obese persons, especially those who wear tight clothing.
  - lesions typically start within 1–2 min of contact as a general redness in the area, replaced within 3–5 min with a welt. Maximal swelling usually occurs within 10–15 min and can last for up to 3 hours, although redness generally regresses within an hour.
  - may be associated with other conditions including parasite infection, insect bites, hormonal changes, thyroid disorders, pregnancy, menopause, diabetes, immunological alterations, drug therapy (during or following), chronic candidiasis, angioedema, or elevated levels of *eosinophils* (another type of white blood cell linked to allergies).
- **Cholinergic urticaria:** the second most common physical urticaria, cholinergic urticaria (commonly called "prickly heat rash") is triggered by three basic

types of stimulus – passive overheating, physical exercise, and emotional stress:

- lesions, which depend upon stimulation of the sweat glands, usually arise within 2–10 min after provocation and last for 30–50 min.
- wheals arise at or between hair follicles, typically on the upper trunk and arms.
- other systemic symptoms may occur including headache, swelling around the eyes, tearing, and burning around the eyes. In less frequent severe reactions, symptoms may include nausea, vomiting, abdominal cramps, diarrhea, dizziness, low blood pressure, and asthma attacks.

- **Cold urticaria:** a skin reaction to contact with cold objects, water, or air, cold urticaria lesions are usually restricted to the area of exposure and develop within a few seconds to minutes after the cold trigger is removed, and the skin warms up:
  - widespread local exposure and generalized hives can be accompanied by flushing, headaches, chills, dizziness, rapid heartbeat, abdominal pain, nausea, vomiting, muscle pain, shortness of breath, wheezing, or unconsciousness.
  - cold urticaria has been observed in conjunction with a variety of clinical conditions including multiple insect bites, penicillin injections, viral infections, parasitic infestations, syphilis, dietary changes, and stress.

Drugs

Drugs are the leading cause of hives in adults. Virtually every drug may cause hives in some persons, but the two most common drugs that produce hives are penicillin and aspirin.

- Drugs are typically composed of small molecules that bind to larger molecules, triggering the immune system to develop allergic antibodies to the larger molecule complex. Alternatively, drugs can interact directly with mast cells to induce the release of histamine.
- Drugs known to cause hives include: acetylsalicylic acid (aspirin), allopurinol, antimony, antipyrines, barbiturates, bismuth, chlorhydrate, chlorpromazine, corticotropin (ACTH), eucalyptus, fluorides, gold, griseofulvin, insulin, iodine, liver extract, menthol, meprobamate, mercury, morphine (opium), para-aminosalicylic acid, penicillin, phenacetin, phenobarbital, pilocarpine, poliomyelitis vaccine, potassium sulfocyanate, procaine, promethazine, quinine, reserpine, saccharin, thiamin chloride, thiouracil.
- **Penicillin:** at least 10% of the general population is thought to be allergic to penicillin, and nearly 25% of these individuals will display hives, angioedema, or *anaphylaxis* (when the swelling of angioedema affects the throat, interfering with a person's ability to breathe) when given penicillin:
  - penicillin and related contaminants can exist undetected in foods, and anaphylactic symptoms have been traced to penicillin in milk, soft drinks, and frozen dinners.
  - milk is especially problematic since penicillin breaks down into more allergenic compounds in milk.
  - in one study of 245 patients with chronic hives, 42 were sensitive to penicillin. Of these 42, 22 improved on a dairy-free diet.

- **Aspirin:** patients with chronic hives are 20 times more likely to be sensitive to aspirin than normal persons without hives. Studies have found that 2–67% of patients with chronic hives are sensitive to aspirin. Aspirin and other NSAIDs (non-steroidal anti-inflammatory drugs) not only directly trigger an immune response, but also dramatically increase gut permeability and thus the absorption of potential allergens from the digestive tract.

Food allergy

Although any food can be the causative agent, in adults the most common offenders are milk, fish (especially shellfish), meat, eggs, beans, and nuts.

- For a food allergy to develop, the allergen must be absorbed through the intestinal barrier into the circulation. Several factors are known to significantly increase gut permeability including:
  - vasoactive amines – compounds found in certain foods such as chocolate, red wine and aged cheese or produced by the action of unfriendly gut bacteria on essential amino acids
  - alcohol
  - NSAIDs
  - many food additives.

Underlying digestive dysfunction

Several investigators have reported alterations in gastric acidity, intestinal motility (contractions of the intestine that propel food through), and other gastric functions in up to 85% of patients with chronic hives.

- Achlorhydria (no gastric acid output) was noted in one study in 24 (31%) of 77 patients with chronic hives.
- Hypochlorhydria was noted in 41 (53%) of patients in this same study.
- Correction of these underlying digestive dysfunctions through supplementation with hydrochloric acid and a vitamin B complex resulted in impressive clinical improvement.

Food additives

Food additives are a major factor in chronic hives in children.

- **Sensitivity:** all of the following have been shown to produce hives in sensitive individuals: colorants (azo dyes, particularly tartrazine, discussed below), flavorings (particularly salicylates, aspartame), preservatives (benzoates, nitrites, sorbic acid), antioxidants (hydroxytoluene, sulfite, gallate), and emulsifiers/stabilizers (polysorbates, vegetable gums).
- **Additive-free diet:** in a recent study of 64 patients with chronic urticaria, within 2 weeks on an additive-free diet, 73% had a significant reduction of symptoms.
- **Tartrazine (FD&C yellow #5):** reported in 1959 to induce hives, tartrazine is one of the most widely used colorants, added to almost every packaged food and to many drugs, including some antihistamines, antibiotics, steroids (including aminophylline, an antiasthma drug), and sedatives:
  - reactions to tartrazine are so common, its use has been banned in Sweden. Numerous studies have shown that diets which eliminate tartrazine, and other azo dyes and food additives, are of great benefit to individuals sensitive to these compounds.
  - in studies, from 5–95% of patients with chronic hives were sensitive to tartrazine.
  - in the US, the average person consumes 15 mg of certified dyes each day, 85% of which is tartrazine; among children, dye consumption is typically much higher.
  - among individuals who are sensitive to aspirin, 20–50% are also sensitive to tartrazine. Both compounds share a mechanism of action – they inhibit the enzyme cyclo-oxygenase. In some individuals, this results in the production of excessive levels of inflammatory compounds called leukotrienes that are 100 times more potent than histamine.
  - the cyclooxygenase enzyme has two forms: one form, COX-2, produces inflammation, while the other form, COX-1, is protective of the mucosal lining of the gut. Like aspirin and other non-steroidal anti-inflammatory drugs that block both COX-1 and COX-2, tartrazine may cause an increase in gut permeability.
  - tartrazine (along with benzoate and aspirin) increases production of another compound (lymphokine leukocyte inhibitory factor) that results in an increase in the number of mast cells throughout the body.
- **Salicylates:** salicylic acid esters, agents whose mechanism of action is similar to aspirin, are used to flavor foods such as cake mixes, puddings, ice cream, chewing gum, and soft drinks:
  - in addition, natural salicylates are found in many foods, and dietary intake may be a significant

contributing factor to hives in sensitive individuals. Average salicylate intake from foods is estimated to range from 10–200 mg q.d.
  - foods containing the highest amounts of salicylates include berries and dried fruits, especially raisins and prunes; candies made of licorice and peppermint; and some herbs and condiments, especially curry powder, paprika, thyme, dill, oregano, and turmeric. Moderate levels of salicylates are found in nuts and seeds.
- **Benzoates:** one reason why adverse reactions to fish and shrimp are so common in patients with hives is that these foods frequently contain extremely high levels of added benzoates.
- **BHT and BHA:** typically, 15% of patients with chronic hives test positive to oral challenge with BHT. BHT and BHA are the primary antioxidants used in prepared and packaged foods.
- **Sulfites:** ubiquitous in foods and drugs, sulfites are added to processed foods to prevent microbial spoilage and to keep them from turning brown or changing color. Sulfites are also sprayed on fresh foods such as shrimp, fruits and vegetables, and used as antioxidants and preservatives in many drugs:
  - although their use on fruits and vegetables has been banned in the US because they caused so many health problems, including asthma and hives, sulfites are still found in many foods, especially wine and beer – two to three glasses of wine or beer provides 10 mg of sulfites.
  - normally, sulfites are metabolized by the enzyme sulfite oxidase into safer sulfates, which are then excreted in the urine. In some individuals, however, sulfite oxidase functions poorly, leading to problems caused by a buildup of sulfites. The enzyme sulfite oxidase is dependent on the trace mineral molybdenum, so supplementation of molybdenum (200 µg q.d.) may be beneficial.
- **Food emulsifiers and stabilizers:** these may also induce hives in sensitive individuals and include polysorbate in ice cream, vegetable gums such as acacia, gum arabic, tragacanth, quince, and carrageenan. Most of the foods that contain these compounds also contain dyes, preservatives, and antioxidants.
- **Infections:** bacteria, viruses, and the yeast *Candida albicans* have all been found to cause hives:
  - bacterial infections contribute to acute hives in children with acute streptococcal tonsillitis, and chronic hives in adults with chronic dental infections.
  - hepatitis B is the most frequent cause of virally induced hives; one study found 15.3% of patients with chronic hives had antibodies to hepatitis B. Hives appear in 5% of individuals with infectious

mononucleosis, and may appear several weeks before mononucleosis manifests.

■ *Candida albicans*: in studies, the number of patients with chronic hives who test positive for Candida antigens ranges from 19–81%. In Candida-sensitive individuals, treatment with the drug nystatin can achieve a cure – although in a study of 49 patients, only 9 responded to a 3-week course of nystatin while 18 became symptom-free only after also adopting a "yeast-free" diet, which excluded bread, buns, sausage, wine, beer, cider, grapes, raisins, vinegar, tomato, ketchup, pickles, and prepared foods containing yeasts.

Stress

In one study of 236 cases of chronic hives, stress was reported to be the most frequent primary cause.

■ Stress disrupts digestive secretions. Psychological factors such as worry, depression, or other stress often reduce gastric acidity. In addition, when levels of stress hormones, i.e., cortisol, increase in the circulation, immune system defenses, many of which involve inflammatory chemicals, are upregulated.

■ Stress decreases intestinal secretory IgA levels. Secreted by the cells of the mucous membranes that line the intestinal tract, secretory IgA is an antibody that binds with any perceived pathogens, preventing their entry into the circulation.

Other diseases

Hives may result from the immune system's response to other diseases including autoimmune disease, dysproteinemias, and cancer, especially leukemia.

Pet allergies

In sensitive individuals, exposure to animals, especially cats, may provoke a histamine reaction.

RISK INCREASES WITH

■ Stress
■ Food allergies
■ Environmental allergies
■ Other infection
■ Use of over-the-counter and prescription medications
■ Consumption of highly processed foods
■ Family history of allergies
■ Obesity

PREVENTIVE MEASURES

■ Identify and avoid those factors – such as foods, food additives, and drugs – that cause the immune system

to trigger the release of histamine and other allergenic compounds.

■ Learn to cope with stress constructively. Learn relaxation techniques such as biofeedback or self-hypnosis, meditate, pray, exercise, seek assistance from a religious or psychological counselor. Taking the time to discover which practices help and to integrate them into a lifestyle will significantly benefit not just skin health, but will improve overall health, joy in living, and longevity.

■ Get a minimum of 7 hours sleep each night.

Expected outcomes

Identification and elimination of clear causative factors, such as food allergies or sensitivities to food additives, will often bring about dramatic improvements within the first 2 weeks of treatment in many cases. In cases where food allergies/sensitivities do not appear to be primary factors, however, improvements will be more subtle and gradual.

TREATMENT

Diet

■ **Elimination diet:** the best diagnostic and therapeutic tool is an elimination diet:

  ■ the strictest elimination diets allow only water, lamb, rice, pears, and vegetables.

  ■ strictly avoid the foods most commonly associated with inducing hives: milk, eggs, chicken, fruits, nuts, and additives.

  ■ even if no direct allergy to them is noted, eliminate foods containing vasoactive amines: cured meat, alcoholic beverages, cheese, chocolate, citrus fruits, and shellfish.

  ■ eliminate food additives; not only do they increase the number of mast cells in the skin, they may also do the same in the small intestine, thereby greatly increasing the risk of injury to the gut wall which may result in a "leaky gut" that allows potential allergens and other immune triggers to leak into the circulation.

Nutritional supplements

■ **Vitamin C:** vitamin C exerts a number of effects against histamine including preventing its secretion by white blood cells and increasing the rate at which it is detoxified. Dosages of at least 2,000 mg daily appear necessary to produce these effects; dosage: 1 g t.i.d.

■ **Vitamin B_{12}:** especially effective in treating sulfite-sensitive individuals, B_{12}, when given orally before challenge, forms a sulfite–cobalamin complex that

blocks sulfite's allergic effect in asthmatic patients:
- in addition, B_{12} plays a critical role in nervous system function and has been anecdotally reported to be of value in the treatment of acute and chronic hives.
  - dosage: 1,000 µg q.d. orally, or by injection, once per week.
- **Quercetin:** a flavonoid, quercetin inhibits the manufacture of histamine and other inflammatory mediators from mast cells and basophils. The anti-allergy drug, *sodium cromoglycate*, which offers excellent protection against the development of hives in response to ingested food allergens, is similar in structure and function to quercetin; dosage: 200–400 mg 20 min before each meal.

Psychological medicine
- ***Perform relaxation techniques daily***: in one study, 15 patients with chronic hives who were given an audiotape and asked to use the relaxation techniques described on the tape at home, all experienced significant benefit. At their follow-up examination 5–14 months later, six patients were free of hives and the remaining seven reported improvement.

Physical medicine
In cases of chronic physical urticaria including cold, cholinergic, and dermographic hives, exposure to ultraviolet light has been shown to be of some benefit. Sunbathe or use a UVA solarium daily for 15–20 min. Those with solar urticaria should **not** sunbathe.

Vaginitis and vulvovaginitis

DESCRIPTION

Vaginitis is an infection of the vaginal tract that causes inflammation of the vaginal lining. In vulvovaginitis, the inflammation extends to the *vulva*, the external genital area, which includes the pubic mound, labia, clitoris, and opening of the urethra, as well as the vaginal tract. Although vaginitis can be caused by a sexually transmitted infectious micro-organism, it is more typically due to a disturbance in the delicate ecology of the vagina that allows organisms normally found in a healthy vagina to overgrow and produce an infection. Symptoms vary somewhat depending upon the causative infectious agent, but all involve increased volume of vaginal secretions; abnormal color, consistency, or odor of vaginal secretions; vaginal and vulval itching, burning or irritation; and painful urination or pain with intercourse.

Almost all women experience vaginitis at some time during their lives. One of the most common reasons women seek medical attention, vaginitis accounts for approximately 7% of all visits to gynecologists. Vaginal infections are six times more common than urinary tract infections, and painful urination is much more likely to indicate a vaginal rather than a urinary tract infection. Since the vagina can become a reservoir of infectious bacteria, recurrent urinary infections are often the result of chronic vaginal infection.

Although over-the-counter medications can be purchased to treat vaginitis, it is important to consult a physician and get a precise diagnosis for several reasons. (1) There are different kinds of vaginitis, and, to be truly effective, treatment should be targeted to the specific microbial cause and to the underlying causes that allowed it to multiply and produce this vaginal infection. (2) Vaginitis may be a symptom of a more serious underlying problem, such as a sexually transmitted disease or *cervicitis* – a chronic inflammation of the cervix, which if untreated, may progress to cervical dysplasia. (3) If not properly treated, the infection may travel up the vagina to deeper tissues and lead to pelvic inflammatory disease – a serious condition that can result in infertility because of scarring of the fallopian tubes.

FREQUENT SIGNS AND SYMPTOMS

Signs and symptoms vary depending upon the causative agent.

- ■ *Candida albicans*:
  - ▪ vulval itching, which can be severe, is the key symptom of a vaginal yeast infection
  - ▪ a thick, curdy, or "cottage cheese" discharge is also common, but a scant discharge or its absence does not rule out Candida infection
  - ▪ pelvic examination will reveal adherent white patches with a reddened border
  - ▪ no odor
  - ▪ pH < 4.5.
- ■ *Trichomonas vaginalis*:
  - ▪ the most frequent symptom of trichomonal infection is a frothy, malodorous (may smell fishy), greenish-yellow vaginal discharge
  - ▪ discharge is accompanied by itching and burning
  - ▪ pelvic examination may show reddened bumps on the cervix or vaginal lining
  - ▪ pH > 5.0.
- ■ *Neisseria gonorrhoeae*:
  - ▪ although *gonorrhea* may be present with no symptoms, during reproductive years, the primary symptom of gonorrhea is severe infection of the cervix with painful, bloody, pus-filled discharge
  - ▪ no odor
  - ▪ pelvic examination will show cervical discharge; may have pelvic tenderness
  - ▪ pH < 4.5.
- ■ *Chlamydia trachomatis*:
  - ▪ *Chlamydia* infects 5–10% of sexually active women, but is usually without symptoms until other infections develop (e.g., in the cervix, fallopian tubes, or urethra), and then may produce symptoms of pelvic inflammatory disease (PID)
  - ▪ no discharge or odor
  - ▪ pelvic examination may show signs of PID
  - ▪ pH < 4.5.
- ■ **Nonspecific vaginitis (NSV):**
  - ▪ key symptoms are the odor and discharge
  - ▪ the odor is fishy, foul or rotten, and the discharge is nonirritating, grey in color, usually of even

consistency, and occasionally frothy, or thick and pasty
- pelvic examination shows no unusual symptoms
- pH > 4.5.
- **Herpes:**
  - primary symptom is small genital blisters (vesicles) or ulcers
  - no discharge or odor
  - pelvic examination shows small, multiple vesicles or ulcers on the cervix or labia
  - pH < 4.5.

CAUSES

Approximately 90% of vulvovaginitis is associated with one of three organisms: *Trichomonas vaginalis, Candida albicans,* or *Gardnerella vaginalis.*

- ***Trichomonas vaginalis:*** a sexually transmitted single-celled organism, *Trichomonas* does not invade tissues and rarely causes serious complications.
- ***Candida albicans:*** vaginal infection with Candida, a yeast that is a normal inhabitant of the gastrointestinal tract, has increased dramatically over the last 40 years, largely because of the frequent use of antibiotics. Antibiotics destroy friendly flora in both the gastrointestinal tract and vagina, allowing Candida to multiply aggressively and encouraging its transmission from the intestinal tract to the vagina. Allergies, which also damage the lining of the gastrointestinal tract, have been reported to cause recurrent Candida overgrowth and vaginal infection, which resolves when the allergies are treated.
- **Nonspecific vaginitis (NSV):** a category defined as "vaginitis not due to *Trichomonas,* gonorrhea, or Candida", NSV is identified by its primary symptoms – a non-irritating grey discharge with a fishy, foul odor. The odor is caused by the breakdown of proteins by bacteria and worsens as the pH level, which is elevated to 5.0–5.5 in most cases, rises:
  - the organism most frequently cited as responsible for NSV is *Gardnerella vaginalis,* which is found in 95% of women with NSV, but is also found in 40% of women without vaginitis.
  - although *Gardnerella* prospers under the conditions of NSV, growing evidence suggests that anerobic bacteria are NSV's primary cause:
    - *Gardnerella* lacks the enzymes to produce the amines characteristic of NSV, and the antibiotic most effective against NSV is more active against anerobes than *Gardnerella.*
- ***Neisseria gonorrhoeae:*** a sexually transmitted organism, *N. gonorrhoeae* is responsible for less than 4% of vaginitis cases:
  - gonorrhea is more common among young girls because the vaginal epithelium is thinner before puberty.
  - gonorrhea, either alone or in combination with other organisms, is cultured in 40–60% of cases of pelvic inflammatory disease, a serious infection that is a major cause of infertility.
- **Herpes simplex:** a sexually transmitted organism, herpes simplex virus, is the most common cause of painful genital ulcers, which may occur on the labia or cervix. However, the key symptoms of other forms of vaginitis – itching, odor and increased vaginal discharge – are not present in herpes simplex infection (for additional information, see the chapter on Herpes simplex).
- ***Chlamydia trachomatis:*** a parasite that lives within human cells, *Chlamydia* rarely causes vaginitis on its own, but is frequently found in association with other causes, such as *Candida albicans.* Identifying and properly treating *Chlamydia* is extremely important:
  - *Chlamydia* is frequently found in cultures of women with pelvic inflammatory disease and is a major cause of infertility because of scarring of the fallopian tubes.
  - during pregnancy, chlamydial infection increases the risk of premature delivery and infant death.
  - if a healthy baby is born to a woman with a chlamydial infection, the child has a 50% risk of developing chlamydial infection of the eyes and a 10% chance of contracting pneumonia.

RISK INCREASES WITH

- **Antibiotic treatment:** antibiotics kill protective friendly organisms in the vagina (particularly *Lactobacillus acidophilus*).
- **Allergies:** the ingestion of allergenic proteins results in damage to the intestinal lining. Breeches in the integrity of the intestinal wall allow not only allergens, but also pathogens and other toxins to enter into the general circulation, placing significant stress on the immune defensc system.
- **High intake of refined carbohydrates**, especially sugars and alcohol.
- **Hot weather and non-ventilating clothing**, particularly pantyhose, that increases moisture, warmth, and darkness – ideal conditions for the growth of infectious organisms.
- **Diabetes mellitus:** the elevation in blood sugar levels results in a less effective immune response and a more favorable environment for infectious organisms.
- **Pregnancy:** the sugar (glycogen) content in vaginal tissues increases during pregnancy, providing a more hospitable environment for Candida overgrowth.

- **Menstruation:** the presence of blood provides a more favorable environment for the growth of some infectious organisms.
- **Oral contraceptives:** birth control pills contain synthetic estrogen, the hormone responsible for the building up of the uterine lining each month. A thicker uterine lining results in more menstrual bleeding when the lining is shed.
- **Immunosuppression** caused by drugs such as steroids or by disease.

PREVENTIVE MEASURES

- Use antibiotics only when truly necessary.
- Identify and eliminate food allergens from the diet.
- Minimize consumption of refined carbohydrates, sugars, and alcohol.
- Consider switching from oral contraceptives to a different form of birth control.
- Practice safe sex: monogamy with a healthy partner or use a latex condom every time for intercourse.
- Avoid tight-fitting, synthetic clothing that traps heat and moisture. Try thigh-high stockings with elasticized tops instead of pantyhose.
- After exercising, get out of hot, sweaty gym clothes promptly. Take at least a quick shower, and towel and air-dry thoroughly before dressing. Wear cotton underwear and clothing made from natural fabrics or synthetic fabrics that wick away moisture.
- In recurrent cases of vaginitis, consider having sexual partners treated.

Expected outcomes

Effective treatment requires proper identification of the cause of vaginitis. After proper evaluation and diagnosis, an effective treatment plan generally produces significant improvement within 1–3 days. However, to ensure full elimination of the infectious organism, it is important to continue with the full course of prescribed treatment even after resolution of signs and symptoms.

TREATMENT

- Consult a physician for an accurate diagnosis.
- Avoid sexual activity during treatment to prevent reinfection and to reduce trauma to inflamed tissues. If this is not possible, at least use a condom.

Diet

- **Eliminate refined and simple sugars:**
  - consuming 75 g (3 oz) of sugar in one sitting in any form (sucrose, honey, fruit juice) depresses white (immune) cell activity by 50% for 1–5 hours.
  - sugar is the chief nutrient for *Candida albicans*.

- on labels, sugar may be listed as fructose, maltose, dextrose, polydextrose, corn syrup, molasses, sorbitol, maltodextrin, honey, or maple syrup. Fruit juice, which concentrates fruit sugars, should also be avoided.
- **Eliminate alcohol:**
  - alcohol damages the liver, raises blood sugar levels, and increases intestinal permeability, allowing infectious agents access to the rest of the body.
- **Eliminate milk and dairy products:**
  - milk's high content of lactose (milk sugar) promotes Candida overgrowth.
  - milk is one of the most common food allergens.
  - milk may contain trace levels of antibiotics.
- **Eliminate mold and yeast-containing foods** including alcoholic beverages, cheeses, dried fruits, melons, and peanuts.
- **Eliminate all known or suspected food allergens** (for more information about how to identify and treat food allergies see the chapter on Food allergy).
- **Consume a health-promoting diet** rich in whole, unprocessed, preferably organic foods, especially plant foods (vegetables, whole grains, beans, nuts [especially walnuts], and seeds), and cold-water fish (for more detailed information, see Appendix 1).

Nutritional supplements

- **A high-potency multiple vitamin and mineral daily supplement** providing all of the known vitamins and minerals. Among those contained in a multiple, the following nutrients are particularly important in vaginal health and should be present in the following amounts:

Vitamin	Amount
Vitamin A	5,000 IU or beta-carotene: 50,000 IU
Vitamin B$_1$ (thiamin)	10–100 mg
Vitamin B$_2$ (riboflavin)	10–50 mg
Niacin	10–100 mg
Niacinamide	10–30 mg
Vitamin B$_6$ (pyridoxine)	25–100 mg
Biotin	100–300 µg
Pantothenic acid	25–100 mg
Folic acid	400 µg
Vitamin B$_{12}$	400 µg
Choline	10–100 mg
Inositol	10–100 mg
Zinc	10–15 mg if zinc picolinate is used; if not, 30–50 mg
Vitamin E	200 IU of mixed tocopherols

Caution: folic acid supplementation should always be accompanied by vitamin B$_{12}$ supplementation to prevent folic acid from masking a vitamin B$_{12}$ deficiency.

- ***Lactobacillus acidophilus*:** this desirable bacterium is an integral component of normal vaginal flora and helps prevent the overgrowth of *Candida albicans* and less desirable bacterial species:
  - *L. acidophilus* promotes vaginal health by (1) producing lactic acid and natural antibiotic substances, and (2) competing with other bacteria and Candida for available glucose (sugar).
  - dosage: an oral dosage of 1–2 billion live organisms q.d., plus douching with an acidophilus-containing solution (discussed below under Topical medicine).

Botanical medicines

- ***Glycyrrhiza glabra* (licorice):** licorice is an effective antiviral, and licorice gel, applied topically, has proven quite helpful in reducing the healing time and pain associated with herpes lesions. In addition, licorice contains isoflavonoids that have been shown effective against Candida:
  - dosage: for herpes lesions, apply licorice gel topically. For Candida, choose one of the following forms and take the recommended dosage t.i.d.:
    - powdered root: 1–2 g
    - fluid extract (1 : 1): 2–4 ml
    - solid (dry powdered) extract (4 : 1): 250–500 mg.
- ***Allium sativum* (garlic):** garlic is antibacterial, antiviral, and antifungal, and has even been shown to be effective against some antibiotic-resistant organisms:
  - dosage: garlic may be added to douching solutions or may be wrapped in gauze and placed as a tampon/suppository for most forms of infectious vaginitis.
- ***Hydrastis canadensis* (goldenseal):** goldenseal is a remarkably safe and effective natural antibiotic. Its most active alkaloid constituent, berberine sulfate, exhibits a broad range of antibiotic action against a wide variety of bacteria (including *Chlamydia*, *Trichomonas*, and *N. gonorrhoeae*), fungi (including Candida), and protozoa. Its action against some of these pathogens is actually stronger than that of commonly used antibiotics, but unlike antibiotic drugs, goldenseal does not destroy the protective bacteria (lactobacilli) in our intestines:
  - when taken internally, berberine enhances immune function, and when used in douching solutions, it offers symptomatic relief by soothing inflamed mucous membranes.
  - berberine is a more effective antimicrobial agent in an alkaline environment. Alkalinity can be increased by consuming fewer animal products and more plant foods, especially fruits. Although most fruits are acidic, digestion uses up their acid components leaving behind an alkaline residue.

- dosage: for internal use, choose one of the following forms and take the recommended dosage t.i.d. (the dosage should be based on berberine content, and standardized extracts are recommended):
  - dried root or as infusion (tea): 2–4 g
  - tincture (1 : 5): 6–12 ml (1.5–3 tsp)
  - fluid extract (1 : 1): 2–4 ml (0.5–1 tsp)
  - solid (dry powdered) extract (4 : 1 or 8–12% alkaloid content): 250–500 mg.
- dosage: as a douche, mix 1 tbsp of the solid (dry powdered) extract noted above into one cup of water and use as a douching solution, once per day for up to 1 week.

Drug–herb interaction cautions

- ***Allium sativum* (garlic):**
  - plus *insulin*: animal studies suggest insulin dose may require adjusting because of the hypoglycemic effects of whole garlic (in rats) and its constituent allicin (in rabbits).
  - plus *warfarin*: the anticoagulant activity of warfarin is enhanced as a result of increased fibrinolytic activity and diminished platelet aggregation caused by garlic components allicin, ajoene, trisulfides, and adenosine.
- ***Glycyrrhiza glabra* (licorice):**
  - plus *digoxin, digitalis*: due to a reduction of potassium in the blood, licorice enhances the toxicity of cardiac glycosides. Interaction with these cardiac glycoside drugs could lead to arrhythmias and cardiac arrest.
  - plus *stimulant laxatives or diuretics* (thiazides, spironolactone or amiloride): licorice should not be used with these drugs because of the additive increase of potassium loss to potentially dangerous levels.

Topical medicine

- Warm sitz baths with Epsom salts may provide quick relief for itching and burning.
- Douches and *pessaries* (saturated tampons) are effective methods of concentrating therapeutic agents in the vagina. While other agents may also be effective, the following are chosen since their effectiveness is well referenced in the medical literature. Choose one or more of the agents discussed below. Do not use them together; the variety is given to provide alternatives for use in resistant cases.
  - *Lactobacillus* spp.: prepare a solution using a high-quality *acidophilus* supplement or active-culture yogurt (read the label carefully since most commercially available yogurts do not contain live

lactobacilli):

- dissolve enough in 10 ml of water to provide one billion organisms. Use a syringe to douche the solution into the vagina.
- since lactobacilli are normal vaginal inhabitants, the douche can be retained as long as desired.

povidone-iodine (Betadine): used topically as a douche, Betadine is effective against a wide range of organisms linked to vaginal infections, including *Trichomonas*, Candida, *Chlamydia*, and non-specific vaginitis. A study published in 1969 showed Betadine effective against 100% of cases of candidial vaginitis, 80% of *Trichomonas*, and 93% of combination infections:

- available at any pharmacy, Betadine has all the advantages of iodine without stinging or staining.
- prepare a douching solution diluted to one part iodine in 100 parts water, and use b.i.d. for 14 days.
- **caution:** avoid excessive use since some iodine will be absorbed into the system and, in sensitive individuals, can cause suppression of thyroid function.

boric acid: capsules of boric acid inserted into the vagina have been used to treat vaginitis due to *Candida albicans* and have been shown to be significantly more effective than nystatin and creams containing the antifungal drugs miconazole, clotrimazole, or butaconazole:

- in a recent study of 92 women with chronic vaginal yeast infection, patients who used boric acid not only eliminated their vaginal infection, but a microscopic examination of their vaginal swabs also revealed normal vaginal cells.
- no patient who received antifungal drugs had a normal microscopic examination; all demonstrated continued presence of yeast, damaged cells lining the vagina, or some other abnormality.
- dosage: 600 mg of boric acid in a vaginal suppository used b.i.d. for 2 weeks.
- **caution:** although side effects from boric acid use are quite rare, if boric acid leaks out of the vagina, it may irritate the labia. If this occurs, reduce the amount of boric acid used or discontinue use.

Varicose veins

DESCRIPTION

Varicose veins are veins that have become swollen, twisted, and tortuous. Veins, the part of the circulatory system that returns blood to the heart, are surprisingly frail structures. Unlike the arteries, which deliver blood to the body effortlessly (the beating of the heart provides all the pumping action necessary), the veins must rely on the expansion and contraction of surrounding muscles to push returning blood along. Since the strength of our other muscles' normal contractions pales in comparison to the heart, veins contain one-way valves every few inches to help blood return against gravity to the heart rather than flowing back. If enough pressure is exerted so that any of these valves fail, however, the blood does fall back, stressing other valves. Eventually, when a number of valves have become damaged, the blood pools, stretching the vein until it becomes swollen, prominent and distorted.

Varicose veins affect nearly 50% of middle-aged adults. The veins most commonly affected are the superficial veins of the legs, largely as a result of the gravitational pressure that standing exerts on the legs. Individuals with occupations that require long periods of standing are at greatest risk for developing varicose veins since standing for long periods of time can increase pressure in the legs up to 10 times! The risk for varicose veins increases with age because of loss of tissue tone and muscle mass, and weakening of the walls of the veins. Varicose veins are four times more common in women than in men. Obesity, an additional gravitational stress, significantly increases risk. Pregnancy may also lead to the development of varicose veins since it increases venous pressure in the legs.

Most varicose veins, although cosmetically unappealing, are not dangerous if the involved vein is near the surface. Significant symptoms are uncommon with superficial varicose veins, although the legs may feel heavy, tight and tired. If the deeper veins of the leg become varicose, however, problems such as thrombophlebitis (severe inflammation of a vein), pulmonary embolism (blood clot in the lungs), heart attack, or stroke are possible outcomes. Ultrasound evaluation is the most accurate method of determining if deep veins are involved.

FREQUENT SIGNS AND SYMPTOMS

- Enlarged, disfiguring, tortuous, bluish veins, which are visible under the skin, especially when standing.
- May be without symptoms or may be associated with fatigue, aching discomfort, feelings of heaviness or pain in the legs.
- The appearance of the veins does not necessarily correspond with the severity of symptoms: some people with many, very obvious varicose veins notice no discomfort, while others with less severe varicosities may experience aching pain.
- Fluid retention (edema), discoloration, and ulceration of the skin may develop due to lack of adequate blood flow to supply nutrients and remove wastes from the area.

CAUSES

- **Genetic weakness of the vein walls or their valves:** weakness of the vein walls resulting from abnormalities in structural components (*proteoglycans*) or excessive release of enzymes that break down proteoglycans, leads to loss of integrity in the vein.
- **Genetic weakness in the ability to break down fibrin:**
  - individuals with varicose veins have a decreased ability to break down fibrin, a compound involved in clot and scar formation. When fibrin is deposited in the tissue near the varicosed veins, the skin becomes hard and lumpy due to the presence of fibrin and fat.
  - decreased fibrinolytic activity also increases the risk of thrombus (blood clot) formation, which may result in thrombophlebitis, heart attack, pulmonary embolism or stroke.
- **Excessive pressure within the vein due to:**
  - prolonged standing
  - constipation/straining during defecation
  - heavy lifting
  - pregnancy
  - obesity.
- **Low-fiber diet:** individuals who consume a low-fiber diet tend to strain more during bowel movements. Straining increases pressure in the abdomen,

obstructing the flow of blood up the legs. Over time, this increased pressure may significantly weaken the vein wall, leading to varicose veins and hemorrhoids:

- in contrast to the US and other developed countries, varicose veins are rarely seen in parts of the world where high-fiber, unrefined diets are consumed.
- a diet rich in vegetables, fruits, legumes, and grains contains many fiber components that attract water and form a gelatinous mass that keeps feces soft, bulky, and easy to pass.

■ **Inflammatory damage to the vein** resulting from vein disease, such as thrombophlebitis.

RISK INCREASES WITH

- **Sex:** women are affected four times as frequently as men
- **Menstruation:** in some women, symptoms worsen before and during menstruation
- **Family history of varicose veins**
- **An occupation that involves prolonged standing or heavy lifting**
- **Pregnancy**
- **Obesity**
- **Lack of regular exercise:** exercise tones and strengthens the muscles and increases circulation
- **Low-fiber diet:** leads to constipation, straining during defecation
- **Age:** the walls of the veins weaken, and muscle mass and tone commonly decrease with age

PREVENTIVE MEASURES

- Where a job involves prolonged periods of standing or sitting, make it a habit to walk around for 5 min every hour.
- Exercise regularly – a minimum of 30 min 5 days a week.
- If obese, shed those excess pounds and maintain a healthy weight (for more information, see the chapter on Obesity).
- Consume a fiber-rich diet high in whole, unprocessed foods, especially plant foods (fruits, vegetables, beans, seeds and nuts, and whole grains) and cold-water fish, and low in animal products and processed foods (for more detailed information, see Appendix 1).
- If pregnant, avoid standing for long periods of time and consider wearing compression stockings to help provide support for the veins during the final 3–4 months of the pregnancy.

Expected outcomes

The natural treatments outlined below are very effective at relieving the symptoms associated with varicose veins.

While small spider veins may resolve entirely, larger, well-defined varicose veins will not disappear. However, the program discussed in this guide does produce results as good as or better than compression stockings in most cases – without the hassle or discomfort. Also, unlike compression stockings, this program will strengthen the walls of the veins, reducing the risk of developing additional varicose veins.

In cases of severe varicose veins, *sclerotherapy* (injection of an agent that causes the walls of the vein to collapse and fuse together, so the vein no longer carries blood) or surgical stripping (the surgical removal of the entire vein), performed by a vascular surgeon or phlebologist (a doctor who specializes in treating varicose veins) are appropriate options. However, other varicose veins may develop as time passes.

TREATMENT

Diet
- **Consume a high-fiber diet:**
  - a good goal for dietary fiber intake is 40–50 g q.d. This can be easily achieved when the diet is based on whole, unprocessed plant foods – vegetables, fruits, whole grains, nuts and seeds.
  - vegetables are excellent sources of fiber:
    - 1 cup of cooked carrots has almost the same amount of fiber as 3 slices of whole wheat bread or 2 cups of oatmeal.
    - all vegetables contain fiber, but the following are especially good sources: peas and Brussels sprouts lead, providing about 8 g of soluble fiber in a 1-cup serving, and broccoli, sweet potatoes, potatoes and artichokes are not far behind in their fiber content.
  - like vegetables, most fruits contain fiber, and the following are exceptionally good sources: apples, mangoes, oranges, blueberries, guavas, kiwis and, of course, prunes.
- **Minimize consumption of processed foods**, especially baked goods (bread, crackers, pasta) made from refined flour:
  - if the first ingredient listed is not *whole* wheat, the product is made primarily from refined, virtually fiberless flour.
- **Add other whole grains to meals**, especially buckwheat:
  - buckwheat contains the bioflavonoid *rutin* that, like the bioflavonoids in blue-red berries (described below), reduces capillary fragility, increases the integrity of the venous wall, inhibits the breakdown of the compounds composing the ground substance, and increases the muscular tone of the vein.

- **Vary whole grain consumption:** in addition to buckwheat, whole grains such as rye bread, brown and wild rice, old-fashioned rather than quick-cooking oats, wheat berries, amaranth, and quinoa provide not only fiber, but also a variety of healthful nutrients along with complex carbohydrates that help provide the lasting energy needed to enjoy regular exercise:
  - those who are overweight will find these whole foods very filling, truly satisfying hunger, and thereby helping with weight loss.
- **Increase consumption of blue-red berries** such as blackberries, cherries, and blueberries:
  - these berries are rich in *proanthocyanidins* and *anthocyanidins*, flavonoid compounds that improve the integrity of support structures of the veins and entire vascular system.
- **Consume garlic, onions, ginger and cayenne** frequently and liberally:
  - individuals with varicose veins have a decreased ability to break down fibrin, a protein involved in blood clot and scar formation that forms deposits near varicosed veins making the skin hard and lumpy, a condition called *lipodermatosclerosis*.
  - these herbs and spices all increase fibrin breakdown.

Nutritional supplements

- **Vitamin C:** vitamin C is necessary for the production of healthy *collagen*, the most abundant protein in the body and the "ground substance" of all types of tissue, including the veins:
  - in addition to strengthening the collagen structures of the veins, vitamin C inhibits platelet aggregation, and regenerates oxidized vitamin E, enabling it to resume its protective activities.
  - dosage: 500–3,000 mg q.d.
- **Bioflavonoids:** supplementation with bioflavonoids, particularly with the *anthocyanosides* (the blue-red pigments found in berries):
  - enhances the effects of vitamin C
  - improves capillary integrity
  - stabilizes the collagen matrix by preventing free radical damage, inhibiting enzymes from cleaving the collagen matrix, and directly cross-linking with collagen fibers to form a more stable collagen matrix
  - increases the muscular tone of the vein
  - dosage: 100–1,000 mg q.d.
- **Vitamin E:** an excellent blood thinner, vitamin E increases the breakdown of fibrin, a protein compound involved in clot and scar formation, and helps to improve circulation, reducing the pain caused by varicose veins; dosage: 200–600 IU mixed tocopherols q.d.
- **Zinc:** a cofactor in many enzymatic reactions, zinc is essential for inflammation control and tissue regeneration; dosage: 15–30 mg q.d. (zinc picolinate, a well-absorbed form, is preferred).
- **Bulking agents:** natural bulking compounds such as psyllium seed, pectin, and guar gum possess mild laxative action as a result of their ability to attract water and form a gelatinous mass. This keeps feces soft and promotes peristalsis, thus reducing straining during defecation. These fibers are preferred since they are less irritating than wheat bran and other cellulose fiber products; dosage: follow instructions given on the product.

Botanical medicines

Extracts of the following botanicals have significant support in the scientific literature for their efficacy as *venotonics* – agents that enhance the structure, function, and tone of veins. Choose one or more of the following:

- ***Aesculus hippocastanum* (horse chestnut):**
  - extracts of horse chestnut standardized for the key compound *escin* have been shown to improve venous tone by increasing the contractile potential of the elastic fibers in the vein wall. Relaxation of the venous wall is a significant contributing factor in the development of varicose veins.
  - escin-standardized extracts inhibit the enzymes that break down the support structures of the vein, thus decreasing capillary permeability by reducing the number and size of the small pores in the capillary walls, and reducing edema and inflammation.
  - in comparison studies, escin-standardized extracts were found to be as effective as leg compression stockings when patients were evaluated by a machine (a *phlethysmograph*) that measures the volume of fluid in the leg.
  - dosage: use extracts that provide a daily dose of 50 mg escin:
    - **caution:** because of the lack of sufficient evaluation, escin preparations should not be used during pregnancy and lactation.
- ***Centella asiatica* (gotu kola):** an extract of *Centella* containing 70% triterpenic acids has demonstrated excellent clinical results in the treatment of varicose veins, venous insufficiency of the lower limbs, and cellulite:
  - *Centella* extracts increase the integrity of the *perivascular sheath* – the connective tissue structure that surrounds the vein – thus giving damaged veins some support. By increasing this support structure's integrity, vein function is improved.
  - dosage: use extracts that provide a daily dose of 30–60 mg triterpenic acids:
    - **caution:** because of the lack of sufficient evaluation, gotu kola preparations should not be used during pregnancy and lactation.

- *Ruscus aculeatus* **(butcher's broom):** ruscogenins, the active ingredients in butcher's broom, exhibit a wide range of beneficial pharmacological actions including anti-inflammatory and vasoconstrictor effects:
  - in Europe, where butcher's broom is used internally and externally to treat varicose veins and hemorrhoids, clinical research has used butcher's broom in combination with hesperidin (a bioflavonoid) and vitamin C.
  - dosage: use extracts standardized to contain 9–11% ruscogenin at a dosage of 100 mg t.i.d.:
    - **caution:** because of the lack of sufficient evaluation, butcher's broom preparations should not be used during pregnancy and lactation.
- *Vaccinium myrtillus* **(bilberry):** bilberry is an especially rich source of proanthocyanidins and anthocyanidins – flavonoids that have been shown to improve the integrity of support structures of the veins and the entire vascular system:
  - dosage: use extracts standardized to contain 25% anthocyanoside: 80–160 mg t.i.d.
- *Vitis vinifera* **(grape seed) or** *Pinus maritima* **(pine bark):** flavonoid extracts from these two botanicals are widely used in Europe as medications for various circulatory conditions, including varicose veins. Extracts of grape seed and pine bark are the most popular and possibly most effective:
  - dosage: use extracts standardized to contain 95% or more procyanidolic oligomers (PCOs or OPCs), 150–300 mg q.d.
- **Bromelain:** a proteolytic enzyme from pineapple, bromelain may help to prevent the development of the hard, lumpy skin (lipodermatosclerosis) that often forms around varicosed veins:
  - bromelain acts in a manner similar to *plasminogen activator* (a component of vein walls) that promotes the breakdown of fibrin.
  - dosage: (1,200–1,800 MCU) 500–750 mg b.i.d.–t.i.d. between meals.

Drug–herb interaction cautions
- *Aesculus hippocastanum* **(horse chestnut):**
  - plus *aspirin or anticoagulants*: it has been speculated that horse chestnut should not be taken with aspirin or anticoagulants because the antithrombin activity of its hydroxycoumarin component, *aesculin*, might cause increased bleeding time.

Physical medicine
- **Exercise regularly:** exercise improves muscle tone, increases circulation, and when done four to five times each week for 30 min or more, helps to promote lasting weight loss.

Viral pharyngitis

DESCRIPTION

Viral pharyngitis is a sore throat or inflammation of the *pharynx* (the medical term for the throat) as a result of viral infection. A wide variety of viruses are capable of infecting the *upper respiratory tract*, which includes the nasal passages, sinuses, and throat. We are all constantly exposed to many of these viruses, but most of us do not succumb to infection and the resulting sore throat (frequently accompanied by a cold) more than once or twice a year. This suggests that lowered resistance due to a decrease in immune function is the primary factor that allows a virus to successfully infect the respiratory tract.

The majority (over 90%) of sore throats are the result of viral infections – against which antibiotics are ineffective, and which typically resolve after a few days of bed rest, extra fluids, and basic immune support (discussed below). However, anyone with a sore throat should consult with a physician to rule out *strep throat*, a sore throat caused by a bacterial infection for which antibiotics may be suggested. Even in strep throat, aggressive treatment with natural therapies that specifically target streptococci may render antibiotics unnecessary, but a definitive diagnosis is essential. If untreated, a strep throat may lead to rheumatic fever or kidney disease. Only a throat culture can accurately diagnose strep throat, but physicians now have swabs that can immediately test for strep, providing a definitive answer in as little as 15 min (for further information see the chapter on Streptococcal pharyngitis).

FREQUENT SIGNS AND SYMPTOMS

Signs suggestive of sore throat due to viral infection
- Gradual onset from mild scratchy throat to uncomfortable sore throat
- Mild difficulty in swallowing
- Cough
- Headache
- Hoarseness
- Throat is typically red and quite dry
- Tonsils may be swollen and may have a white coating
- Watery nasal discharge followed by thicker secretions containing mucus (if a cold accompanies the sore throat)
- Sneezing
- Mild to moderate fever, if any

Signs suggestive of sore throat due to strep infection
- Sudden onset
- Very painful sore throat
- Tender, swollen lymph nodes in the neck
- Much difficulty in swallowing
- Appetite loss
- General ill feeling
- Headache, stomach pain, vomiting
- Red swollen tonsils, with white splotches (pus)
- Fever of 102°F or higher

Signs suggestive of sore throat due to allergies
- Symptoms are similar to viral sore throat, except:
  - no fever occurs
  - there is no evidence of infection
  - there is usually a history of seasonal allergic episodes.

Signs suggestive of sore throat due to influenza
- Symptoms are much more severe
- Influenza usually occurs in epidemics, so contact the local Public Health Department

Caution: if you are recovering from a sore throat and develop fever, joint pain, all-over aches and pain, a rash or muscle spasms, call a physician immediately. These may be signs of rheumatic fever.

CAUSES

- **Viral infection:** although a wide variety of viruses are capable of infecting the upper respiratory tract and producing a sore throat, their ability to do so is dependent upon lowered host resistance. Factors that impair resistance are outlined below.

RISK INCREASES WITH

- **Cold, wet, weather:** sore throats occur more often in late winter and early spring.
- **Illness** that has lowered resistance.

- **Fatigue or overwork:** during the deepest levels of sleep, potent immune-enhancing compounds are released and many immune functions are greatly increased:
  - inadequate rest (less than 7 hours sleep per night) compromises immune function.
  - overwork exacerbates stress, which, if excessive or unrelieved, also depresses immune function.
- **Stress:** stress increases levels of adrenal gland hormones, including adrenaline and corticosteroids, which inhibit white blood cell formation and function, and cause the thymus gland (the master gland of the immune system) to shrink:
  - stress also stimulates the sympathetic nervous system – the part of the autonomic nervous system responsible for the fight-or-flight response.
  - the immune system functions better under the other arm of the autonomic nervous system – the parasympathetic nervous system – which assumes control over the body during periods of rest, relaxation, meditation, and sleep.
- **Smoking:** both smoking and exposure to cigarette smoke increase susceptibility to a sore throat via several mechanisms:
  - exposure to cigarette smoke depletes the body's vitamin C stores.
  - nicotine causes the body to produce cortisol, a hormone that suppresses the immune system.
  - cigarette smoke is a local irritant, damaging the protective mucous membranes lining the throat.
- **Alcohol consumption:** studies of human white cells show a profound depression in the rate of mobilization into areas of infection after people consume alcohol.
- **Frequent consumption of sugar, refined foods:** consuming 75 g (3 oz) of sugar in one sitting in any form (sucrose, honey, fruit juice) depresses white (immune) cell activity by 50% for 1–5 hours.
- **Local irritation:** a variety of factors can damage the throat's protective mucosal lining, the body's first line of defense that prevents pathogens from entering:
  - the mucus secreted by the cells of these membranes is a sticky substance that traps the pathogens and moves them out, either through the nose or into the intestines where they are destroyed by stomach acid.
  - mucus also contains an antibody called secretory IgA that binds to the pathogens, preventing them from penetrating the mucous membranes.
  - the mucous membranes form a mechanical barrier to the invader.
  - factors that can damage the mucosal membrane include: overuse of the *larynx* (the voice box); inhaled environmental pollutants, e.g., gasoline fumes, pesticides; chemicals used in the workplace, e.g., copy machines, beauty salon hair and nail products, car cleaning products, painting supplies; cigarette smoke, smoke from burning leaves or wood-burning fireplaces; house cleaning products; dust, and dry winter air.
- **Nutrient deficiency:** an overwhelming number of clinical and experimental studies show that a deficiency of any single nutrient (especially folic acid, pantothenic acid, pyridoxine, riboflavin, vitamins A, B_{12}, and C, and the trace minerals copper and zinc) can profoundly impair immune function.
- **Standard American Diet:** immune function is directly related to the quality of foods routinely eaten. The Standard American Diet, which is based on processed foods, is high in fats and sugars (both of which depress immune function), and leads to obesity, which has also been linked to suppressed immune function.
- **Obesity:** in overweight individuals, the production of antibodies and the ability of white blood cells to destroy bacteria are decreased.
- **Food allergy:** the typical upper respiratory tract symptoms of chronic delayed food allergy include chronic sore throat, runny nose, sinusitis, tonsillitis, and laryngitis. When allergenic foods are consumed, immune defenses are deployed against food particles rather than invading microbes, resulting in increased susceptibility to infection.
- **Excessive exercise:** the increased levels of free radicals generated use up immune defenses.
- **Drugs:** many drugs, including aspirin, acetaminophen, ibuprofen, and corticosteroids, decrease antibody production and suppress a wide variety of immune defense mechanisms. Chronic antibiotic use causes general immune impairment and promotes the development of resistant organisms.

PREVENTIVE MEASURES

- Minimize consumption of sugars, and refined foods: consuming 75 g (3 oz) of sugar in one sitting in any form (sucrose, honey, fruit juice) depresses white (immune) cell activity by 50% for 1–5 hours.
- A high-potency multiple vitamin and mineral supplement including 400 µg of folic acid, 400 µg of vitamin B_{12}, and 50–100 mg of vitamin B_6. (Folic acid supplementation should always be accompanied by vitamin B_{12} supplementation to prevent folic acid from masking a vitamin B_{12} deficiency.) A daily multiple providing all of the known vitamins and minerals provides basic immune support.

- If food allergies are suspect, see the chapter on Food allergy, for additional information on identifying and removing dietary allergens.
- Consume a balanced diet composed of whole, unprocessed, preferably organic foods, especially plant foods (fruits, vegetables, whole grains, beans, nuts [especially walnuts], and seeds), and cold-water fish (for more detailed information, see Appendix 1).
- Get a minimum of 7 hours sleep each night.
- Don't smoke and avoid exposure to second-hand smoke.
- Minimize alcohol consumption.
- Use drugs only when truly medically necessary.
- Learn to cope with stress constructively. Relaxation techniques such as biofeedback or self-hypnosis, meditation, prayer, and moderate exercise can all significantly reduce stress. Taking the time to discover which practices help and to integrate them into a lifestyle will significantly improve overall health, joy in living, and longevity.
- Maintain a healthy weight.
- To minimize exposure to irritating chemicals use "natural" housecleaning products and always open windows for good ventilation. If using a wood-burning stove, be sure to ventilate the house for several hours each day.
- Drink at least eight 240 ml (8 US fl oz) glasses of water, herb tea, or fruit juice diluted at least 50% with water daily.
- If suffering from environmental allergies, consider purchasing a HEPA filter for regularly used rooms.

Expected outcomes

Sore throats due to viral infections are self-limiting diseases that should resolve within a week or less. With a healthy, functioning immune system, viral pharyngitis should not last more than 3–4 days at most.

Once those factors contributing to immune suppression have been identified and appropriate measures (described in Preventive Measures and Treatment) have been instituted, sore throats due to viral infection should rarely be a problem.

TREATMENT

Fever is a natural immune defense mechanism and should be supported, rather than suppressed by using drugs – unless the body temperature approaches 104°F, at which point the body's ability to control temperature becomes impaired.

Diet

- Eliminate all sources of concentrated simple sugars: sugar, honey, fruit juice, dried fruit, candy, cake, cookies, baked goods, ice cream, popsicles, etc.

- Even fruit and fruit juice consumption should be limited so that no more than 50 g of fruit sugar are ingested q.d.
- Eliminate refined carbohydrates, which are quickly broken down into sugars in the digestive tract. Products made from refined flour (white or wheat – rather than whole wheat – flour) include bread, cereals, crackers, chips, and pasta. Use whole wheat or whole grain versions of these products.
- Minimize consumption of dairy products. A common allergen, dairy also increases mucus production in some people.
- Increase fluid intake to 240 ml (8 US fl oz) per hour, using filtered water and the herbal teas listed below.
- Follow food recommendations given in Preventive Measures.
- Eliminate all suspected food allergens from the diet (for additional information see the chapter on Food allergy).

Nutritional supplements

- **Vitamin A:** often called the anti-infective vitamin, vitamin A exerts antiviral effects and is essential for the health of the mucous membranes:
  - when vitamin A levels are inadequate, keratin is secreted in these membranes, transforming them from their normally pliable, moist condition into stiff dry tissue that is unable to carry out its functions, and leading to breaches in mucosal integrity that significantly increase susceptibility to infection and the development of allergy.
  - dosage: 50,000 IU q.d. for up to 2 days in infants and up to 1 week in adults, or beta-carotene: 200,000 IU q.d.
  - **caution:** at high doses, vitamin A has been linked to birth defects. Women of childbearing age who are pregnant or at risk for pregnancy should **not** use vitamin A. For these women, beta-carotene, also called pro-vitamin A since it can be converted in the body to vitamin A, is a safe and effective alternative.
- **Vitamin C:** the body's primary water-soluble anti-oxidant, vitamin C is directly antiviral and antibacterial, but its most potent protective benefits are the result of its amplification of immune function via numerous mechanisms including improving the integrity of the lining of the mucous membranes, enhancing white blood cell response and function, increasing interferon levels (a special chemical factor that fights viral infection and cancer), and increasing the secretion of thymic hormones (the thymus is the master gland of the immune system):
  - dosage: 500–1,000 mg every 2 waking hours (if this amount produces excessive gas [flatulence] or

diarrhea, decrease the dosage to 100–250 mg, but continue to take vitamin C every 2 hours).

- **Bioflavonoids:** a group of plant pigments largely responsible for the colors of fruits and flowers, bioflavonoids are powerful antioxidants in their own right, and, when taken with vitamin C, significantly enhance both its absorption and effectiveness; dosage: 1,000 mg q.d.
- **Zinc:** the most critical mineral for immune function, zinc promotes the destruction of foreign particles and micro-organisms, protects against free radical damage, acts synergistically with vitamin A, is required for proper white cell function, and is necessary for the activation of serum thymic factor – a thymus hormone with profound immune-enhancing actions:
  - zinc taken in the form of lozenges is especially helpful against viral pharyngitis since it inhibits replication of several viruses, including those that cause the common cold:
    - several double-blind, placebo-controlled studies have demonstrated that the use of zinc lozenges significantly reduces duration and severity of symptoms associated with the common cold.
    - in the most recent study, complete recovery was achieved in 4.4 days with zinc compared to 7.6 days for placebo. For sore throat, specifically, duration was only 1 day in those given zinc and 3 days in those receiving placebo.
  - dosage: use lozenges that supply 15–25 mg of elemental zinc (gluconate form with no citrate, mannitol or sorbitol):
    - in order for zinc to be effective, it must first be ionized in the saliva. When various zinc lozenges were tested, 90% of the zinc was ionized when the lozenges contained zinc gluconate (a form in which glycine is added as a sweetening agent). However, virtually none of the zinc was ionized when the lozenges contained citrate, mannitol or sorbitol.
    - dissolve one lozenge in the mouth every 2 waking hours after an initial double dose.
    - continue for up to 7 days.
    - supplementation at this dosage is **not** recommended for more than 1 week as it may lead to suppression of the immune system.

Botanical medicines

- ***Echinacea* spp. (*Echinacea angustifolia* and *Echinacea purpurea*):** both of these widely used species of *Echinacea* exert profound immune-enhancing effects that result in increased activity of many key immune functions including production of T cells, macrophage phagocytosis, antibody binding, natural killer cell activity, and levels of circulating neutrophils:
  - more than 300 scientific studies demonstrate the immune-enhancing effects of echinacea. In one recent study, 108 patients with colds were given either a placebo or an extract of fresh-pressed *E. purpurea* juice (4 ml b.i.d.) or a placebo for 8 weeks with the following results:
    - 32.5% of those receiving *Echinacea* remained healthy vs. 25.9% of those given placebo.
    - length of time between infections was 40 days for those given *Echinacea*, 25 days for those given placebo.
    - when infections occurred, they were less severe and resolved more quickly in those given *Echinacea*.
    - patients who showed evidence of a weakened immune system (helper to suppressor cell ratio less than 1.5) showed the most benefit from *Echinacea*.
  - dosage: choose one of the following forms and take the recommended dosage t.i.d.:
    - dried root (or as tea): 0.5–1 g
    - freeze-dried plant: 325–650 mg
    - juice of aerial portion of *E. purpurea* stabilized in 22% ethanol: 2–3 ml
    - tincture (1 : 5): 2–4 ml
    - fluid extract (1 : 1): 2–4 ml
    - solid (dry powdered) extract (6.5 : 1 or 3.5% echinacoside): 150–300 mg.

Drug–herb interaction cautions
None.

Topical medicine
- **Gargle with salt water b.i.d.:** 1 tbsp of salt dissolved in 240 ml (8 US fl oz) of warm water.
- ***Zingiber officinale* (ginger) tea:** fresh ginger has analgesic properties, so a strong ginger tea is helpful in relieving throat irritation. To prepare an analgesic tea, dice several thin slices of fresh ginger root, place in a teacup or mug, pour in boiling water, and let steep for 5–10 min.

Appendix 1: A health-promoting diet

CONSUME A DIET BASED ON PLANT FOODS

A tremendous amount of evidence shows that deviating from a predominantly plant-based diet is a major factor in the development of heart disease, cancer, strokes, arthritis, and many other chronic degenerative diseases. Numerous health and medical organizations recommend that the human diet be primarily composed of plant foods: vegetables, fruits, grains, legumes, nuts and seeds. A diet primarily composed of plant foods is high in dietary fiber. In addition, a plant-based diet is low in saturated fat, high in essential fatty acids, and high in antioxidant nutrients and phytochemicals.

A good daily goal for dietary fiber intake is 35 g. This amount can easily be consumed when the diet is based on whole, unprocessed plant foods and provides numerous health-protective benefits including:

■ decreased intestinal transit time
■ delayed stomach emptying, preventing excessive blood sugar elevation after meals
■ increased feeling of fullness
■ increased secretion of digestive enzymes
■ increased stool weight
■ more advantageous intestinal microflora
■ increased production of short chain fatty acids, the preferred food of intestinal cells
■ decreased levels of fats in the blood
■ more soluble bile (bile aids in the absorption of fats and fat-soluble vitamins and the excretion of toxins from the body).

As demonstrated by the list of selected foods below, vegetables are excellent sources of fiber. Just 1 cup of cooked carrots has almost the same amount of fiber as 3¹/₂ slices of whole wheat bread or 2¹/₄ cups of oatmeal.

Dietary fiber content of selected foods

Food	Serving	Calories	Grams of fiber
Fruits			
Apple (with skin)	1 medium	81	3.5
Banana	1 medium	105	2.4
Orange	1 medium	62	2.6
Pear (with skin)	¹/₂ large	61	3.1
Prunes	3	60	3.0

Food	Serving	Calories	Grams of fiber
Raisins	¹/₄ cup	106	3.1
Raspberries	¹/₂ cup	35	3.1
Vegetables, raw			
Celery, diced	¹/₂ cup	10	1.1
Lettuce	1 cup	10	0.9
Mushrooms	¹/₂ cup	10	1.5
Pepper, green	¹/₂ cup	9	0.5
Tomato	1 medium	20	1.5
Vegetables, cooked			
Beans, green	1 cup	32	3.2
Broccoli	1 cup	40	4.4
Cabbage, red	1 cup	30	2.8
Carrots	1 cup	48	4.6
Cauliflower	1 cup	28	2.2
Corn	¹/₂ cup	87	2.9
Potato (with skin)	1 medium	106	2.5
Spinach	1 cup	42	4.2
Sweet potato	1 medium	160	3.4
Zucchini	1 cup	22	3.6
Legumes			
Baked beans	¹/₂ cup	155	8.8
Dried peas, cooked	¹/₂ cup	115	4.7
Kidney beans, cooked	¹/₂ cup	110	7.3
Lima beans, cooked	¹/₂ cup	64	4.5
Lentils, cooked	¹/₂ cup	97	3.7
Navy beans, cooked	¹/₂ cup	112	6.0
Rice, breads, pastas, and flour			
Bran muffins	1 muffin	104	2.5
Bread, whole wheat	1 slice	61	1.4
Crisp bread, rye	2 crackers	50	2.0
Rice, brown, cooked	¹/₂ cup	97	1.0
Spaghetti, whole wheat, cooked	¹/₂ cup	155	3.9

table continues

Dietary fiber content of selected foods (continued)

Food	Serving	Calories	Grams of fiber
Breakfast cereals			
All-Bran	1/3 cup	71	8.5
Bran Chex	2/3 cup	91	4.6
Corn Bran	2/3 cup	98	5.4
Grape-Nuts	1/4 cup	101	1.4
Oatmeal	3/4 cup	108	1.6
Raisin Bran-type	2/3 cup	115	4.0
Shredded Wheat	2/3 cup	102	2.6
Nuts			
Almonds	10 nuts	79	1.1
Filberts	10 nuts	54	0.8
Peanuts	10 nuts	105	1.4

Try to consume three to five servings of fruit and five to seven servings of vegetables each day. Minimal consumption should not drop below two to three servings of fruit and three to five servings of vegetables per day.

Plants provide protective antioxidants and phytochemicals

Numerous population studies have repeatedly demonstrated that a high intake of carotene-rich and flavonoid-rich fruits and vegetables reduces the risk of cancer, heart disease and strokes. The best dietary sources of carotenes are green leafy vegetables and yellow-orange colored fruits and vegetables, e.g., carrots, apricots, mangoes, yams, and squash. Red and purple vegetables and fruits – such as tomatoes, red cabbage, berries, and plums – contain a large portion of non-vitamin A active pigments, including flavonoids. Legumes, grains, and seeds are also significant sources of carotenoids. Good dietary sources of flavonoids include citrus fruits, berries, onions, parsley, legumes, green tea, and red wine.

REDUCE INTAKE OF SATURATED FATS, BALANCE INTAKE OF POLYUNSATURATED FATS, AND USE MONOUNSATURATED FATS FOR COOKING

A diet high in saturated fat and cholesterol, or excessively high in a type of polyunsaturated fatty acid called omega-6 fatty acids, has been linked to numerous cancers, heart disease, and strokes. Saturated fats and cholesterol are derived from animal products, so the best way to reduce intake of saturated fat and cholesterol is to limit consumption of animal products to no more than

110–175 g (4–6 oz) q.d. and choose fish, skinless poultry and lean cuts rather than fat-laden meats.

Omega-6 essential fatty acids, derived primarily from polyunsaturated vegetable oils but also from animal products, are, as their name implies, essential to health. However, they must be consumed in proper ratio to omega-3 essential fats, whose actions counterbalance theirs. The suggested ratio of omega-6 to omega-3 fatty acids ranges from three to six times more omega-6 than omega-3 or a maximum ratio of 6:1. Unfortunately, because animal products and the most frequently consumed vegetable oils – corn, peanut, safflower, sesame, soy, and sunflower oils – contain excessively high amounts of omega-6 fats in comparison to omega-3 fats, a typical diet in the United States provides a ratio of omega-6 to omega-3 fats of 10:1.

Ratio of omega-6 to omega-3 fats

Fat	Ratio
Canola oil	2:1
Cod liver oil	1:10
Corn oil	29:1
Flaxseed oil	1:4
Peanut oil	32:1
Safflower oil	74:less than 1
Salmon	1:15
Sesame oil	41:less than 1
Soy oil	7.5:1
Sunflower oil	19:1
Walnut oil	5:1

The omega-6 and omega-3 essential fatty acids are used by the body to produce different types of hormone-like molecules called prostaglandins, so the end result of this imbalance is the production of too much of the type of prostaglandin derived from the omega-6 fats, the series 2 prostaglandins. Prostaglandins of the 1 and 3 series, derived from omega-3 fats, are generally viewed as "good" prostaglandins while prostaglandins of the 2 series are viewed as "bad", but this is an oversimplification. Each type of prostaglandin plays a necessary role. Problems only arise when the balance between them is disturbed.

One example of the negative effects of an imbalance between prostaglandins can be seen by looking at their effects on platelets. Prostaglandins of the 2 series promote platelet stickiness, an action without which blood would not clot when necessary. Too much platelet stickiness, however, leads to hardening of the arteries, heart disease, and strokes. When the system is in balance, the 1 and 3 series prostaglandins prevent excessive platelet adhesiveness, improve blood flow, and reduce inflammation.

Prostaglandin metabolism can be brought back into healthful balance by restricting the intake of animal foods and high-omega-6 oils, while increasing that of foods containing a health-promoting ratio of omega-6 to omega-3 fats such as canola oil, and flaxseed, walnuts, and the oils derived from them. Those who are not vegetarian should also increase their intake of cold-water fish such as salmon, cod, mackerel, and herring. Conditions improved by balancing essential fatty acid ratios include atherosclerosis, multiple sclerosis, psoriasis, eczema, menstrual cramps, rheumatoid arthritis, and many other allergic or inflammatory conditions.

Margarine and the shortenings used in processed foods, which contain trans *fatty acids (also called partially hydrogenated oils), should be eliminated from the diet. Trans* fatty acids interfere with the body's ability to utilize essential fatty acids, thus disrupting prostaglandin metabolism. In addition, margarine and other hydrogenated vegetable oils not only raise low density lipoprotein (LDL) cholesterol, they also lower the protective high density lipoprotein (HDL) cholesterol level, and are suspected of contributing to the occurrence of certain cancers (including breast cancer).

ELIMINATE REFINED SUGAR

When high sugar foods are eaten alone, blood sugar levels rise too quickly, producing a heightened release of insulin. Eating foods high in simple sugars severely taxes the body's blood sugar control mechanisms, and is especially harmful in hypoglycemics and diabetics whose ability to regulate blood sugar levels is already impaired. Sugar, especially when combined with caffeine, also has a detrimental effect on mood, premenstrual syndrome, and many other health conditions.

Currently, more than half of the carbohydrates consumed by most Americans are in the form of sugars being added to foods as sweetening agents. Read food labels carefully. If the words sucrose, glucose, maltose, lactose, fructose, corn syrup, or white grape juice concentrate appear on the label, extra sugar has been added.

REDUCE EXPOSURE TO PESTICIDES AND HERBICIDES

In the US each year, over 1.2 billion pounds of pesticides and herbicides are sprayed or added to crops. That is roughly 10 pounds of pesticides for each man, woman, and child. Most pesticides in use are synthetic chemicals of questionable safety. The major long-term health risks include the potential to cause cancer and birth defects,

while the major immediate health risks of acute intoxication include vomiting, diarrhea, blurred vision, tremors, convulsions, and nerve damage.

Pesticides are found in many crops, but those of greatest concern in descending order are tomatoes, beef, potatoes, oranges, lettuce, apples, peaches, pork, wheat, soybeans, beans, carrots, chicken, corn, and grapes. Many of the pesticides penetrate the entire fruit or vegetable and cannot be washed off, which is why organic produce is highly recommended. If organic produce is not available, however, the presence of pesticides in fruits and vegetables should not be a deterrent to eating a diet high in these foods. Concentrations in fruits and vegetables are much lower than the levels found in animal fats, meat, cheese, whole milk, and eggs. Furthermore, the various antioxidants in fruits and vegetables help the body detoxify the pesticides.

To minimize exposure to pesticides, waxes, fungicides, and fertilizers from produce:
1. avoid non-organic animal fat, meat, eggs, cheese, and milk; pesticide residues are concentrated in these foods
2. buy organic produce
3. try to buy local produce that is in season if organic produce is not readily available
4. remove surface pesticide residues, waxes, fungicides, and fertilizers by soaking the produce in a mild solution of additive-free soap like Ivory or pure castille soap from the health food store. All-natural, biodegradable cleansers are also available at most health food stores. Simply spray the produce with the cleanser, gently scrub, then rinse off.
5. peel off the skin or remove the outer layer of leaves. The downside here is that many of the nutritional benefits are concentrated in the skin and outer layers.

ELIMINATE THE INTAKE OF FOOD ADDITIVES AND COLORING AGENTS

Numerous synthetic food additives still in use are being linked to such diseases as depression, asthma or other allergy, hyperactivity or learning disabilities in children, and migraine headaches. Obviously, the most sensible approach is to focus on whole, fresh, natural foods and avoid foods that are highly processed.

KEEP SALT INTAKE LOW, POTASSIUM INTAKE HIGH

Excessive salt (sodium chloride) consumption, coupled with diminished dietary potassium, greatly stresses the kidneys' ability to maintain proper fluid volume. As a result some people are "salt-sensitive" in that high salt intake causes high blood pressure or, in other cases, water retention. Read labels carefully to keep the total daily sodium intake below 1,800 mg.

Most Americans have a potassium-to-sodium (K : Na) ratio of less than 1 : 2. Researchers recommend a dietary potassium-to-sodium ratio of greater than 5 : 1 to maintain health. A plant-based diet is again the answer to this problem as most fruits and vegetables have a K : Na ratio of at least 50 : 1.

If the taste of salt is essential, use the so-called salt substitutes such as the popular brands No-Salt and Nu-Salt. These products are composed of potassium chloride, which tastes very similar to sodium chloride.

DRINK 2+ L OF CLEAN WATER DAILY

Each day our body requires an intake of 2+ L of water to function optimally. About 1 L each day is provided in the foods we eat. This means that we need to drink at least 1 L of liquids each day to maintain good water balance. More liquids are needed in warmer climates or for physically active people. Not drinking enough liquids puts a great deal of stress on the body. Kidney function is likely to be affected, gallstones and kidney stones are likely to form, and immune function will be impaired.

To ensure that the drinking water is safe, contact the local water company; most cities have quality assurance programs that perform routine analyses. Simply ask for the most recent analysis. In addition, a quick look in the yellow pages of the phone book under "Water Purification & Filter Equipment" will list local companies selling water purification units. Many of their advertisements will state free water testing. Make sure the company being called is a certified water treatment specialist.

IDENTIFY AND ADDRESS FOOD ALLERGIES

The importance of identifying and addressing food allergies and sensitivities is discussed in the chapter on Food allergy.

USE THE HEALTHY EXCHANGE SYSTEM TO CONSTRUCT A HEALTH-PROMOTING DIET

The following exchange system emphasizes healthy food choices and focuses on unprocessed, whole foods. Simply choose the number of exchanges allowed per list to plan a day's meals. There are seven exchange lists; however, the milk and meat lists should be considered optional.

The healthy exchange system

- List 1 – Vegetables
- List 2 – Fruits
- List 3 – Breads, cereals, and starchy vegetables
- List 4 – Legumes (beans)
- List 5 – Fats and oils
- List 6 – Milk
- List 7 – Meats, fish, cheese, and eggs

Because all food portions within each exchange list provide approximately the same calories, proteins, fats, and carbohydrates per serving, it is easy to construct a diet consisting of the recommended percentages of:

- carbohydrates: 60–70% of total calories
- fats: 15–25% of total calories
- protein: 15–20% of total calories
- dietary fiber: at least 35 g.

Of the carbohydrates ingested, 90% should be complex carbohydrates or naturally occurring sugars. Intake of refined carbohydrate and concentrated sugars (including honey, pasteurized fruit juices, and dried fruit, as well as sugar and white flour) should be limited to less than 10% of the total calorie intake.

Examples of exchange recommendations

1,500 calorie vegan diet

List 1 – Vegetables: 5 servings
List 2 – Fruits: 2 servings
List 3 – Breads, cereals, and starchy vegetables: 9 servings
List 4 – Beans: 2.5 servings
List 5 – Fats: 4 servings

This recommendation would result in an intake of approximately 1,500 calories, of which 67% are derived from complex carbohydrates and naturally occurring sugars, 18% from fat, and 15% from protein. The protein intake is entirely from plant sources, but still provides approximately 55 g, an amount well above the recommended daily allowance of protein intake for someone requiring 1,500 calories. At least one-half of the fat servings should be from nuts, seeds, and other whole foods from the fats exchange list. The dietary fiber intake would be approximately 31–74.5 g:

- percentage of calories as carbohydrates: 67%
- percentage of calories as fats: 18%
- percentage of calories as protein: 15%
- protein content: 55 g
- dietary fiber content: 31–74.5 g

1,500 calorie omnivore diet

List 1 – Vegetables: 5 servings
List 2 – Fruits: 2.5 servings

List 3 – Breads, cereals, and starchy vegetables: 6 servings
List 4 – Beans: 1 serving
List 5 – Fats: 5 servings
List 6 – Milk: 1 serving
List 7 – Meats, fish, cheese, and eggs: 2 servings
- percentage of calories as carbohydrates: 67%
- percentage of calories as fats: 18%
- percentage of calories as protein: 15%
- protein content: 61 g (75% from plant sources)
- dietary fiber content: 19.5–53.5 g

2,000 calorie vegan diet
List 1 – Vegetables: 5.5 servings
List 2 – Fruits: 2 servings
List 3 – Breads, cereals, and starchy vegetables: 11 servings
List 4 – Beans: 5 servings
List 5 – Fats: 8 servings
- percentage of calories as carbohydrates: 67%
- percentage of calories as fats: 18%
- percentage of calories as protein: 15%
- protein content: 79 g
- dietary fiber content: 48.5–101.5 g

2,000 calorie omnivore diet
List 1 – Vegetables: 5 servings
List 2 – Fruits: 2.5 servings
List 3 – Breads, cereals, and starchy vegetables: 13 servings
List 4 – Beans: 2 servings
List 5 – Fats: 7 servings
List 6 – Milk: 1 serving
List 7 – Meats, fish, cheese, and eggs: 2 servings
- percentage of calories as carbohydrates: 66%
- percentage of calories as fats: 19%
- percentage of calories as protein: 15%
- protein content: 78 g (72% from plant sources)
- dietary fiber content: 32.5–88.5 g

2,500 calorie vegan diet
List 1 – Vegetables: 8 servings
List 2 – Fruits: 3 servings
List 3 – Breads, cereals, and starchy vegetables: 17 servings
List 4 – Beans: 5 servings
List 5 – Fats: 8 servings
- percentage of calories as carbohydrates: 69%
- percentage of calories as fats: 15%
- percentage of calories as protein: 16%
- protein content: 101 g
- dietary fiber content: 33–121 g

2,500 calorie omnivore diet
List 1 – Vegetables: 8 servings
List 2 – Fruits: 3.5 servings
List 3 – Breads, cereals, and starchy vegetables: 17 servings
List 4 – Beans: 2 servings
List 5 – Fats: 8 servings
List 6 – Milk: 1 serving
List 7 – Meats, fish, cheese, and eggs: 3 servings
- percentage of calories as carbohydrates: 66%
- percentage of calories as fats: 18%
- percentage of calories as protein: 16%
- protein content: 102 g (80% from plant sources)
- dietary fiber content: 40.5–116.5 g

3,000 calorie vegan diet
List 1 – Vegetables: 10 servings
List 2 – Fruits: 4 servings
List 3 – Breads, cereals, and starchy vegetables: 17 servings
List 4 – Beans: 6 servings
List 5 – Fats: 10 servings
- percentage of calories as carbohydrates: 70%
- percentage of calories as fats: 16%
- percentage of calories as protein: 14%
- protein content: 116 g
- dietary fiber content: 50–84 g

3,000 calorie omnivore diet
List 1 – Vegetables: 10 servings
List 2 – Fruits: 3 servings
List 3 – Breads, cereals, and starchy vegetables: 20 servings
List 4 – Beans: 2 servings
List 5 – Fats: 10 servings
List 6 – Milk: 1 serving
List 7 – Meats, fish, cheese, and eggs: 3 servings
- percentage of calories as carbohydrates: 67%
- percentage of calories as fats: 18%
- percentage of calories as protein: 15%
- protein content: 116 g (81% from plant sources)
- dietary fiber content: 45–133 g

(*Note*: these recommendations can be used as the basis for calculating other calorie diets. For example, for a 4,000 calorie diet add the 2,500 to the 1,500. For a 1,000 calorie diet divide the 2,000 calorie diet in half.)

The healthy exchange lists

Exchange List 1 – Vegetables

The list below shows the vegetables to use for one vegetable exchange. One exchange equals one cup cooked vegetables or fresh vegetable juice, or 2 cups raw vegetables. (Starchy vegetables like potatoes and yams are included in Exchange List 3 – Breads, cereals, and starchy vegetables.)

Artichoke (1 medium)
Asparagus
Bean sprouts
Beets
Broccoli
Brussels sprouts
Carrots
Cauliflower
Eggplant
Greens:
    Beet
    Chard
    Collard
    Dandelion
    Kale
    Mustard
    Spinach
    Turnip
Mushrooms
Okra
Onions
Rhubarb
Rutabaga
Sauerkraut
String beans, green or yellow
Summer squash
Tomatoes, tomato juice, vegetable juice cocktail
Zucchini

The following vegetables may be used as often as desired, especially in their raw form:
Alfalfa sprouts
Bell peppers
Bok choy
Cabbage
Chicory
Celery
Chinese cabbage
Cucumber
Endive
Escarole
Lettuce
Parsley
Radishes
Spinach
Turnips
Watercress

Exchange List 2 – Fruits
Each of the following equals one exchange:

Fresh Juice	1 cup (240 ml)
Pasteurized Juice	$2/_3$ cup
Apple	1 large
Apple sauce (unsweetened)	1 cup
Apricots, fresh	4 medium
Apricots, dried	8 halves
Banana	1 medium
Berries:	
Blackberries	1 cup
Blueberries	1 cup
Cranberries	1 cup
Raspberries	1 cup
Strawberries	$1^1/_2$ cups
Cherries	20 large
Dates	4
Figs, fresh	2
Figs, dried	2
Grapefruit	1
Grapes	20
Mango	1 small
Melons:	
Cantaloupe	$1/_2$ small
Honeydew	$1/_4$ medium
Watermelon	2 cups
Nectarine	2 small
Orange	1 large
Papaya	$1^1/_2$ cups
Peach	2 medium
Persimmon, native	2 medium
Pineapple	1 cup
Plums	4 medium
Prunes	4 medium
Prune juice	$1/_2$ cup
Raisins	4 tbsp
Tangerine	2 medium

Additional fruit exchanges (no more than one per day):

Honey	1 tbsp
Jams, jellies, preserves	1 tbsp
Sugar	1 tbsp

Exchange List 3 – Breads, cereals, and starchy vegetables
One of the following equals one exchange:

Breads:	
Bagel, small	$1/_2$
Dinner roll	1
Dried breadcrumbs	3 tbsp
English muffin, small	$1/_2$
Tortilla (6″)	1
Whole wheat, rye or	
pumpernickel	1 slice
Cereals:	
Bran flakes	$1/_2$ cup

Cornmeal (dry)	2 tbsp
Cereal (cooked)	1/2 cup
Flour	2 1/2 tbsp
Grits (cooked)	1/2 cup
Pasta (cooked)	1/2 cup
Puffed cereal (unsweetened)	1 cup
Rice or barley (cooked)	1/2 cup
Wheat germ	1/4 cup
Other unsweetened cereal	3/4 cup

Crackers:

Arrowroot	3
Graham (2 1/2" square)	2
Matzo (4" × 6")	1/2
Rye wafers (2" × 3 1/2")	3
Saltines	6

Starchy vegetables:

Corn	1/3 cup
Corn on cob	1 small
Parsnips	2/3 cup
Potato, mashed	1/2 cup
Potato, white	1 small
Squash: winter, acorn, or butternut	1/2 cup
Yam or sweet potato	1/4 cup

Prepared foods:

Biscuit, 2" diameter (omit 1 fat exchange)	1
Corn bread, 2" × 2" × 1" (omit 1 fat exchange)	1
French fries, 2–3" long (omit 1 fat exchange)	8
Muffin, small (omit 1 fat exchange)	1
Potato or corn chips (omit 2 fat exchanges)	15
Pancake, 5" × 1/2" (omit 1 fat exchange)	1
Waffle, 5" × 1/2" (omit 1 fat exchange)	1

Exchange List 4 – Legumes (beans)

One half cup of the following cooked or sprouted beans equals one exchange:

Black-eyed peas
Chick peas (also called garbanzo beans)
Kidney beans
Lentils
Lima beans
Pinto beans
Soybeans, including tofu (omit 1 fat exchange)
Split peas
Other dried beans and peas

Exchange List 5 – Fats and oils

It is strongly recommended by most nutritional experts that the total fat intake be kept below 30% of the total calories. It is also recommended that at least twice as much unsaturated fat be consumed compared to saturated fats. In addition, the unsaturated fats should contribute a ratio of no more than 6 : 1 omega-6 to omega-3 essential fatty acids. Although they sound complicated, these recommendations can be followed by simply reducing the amount of animal products in the diet, increasing the amount of nuts and seeds consumed (particularly flaxseed and walnuts), and using natural flaxseed, walnut, and canola oils. These oils, however, are easily oxidized, so they should not be heated. Virgin olive oil, the oil most resistant to oxidation from heat, is the best oil to use for cooking, and since it contains monounsaturated fat, it does not adversely impact on the dietary ratio of omega-6 to omega-3 fatty acids. In addition, virgin olive oil, which contains oleic acid, lowers (bad) LDL cholesterol but not (protective) HDL cholesterol.

Each of the following equals one exchange:

Polyunsaturated

Vegetable Oils:	1 tsp
Canola	
Flax (highest in omega-3s)	
Walnut	
Avocado (4" diameter)	1/8
Almonds	10 whole
Pecans	2 large
Peanuts:	
Spanish	20 whole
Virginia	10 whole
Peanut butter	1 tbsp
Seeds:	1 tbsp
Flax	
Pumpkin	
Sesame	
Sunflower	
Walnuts	6 small

Monounsaturated

| Olive oil | 1 tsp |
| Olives | 5 small |

Saturated (use sparingly):

Butter	1 tsp
Bacon	1 slice
Cream, light or sour	2 tbsp
Cream, heavy	1 tbsp
Cream cheese	1 tbsp
Salad dressings	2 tsp
Mayonnaise	1 tsp

Exchange List 6 – Milk

Many people are allergic to cow's milk or lack the enzymes necessary to digest it. Even if cow's milk is tolerated, consumption should be limited to no more than one or two servings per day. Soy milk, which provides health-promoting phytochemicals along with protein and, if fortified, calcium, is a better choice.

One cup equals one exchange:
Non-fat cow's milk or yogurt
Non-fat soy milk
Soy milk (omit 1 fat exchange)
2% milk (omit 1 fat exchange)
Cottage cheese, low fat (omit 1 fat exchange)
Low-fat yogurt (omit 1 fat exchange)
Whole milk (omit 2 fat exchanges)
Yogurt (omit 2 fat exchanges)
1 oz of cheese equals 1 milk exchange and 1 fat exchange

Exchange List 7 – Meats, fish, cheese, and eggs

Choose primarily from the low fat group and remove the skin of poultry to keep the amount of saturated fat low. Use these foods in small amounts as "condiments" in the diet rather than as mainstays. Definitely stay away from cured meats like bacon, pastrami, etc.; these foods are rich in compounds that can lead to the formation of cancer-causing nitrosamines.

A possible exception to the recommendation of reducing the intake of animal foods are cold-water fish such as salmon, mackerel and herring which are excellent sources of omega-3 essential fatty acids. These beneficial fats lower cholesterol and triglyceride levels, thereby reducing the risk for heart disease and strokes, and are also recommended to treat or prevent high blood pressure, other cardiovascular diseases, cancer, autoimmune diseases like multiple sclerosis and rheumatoid arthritis, allergies and inflammation, eczema, psoriasis, and many other diseases.

Each of the following equals one exchange:
Low fat (less than 15% fat content)

Beef: baby beef, chipped beef, chuck, steak (flank, plate), tenderloin plate ribs, round (bottom, top), all cuts rump, spare ribs, tripe	1 oz
Fish	1 oz
Lamb: leg, rib, sirloin, loin (roast and chops), shank, shoulder	1 oz
Poultry: chicken or turkey without skin	1 oz
Veal: Leg, loin, rib, shank, shoulder, cutlet	1 oz

Medium fat (for each omit 1/2 fat exchange)

Beef: ground (15% fat), canned corned beef, rib eye, round (ground commercial)	1 oz
Cheese: mozzarella, ricotta, farmer's, Parmesan	1 oz
Eggs	1
Organ meats	1 oz
Pork: loin (all tenderloin), picnic and boiled ham, shoulder, Boston butt, Canadian bacon	1 oz

High fat (for each exchange omit 1 fat exchange)

Beef: brisket, corned beef, ground beef (more than 20% fat), hamburger, roasts (rib), steaks (club and rib)	1 oz
Duck or goose	1 oz
Lamb: breast	1 oz
Pork: spareribs, loin, ground pork, country-style ham, deviled ham	1 oz

Appendix 2: High-potency multiple vitamin and mineral supplements

The recommendations below provide an optimal daily intake range of known vitamins and minerals and can be used in selecting a high-potency multiple.

Vitamin/mineral	Range for adults
Vitamin	
Vitamin A (retinol)	5,000 IU*
Vitamin A (from beta-carotene)	5,000–25,000 IU
Vitamin D	100–400 IU[†]
Vitamin E (D-alpha-tocopherol)	100–800 IU[††]
Vitamin K (phytadione)	60–300 µg
Vitamin C (ascorbic acid)	100–1,000 mg[§]
Vitamin B_1 (thiamin)	10–100 mg
Vitamin B_2 (riboflavin)	10–50 mg
Niacin	10–100 mg
Niacinamide	10–30 mg
Vitamin B_6 (pyridoxine)	25–100 mg
Biotin	100–300 µg
Pantothenic acid	25–100 mg
Folic acid	400 µg
Vitamin B_{12}	400 µg
Choline	10–100 mg
Inositol	10–100 mg
Minerals	
Boron	1–6 mg
Calcium	250–1,500 mg[#]
Chromium	200–400 µg[##]
Copper	1–2 mg
Iodine	50–150 µg
Iron	15–30 mg**
Magnesium	250–500 mg[†††]
Manganese	10–15 mg
Molybdenum	10–25 µg
Potassium	200–500 mg
Selenium	100–200 µg
Silica	1–25 mg
Vanadium	50–100 µg
Zinc	15–45 mg

* Women of childbearing age should not take more than 5,000 IU of retinol daily if becoming pregnant is a possibility, due to the risk of birth defects.

[†] Elderly people who live in northern latitudes should supplement at the high end of the range.

[††] It may be more cost-effective to take vitamin E separately.

[§] It may be easier to take vitamin C separately.

[#] Taking a separate calcium supplement may be necessary in women at risk or suffering from osteoporosis.

[##] For diabetes and weight loss, dosages of 600 µg can be used.

** Men and postmenopausal women rarely need supplemental iron. Persons with hepatitis C should not take iron.

[†††] When magnesium therapy is indicated, take a separate magnesium supplement.

Index